Acta Neurochirurgica Supplement 126

Series Editor:
Hans-Jakob Steiger

More information about this series at http://www.springer.com/series/4

Thomas Heldt
Editor

Intracranial Pressure & Neuromonitoring XVI

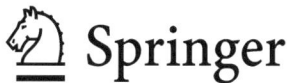

Springer

Editor
Thomas Heldt
Institute for Medical Engineering & Science
Massachusetts Institute of Technology
Cambridge
Massachusetts
USA

ISSN 0065-1419   ISSN 2197-8395   (electronic)
Acta Neurochirurgica Supplement
ISBN 978-3-319-65797-4   ISBN 978-3-319-65798-1   (eBook)
https://doi.org/10.1007/978-3-319-65798-1

Library of Congress Control Number: 2018930544

© Springer International Publishing AG 2018
This work is subject to copyright. All rights are reserved by the Publisher, whether the whole or part of the material is concerned, specifically the rights of translation, reprinting, reuse of illustrations, recitation, broadcasting, reproduction on microfilms or in any other physical way, and transmission or information storage and retrieval, electronic adaptation, computer software, or by similar or dissimilar methodology now known or hereafter developed.
The use of general descriptive names, registered names, trademarks, service marks, etc. in this publication does not imply, even in the absence of a specific statement, that such names are exempt from the relevant protective laws and regulations and therefore free for general use.
The publisher, the authors and the editors are safe to assume that the advice and information in this book are believed to be true and accurate at the date of publication. Neither the publisher nor the authors or the editors give a warranty, express or implied, with respect to the material contained herein or for any errors or omissions that may have been made. The publisher remains neutral with regard to jurisdictional claims in published maps and institutional affiliations.

Printed on acid-free paper

This Springer imprint is published by Springer Nature
The registered company is Springer International Publishing AG
The registered company address is: Gewerbestrasse 11, 6330 Wien, Switzerland

Preface

The International Conference on Intracranial Pressure and Neuromonitoring ("ICP Conference") is dedicated to the exchange of ideas and research results in multimodality neuromonitoring and management of diseases of the central nervous system. To achieve its goals, the ICP Conference brings together a diverse group of clinicians—including neurosurgeons, neurologists, neurointensivists, and anesthesiologists—as well as scientists, engineers, informaticists, and mathematicians.

Since its inception in 1972 at Hannover Medical School in Germany, the ICP Conference has maintained a special focus on the measurement of intracranial pressure in trauma, stroke, hydrocephalus, and during administration of anesthesia, as well as the interpretation of the associated recordings. With the increasing complexity of patient monitoring in perioperative and neurocritical care, and the ability to archive and retrospectively analyze the multimodal and multivariate monitoring data streams, the scope of the ICP Conference has expanded to include all monitoring modalities in neurological, neurocritical, and neurosurgical care.

The 16th ICP Conference was held in Cambridge, Massachusetts, from June 28 through July 2, 2016, and continued the long tradition of bringing together diverse groups of clinicians and researchers to advance the field of neuromonitoring. We are particularly pleased to have been joined by the Cerebral Autoregulation Research Network (CARNet), whose sixth annual meeting was co-hosted with the 2016 ICP Conference and thereby significantly expanded the breadth and richness of the meeting.

The conference attracted over 300 attendees, including 81 trainees, from 28 countries across six continents. It featured 235 contributed presentations as well as 15 keynote lectures and panel discussions from leading experts in the fields of traumatic brain injury, neurocritical care informatics, cerebrovascular autoregulation, hydrocephalus, visual impairment and intracranial hypertension, spreading depolarizations, and craniosynostosis. The 61 papers contained in this volume represent a cross section of the work presented at the conference and provide a glimpse into the current state-of-the-art in neuromonitoring. They also serve as a reminder that many important questions in these domains remain to be resolved to the full benefit of patients with brain injuries and neurological disorders. We look forward to the 17th ICP Conference in 2019 in Leuven, Belgium, with the hope that some of the pressing questions may be addressed by then.

I wish to thank the members of the Local Scientific Steering Committee and the International Advisory Committee for their help and guidance. Additionally, I wish to acknowledge the unwavering administrative support of Ms. Caitlin Vinci, whose help and support made the conference and this book possible.

Cambridge, MA   Thomas Heldt, Ph.D.

Contents

Traumatic Brain Injury

Cerebral Perfusion Pressure Variability Between Patients and Between Centres 3
B. Depreitere, F. Güiza, I. Piper, G. Citerio, I. Chambers, P. A. Jones, T-Y. M. Lo,
P. Enblad, P. Nilsson, B. Feyen, P. Jorens, A. Maas, M. U. Schuhmann,
R. Donald, L. Moss, G. Van den Berghe, and G. Meyfroidt

Pre-hospital Predictors of Impaired ICP Trends in Continuous Monitoring of Paediatric Traumatic Brain Injury Patients 7
A. M. H. Young, J. Donnelly, X. Liu, M. R. Guilfoyle, M. Carew, M. Cabeleira,
D. Cardim, M. R. Garnett, H. M. Fernandes, C. Haubrich, P. Smielewski,
M. Czosnyka, P. J. Hutchinson, and S. Agrawal

Prognosis of Severe Traumatic Brain Injury Outcomes in Children 11
S. V. Meshcheryakov, Z. B. Semenova, V. I. Lukianov, E. G. Sorokina, and
O. V. Karaseva

Do ICP-Derived Parameters Differ in Vegetative State from Other Outcome Groups After Traumatic Brain Injury? 17
M. Czosnyka, J. Donnelly, L. Calviello, P. Smielewski, D. K. Menon, and
J. D. Pickard

Cerebral Arterial Compliance in Traumatic Brain Injury 21
M. Dobrzeniecki, A. Trofimov, and D. E. Bragin

The Cerebrovascular Resistance in Combined Traumatic Brain Injury with Intracranial Hematomas 25
A. O. Trofimov, G. Kalentyev, O. Voennov, M. Yuriev, D. Agarkova,
S. Trofimova, and V. Grigoryeva

Computed Tomography Indicators of Deranged Intracranial Physiology in Paediatric Traumatic Brain Injury 29
A. M. H. Young, J. Donnelly, X. Liu, M. R. Guilfoyle, M. Carew, M. Cabeleira,
D. Cardim, M. R. Garnett, H. M. Fernandes, C. Haubrich, P. Smielewski,
M. Czosnyka, P. J. Hutchinson, and S. Agrawal

Mean Square Deviation of ICP in Prognosis of Severe TBI Outcomes in Children 35
Z. B. Semenova, V. I. Lukianov, S. V. Meshcheryakov, and L. M. Roshal

KidsBrainIT: A New Multi-centre, Multi-disciplinary, Multi-national Paediatric Brain Monitoring Collaboration 39
T. Lo, I. Piper, B. Depreitere, G. Meyfroidt, M. Poca, J. Sahuquillo, T. Durduran,
P. Enblad, P. Nilsson, A. Ragauskas, K. Kiening, K. Morris, R. Agbeko, R. Levin,
J. Weitz, C. Park, P. Davis, and on Behalf of BrainIT

Increased ICP and Its Cerebral Haemodynamic Sequelae 47
J. Donnelly, M. Czosnyka, S. Harland, G. V. Varsos, D. Cardim,
C. Robba, X. Liu, P. N. Ainslie, and P. Smielewski

What Determines Outcome in Patients That Suffer Raised Intracranial Pressure After Traumatic Brain Injury? 51
S. P. Klein and B. Depreitere

Visualisation of the 'Optimal Cerebral Perfusion' Landscape in Severe Traumatic Brain Injury Patients 55
A. Ercole, P. Smielewski, M. J. H. Aries, R. Wesselink, J. W. J. Elting,
J. Donnelly, M. Czosnyka, and N. M. Maurits

Is There a Relationship Between Optimal Cerebral Perfusion Pressure-Guided Management and PaO_2/FiO_2 Ratio After Severe Traumatic Brain Injury? 59
M. Moreira, D. Fernandes, E. Pereira, E. Monteiro, R. Pascoa, and C. Dias

Cognitive Outcomes of Patients with Traumatic Bifrontal Contusions 63
G. K. C. Wong, K. Ngai, W. S. Poon, V. Z. Y. Zheng, and C. Yu

Brain Monitoring Technology

Non-invasive Intracranial Pressure Assessment in Brain Injured Patients Using Ultrasound-Based Methods 69
C. Robba, D. Cardim, T. Tajsic, J. Pietersen, M. Bulman, F. Rasulo,
R. Bertuetti, J. Donnelly, L. Xiuyun, Z. Czosnyka, M. Cabeleira,
P. Smielewski, B. Matta, A. Bertuccio, and M. Czosnyka

Analysis of a Minimally Invasive Intracranial Pressure Signals During Infusion at the Subarachnoid Spinal Space of Pigs 75
G. Frigieri, R. A. P. Andrade, C. C. Wang, D. Spavieri Jr., L. Lopes, R. Brunelli,
D. A. Cardim, R. M. M. Verzola, and S. Mascarenhas

Comparison of Different Calibration Methods in a Non-invasive ICP Assessment Model 79
B. Schmidt, D. Cardim, M. Weinhold, S. Streif, D. D. McLeod, M. Czosnyka, and
J. Klingelhöfer

An Embedded Device for Real-Time Noninvasive Intracranial Pressure Estimation 85
J. M. Matthews, A. Fanelli, and T. Heldt

Transcranial Bioimpedance Measurement as a Non-invasive Estimate of Intracranial Pressure 89
C. Hawthorne, M. Shaw, I. Piper, L. Moss, and J. Kinsella

Pulsed Electromagnetic Field (PEMF) Mitigates High Intracranial Pressure (ICP) Induced Microvascular Shunting (MVS) in Rats 93
D. E. Bragin, O. A. Bragina, S. Hagberg, and E. M. Nemoto

Volumetric Ophthalmic Ultrasound for Inflight Monitoring of Visual Impairment and Intracranial Pressure 97
A. Dentinger, M. MacDonald, D. Ebert, K. Garcia, and A. Sargsyan

**Does the Variability of Evoked Tympanic Membrane Displacement
Data (V_m) Increase as the Magnitude of the Pulse Amplitude Increases?** 103
S. J. Sharif, C. M. Campbell-Bell, D. O. Bulters, R. J. Marchbanks, and A. A. Birch

**Analysis of a Non-invasive Intracranial Pressure Monitoring
Method in Patients with Traumatic Brain Injury** 107
G. Frigieri, R. A. P. Andrade, C. Dias, D. L. Spavieri Jr., R. Brunelli,
D. A. Cardim, C. C. Wang, R. M. M. Verzola, and S. Mascarenhas

A Wearable Transcranial Doppler Ultrasound Phased Array System 111
S. J. Pietrangelo, H-S. Lee, and C. G. Sodini

**Quantification of Macrocirculation and Microcirculation in Brain
Using Ultrasound Perfusion Imaging** 115
E. J. Vinke, J. Eyding, C. de Korte, C. H. Slump, J. G. van der Hoeven, and
C. W. E. Hoedemaekers

**HDF5-Based Data Format for Archiving Complex Neuro-monitoring
Data in Traumatic Brain Injury Patients** 121
M. Cabeleira, A. Ercole, and P. Smielewski

Neurocritical Care Informatics

**Are Slow Waves of Intracranial Pressure Suppressed by
General Anaesthesia?** 129
D. A. Lalou, M. Czosnyka, J. Donnelly, A. Lavinio, J. D. Pickard,
M. Garnett, and Z. Czosnyka

**Critical Closing Pressure During a Controlled Increase
in Intracranial Pressure** 133
K. Kaczmarska, M. Kasprowicz, A. Grzanka, W. Zabołotny, P. Smielewski,
D. A. Lalou, G. Varsos, M. Czosnyka, and Z. Czosnyka

**Effect of Mild Hypocapnia on Critical Closing Pressure and Other
Mechanoelastic Parameters of the Cerebrospinal System** 139
P. Smielewski, L. Steiner, C. Puppo, K. Budohoski, G. V. Varsos, and M. Czosnyka

Occurrence of CPPopt Values in Uncorrelated ICP and ABP Time Series 143
M. Cabeleira, M. Czosnyka, X. Liu, J. Donnelly, and P. Smielewski

**Simultaneous Transients of Intracranial Pressure and Heart Rate
in Traumatic Brain Injury: Methods of Analysis** 147
G. M. Dimitri, S. Agrawal, A. Young, J. Donnelly, X. Liu, P. Smielewski,
P. Hutchinson, M. Czosnyka, P. Lio, and C. Haubrich

**Increasing the Contrast-to-Noise Ratio of MRI Signals for
Regional Assessment of Dynamic Cerebral Autoregulation** 153
J. L. Jara, N. P. Saeed, R. B. Panerai, and T. G. Robinson

**Comparing Models of Spontaneous Variations, Maneuvers and
Indexes to Assess Dynamic Cerebral Autoregulation** 159
M. Chacón, S. Noh, J. Landerretche, and J.L. Jara

ICP and Antihypertensive Drugs 163
C. Rouzaud-Laborde, P. Lafitte, L. Balardy, Z. Czosnyka, and E. A. Schmidt

ICP: From Correlation to Causation 167
E. A. Schmidt, O. Maarek, J. Despres, M. Verdier, and L. Risser

A Waveform Archiving System for the GE Solar 8000i Bedside Monitor 173
A. Fanelli, R. Jaishankar, A. Filippidis, J. Holsapple, and T. Heldt

**Deriving the PRx and CPPopt from 0.2-Hz Data:
Establishing Generalizability to Bedmaster Users** 179
M. Megjhani, K. Terilli, A. Martin, A. Velazquez, J. Claassen, D. Roh,
S. Agarwal, P. Smielewski, A. K. Boehme, J. M. Schmidt, and S. Park

**Medical Waveform Format Encoding Rules Representation
of Neurointensive Care Waveform Data** 183
I. Piper, M. Shaw, C. Hawthorne, J. Kinsella, and L. Moss

**Multi-Scale Peak and Trough Detection Optimised for Periodic
and Quasi-Periodic Neuroscience Data** 189
Steven M. Bishop and Ari Ercole

Room Air Readings of Brain Tissue Oxygenation Probes 197
S. Wolf, L. Schürer, and D. C. Engel

What Do We Mean by Cerebral Perfusion Pressure? 201
B. Depreitere, G. Meyfroidt, and F. Güiza

**Investigation of the Relationship Between the Burden of Raised
ICP and the Length of Stay in a Neuro-Intensive Care Unit** 205
M. Shaw, L. Moss, C. Hawthorne, J. Kinsella, and I. Piper

**Pressure Reactivity-Based Optimal Cerebral Perfusion Pressure
in a Traumatic Brain Injury Cohort** 209
J. Donnelly, M. Czosnyka, H. Adams, C. Robba, L. A. Steiner, D. Cardim,
B. Cabella, X. Liu, A. Ercole, P. J. Hutchinson, D. K. Menon, M. J. H. Aries,
and P. Smielewski

Hydrocephalus and CSF Biophysics

**Spaceflight-Induced Visual Impairment and Globe Deformations
in Astronauts Are Linked to Orbital Cerebrospinal Fluid Volume Increase** 215
N. Alperin and A. M. Bagci

**Ventriculomegaly in the Elderly: Who Needs a Shunt? A MRI
Study on 90 Patients** 221
M. Baroncini, O. Balédent, C. E. Ardi, V. D. Delannoy, G. Kuchcinski,
A. Duhamel, G. S. Ares, J. Lejeune, and J. Hodel

**Is There a Link Between ICP-Derived Infusion Test Parameters
and Outcome After Shunting in Normal Pressure Hydrocephalus?** 229
E. Nabbanja, M. Czosnyka, N. C. Keong, M. Garnett, J. D. Pickard,
D. A. Lalou, and Z. Czosnyka

Mathematical Modelling of CSF Pulsatile Flow in Aqueduct Cerebri 233
Z. Czosnyka, D-J. Kim, O. Balédent, E. A. Schmidt, P. Smielewski, and M. Czosnyka

**Cerebrospinal Fluid and Cerebral Blood Flows in Idiopathic
Intracranial Hypertension** 237
C. Capel, M. Baroncini, C. Gondry-Jouet, R. Bouzerar, M. Czosnyka,
Z. Czosnyka, and O. Balédent

Significant Association of Slow Vasogenic ICP Waves with Normal Pressure Hydrocephalus Diagnosis 243
A. Spiegelberg, M. Krause, J. Meixensberger, B. Seifert, and V. Kurtcuoglu

ICP Monitoring and Phase-Contrast MRI to Investigate Intracranial Compliance 247
A. Lokossou, O. Balédent, S. Garnotel, G. Page, L. Balardy,
Z. Czosnyka, P. Payoux, and E. A. Schmidt

Numerical Cerebrospinal System Modeling in Fluid-Structure Interaction 255
S. Garnotel, S. Salmon, and O. Balédent

Cerebrovascular Autoregulation

Differential Systolic and Diastolic Regulation of the Cerebral Pressure-Flow Relationship During Squat-Stand Manoeuvres 263
J. D. Smirl, A. D. Wright, P. N. Ainslie, Y-C. Tzeng, and P. van Donkelaar

Normative Ranges of Transcranial Doppler Metrics 269
S. Krakauskaite, C. Thibeault, J. LaVangie, M. Scheidt, L. Martinez,
D. Seth-Hunter, A. Wu, M. O'Brien, F. Scalzo, S. J. Wilk, and R. B. Hamilton

Autoregulating Cerebral Tissue Selfishly Exploits Collateral Flow Routes Through the Circle of Willis 275
F. A. K. McConnell and S. J. Payne

ICP Monitoring by Open Extraventricular Drainage: Common Practice but Not Suitable for Advanced Neuromonitoring and Prone to False Negativity 281
K. Hockel and M. U. Schuhmann

Comparison of Intracranial Pressure and Pressure Reactivity Index Obtained Through Pressure Measurements in the Ventricle and in the Parenchyma During and Outside Cerebrospinal Fluid Drainage Episodes in a Manipulation-Free Patient Setting 287
S. P. Klein, D. Bruyninckx, I. Callebaut, and B. Depreitere

Visualizing Cerebrovascular Autoregulation Insults and Their Association with Outcome in Adult and Paediatric Traumatic Brain Injury 291
M. Flechet, G. Meyfroidt, I. Piper, G. Citerio, I. Chambers, P. A. Jones,
T. M. Lo, P. Enblad, P. Nilsson, B. Feyen, P. Jorens, A. Maas, M. U. Schuhmann,
R. Donald, L. Moss, G. V. den Berghe, B. Depreitere, and F. Güiza

Assessing Cerebral Hemodynamic Stability After Brain Injury 297
B. Pineda, C. Kosinski, N. Kim, S. Danish, and W. Craelius

Systolic and Diastolic Regulation of the Cerebral Pressure-Flow Relationship Differentially Affected by Acute Sport-Related Concussion 303
A. D. Wright, J. D. Smirl, K. Bryk, and P. van Donkelaar

Induced Dynamic Intracranial Pressure and Cerebrovascular Reactivity Assessment of Cerebrovascular Autoregulation After Traumatic Brain Injury with High Intracranial Pressure in Rats 309
D. E. Bragin, G. L. Statom, and E. M. Nemoto

Prediction of the Time to Syncope Occurrence in Patients Diagnosed with Vasovagal Syncope.. 313
K. Kostoglou, R. Schondorf, J. Benoit, S. Balegh, and G. D. Mitsis

Statistical Signal Properties of the Pressure-Reactivity Index (PRx)............. 317
S. Kelly, S. M. Bishop, and A. Ercole

Author Index... 321

Subject Index.. 325

Traumatic Brain Injury

Cerebral Perfusion Pressure Variability Between Patients and Between Centres

Bart Depreitere, Fabian Güiza, Ian Piper, Giuseppe Citerio, Iain Chambers, Patricia A. Jones, Tsz-Yan M. Lo, Per Enblad, Pelle Nilsson, Bart Feyen, Philippe Jorens, Andrew Maas, Martin U. Schuhmann, Rob Donald, Laura Moss, Greet Van den Berghe, and Geert Meyfroidt

Abstract *Introduction*: The aim of this analysis was to investigate to what extent median cerebral perfusion pressure (CPP) differs between severe traumatic brain injury (TBI) patients and between centres, and whether the 2007 change in CPP threshold in the Brain Trauma Foundation guidelines is reflected in patient data collected at several centres over different time periods.

Methods: Data were collected from the Brain-IT database, a multi-centre project between 2003 and 2005, and from a recent project in four centres between 2009 and 2013. For patients nursed with their head up at 30° and with the blood pressure transducer at atrium level, CPP was corrected by 10 mmHg. Median CPP, interquartile ranges and total CPP ranges over the monitoring time were calculated per patient and per centre.

Results: Per-centre medians pre-2007 were situated between 50 and 70 mmHg in 6 out of 16 centres, while 10 centres had medians above 70 mmHg and 4 above 80 mmHg. Post-2007, three out of four centres had medians between 60 and 70 mmHg and one above 80 mmHg. One out of two centres with data pre- and post-2007 shifted from a median CPP of 76 mmHg to 60 mmHg, while the other remained at 68–67 mmHg.

Conclusions: CPP data are characterised by a high inter-individual variability, but the data also suggest differences in CPP policies between centres. The 2007 guideline change may have affected policies towards lower CPP in some centres. Deviations from the guidelines occur in the direction of CPP > 70 mmHg.

Keywords Severe traumatic brain injury · Cerebral perfusion pressure · Brain Trauma Foundation · Guidelines · Pressure variability

B. Depreitere (✉) · F. Güiza · G. Van den Berghe · G. Meyfroidt
University Hospitals Leuven, Leuven, Belgium
e-mail: bart.depreitere@uzleuven.be

I. Piper · L. Moss
Southern General Hospital, Glasgow, UK

G. Citerio
San Gerardo Hospital, Monza, Italy

I. Chambers
James Cook University Hospital, Middlesborough, UK

P.A. Jones · T.-Y. M. Lo
Royal Hospital for Sick Children, Edinburgh, UK

P. Enblad · P. Nilsson
Uppsala University Hospital, Uppsala, Sweden

B. Feyen · P. Jorens · A. Maas
University Hospital Antwerp, Antwerp, Belgium

M.U. Schuhmann
Universitätsklinikum Tübingen, Tübingen, Germany

R. Donald
University of Glasgow, Glasgow, UK

Introduction

The recommendation for targeting cerebral perfusion pressure (CPP) in the Brain Trauma Foundation (BTF) guidelines on the management of severe traumatic brain injury (TBI) has changed from keeping CPP above 70 mmHg in the 1996 edition [1] to 50–70 mmHg in the 2007 edition [2]. The change to recommending lower CPP was mainly inspired by the non-beneficial effect of keeping CPP above 70 mmHg by administering high doses of vasopressors in the randomised controlled trial performed by Robertson et al. [3]. This was later confirmed in the post hoc analysis of the Selfotel data [4]. As it has been demonstrated that adherence to the BTF guidelines effectively had a positive effect on outcomes in severe TBI [5, 6], one would expect such change in recommendation to be followed, and hence to lead to alterations in CPP policy across centres. Our study on the visualisation of pressure and time burden of intracranial hypertension in TBI included patients who were collected from data-capture initiatives in several centres over different periods of time [7]. The aim of this analysis was to investigate to what extent median CPP differed between patients and between centres and whether the change in guideline with respect to CPP target in 2007 was reflected in the clinical data.

Methods

The adult group of the study cohort consisted of 261 patients with severe TBI. Of these, 166 patients were included from the Brain-IT database, a European multi-centre data collection made between March 2003 and July 2005 [7, 8]. The Multi-Centre Research Ethics Committee for Scotland MREC/02/0/9 granted the use of these data for scientific purposes on 14 February 2002. The data of the remaining 95 adult patients were collected from four centres between 2009 and 2013 [7]: San Gerardo Hospital Monza (Italy), University Hospitals Leuven (Belgium), University Hospital Antwerp (Belgium) and University Hospital Tübingen (Germany). Local Ethics Committee approval to use the anonymised data for this analysis was obtained in all four centres. Two centres delivered data to both the early and later cohort. For patients nursed head up at 30° and with the blood pressure transducer at atrium level, CPP was corrected by subtracting 10 mmHg. Median CPP, interquartile range and total CPP range over the patients' monitoring time were calculated per patient and per centre, a similar analysis was done for patients' median CPPs.

Results

Over the entire cohort, the median CPP per patient varied between 27 and 96 mmHg, while the global CPP range extended from 0 to >140 mmHg. The per-centre median of patients' medians varied between 58 and 87 mmHg. Overall, inter-individual variability exceeded inter-centre variability. CPP variability was independent of intracranial pressure, and hence was also reflected in mean arterial pressure (MAP) variability. In line, CPP strongly correlated with MAP, and this analysis expressed different centre policies. Per-centre medians pre-2007 were situated between 50 and 70 mmHg in 6 out of 16 centres, while 10 centres had medians above 70 mmHg and 4 above 80 mmHg (Fig. 1). Centre comparison post-2007 demonstrates that three centres had their median CPP between 50 and 70 mmHg, while one was above 80 mmHg (Fig. 1). The post-2007 patient data grouped per centre clearly suggest an effect of centre CPP policy in addition to inter-individual CPP variability (Fig. 2).

With respect to the potential effect of guideline change in 2007, the overall mean CPP dropped from 71.1 (± 10.4) mmHg before 2007 to 61.1 (± 14.5) mmHg after 2007 ($p = 0.001$). One of the two centres with data pre- and post-2007 shifted from a centre median CPP of 76 to 60 mmHg before and after 2007, while the other remained at 68–67 mmHg.

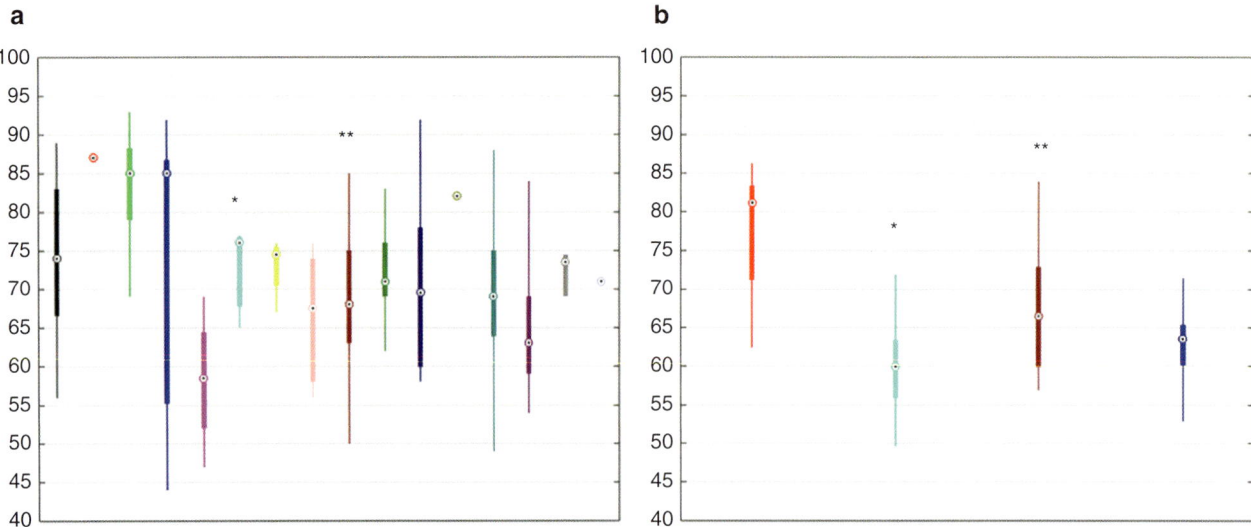

Fig. 1 Per-centre CPPs (median, interquartile range and total range of patients' medians). (**a**) Study cohort 2003–2005. (**b**) Study cohort 2009–2013. *Each colour* represents a centre; * and ** indicate centres appearing in both cohorts

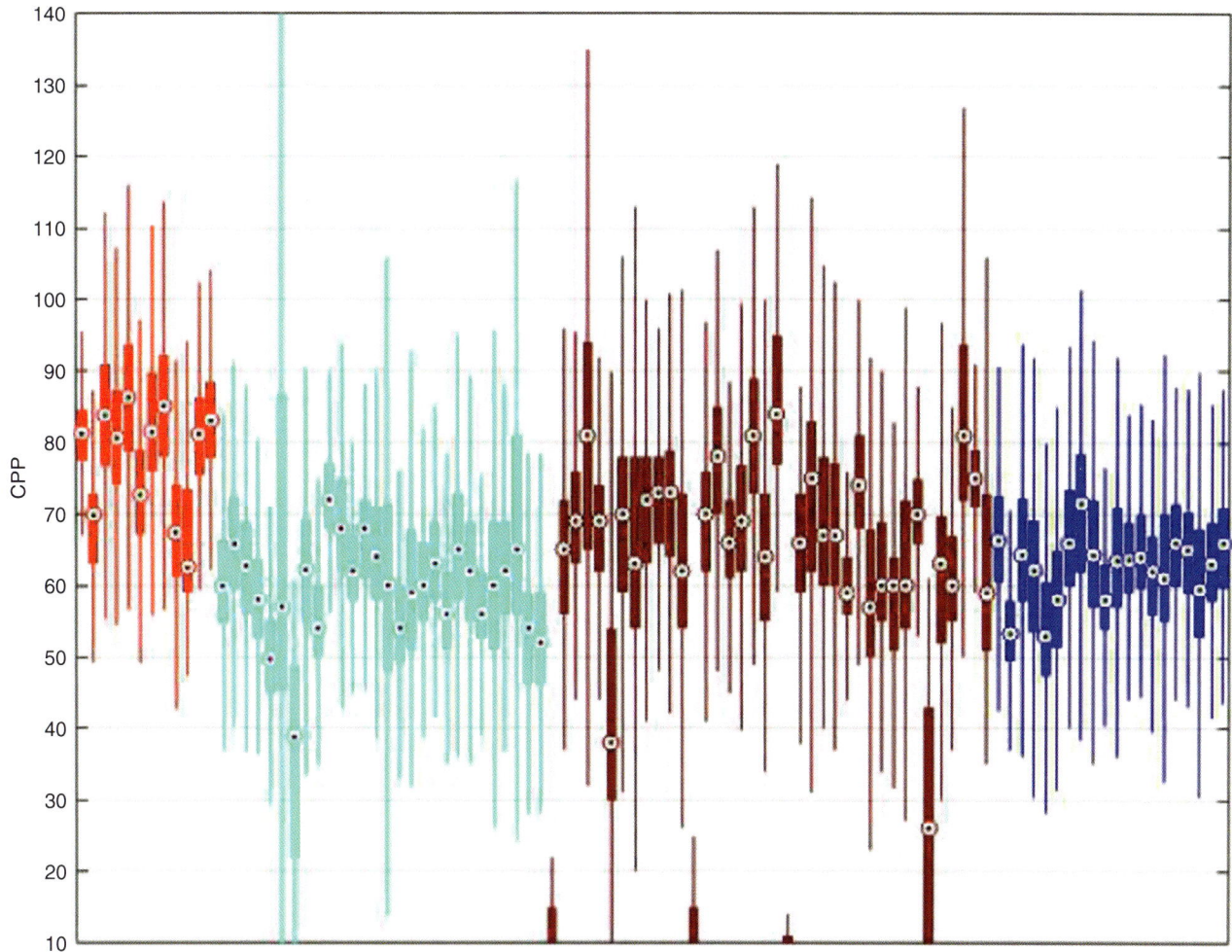

Fig. 2 Per-patient CPPs (median, interquartile range and total range) for the 2009–2013 study cohort. *Each colour* represents a centre

Discussion

The current analysis demonstrates that in the patient cohorts studied, the inter-individual CPP variability exceeds the inter-centre variability as expressed in interquartile ranges and total ranges. However, it is still possible to discern an effect of centres' CPP target policies in the data. The change in CPP thresholds in the BTF guidelines in 2007 did affect one of the two centres where this could be measured, while the rate of 75% post-2007 having median CPP below 70 mmHg may also mean that an effort was made to follow the BTF guidelines. When looking at individual data, though, it can be stated that deviations from the BTF guidelines occurred more frequently to the right, i.e. to higher CPPs, than to the left, i.e. to lower CPPs. To the best of our knowledge, this is the first study specifically documenting CPP adherence and variability.

When studying CPP variability across centres and patients, two questions emerge. The first question is how accurately CPP can effectively be steered towards specific values or ranges in the everyday clinical setting, given that it is influenced by ICP variability, MAP variability including systemic events and responses to drugs, and by responses to therapeutic actions intended to decrease raised ICP. This question is particularly relevant in light of the recommended CPP range being narrowed down to 60–70 mmHg in the latest version of the BTF guidelines issued this year [9], as well as in light of the emerging concept of dynamic individual CPP targets influenced by autoregulation capacity [10, 11]. The second question is whether deviations to the right (higher CPPs) originate from the fear of too low CPP and possible associated ischaemia, while the effects of too high CPP are less well documented or feared. In fact, the higher incidence of acute respiratory distress syndrome (ARDS) reportedly associated with vasopressors in the CPP > 70 mmHg group in the trial by Robertson et al. [3] does not seem to be that much of a concern in clinical practice.

The current analysis is a spin-off of another study for which the current data were brought together [7]. Hence, it is limited by its retrospective nature. Moreover, only four centres contributed data in the post-2007 cohort. Different centres used different CPP methodology, i.e. they had the arterial blood pressure transducer at tragus or at atrium height and nursed patients flat or with their head up at 30°. For patients with the transducer at atrium height and being nursed at 30° head up, the CPP was corrected by subtracting 10 mmHg [estimation of tragus-atrium distance × sin(30°) × 0.76 mmHg/cmH$_2$O]. When we repeated the analysis without this correction, all conclusions stated in the first paragraph of the discussion section remained valid.

While it may be irrelevant to issue CPP targets that are expected to be universally valid in all patients at all times, it may be useful to produce CPP safety limits. The current study demonstrated that centres' CPP policies do have some effect, but that it is exceeded by intra- and inter-individual CPP variability.

Conflicts of interest statement We declare that we have no conflict of interest.

References

1. Brain Trauma Foundation; American Association of Neurological Surgeons; Joint Section on Neurotrauma and Critical Care, et al. Guidelines for cerebral perfusion pressure. J Neurotrauma. 1996;13:693–697.
2. Brain Trauma Foundation, American Association of Neurological Surgeons, Congress of Neurological Surgeons, Joint Section on Neurotrauma and Critical Care, AANS/CNS, et al. Guidelines for the management of severe traumatic brain injury. IX. Cerebral perfusion thresholds. J Neurotrauma. 2007;24(Suppl 1):S59–64.
3. Robertson CS, Valadka AB, Hannay HJ, Contant CF, Gopinath SP, Cormio M, et al. Prevention of secondary ischemic insults after severe head injury. Crit Care Med. 1999;27:2086–95.
4. Juul N, Morris GF, Marshall SB, Marshall LF. Intracranial hypertension and cerebral perfusion pressure: influence on neurological deterioration and outcome in severe head injury. The Executive Committee of the International Selfotel Trial. J Neurosurg. 2000;92:1–6.
5. Cnossen MC, Scholten AC, Lingsma HF, Synnot A, Tavender E, Gantner D, et al. Adherence to guidelines in adult patients with traumatic brain injury: a living systematic review. J Neurotrauma. 2016. doi:10.1089/neu.2015.4121.
6. Gupta D, Sharma D, Kannan N, Prapruettham S, Mock C, Wang J, et al. Guideline adherence and outcomes in severe adult traumatic brain injury for the CHIRAG (Collaborative Head Injury and Guidelines) study. World Neurosurg. 2016;89:169–79.
7. Güiza F, Depreitere B, Piper I, Citerio G, Chambers I, Jones PA, et al. Visualizing the pressure and time burden of intracranial hypertension in adult and paediatric traumatic brain injury. Intensive Care Med. 2015;41:1067–76.
8. Piper I, Citerio G, Chambers I, Contant C, Enblad P, Fiddes H, et al. The Brain-IT group: concept and core dataset definition. Acta Neurochir. 2003;145:615–28.
9. Carney N, Totten AM, O'Reilly C, Ullman JS, Hawryluk GW, Bell MJ, et al. Guidelines for the management of severe traumatic brain injury. 4th ed. Neurosurgery. 2017;80:6–15.
10. Steiner LA, Czosnyka M, Piechnik K, Smielewski P, Chatfield D, Menon DK, et al. Continuous monitoring of cerebrovascular pressure reactivity allows determination of optimal cerebral perfusion pressure in patients with traumatic brain injury. Crit Care Med. 2002;30:733–8.
11. Aries MJ, Czosnyka M, Budohoski KP, Steiner LA, Lavinio A, Kolias AG, et al. Continuous determination of optimal cerebral perfusion pressure in traumatic brain injury. Crit Care Med. 2012;40:2456–63.

Pre-hospital Predictors of Impaired ICP Trends in Continuous Monitoring of Paediatric Traumatic Brain Injury Patients

Adam M.H. Young[†], Joseph Donnelly[†], Xiuyun Liu, Mathew R. Guilfoyle, Melvin Carew, Manuel Cabeleira, Danilo Cardim, Matthew R. Garnett, Helen M. Fernandes, Christina Haubrich, Peter Smielewski, Marek Czosnyka, Peter J. Hutchinson, and Shruti Agrawal

Abstract *Objective*: Although secondary insults such as raised intracranial pressure (ICP) or cardiovascular compromise strongly contribute to morbidity, a growing interest can be noticed in how the pre-hospital management can affect outcomes after traumatic brain injury (TBI). The objective of this study was to determine whether pre-hospital co-morbidity has influence on patterns of continuously measured waveforms of intracranial physiology after paediatric TBI.

Materials and methods: Thirty-nine patients (mean age, 10 years; range, 0.5–15) admitted between 2002 and 2015 were used for the current analysis. Pre-hospital motor score, pupil reactivity, pre-hospital hypoxia ($SpO_2 < 90\%$) and hypotension (mean arterial pressure < 70 mmHg) were documented. ICP and arterial blood pressure (ABP) were monitored continuously with an intraparenchymal microtransducer and an indwelling arterial line. Pressure monitors were connected to bedside computers running ICM+ software. Pressure reactivity was determined as the moving correlation between 30 10-s averages of ABP and ICP (PRx). The mean ICP and PRx were calculated for the whole monitoring period for each patient.

Results: Those with pre-hospital hypotension were susceptible to higher ICP [20 (IQR 8) vs 13 (IQR 6) mmHg; $p = 0.01$] and more frequent ICP plateau waves [median = 0 (IQR 1), median = 4 (IQR 9); $p = 0.001$], despite having similar MAP, CPP and PRx during monitoring. Those with unreactive pupils tended to have higher ICP than those with reactive pupils (18 vs 14 mmHg, $p = 0.08$). Pre-hospital hypoxia, motor score and pupillary reactivity were not related to subsequent monitored intracranial or systemic physiology.

Conclusion: In paediatric TBI, pre-hospital hypotension is associated with increased ICP in the intensive care unit.

Keywords Brain · Injury · Pre-hospital · ICP

Introduction

Traumatic brain injury is a major cause of morbidity, particularly in children. After the initial injury, secondary injuries, such as raised intracranial pressure (ICP), decreased cerebral perfusion pressure (CPP), impaired cerebral blood flow regulation or hyperthermia, contribute to further intracranial and systemic insult and, importantly, represent a potential avenue for therapy [1]. Thus, in adults and children, prevention of secondary injury forms an integral part of the intensive care management.

Monitoring of ICP affords the opportunity to detect evolving intracranial pathology and monitor the efficacy of ICP-lowering therapies. However, deciding which patients may benefit from ICP monitoring is uncertain, particularly in children. Current guidelines from adults indicate that ICP monitoring should be considered in those with a Glasgow Coma Score of 8 or less, or with an abnormal computed tomography (CT) scan [2].

At the scene of the brain trauma, several features are available that can indicate impaired oxygen delivery to the

---

[†]Adam Young and Joseph Donnelly contributed equally to this work.

A.M.H. Young (✉) · M.R. Guilfoyle · M.R. Garnett
H.M. Fernandes · P.J. Hutchinson
Division of Academic Neurosurgery, Department of Clinical Neurosciences, Cambridge University Hospitals, University of Cambridge, Cambridge, UK
e-mail: ay276@cam.ac.uk

J. Donnelly · X. Liu · M. Cabeleira · D. Cardim · C. Haubrich
P. Smielewski · M. Czosnyka
Brain Physics Laboratory, Division of Neurosurgery, Department of Clinical Neuroscience, Cambridge University Hospitals, University of Cambridge, Cambridge, UK

M. Carew · S. Agrawal
Department of Paediatric Intensive Care, Cambridge University Hospitals, Cambridge, UK

brain, such as systemic hypoxia and systemic hypotension, or provide an early indication of secondary cerebral dysfunction such as impaired pupillary reactivity or impaired motor response to painful stimuli. How these early clinical features relate to the intracranial variables subsequently monitored on the intensive care unit, such as ICP, cerebral pressure reactivity (PRx), CPP and mean arterial pressure (MAP), is unknown.

Methods

Patients

Thirty-nine patients were recruited from the paediatric intensive care unit at Addenbrooke's Hospital, Cambridge, UK, between the years of 2002 and 2015. The data are routinely collected for clinical purposes and guides the management of patients. The analysis of data within this study for the purposes of service evaluation was approved by the Cambridge University Hospital NHS Trust, Audit and Service Evaluation Department (Ref. 2143) and did not require ethical approval or patient consent. Patients were included in this cohort if they had a clinical need for ICP monitoring. Patients were treated according to current paediatric traumatic brain injury guidelines [3], which aim to keep the ICP below 20 mmHg through a stepwise regime, including: positioning, sedation, paralysis, osmotic agents, ventriculostomy and induced hypothermia. Pre-hospital clinical features—hypotension (age adjusted [4]), hypoxia ($SpO_2 < 90\%$), pupil reactivity and motor score—were extracted from the pre-hospital phase of management (first recorded measure).

Data Acquisition and Analysis

Arterial blood pressure (ABP) was measured at the radial or femoral artery, zeroed at the level of the heart (Baxter Healthcare, Westlake Village, CA, USA; Sidcup, UK). ICP was measured with an intraparenchymal microsensor in the frontal cortex (Codman ICP Micro-Sensor; Codman & Shurtleff, Raynham, MA, USA). ICP and ABP data were collected at 100 Hz with an analogue to digital converter (DT9801, Data Translation, Marlboro, MA, USA) coupled with a laptop computer running ICM+ software (University of Cambridge, Cambridge Enterprise, Cambridge, UK, http://www.neurosurg.cam.ac.uk/icmplus). Pressure reactivity index (PRx) was calculated as the moving correlation between 10-s averages of ICP and ABP. Patients ICP, PRx, mean arterial pressure (MAP) and CPP were then averaged over the first 72 h of their intensive care unit stay.

Statistical Analysis

Mean ICP, PRx, CPP and MAP over the first 3 days of monitoring were calculated. The influence of the presence or absence of prehospital factors (hypotension, hypoxia, more than one unreactive pupil, motor score 3 or less) on subsequent ICP and PRx were tested using a non-parametric Wilcoxon test. All data manipulations and analysis were performed using R language and software environment for statistical computation (version 2.12.1) [5].

Results

The median age was 12 years (range, 0.5–15). Of the 39 patients, 14 were female, 15 had pre-hospital hypoxia, 9 had pre-hospital hypotension, 7 had at least one unreactive pupil and 12 had a motor score of 3 or less. Those with pre-hospital hypotension had a higher mean ICP over the first 3 days of monitoring (median 13.7, IQR 6.33 vs 20.6, IQR 8.33 mmHg $p = 0.01$; Fig. 1). Those with unreactive pupils tended to have higher ICP than those with reactive pupils (18.02 vs 13.68 mmHg, $p = 0.08$). Those with pre-hospital hypotension had more plateau waves, and tended to have a lower power of slow waves of ICP. Pre-hospital clinical factors did not influence subsequently monitored PRx (Table 1), MAP or CPP (data not shown).

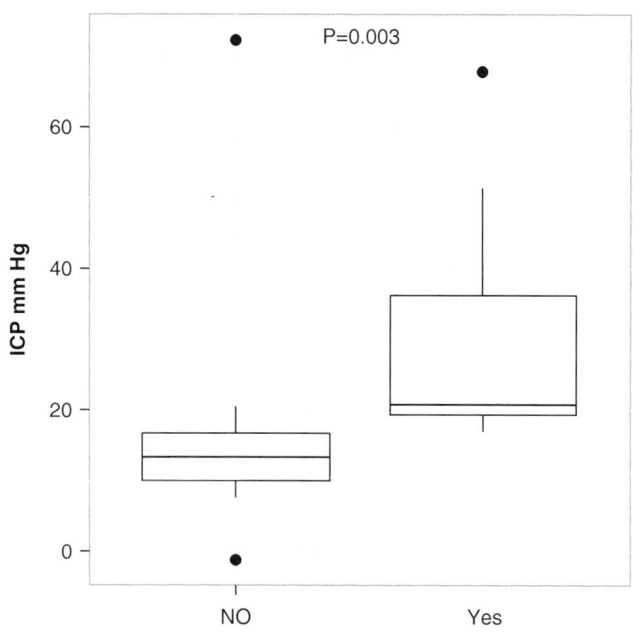

Fig. 1 Relationship between pre-hospital hypotension and mean ICP after TBI ($n = 33$). Paediatric TBI patients with pre-hospital hypotension (MAP less than 70 mmHg) had higher mean ICP during subsequent multimodality monitoring

Table 1 Relationships of early clinical factors with ICP over the first 72 h of monitoring

		ICP (mmHg)				PRx (a.u.)			
		Median	IQR	W	p value	Median	IQR	W	p value
Hypotension	Present	20.62	8.48	62	0.014	0.01	0.34	114	0.96
	Absent	13.68	6.33			−0.02	0.31		
Hypoxia	Present	13.61	7.29	179	0.99	0	0.38	175	0.56
	Absent	15.02	6.76			−0.08	0.36		
Unreactive pupils	Present	18.02	7.21	63	0.08	−0.17	0.38	121	0.26
	Absent	13.68	7.12			−0.01	0.3		
Motor score <4	Present	15.27	8.25	193	0.35	−0.11	0.44	133	0.76
	Absent	13.75	6.83			−0.01	0.28		

ICP intracranial pressure, *PRx* cerebrovascular auto regulation, *IQR* interquartile range, *W* Wilcoxon statistic

Discussion

In this study, we investigated the relationship between pre-hospital clinical factors and subsequent intracranial physiology after severe traumatic brain injury in children. Children with pre-hospital hypotension went on to develop higher ICP. Pre-hospital hypotension should alert the clinician to the potential for subsequent problems with ICP control.

Pre-hospital hypotension in the setting of traumatic brain injury can have many causes, including blood loss, obstructive shock or a systemic inflammatory response, and its presence has been shown to be an indicator of poor prognosis in both adults and children [6]. After brain trauma, any systemic hypotension reduces cerebral perfusion pressure and thus potentially causes cerebral hypoperfusion and ischaemia.

Against this context, our finding of increased ICP following hypotension could have a variety of causes. It is possible that an early cerebral ischaemia triggers a cascade of events that result in cerebral swelling and raised ICP. In support of this, Marmarou et al. [7] examined the combined effects of hypoxia and hypotension on subsequent brain swelling and found an increased ICP with the combination of early insults.

The tendency of unreactive pupils to be related to ICP is consistent with the thesis that raised intracranial pressure can disrupt the function of the oculomotor nerve. Pre-hospital hypoxia and impaired motor response to pain did not seem to influence subsequent ICP. No pre-hospital factors were related to subsequently monitored PRx, MAP or CPP, perhaps indicating that these factors are more closely related to insults occurring in the intensive care unit rather than before admission to the hospital.

Implications

Early prediction of raised ICP has the potential to facilitate the management of traumatic brain injury patients by alerting the clinicians to patients who require more intensive monitoring or perhaps a lower threshold for ICP treatment. However, prediction remains difficult and is usually confined to analysis of high-frequency ICP waveforms [8]. Thus, the current preliminary findings, if confirmed, could enhance existing ICP prediction tools. In addition, the current data potentially indicate that enhanced pre-hospital care may aid in avoiding secondary insults occurring up to 72 h after admission to hospital. Furthermore, the finding of a relationship between pre-hospital hypotension and subsequent ICP highlights the need to include pre-hospital factors in the analyses between physiological variables and patient outcome.

Limitations

As this current analysis is from quite a small dataset, we cannot exclude that more subtle relationships between pre-hospital factors and ICP or PRx may emerge with a larger dataset [9].

Conclusion

After severe paediatric traumatic brain injury, those patients with pre-hospital hypotension go on to develop higher ICP.

Conflicts of interest statement We declare that we have no conflict of interest.

References

1. Kolias A, Guilfoyle M, Helmy A, et al. Traumatic brain injury in adults. Pract Neurol. 2013;13:228–35.
2. Brain Trauma Foundation. Guidelines for the management of severe traumatic brain injury, 3rd edition. J Neurotrauma. 2007;24(Suppl 1):S37–44.

3. Kochanek PM, Carney NA, Adelson PD, et al. Guidelines for the acute medical management of severe traumatic brain injury in infants, children, and adolescents—second edition. Pediatr Crit Care Med. 2012;13(Suppl):S1–82.
4. Kleinman ME, Chameides L, Schexnayder SM, et al. Part 14: pediatric advanced life support: 2010 American Heart Association Guidelines for Cardiopulmonary Resuscitation and Emergency Cardiovascular Care. Circulation. 2010;122(18 Suppl 3):S876–908. doi:https://doi.org/10.1161/CIRCULATIONAHA.110.971101
5. R Core Team. R: a language and environment for statistical computing. Vienna: R Foundation for Statistical Computing; 2015. http://www.r-project.org/.
6. Pigula FA, Wald SL, Shackford SR, Vane DW. The effect of hypotension and hypoxia on children with severe head injuries. J Pediatr Surg. 1993;28:310–6.
7. Kita H, Marmarou A. The cause of acute brain swelling after the closed head injury in rats. Acta Neurochir Suppl (Wien). 1994;60:452–5.
8. Hu X, Xu P, Asgari S, Vespa P, Bergsneider M. Forecasting ICP elevation based on prescient changes of intracranial pressure waveform morphology. IEEE Trans Biomed Eng. 2010;57:1070–8.
9. Cabella B, Donnelly J, Cardim D, Liu X, Cabeleira M, Smielewski P, Haubrich C, Hutchinson P, Kim DJ, Czosnyka M. An association between ICP-derived data and outcome in TBI patients: the role of sample size. Neurocrit Care. 2017;27(1):103–7.

Prognosis of Severe Traumatic Brain Injury Outcomes in Children

Semen V. Meshcheryakov, Zhanna B. Semenova, Valery I. Lukianov, Elena G. Sorokina, and Olga V. Karaseva

Abstract *Objectives*: We aimed to determine prognostic factors that can influence the outcome of severe traumatic brain injury (TBI) in children.

Materials and methods: One hundred and sixty-nine patients with severe TBI were included. Consciousness was evaluated using the Glasgow Coma Scale (GCS). Severity of concomitant injuries was evaluated using the Injury Severity Score (ISS). Computer tomography (CT) scanning was used on admission and later. Intracranial injuries were classified using the Marshall CT scale. Intracranial pressure (ICP) monitoring took place in 80 cases. Serum samples of 65 patients were tested for S-100β protein and of 43 patients for neuron specific enolase (NSE). Outcomes were evaluated 6 months after trauma using the Glasgow Outcome Scale (GOS). Statistical and mathematical analysis was conducted. The accuracy of our prognostic model was defined in another group of patients ($n = 118$).

Results: GCS, pupil size and photoreaction, ISS, hypotension and hypoxia are significant predictors of outcome of severe TBI in children. CT results complement the forecast significantly. The accuracy of surviving prognosis came to 76% (0.76) in case of S-100β protein level $\leq$ 0.25 μg/l and NSE level < 19 μg/l. A mathematical model of outcome prognosis was based on discriminant function analysis. The model of prognosis was tested on the control group. The accuracy of prognosis was 86%.

Conclusions: A personalised prognostic model makes it possible to predict the outcome of severe TBI in children on the first day after trauma.

Keywords Severe brain injury · Outcomes · Prognosis · Intracranial hypertension · Math model

Introduction

In Moscow, a 1.5-times increase in patients with traumatic brain injury (TBI) has been observed in the past 5 years. Total mortality amounts to 5–10%, but in the case of severe TBI this rate goes to 41–85% [1, 2]. Recent medical achievements make it possible to decrease the mortality rate, but the frequency of severe disability and persistent vegetative state in such patients is still high [3–5]. Economic losses for government include not only treatment expenses and supplies for the disabled, but missed profits and future potential labour losses as well. Further technology development and implementation of new health care standards are expected to lead not only to improved treatment results but also to increases in health care costs. So, the choice of most efficient and economically profitable treatment should unavoidably become a key issue. Prognosis may be very useful in this case. Perel et al. [6] reported that despite a great amount of evidence there is no universal application of prognostic abilities. Nowadays most doctors are prone to be either excessively optimistic or too pessimistic. It seems to be attributed to differences in material and technical equipment as well as in medical staff qualifications [6]. A variety of clinical, radiological and laboratory investigations were determined to be independent predictors of TBI outcome [1, 4, 5, 7]. The development of multifactor models using these predictors allows prognosis to be personalised. The most available personalised models of TBI prognosis in adults are

S.V. Meshcheryakov (✉)
Children's Clinical and Research Institute of Emergency Surgery and Trauma, Moscow, Russia

Department of Neurosurgery, Children's Clinical and Research Institute of Emergency Surgery and Trauma,
St. Bolshaya Polyanka 22, 119180 Moscow, Russia
e-mail: msaemon@rambler.ru

Z.B. Semenova • V.I. Lukianov • O.V. Karaseva
Children's Clinical and Research Institute of Emergency Surgery and Trauma, Moscow, Russia

E.G. Sorokina
Federal State Autonomous Institution "Scientific Center of Children's Health" of the Ministry of Health of the Russian Federation, Moscow, Russia

prognosis calculators based on crash and impact studies. Unfortunately, no such research has been done for children.

Methods and Materials

We retrospectively reviewed 169 cases of severe TBI [Glasgow Coma Scale (GCS) ≤8] in children who were admitted to our clinic in a 7-year period (from 2004 to 2011). Level of consciousness was evaluated using GCS. The frequency and severity of concomitant injuries in children are usually due to so-called high-energy trauma [2, 5]. Severity of concomitant injuries was evaluated using the Injury Severity Score (ISS). Computed tomography (CT) remains the leading method of objective diagnostics. All children underwent brain CT. We used the Marshall CT scale for brain injury classification (Fig. 1). We also monitored intracranial pressure (ICP). The rising interest in serum brain injury marker usage is related to the development of modern immunology and biochemistry and to their commercial availability [7–10]. The dynamics of S-100β protein and neuron specific enolase (NSE) levels was analysed. We evaluated serum samples for S-100β protein level in 65 patients on days 1–3, 6–8, 14–15 and 20–23 after injury. In 43 patients, the serum level of NSE was analysed.

We estimated the outcomes of severe TBIs using the Glasgow Outcome Scale (GOS). Patients with good recovery and mild disability (GOS 4–5) were included in the positive outcome group; patients with severe disability and persistent vegetative state (GOS 2–3), in negative outcome group. The third group consisted of patients with lethal outcome (GOS 1).

A mathematical model approach is meant to be the most informative for prognosis. Widespread personal computer usage for creating databases and availability of applicable programs for mathematical calculations have become a background for the creation of multifactor prognosis models. On the basis of discriminant function analysis, a personalised model of severe TBI outcome prognosis in children has been designed. The basic model is founded on seven signs, which can be observed during pre-hospital period and after patient's admission: age, hypoxia during the pre-hospital period, GCS level, size and reaction of pupils, presence of concomitant injury, ISS level, type of damage according to Marshall CT scale. For GCS and ISS levels, numerical values were used. For other predictors, gradations of values are given in Table 1. All the signs were classified and the classificatory matrix, that is reflective for weighting coefficients and constants for each outcome variant, was made, Table 2. Using this classificatory matrix of basic model, it is possible to calculate the discriminant function value for each outcome by applying this formula:

Table 1 Predictors of outcome and their meanings

Predictor	Value
Age (F1)	1 – <4 years 2 – ≥4 to <8 years 3 – ≥8 to <13 years 4 – >13 years
Pre-hospital hypoxia (F2)	0 – no, 1, – yes
GCS (F3)	Points
Pupillary diameter @ light reflex (F4)	1 – normal 2 – anisocoria 3 – midriasis
Presence of concomitant injury (F5)	1 – no, 2 – yes
ISS scale (F6)	Points
Marshall CT scale (F7)	1 – (I), 2 – (II), 3 – (III), 4 – IV, 5 – (V), 6 – (VI)

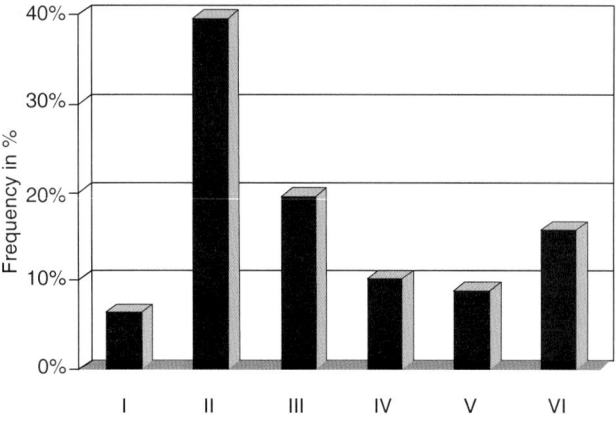

Fig. 1 Marshall CT scale on admission the first day after injury

Table 2 The classification matrix of outcomes. Recorded weight values for all predictors in each outcome group

Predictor		Coefficient		
		GOS 1	GOS 2, 3	GOS 4, 5
Age	k1	1.39	1.02	1.63
Prehospital hypoxia	k2	10.15	7.66	8.23
GCS	k3	7.25	7.62	7.65
Pupillary diameter @ light reflex	k4	14.08	12.02	9.71
Presence of concomitant injury	k5	4.62	4.85	5.72
ISS scale	k6	0.50	0.49	0.32
Marshall CT scale	k7	2.02	1.85	1.51
Constant		−56.99	−52.18	−45.78

$$DF = (k1 \times F1) + (k2 \times F2) + (k3 \times F3) + (k4 \times F4)$$
$$+ (k5 \times F5) + (k6 \times F6) + (k7 \times F7) + C$$

where DF is the discriminant function value, $k1$–7 are weighting coefficients of predictors, $F1$–7 are predictor values and C is a constant.

The largest discriminant function value accords with the most probable outcome. The accuracy of positive outcome prognosis (GOS 4–5) is more than 90%, and for lethal outcome prognosis (GOS 1) the accuracy is more than 80%.

In our study, we used analysis of variance, log-regression analysis, cluster analysis and non-parametric statistic methods—Spearman's Rank Correlation Index and the Gamma Index in particular. The mathematical model of severe TBI outcome prognosis was based on discriminant function analysis.

Results

Among 169 cases of severe TBI admitted, boys accounted for 66.1% and girls for 33.9%. Average age was 8.9 ± 5 years. Most of the patients (64.2%) were injured in road traffic accidents; 18.8% of injuries were caused by falling from height; in 10% it was an injury resulting from the fall of a heavy object on their head; in 3.8%, forced trauma; in 3.1%, gunshot wound.

Trauma mechanism and outcomes differ in age groups (Fig. 2). Infants ($n = 7$) were shown to have forced brain trauma frequently; in this group, we saw lethal outcomes in 43% of cases and positive outcomes in 43% of cases, respectively. Children 1–3 years old ($n = 23$) were injured in road traffic accidents more often and by falling from a height less frequently. The mortality rate in this group was 21.7%; positive outcomes were seen in 47.8% of cases. The leading cause of brain injury in children of 4–17 years old was road traffic accidents and more rarely they were injured by falling from a height. Gunshot wounds were seen only in several patients and were connected to careless handling of firearms.

Statistical analysis showed that positive outcomes of severe TBI were more frequent in elder children, and lethal outcomes were seen more often in infants. There was no statistically reliable difference in outcome for children of different age ($p = 0.1$). Six months after injury, we estimated that 47.9% of patients had positive outcome and total mortality rate was 27.8%.

In 48% of patients ($n = 81$) the GCS score was 7–8, while in 35% ($n = 59$) the GCS score was 5–6, and the consciousness level of 17% of patients ($n = 29$) was estimated as 3–4 by GCS. Patients with GCS 7–8 were shown to have positive outcomes more often (in 65.9% of cases), and lethal outcomes in this group accounted for only 6.1%. In the group of patients with GCS 5–6, positive outcomes were seen more rarely (in 35.6% of cases), but negative and lethal outcomes prevailed and accounted for 28.8% and 35.6% respectively. Outcomes in children with GCS 3–4 at 6 months after injury were mostly negative, and the mortality rate came to 82.1%. The outcome of TBI in children depends on level of consciousness: positive outcomes were seen statistically more often in patients with higher GCS level. A strong correlation was determined (Gamma Index = 0.6663, $p < 0.05$).

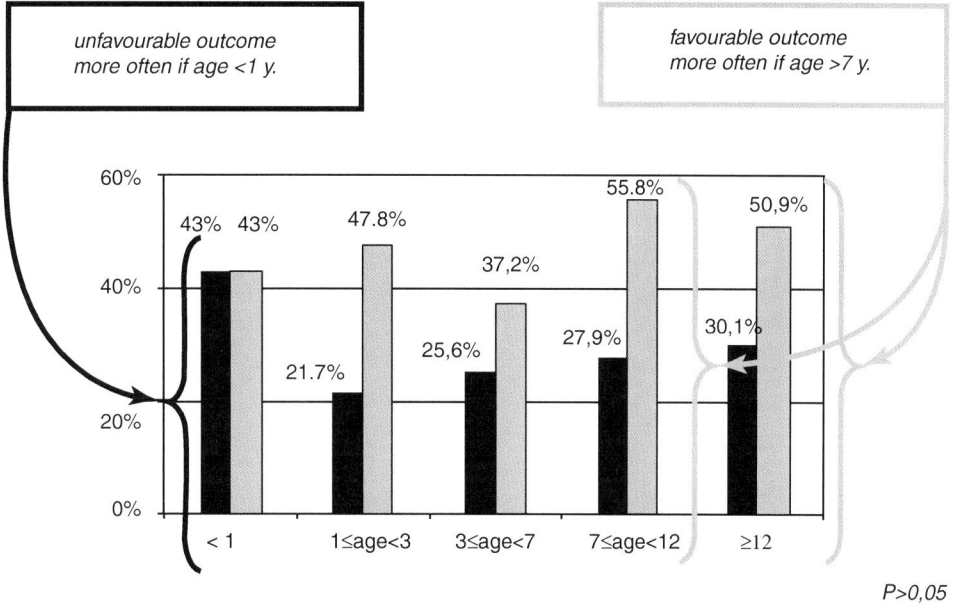

Fig. 2 Frequency of unfavourable and favourable outcomes of severe TBI in children of different ages

TBI was associated with concomitant injuries in 63.3% of cases ($n = 107$). The average ISS for concomitant injuries was 32.8 ± 9.7. Chest trauma prevailed (63.5%) among concomitant injuries; abdominal cavity and retroperitoneal organs were damaged in 53% of patients; orthopaedic trauma was registered in 53% of cases, vertebral column injury in 13% of cases and craniofacial trauma in 24% of cases.

It was shown for children with GCS > 5 that outcome depended mostly on TBI severity and that ISS level did not play a significant role for prognosis. In contrast, for children with GCS < 5 the probability of positive or negative outcome correlated with ISS level. In the case of ISS ≤ 32, we saw positive outcomes statistically more frequently. In the case of ISS > 40, the same conclusion was true for negative outcomes. Moderate correlation was determined between severe TBI (GCS 6–8) outcome and ISS level in case of concomitant injuries (Gamma Index = 0.476, $p < 0.05$).

Intracranial pressure (ICP) monitoring was instrumented in 80 patients (47.3%). Neurosurgical procedures were performed in 31% ($n = 53$) of children with severe TBI: in 9% ($n = 15$) of cases, there was craniotomy accompanied by haematoma removal and depressed fracture reposition; in 22.5% ($n = 38$) of cases, decompressive craniectomy was done.

Statistical analysis showed moderate correlation between GCS level and type of brain injury by Marshall CT scale, size of pupils and photoreaction. Type II diffuse brain injury occurred in patients with GCS 6–8 statistically more frequently and type IV in patients with GCS 3–5. Anisocoria was seen reliably more often in patients with GCS 5–6 and accounted for 24.3%. Photoreaction loss and mydriasis occurred in patients with GCS 3–4 and came to 15.9%. A moderate correlation was determined (Gamma Index = 0.5377, $p < 0.05$). Negative outcomes in children with mydriasis and photoreaction loss were determined in 89% of cases; among them, lethal outcomes amounted to 74%. In case of anisocoria, we saw negative outcomes in 61% of patients; among them, lethal outcomes were registered in 24.4%. In case of safe photoreaction, 62% of outcomes were positive and mortality rate came to only 17.8%.

Non-parametric analysis showed statistically reliable moderate correlation between severe TBI outcome in children and level of cisterna ambiens compression (Gamma Index = 0.6501, $p < 0.05$), and low correlation in case of subarachnoid haemorrhage and midline shift (Gamma Index = −0.329 and 0.027 respectively, $p < 0.05$). Outcomes differed due to Marshall CT scale variants of injury (Fig. 3). Positive outcomes (68.5%) occurred more often in patients with type I–II diffuse brain injury. Negative (43%) and lethal (43%) outcomes were observed in case of type III–IV diffuse brain injury. Strong correlation was determined (Gamma Index = −0.711, $p < 0.05$). In patients after mass-effect removal procedures (type V by Marshall CT scale), positive outcomes were seen in 46% of cases. When mass effect persisted continuously (type VI), we observed lethal outcomes more frequently (in 45% of patients). Moderate correlation was determined (Gamma Index = −0.501, $p < 0.05$).

Hypotension and hypoxia were detected in every third patient. Negative outcomes in children with hypotension and hypoxia were shown in more than 70% of cases and were statistically more frequent ($p = 0.015$).

We considered 0.090–0.125 µg/l as the upper normal serum level for S-100β protein and 13 µg/l for NSE

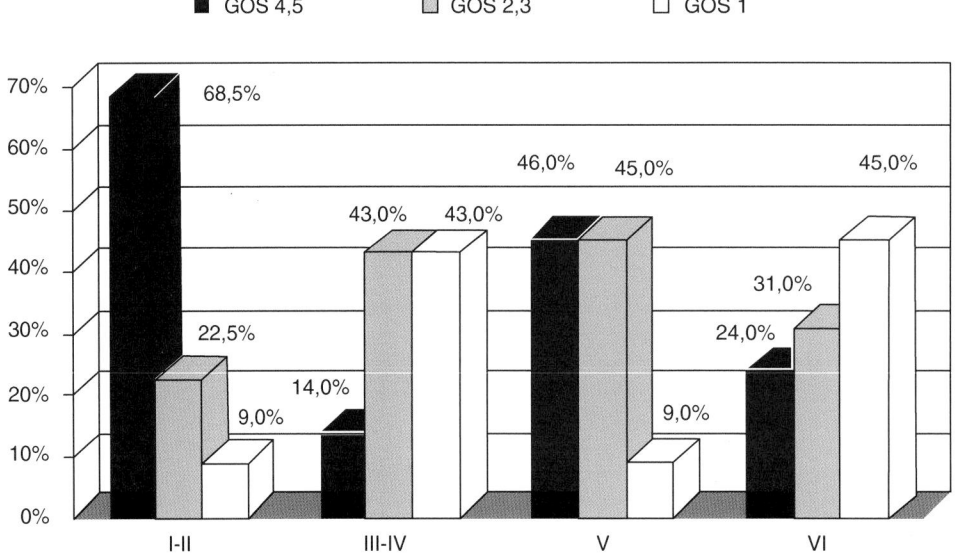

Fig. 3 Frequency outcomes in various brain injury (Marshall CT scale)

respectively. In case of positive outcome, the S-100β protein and NSE levels were high at 1 day after brain injury and then they decreased to normal values after 2–3 days. In case of negative outcome, the S-100β protein and NSE levels stayed high for 10 days on average and then showed a tendency to decrease. In case of lethal outcome, S-100β protein and NSE levels remained high until the patient's death. The highest level of S-100β protein was observed in children with negative outcomes of severe TBI in combination with concomitant injuries, and it was explained in recent scientific publications that other tissues could produce this protein as well in case of injury [1, 6, 9]. The S-100β protein and NSE levels differed statistically reliably in the group of survivors and in the group of children with lethal outcomes ($p = 0.038$). By contrast, we observed that there was no correlation between these levels in patients with positive outcome (GOS 4–5) and in patients with negative outcome (GOS 2–3). The accuracy of surviving prognosis in children with severe TBI came to 76% (0.76) in case of S-100β protein level ≤ 0.25 µg/l and NSE level <19 µg/l.

The accuracy of our prognostic model was defined in the group of patients ($n = 118$) that were admitted to our clinic in 2012–2015. Boys accounted for 63.5% ($n = 75$), girls for 36.5% ($n = 43$). Average age was 10.2 ± 5 years. Level of consciousness was estimated as GCS 7–8 in 50% of patients ($n = 59$), as GCS 5–6 in 35.6% of patients ($n = 42$) and as GCS 3–4 in 14.4% of patients ($n = 17$). In that group, children had concomitant injuries in 85% of cases ($n = 100$), and the severity of concomitant injuries was estimated as 28.2 ± 7.5 by ISS scale. Positive outcomes (GOS 4–5) were seen in 65.3% of patients ($n = 17$), negative outcomes (GOS2–3) in 17.8% of patients ($n = 21$) and lethal outcomes (GOS = 1) in 16.9% of patients ($n = 20$). The personalised model of severe TBI outcome prognosis was tested on a control group of patients, which consisted of children with severe TBI had been admitted to our clinic in 2012–2015. The accuracy of prognosis (total right prognosis) was 86%.

Discussion

The prognostic value of age as a predictor of severe TBI outcome was confirmed in adult patients [1–4, 8]. The increase of negative outcomes in elderly patients is mostly due to health decrement and escalation of the frequency of complications. It is thought that children of tender age have more compensation abilities, and so they can show better recovery after severe TBI [5]. But some anatomical and physiological aspects of children's metabolism increase the risk of severe primary brain injury in comparison with adults. Moreover, physiological brain sensitivity makes children more prone to secondary brain injury. So, age cannot be considered as independent and statistically reliable predictor of severe TBI outcome in children, but it may determine the mechanism of trauma and the structure of brain injury. Hypotension and hypoxia are still the leading factors of secondary brain injury [4, 11].

CGS level still can be considered as a strong predictor of TBI outcome, and it is used in most prognostic scales and models [1, 4, 6, 11, 12].

Size of pupils and photoreaction can be assessed easily and accurately at any moment after injury. These predictors still remain as principal and common prognostic factors of TBI outcome: they are included in 85% of prognostic models [6].

The severity of concomitant injuries (ISS) has an influence on severe TBI outcome in children at a greater degree in case of GCS level more than 5, but for children with 3–5 GCS level this influence is not statistically reliable. On the one hand, concomitant injuries induce the development of such pathophysiological processes as hypoxia or hypotension, which can lead to secondary brain damage. On the other hand, in most cases we can control concomitant injuries, so secondary brain damage can be avoided completely. The situation when ISS level can influence the TBI outcome is mostly in the group with higher GCS level. For example, brachial plexus injury can decrease the quality of life significantly in patients with good consciousness recovery, and in cases of permanent vegetative state such recovery may be considered as inessential.

Marshall CT scale can be useful not just for brain injury classification [12]. Using this scale, we can predict either the risk of ICP increase or the possible outcome of severe TBI in children.

There is not enough evidence about the role of neurospecific biomarkers in the prognosis of functional outcome of severe TBI, but their serum levels can be useful for prediction of survival and lethal outcomes in such patients [7–10].

An internal check of the proposed mathematical model's prognostic accuracy showed optimistic results—total accuracy came to 86%. However, it seems to be necessary to perform an external test based on similar children in neurosurgery departments in other Russian clinics.

Conclusions

Hypoxia and hypotension were shown to deteriorate the outcome and to be non-positive prognostic factors for severe TBI in children. GCS level, size of pupils, photoreaction, type of injury by Marshall CT classification and ISS level were proved to be statistically reliable predictors of severe TBI outcome in children. By contrast, we determined that the severity of concomitant injuries (ISS level) did not influence severe

TBI outcome in case of GCS 3–5. S100β and NSE serum levels can be useful to predict survival or lethal outcome. A personalised prognostic model makes it possible to predict the severe TBI outcome in children at first day after trauma.

Conflicts of interest statement We declare that we have no conflict of interest.

References

1. Potapov AA, Lihterman LB, Kravchuk AD, et al. Modern approaches to the study and treatment of traumatic brain injury. Ann Clin Exp Neurol. 2010;4(1):4–12.
2. Puras YuV, Talipov AE, Krilov VV, et al. Risk factors for poor outcome in the surgical treatment of severe traumatic brain injury. Russian J Neurosurg. 2013;(2):C.8–16.
3. Andriessen TM, Horn J, Franschman G, et al. Epidemiology, severity classification, and outcome of moderate and severe traumatic brain injury: a prospective multicenter study. J Neurotrauma. 2011;28(10):2019–31.
4. Brain Trauma Foundation, American Association of Neurological Surgeons, Congress of Neurological Surgeons. BTF guidelines for the management of severe traumatic brain injury (3rd edition). J Neurotrauma. 2007;24(Suppl):1–106.
5. Kan CH, Saffari M, Khoo TH. Prognostic factors of severe traumatic brain injury outcome in children aged 2–16 years at a major neurosurgical referral centre. Malays J Med Sci. 2009;16(4):25–33.
6. Perel P, Edwards P, Wentz R, et al. Systematic review of prognostic models in traumatic brain injury. BMC Med Inform Decis Mak. 2006;6:38.
7. Berger RP. The use of serum biomarkers to predict outcome after traumatic brain injury in adults and children. J Head Trauma Rehabil. 2006;21(4):315–33.
8. Bettermann K, Slocomb JE. Clinical relevance of biomarkers for traumatic brain injury. In: Dambinova S, Hayes RL, Wang KKW, editors. Biomarkers for traumatic brain injury. Cambridge: Royal Society of Chemistry; 2012. p. 1–18.
9. Pinelis VG, Sorokina EG, ZhB S, Reutov VP, Meshcheryakov SV, et al. Biomarkers of brain damage due to traumatic brain injury in children. Zhurnal nevrologii i psikhiatrii imeni S.S. Korsakova. 2015;115(8):66–72.
10. Sorokina EG, Semenova ZB, Reutov VP, Meshcheryakov SV. Autoantibodies to glutamate receptors and products of nitric oxide metabolism in serum in children in the acute phase of craniocerebral trauma. Neurosci Behav Physiol. 2009;39(4):329–34.
11. Kochanek PM, Carney N, David AP, et al. Guidelines for the acute medical management of severe traumatic brain injury in infants, children and adolescents, second edition. Pediatr Crit Care Med. 2012, 131;(Suppl):S1–82.
12. Marshall L, Gautille T, Klauber M, Eisenberg H, Jane J, Luerssen T, et al. The outcome of severe closed head injury. Special Supplements. 1991;75(1S):S28–36.

Do ICP-Derived Parameters Differ in Vegetative State from Other Outcome Groups After Traumatic Brain Injury?

Marek Czosnyka, Joseph Donnelly, Leanne Calviello, Peter Smielewski, David K. Menon, and John D. Pickard

Abstract *Objective*: In nearly 1,000 traumatic brain injury (TBI) patients monitored in the years 1992–2014, we identified 18 vegetative state (VS) cases. Our database provided access to continuous computer-recorded signals, which we used to compare primary signals, intracranial pressure (ICP)-derived indices and demographic data between VS patients, patients who survived but who were not VS (S), and patients who died (D).

Method: Mean values of ICP, arterial blood pressure (ABP) and cerebral perfusion pressure (CPP) from the whole monitoring periods were compared between the different outcome groups. Secondary indices included pressure reactivity index (PRx), the magnitude of slow ICP vasogenic waves, the pulse amplitude of the first harmonic component of the ICP waveform and heart rate (HR).

Results: Mean blood pressure was lowest in the VS group—significantly in comparison to those who died ($p = 0.02$) and almost significantly ($p = 0.1$) in comparison to the patients who survived. Mean ICP in VS patients was lower than those who died (VS, 13 ± 5 mmHg; D, 22 ± 14 mmHg; $p < 0.001$), but not significantly different from those who survived ($p > 0.05$). The magnitude of slow vasogenic ICP waves was the same in VS patients and those who died, but significantly lower than in those who survived (S, 1.04 ± 0.57 mmHg; VS, 0.74 ± 0.45; $p = 0.01$).

Conclusion: Patients who progress to a VS differ from non-VS survivors in displaying decreased power of slow vasogenic waves and from those who die by not experiencing as high a burden of intracranial hypertension.

Keywords Vegetative state · Brain injury · Outcome · Intracranial pressure · Slow waves

Introduction

Brain monitoring following traumatic brain injury (TBI) nowadays includes multiple modalities. Intracranial pressure (ICP) is one of the essential signals. Along with arterial blood pressure (ABP), it permits the calculation of cerebral perfusion pressure (CPP), which in turn is necessary for conducting CPP-oriented management [1]. However, high ICP itself is associated with increased mortality [2]. Therefore, contemporary management protocols combine the lower threshold of CPP (CPP is usually >60–70 mmHg) and the upper thresholds for ICP (20–25 mmHg). The individualisation of thresholds for CPP and ICP has been proposed recently [3, 4]; however, these proposals still await confirmation using prospective randomised multi-centre trials.

Monitoring of ICP cannot by itself improve outcome after TBI [5], unless it is associated with an efficient protocol targeting the prevention of its elevation [6]. As ICP can be affected by multiple mechanisms (arterial blood inflow, venous outflow, cerebrospinal fluid circulation, volumetric brain/lesion changes), the information included in pressure waveforms is very complex and can be processed and presented in a multitude of ways [7]. Simple time-averaging is a crude but efficient method.

A vegetative state (VS) is fortunately uncommon after TBI. In nearly 1,000 TBI patients monitored in the years 1992–2014, we identified only 18 such cases. Our long-established

M. Czosnyka (✉) · J. Donnelly · L. Calviello · P. Smielewski
Brain Physics Lab, Division of Neurosurgery, Cambridge University Hospital, Addenbrookes Hospital, Box 167, Cambridge CB20QQ, UK
e-mail: mc141@medschl.cam.ac.uk

D.K. Menon
Department of Anaesthesiology, Cambridge University Hospital, Cambridge, UK

J.D. Pickard
NIHR Brain Injury Healthcare Technology Co-operative, Cambridge, UK

database provided access to continuous computer-recorded brain monitoring modalities (from 1992 to 2003, 1-min averages; from 2003 to 2014, high-resolution ABP and ICP signals), which we used to compare primary monitored signals, ICP-derived indices and demographic data between VS patients, patients who survived but who were not in a VS (S) and patients who died (D).

Material and Method

All patients were sedated, intubated and mechanically ventilated. A CPP/ICP-oriented protocol for TBI management was used, which targeted maintenance of CPP above 65 mmHg and ICP below 25 mmHg [8]. Anonymised digital recordings were deposited in a computer database. The baseline neurological status of each patient was determined using the Glasgow Coma Score (GCS) collected on scene, before intubation. The clinical outcome was assessed at 6 months using the Glasgow Outcome Scale (GOS). All data were recorded as a part of standard clinical care. Data were averaged for the whole time of stay in the Neuro-Critical Care Unit (NCCU) of Addenbrooke's Hospital in Cambridge, UK. All patients were managed according to NCCU management protocol, and monitored under approval of both the Ethics (REC97/291) and the NCCU Users Committees.

Mean arterial pressure (MAP) was monitored invasively through the radial or femoral artery using a standard pressure monitoring kit (Baxter Healthcare, CardioVascular Group, Irvine, CA, USA). The blood pressure transducer was zeroed at the right atrial level. ICP was monitored using an intraparenchymal probe (Codman ICP MicroSensor; Codman & Shurtleff Inc., Raynham, MA, USA) inserted into the frontal cortex. Mean values of ICP, ABP and cerebral perfusion pressure (CPP) were compared between the different outcome groups (numbers of patients in each group: VS, 18; D, 222; S, 712). Secondary indices included pressure reactivity index (PRx), the cerebrospinal compensatory reserve index (RAP—the 5-min correlation coefficient between 10-s averages of pulse amplitude of ICP and mean ICP), the magnitude of slow ICP vasogenic waves (the square root of the ICP power spectrum within frequency limits 0.005 and 0.05 Hz), the pulse amplitude of the first harmonic component of ICP pulse waveforms and heart rate (HR). Bedside computers running ICM (until 2003) and ICM+ (from 2003 onward) software were used. Non-parametric comparison tests were used.

Results

Typical trends of ICP and CPP in the VS and D groups are presented in Fig. 1. Mean blood pressure was lowest in the VS group—significantly in comparison to those who died ($p = 0.02$) and almost significantly ($p = 0.1$) in comparison to the patients who survived. The distributions of mean ICP and slow vasogenic waves in different outcome groups are given in Fig. 2. Mean ICP in VS patients was lower than those who died (VS, 13 ± 5 mmHg; D, 22 ± 14 mmHg; $p < 0.001$), but not significantly different from those who survived but were not VS (VS, 13 ± 5 mmHg; S, 14.7 ± 5.3 mm Hg; $p > 0.05$). Remarkably, the magnitude of slow vasogenic ICP waves was the same in VS patients and those who died, but significantly lower than in those who survived (S, 1.04 ± 0.57 mm Hg; VS, 0.74 ± 0.45; $p = 0.01$). There was a trend ($p = 0.1$) for better cerebrovascular reactivity in VS patients than in those who died. CPP, cerebrospinal compensatory reserve, heart rate and pulse amplitude of ICP were not significantly different between the groups.

Discussion

With the exceptions of brain imaging studies [9] and electrophysiological investigations [10], there is little known about the physiology of VS. Links between specific profiles of brain monitoring in acute periods and outcome are very rarely discussed.

Patients who progress to the VS differ from non-VS survivors in displaying decreased power of slow vasogenic waves, and from those who died by not experiencing as high a burden of intracranial hypertension. There was a trend in patients with VS to have better cerebral autoregulation than in patients who died. Due to the low number of VS patients, the standard error of PRx was too high in the VS group to classify this difference as significant.

These data reinforce the view that ICP has a critical role in driving survival in TBI, but that the quality of survival is more strongly associated with autoregulatory indices and dynamics of the ICP signal, which discriminate between survivors who do and do not recover consciousness.

Raised dynamics of the ICP signal may be also estimated using entropy measures. Recently, low entropy (complexity) of ICP was reported to be associated with increased mortality after TBI [11]. The complexity of ICP in patients with VS should be analysed—and this will be done in the future, when we have a larger number of cases with raw data recordings.

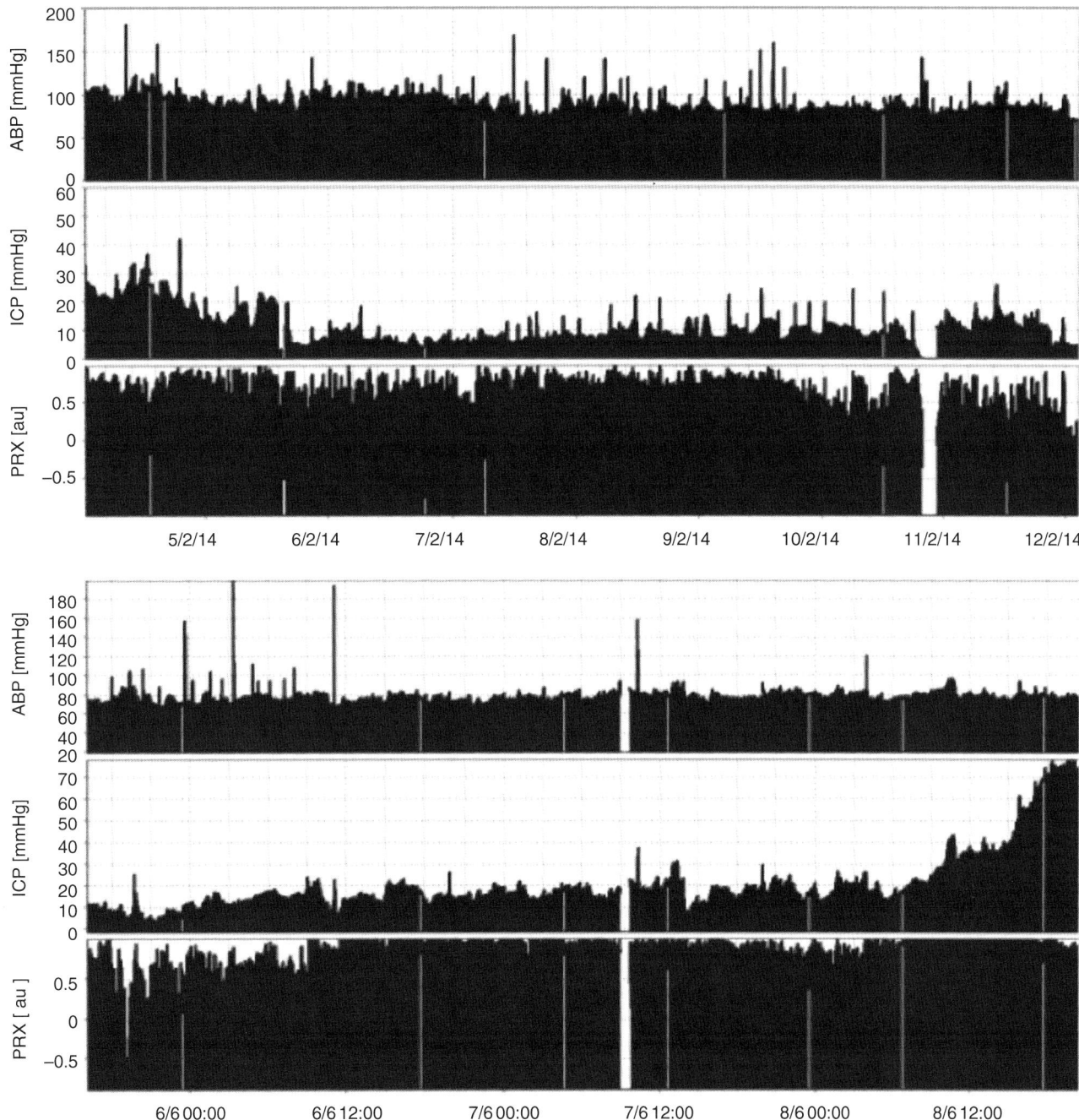

Fig. 1 A few days of monitoring of ICP, ABP and pressure reactivity (PRx) in a patient with VS (*upper*) outcome and in a patient who died (*lower*). Most of the time, ICP was below 20 mmHg in both patients (although the patient who died had a final refractory increase in ICP to 70 mmHg). In both cases, pressure reactivity was most frequently impaired. The *x*-axis shows time in the format of date, hours: minutes

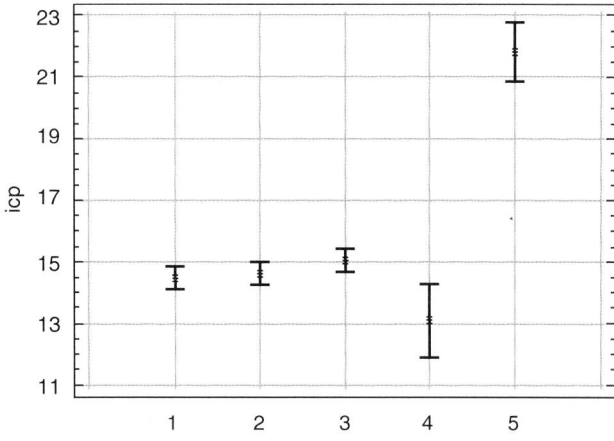
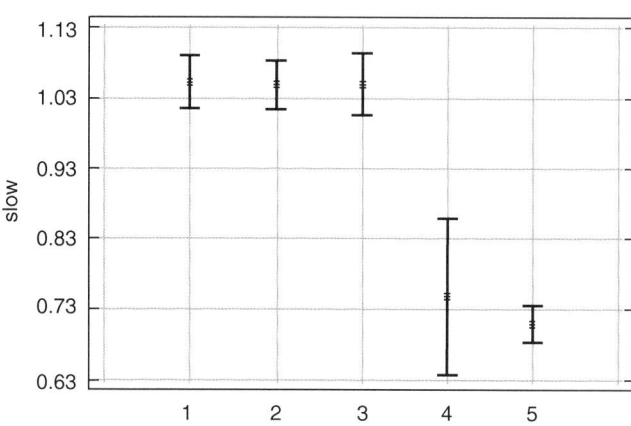
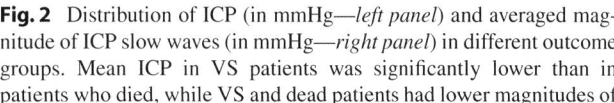

Fig. 2 Distribution of ICP (in mmHg—*left panel*) and averaged magnitude of ICP slow waves (in mmHg—*right panel*) in different outcome groups. Mean ICP in VS patients was significantly lower than in patients who died, while VS and dead patients had lower magnitudes of slow waves than patients who survived after TBI. Mean values and 95% confidence limits for mean. Labels on x-axis denote GOS categories: 1- good, 2- moderate disability, 3- severe disability, 4- vegetative state, 5- dead

Conflicts of interest statement We declare that PS and MC have financial interest in part of licensing fee fro ICM+ software (Cambridge Enterprise Ltd, UK).

References

1. Rosner MJ, Rosner SD, Johnson AH. Cerebral perfusion pressure: management protocol and clinical results. J Neurosurg. 1995;83(6):949–62.
2. Miller JD, Becker DP, Ward JD, Sullivan HG, Adams WE, Rosner MJ. Significance of intracranial hypertension in severe head injury. J Neurosurg. 1977;47(4):503–16.
3. Aries MJ, Czosnyka M, Budohoski KP, Steiner LA, Lavinio A, Kolias AG, Hutchinson PJ, Brady KM, Menon DK, Pickard JD, Smielewski P. Continuous determination of optimal cerebral perfusion pressure in traumatic brain injury. Crit Care Med. 2012;40(8):2456–63.
4. Lazaridis C, DeSantis SM, Smielewski P, Menon DK, Hutchinson P, Pickard JD, Czosnyka M. Patient-specific thresholds of intracranial pressure in severe traumatic brain injury. J Neurosurg. 2014;120(4):893–900.
5. Chesnut RM, Temkin N, Carney N, Dikmen S, Rondina C, Videtta W, Petroni G, Lujan S, Pridgeon J, Barber J, Machamer J, Chaddock K, Celix JM, Cherner M, Hendrix T, Global Neurotrauma Research Group. A trial of intracranial-pressure monitoring in traumatic brain injury. N Engl J Med. 2012;367(26):2471–81.
6. Hutchinson PJ, Kolias AG, Timofeev IS, Corteen EA, Czosnyka M, Timothy J, Anderson I, Bulters DO, Belli A, Eynon CA, Wadley J, Mendelow AD, Mitchell PM, Wilson MH, Critchley G, Sahuquillo J, Unterberg A, Servadei F, Teasdale GM, Pickard JD, Menon DK, Murray GD, Kirkpatrick PJ, RESCUEicp Trial Collaborators. Trial of decompressive craniectomy for traumatic intracranial hypertension. N Engl J Med. 2016;375(12):1119–30.
7. Miller JD, Dearden NM, Piper IR, Chan KH. Control of intracranial pressure in patients with severe head injury. J Neurotrauma. 1992;9(Suppl 1):S317–26.
8. Patel HC, Menon DK, Tebbs S, Hawker R, Hutchinson PJ, Kirkpatrick PJ. Specialist neurocritical care and outcome from head injury. Intensive Care Med. 2002;28(5):547–53.
9. Owen AM, Coleman MR, Menon DK, Johnsrude IS, Rodd JM, Davis MH, Taylor K, Pickard JD. Residual auditory function in persistent vegetative state: a combined PET and fMRI study. Neuropsychol Rehabil. 2005;15(3–4):290–306.
10. Owen AM. Using functional magnetic resonance imaging and electroencephalography to detect consciousness after severe brain injury. Handb Clin Neurol. 2015;127:277–93.
11. Lu CW, Czosnyka M, Shieh JS, Smielewska A, Pickard JD, Smielewski P. Complexity of intracranial pressure correlates with outcome after traumatic brain injury. Brain. 2012;135(Pt 8):2399–408.

Cerebral Arterial Compliance in Traumatic Brain Injury

Michael Dobrzeniecki, Alex Trofimov, and Denis E. Bragin

Abstract *Objective*: The main role of the cerebral arterial compliance (cAC) is to maintain the stiffness of vessels and protect downstream vessels when changing cerebral perfusion pressure. The aim was to examine the flexibility of the cerebral arterial bed based on the assessment of the cAC in patients with traumatic brain injury (TBI) in groups with and without intracranial hematomas (IHs).

Materials and Methods: We examined 80 patients with TBI (mean age, 35.7 ± 12.8 years; 42 men, 38 women). Group 1 included 41 patients without IH and group 2 included 39 polytraumatized patients with brain compression by IH. Dynamic electrocardiography (ECG)-gated computed tomography angiography (DHCTA) was performed 1–14 days after trauma in group 1 and 2–8 days after surgical evacuation of the hematoma in group 2. Amplitude of arterial blood pressure (ABP), as well as systole and diastole duration were measured noninvasively. Transcranial Doppler was measured simultaneously with DHCTA. The cAC was calculated by the formula proposed by Avezaat.

Results: The cAC was significantly decreased ($p < 0.001$) in both groups 1 and 2 compared with normal data. The cAC in group 2 was significantly decreased compared with group 1, both on the side of the former hematoma ($p = 0.017$).

Conclusion: The cAC in TBI gets significantly lower compared with the conditional norm ($p < 0.001$). After removal of the intracranial hematomas, compliance in the perifocal zone remains much lower ($p = 0.017$) compared with compliance of the other brain hemisphere.

Keywords Brain injury · Intracranial hematoma · Cerebral arterial compliance

Introduction

The secondary insults to patients with traumatic brain injury (TBI) are greatly affected by changes in the compliance and stiffness of cerebral vessels. The walls of downstream vessels have no external elastic membrane; therefore, the cerebral capillary network becomes vulnerable to intracranial and intravascular pressure surges [1].

One of the features characterizing the flexibility of the vascular network and its resistance to the said changes is the cerebral arterial compliance (cAC) [2]. The state of the cAC is of great importance for the brain microcirculation. Because the brain is located within an inextensible cranial cavity and is surrounded by an incompressible fluid, the compensation of intracranial pressure surges caused by the pulse wave passage through the brain blood vessels occurs also through the reciprocal changes in arterial lumens [3]. Thus, the higher the cAC, the greater the compliance of a vascular wall and, respectively, the better is the capacity of a vessel to change its lumen (i.e., the vasomotion phenomenon), and thereby to maintain the adequate capillary bed perfusion [4].

Information on the compliance and stiffness of the cerebral vascular bed in the damaged brain is currently rather inconsistent [2, 5], and aspects of the cAC reaction to the intracranial hematoma (IH) development and the disturbed cerebral blood flow (CBF) in the case of TBI remain underinvestigated [3, 6]. The main objective of this study was to examine the flexibility of the cerebral arterial bed based on the assessment of the cAC in TBI groups with and without IH.

Materials and Methods

The study complies with the Declaration of Helsinki [adopted in June 1964 (Helsinki, Finland) and revised in October 2000 (Edinburgh, Scotland)] and was approved by the local ethics committee. All the patients gave informed consent to participate in the study. We examined 80 TBI patients who were treated at the Departments of Neurosurgery in 2013–2016. All patients were divided into two groups. Group 1 included 41 patients with TBI without the development of IH; group 2 included 39 patients with TBI and IH.

Dynamic Helical Computed Tomography Angiography

All patients were subjected to dynamic helical computed tomography angiography (DHCTA) [7] using a Philips Ingenuity CT (Philips Medical Systems, Cleveland, OH, USA). DHCTA was performed 1–12 days after TBI (mean 4 ± 3 days) in group 1 and 2–8 days (mean, 4 ± 2 days) after trauma and surgery of the hematoma in group 2.

DHCTA was performed on 16 volumes of data, 160 mm in thickness, within 60 s of administration of contrast agent (Ultravist 370; Schering, Berlin, Germany) [7]. During or immediately after DHCTA, the monitoring of the transcranial Doppler (TCD) of the MCA was recorded bilaterally with 2-MHz probes within 10 min [8].

Amplitude of arterial blood pressure (ABPamp) and electrocardiography (ECG)-gated duration of the systole (T_{sys}) and the diastole (T_{dia}) were measured noninvasively (IntelliView MP5; Philips Medizin Systeme, Hamburg, Germany). The system appearance is shown in Fig. 1.

The data volume was transferred to the workstation [Philips Extended Brilliance Workspace (Philips HealthCare, Best, The Netherlands) and MATLAB 2013b (The MathWorks, Natick, MA, USA)].

The CBF and cerebral blood volumes (CBVs) were calculated from the DHCTA data with complex mathematical procedures, using the "direct flow model" algorithm [9].

The systolic–diastolic values of the middle cerebral artery (MCA) diameters (D_{sys} and D_{dia}) were determined in CTA series in the proximal part of the M1 of both MCAs.

The amplitude of regional CBV oscillation (ΔCBV) was calculated as the difference between CBVs which flowed through the MCA in systole (CBV_{sys}), and diastole (CBV_{dia}). We used the formulas (1, 2 and 3) proposed by de Jong, Alexandrov and Avezaat [8–10].

$$\Delta CBV = CBV_{sys} - CBV_{dia} \quad (1)$$

$$\Delta CBV = \frac{\pi}{4} \times D_{sys}^2 \times CBFV_{sys} \times T_{sys} - \frac{\pi}{4} \times D_{dia}^2 \times CBFV_{dia} \times T_{dia} \quad (2)$$

$$cAC = \Delta CBV \div ABP_{amp} \quad (3)$$

Reference range cAC was chosen according to Ikdip [11] as 0.105 ± 0.043 cm^3/mmHg.

Statistical Analysis

The t-test for dependent samples was utilized to analyze differences in means of parameters between the ipsilateral and contralateral sides of the temporal lobes. The program Statistica 7.0 (StatSoft, Tulsa, OK, USA) was used for the analysis. Data are presented as mean ± SEM. A significance level was preset to $p < 0.05$.

Results

Sex distribution had a male predominance (38 women, 42 men). Mean age was 35.7 ± 12.8 years (range, 17–87). The wakefulness level according to GCS averaged 9.7 ± 2.5 in group 1 and 10.1 ± 2.5 in group 2.

The acquired and analyzed data are summarized in Table 1.

The cAC was significantly decreased ($p < 0.001$) in both groups 1 and 2 (TBIs without or with IH, respectively) in comparison with normal data ($p < 0.001$).

The cAC in group 2 was significantly decreased compared with group 1, both on the side of the former hematoma ($p = 0.017$).

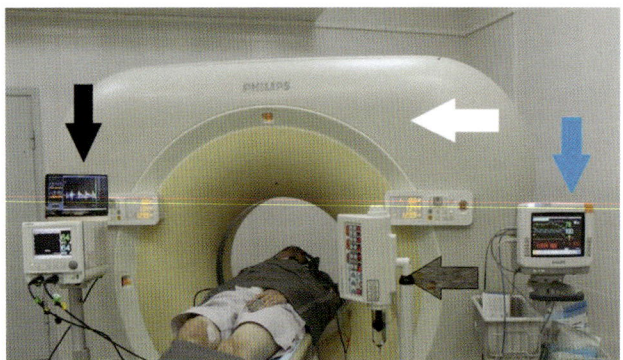

Fig. 1 The investigation system appearance. A *white arrow* indicates a computer tomograph, a *black arrow* shows a TCD, a *blue arrow* shows ECG-ABP monitor and a *gray arrow* marks a syringe-injector

Table 1 Comparison of the analyzed parameters

		Amplitude ABP (mmHg)	ΔCBV_{MCA} (cm^3)	cAC (cm^3/mmHg)
1	Group 1	63.9 ± 11.5	2.7 ± 0.9	0.049 ± 0.035
2	Group 2 (ipsilateral sides)	65.3 ± 12.2	2.6 ± 1.8	0.026 ± 0.017
3	Group 2 (contralateral sides)	65.3 ± 12.2	2.9 ± 1.4	0.037 ± 0.03
	P (1–2)	0.539	0.756	0.017[a]
	P (1–3)	0.427	0.351	0.172
	P (2–3)	0.166	0.62	0.116

[a]Significant difference ($p < 0.01$)

There was no significant difference in cAC between the perifocal zone of the former hematoma and the same locus of the contralateral hemisphere ($p = 0.172$).

Discussion

It is currently shown that the disturbed microcirculation plays a key role in the development of hypoperfusion episodes in patients with TBI. The cAC is deemed to be one of the most important indices, which reflects the degree of the compliance and resistance to deformation of the arterial network in response to spontaneous fluctuations in systemic hemodynamics [12].

The dynamics of the cAC in TBI remains to date poorly studied. At the same time, cAC assessment is required as it may serve as a predictor for an ischemic brain injury [2].

In our study, we have shown that the cAC in TBI is significantly and statistically reliably reduced compared with the norm.

In our opinion, there may be several reasons for such cAC dynamics, but all of them are associated, more or less, with the development of a brain edema [1].

Firstly, the development of a mixed cerebral edema increases the arterial wall stiffness, which affects the cAC [13].

Secondly, an edema development causes the diastolic compression of a pial bed; thus, significantly reducing the capillary bed capabilities to retain its lumen, and accordingly, to maintain the vasomotor activity [9].

It should be noted that the development of the IH changes even more the cAC value.

Here we have shown that even after the removal of an IH, the cAC in the perifocal zone remained significantly lower compared to TBI without IH development.

This effect may be explained by the data of Behzadi [14], which have shown that the CBF is dependent not only on cAC but also on the diameter of blood vessels, which may considerably vary in case of TBI because of the macrovascular and microvascular vasospasm.

To our knowledge, it is impossible to carry out the dynamic assessment of the cAC without a repeated DHCTA. In our study, we failed to eliminate a mathematical error associated with the measurement of the MCA diameters [8].

Thus, our results enable us to conclude that in the early period of TBI some pronounced changes in the cAC and cerebral microcirculation are observed, which are exacerbated by the development of enveloped hematomas.

Our findings may have certain practical significance for optimizing the brain edema therapy, which would prevent the development of cerebral perfusion disorders in patients with TBI.

Conclusion

The cAC in TBI gets significantly lower compared with the normal condition ($p < 0.001$). After removal of the intracranial hematomas, the compliance in the perifocal zone remains much lower ($p = 0.017$) compared with compliance of the other brain hemisphere.

Acknowledgments DB was supported by NIH NIGMS P20GM109089 and RSF No 17-15-01263.

Conflicts of interest statement We declare that we have no conflict of interest.

References

1. Nichols W, O'Rourke M. McDonald's blood flow in arteries: theoretical, experimental and clinical principles. Oxford: University Press; 2005.
2. Esther A, Warnert H. Noninvasive assessment of arterial compliance of human cerebral arteries with short inversion time arterial spin labeling. J Cereb Blood Flow Metab. 2015;35:461–8.
3. O'Rourke MF. Pulse wave form analysis and arterial stiffness: realism can replace evangelism and scepticism. J Hypertens. 2004;22:1633–4.
4. Berne R, Levy M. Physiology. 3rd ed. St Louis: Mosby; 1999.
5. Carrera E, Kim DJ, et al. Effect of hyper- and hypocapnia on cerebral arterial compliance in normal subjects. J Neuroimaging. 2011;21:121–5.

6. Pannier B. Methods and devices for measuring arterial compliance in humans. Am J Hypertens. 2002;15:743–53.
7. Pekkola J. Imaging of blood flow in cerebral arteries with dynamic helical computed tomography angiography (DHCTA) using a 64-row CT scanner. Acta Radiol. 2009;50(7):798–805.
8. Alexandrov AV. Neurovascular examination: the rapid evaluation of stroke patients using ultrasound waveform interpretation. Oxford: Blackwell Publishing Ltd.; 2013.
9. Jong de S. Quantifying cerebral blood flow of both the micro- and macrovascular system using perfusion computed tomography. Nijmegen: Twente; 2015.
10. Avezaat CJJ. Cerebrospinal fluid pulse pressure and craniospatial dynamics. A theoretical, clinical and experimental study. Rotterdam: Erasmus University; 1984.
11. Ikdip K. Exploring differences in vascular aging and cerebrovascular hemodynamics between older adults of White Caucasian and South Asian origin. Ontario: Waterloo; 2014.
12. Itoh T, et al. Rate of successful recording of blood flow signals in the middle cerebral artery using transcranial Doppler sonography. Stroke. 1993;24:1192–5.
13. Marmarou A. A review of progress in understanding the pathophysiology and treatment of brain edema. Neurosurg Focus 2007;22:1–12.
14. Behzadi Y. An arteriolar compliance model of the cerebral blood flow response to neural stimulus. NeuroImage. 2005;25:1100–11.

The Cerebrovascular Resistance in Combined Traumatic Brain Injury with Intracranial Hematomas

Alex O. Trofimov, George Kalentyev, Oleg Voennov, Michail Yuriev, Darya Agarkova, Svetlana Trofimova, and Vera Grigoryeva

Abstract *Objective*: The aim was to evaluate changes in cerebrovascular resistance (CVR) in combined traumatic brain injury (CTBI) in groups with and without intracranial hematomas (IH).

Materials and Methods: Treatment outcomes in 70 patients with CTBI (42 males and 28 females) were studied. Mean age was 35.5 ± 14.8 years (range, 15–73). The patients were divided into two groups: group 1 included 34 CTBI patients without hematomas; group 2 comprised 36 patients with CTBI and IH. The severity according to the Glasgow Coma Scale averaged 10.4 ± 2.6 in group 1, and 10.6 ± 2.8 in group 2. All patients underwent perfusion computed tomography (CT) and transcranial Doppler of both middle cerebral arteries. Cerebral perfusion pressure and CVR were calculated.

Results: The mean CVR values in each group (both with and without hematomas) appeared to be statistically significantly higher than the mean normal value. Intergroup comparison of CVR values showed statistically significant increase in the CVR level in group 2 on the side of the removed hematoma ($p = 0.037$). CVR in the perifocal zone of the removed hematoma remained significantly higher compared with the symmetrical zone in the contralateral hemisphere ($p = 0.0009$).

Conclusion: CVR in patients with CTBI is significantly increased compared to the normal value and remains elevated after evacuation of hematoma in the perifocal zone compared to the symmetrical zone in the contralateral hemisphere. This is indicative of certain correlation between the mechanisms of cerebral blood flow autoregulation and maintaining CVR.

Keywords Combined traumatic brain injury · Intracranial hematoma · Cerebrovascular resistance

Introduction

The optimum cerebral perfusion can be determined using simultaneously several methods of evaluating cerebral macrocirculation and microcirculation—for example, transcranial Doppler (TCD) studies done simultaneously with perfusion computed tomography (PCT), with subsequent calculation of "secondary" surrogate indices [1]. Such an approach is widely used in studying cerebral blood flow (CBF) [2]. The use of this approach provides the opportunity to assess the status of the cerebral microcirculatory bed [1] and to calculate the indices of cerebral hemodynamics with high accuracy [3]. One of these parameters is cerebrovascular resistance (CVR) [4]. It has been established that CVR provides constant brain perfusion in conditions of changing blood pressure (BP), which prevents vasogenic brain edema development. Such an effect of CVR occurs within the same BP interval in which the mechanisms of CBF autoregulation operate. It speaks of a definite correlation between the mechanisms of CBF autoregulation and maintaining CVR [5]. Change in CVR occurs mainly through changing smooth muscle tonus of the whole microcirculatory bed—namely, small arterioles and capillaries, which account for 50% of total vascular resistance [6, 7]. Thus, CVR reflects the status of all bloodstream components and is of great importance for

A.O. Trofimov, M.D. (✉)
Department of Neurosurgery, Nizhniy Novgorod State Medical Academy, 1, Minin Sq., Nizhniy Novgorod 603950, Russia

Department of Polytrauma, Nizhniy Novgorod Regional Hospital, named after N.A. Semashko, 190, Rodionov Str., Nizhniy, Novgorod 603126, Russia
e-mail: alexeytrofimov1975@gmail.com, xtro7@mail.ru

G. Kalentyev • O. Voennov • M. Yuriev • V. Grigoryeva
Department of Neurosurgery, Nizhniy Novgorod State Medical Academy, 190, Rodionov Str., Nizhniy Novgorod 603950, Russia

D. Agarkova • S. Trofimova
Department of Polytrauma, Nizhniy Novgorod Regional Hospital named after N.A. Semashko, 190, Rodionov Str., Nizhniy Novgorod 603126, Russia

understanding the physiology of vascular disturbances after brain injury [8]. It has been established that CVR increase is a predictive sign of cerebral vasospasm and delayed ischemia development [9]. Therefore, understanding microcirculatory reaction, particularly in conditions of combined traumatic brain injury (CTBI) against the background of intracranial hematoma (IH) formation, allows the development of CBF impairment to be predicted. The aim was to evaluate changes in CVR in severe CTBI in groups with and without IH.

Materials and Methods

The study complies with the Declaration of Helsinki and was approved by the local Ethics Committee of Nizhny Novgorod Regional Clinical Hospital N.A. Semashko. All the patients gave informed consent to participate in the study. Seventy patients with CTBI were treated at the Regional Trauma Center in 2012–2015. The mean age of the patients was 35.5 ± 14.8 years (range, 15–73). There were 28 women and 42 men. The patients were divided into two groups: group 1 included 34 CTBI patients without hematomas; group 2 comprised 36 patients with CTBI and IH (6 epidural, 26 subdural, 4 multiple). The groups were comparable in age and severity of TBI and concomitant lesions. The severity of condition according to the Glasgow Coma Scale (GCS) in group 1 averaged 10.4 ± 2.6; in group 2 it was 10.6 ± 2.8. The severity of injuries according to the Injury Severity Score scale in group 1 averaged 32 ± 8 and was 31 ± 11 in group 2. All patients underwent surgery within the first 3 days.

Perfusion Computed Tomography

All the patients underwent a PCT examination of the brain on a multislice tomograph (Toshiba Aquilion TSX-101A; Toshiba Medical Systems, Zoetermeer, The Netherlands). In group 1, PCT examination of the brain was performed within the first 14 days after injury (average of 4 ± 3 days); in group 2, it was done within 2–8 days after surgical procedure (average of 4 ± 2 days). All the patients breathed spontaneously, and required no BP support. The data were transferred to a Vitrea 2 workstation (Vital Imaging, Salt Lake City, UT, USA). The regions of interest (ROIs) were established symmetrically subcortically in the temporal lobes on the level of the middle temporal gyrus, which corresponded to the vascular supply area of the middle cerebral artery (MCA). In patients of group 2, the ROI located on the side of the removed hematoma corresponded to the perifocal zone of microcirculatory changes. Assessment of the mean arterial pressure (MAP) was performed (MAP-03; Cardex, Nizhny Novgorod, Russia) simultaneously with PCT and was immediately followed by TCD of both MCAs (Sonomed 300 M; Spectromed, Moscow, Russia) to provide consistent conditions for the study of CBF. Cerebral perfusion pressure (CPP) was calculated using the formula modified by Czosnyka et al. [10]:

$$\text{Calculated CPP} = \text{MAP} \times V_d \div V_m + 14$$

where V_d is diastolic velocity, V_m is mean velocity.

In PCT study we also calculated the values of regional CBF. To calculate CVR the following formula was used [11]:

$$CVR = CPP \div rCBF$$

The mean normal CVR value (the conditional norm) was estimated as follows [11]:

$$1.31 \pm 0.24 \, \text{mmHg} \times 100 \, \text{g} \times \text{min/ml}.$$

Statistical Analysis

The obtained data had a normal distribution, so they were presented as the average ± standard deviation. Comparisons between the groups were performed using the Student t-test. The level of significance was taken as $p < 0.05$.

Results

Analysis of the studied parameters in the groups (Table 1) showed that the mean CVR values in each group CTBI (both with and without IH) appeared to be statistically significantly higher than the mean normal value. Intergroup comparison of CVR values showed statistically significant increase in the CVR level in group 2 on the side of removed IH compared with group 1 ($p = 0.037$).

The most significant differences were revealed in patients of group 2: the mean CVR in the perifocal zone of removed IH remained significantly higher compared to that in the symmetrical zone of the contralateral hemisphere ($p = 0.0009$). Besides, diastolic and mean CBF velocity as well as CPP differed significantly in the above zones ($p = 0.005$, $p = 0.001$ and $p = 0.0000001$, respectively). Analysis of CVR values in various types of IH showed no statistically significant differences ($p > 0.05$).

Discussion

The evaluation of CVR status is necessary since it can serve as a predictor of posttraumatic vasospasm and secondary brain damage development [4, 12]. It has been demonstrated that CVR in CTBI statistically significantly

Table 1 Values of studied parameters in groups

Groups	Mean AP (mmHg)	V_d (cm/s)	V_m (cm/s)	rCBF (ml/100 g × min)	CPP (mmHg)	CVR (mmHg × 100 g × min/ml)
Group 1 (1)	98.5 ± 15.7	34.0 ± 14.2	46.1 ± 13.8	31.7 ± 10.0	85.3 ± 25.5	2.94 ± 2.2
Group 2 (on the side of former hematoma) (2)	99.9 ± 14.7	32.5 ± 11.5	36.8 ± 12.8	32.3 ± 17.7	109.4 ± 36.0	4.06 ± 2.2
Group 2 (on the side opposite to former hematoma) (3)	99.9 ± 14.7	25.5 ± 9.9	48.7 ± 17.7	28.4 ± 11.1	67.5 ± 17.2	2.7 ± 1.1
P_{1-2}	0.701	0.631	0.005*	0.138	0.002*	0.037*
P_{1-3}	0.701	0.004*	0.5	0.194	0.001*	0.561
P_{2-3}	1	0.005*	0.001*	0.247	0.0000001*	0.0009*

*$p < 0.05$ (difference is statistically significant)

increases compared with the norm. One of the reasons for this increase is development of mixed brain edema [12], resulting in compression of pial vessels. CT signs of brain edema were found in all 70 patients and indirectly confirm this hypothesis. Another reason may be regional microvascular vasospasm due to a high concentration of blood degradation products trapped in the subarachnoid spaces. This effect results from oxidation of oxyhemoglobin to methemoglobin with release of ferrum ions. Moreover, superoxides are supposed to change NO concentration, which leads to development of microvascular vasospasm [9]. In our study, TCD revealed no signs of vasospasm in those who suffered CTBI. In contrast to laser Doppler flowmetry, this method does not provide the possibility to evaluate microvascular spasm. Also, compression of microvasculature can develop due to astrocytic endfeet swelling directly adjacent to the capillary wall [13]. The compression of pial vessels is associated with dysfunction of pericytes, the cells embedded in the basement membrane of capillaries. It has been reported that narrowing of arterioles and capillaries in TBI occurs due to impaired expression of endothelin-1 and its pericytic receptors type A and B; this is caused by migration of more than 40% of pericytes from basement membrane [14]. It should be noted that brain compression by IH changes CVR even more. Thus, we have found that even after IH evacuation, CVR in its perifocal zone remained significantly higher than in the symmetrical zone of the contralateral hemisphere. Some researchers point out that compression of the capillary system in the perifocal zone of hematoma can reach such values at which blood flow in arterioles stops [4]. Such a situation leads to reduction in the number of functioning capillaries and CVR increase on the side of compression. In these conditions, temporary microvascular shunts open, and supracapillary and intercapillary shunting phenomena develop to maintain perfusion in the perifocal zone [14]. Probably, the development of capillary shunting syndrome explains the daunting result obtained in our study, when predicted CVR value on the side of the removed hematoma appeared to be higher than MAP. Thus, the obtained findings enable us to conclude that in the early stage of CTBI, marked changes in CVR and cerebral microcirculation occur, which are exacerbated by development of ICH.

Conclusion

CVR at CTBI is significantly increased compared to the normal value. After evacuation of hematoma in the former perifocal zone, CVR remains significantly elevated compared to the symmetrical zone in the opposite hemisphere. The analysis of CVR status offers the possibility to distinguish a group of patients with high risk of cerebral vasospasm and secondary insult development.

Conflicts of interest statement We declare that we have no conflict of interest.

References

1. Rhee C. The ontogeny of cerebrovascular pressure autoregulation in premature infants. Acta Neurochir Suppl. 2016;122: 151–5.
2. Westermaier T. Value of transcranial Doppler, perfusion-CT and neurological evaluation to forecast secondary ischemia after aneurysmal SAH. Neurocrit Care. 2014;20(3):406–12.
3. Trofimov A. Intrahospital transfer of patients with traumatic brain injury: increase in intracranial pressure. Acta Neurochir Suppl. 2016;122:125–7.
4. Dewey R. Experimental cerebral hemodynamics. Vasomotor tone, critical closing pressure, and vascular bed resistance. J Neurosurg. 1974;41(5):597–606.

5. Sharples PM. Cerebral blood flow and metabolism in children with severe head injuries. Part 2: cerebrovascular resistance and its determinants. J Neurol Neurosurg Psychiatry. 1995;58(2):153–9.
6. Daley M. Model-derived assessment of cerebrovascular resistance and cerebral blood flow following traumatic brain injury. Exp Biol Med (Maywood). 2010;235(4):539–45.
7. Smirl JD. Influence of cerebrovascular resistance on the dynamic relationship between blood pressure and cerebral blood flow in humans. J Appl Physiol. 2014;116(12):1614–22.
8. Bragin DE. High intracranial pressure effects on cerebral cortical microvascular flow in rats. J Neurotrauma. 2011;28(5):775–85.
9. Pluta RM. Delayed cerebral vasospasm and nitric oxide: review, new hypothesis, and proposed treatment. Pharmacol Ther. 2005;105(1):23–56.
10. Czosnyka M, Smielewski P, et al. Continuous assessment of the cerebral vasomotor reactivity in head injury. Neurosurgery. 1997;41(1):11–9.
11. Scheinberg P. The cerebral blood flow in male subjects as measured by the nitrous oxide technique. Normal values for blood flow, oxygen utilization, glucose utilization, and peripheral resistance, with observations on the effect of tilting and anxiety. J Clin Invest. 1949;28(5):1163–71.
12. Marmarou A. A review of progress in understanding the pathophysiology and treatment of brain edema. Neurosurg Focus. 2007;22(5):E1.
13. Bullock R. Glial swelling following human cerebral contusion: an ultrastructural study. J Neurol Neurosurg Psychiatry. 1991;54(5):427–34.
14. Hall CN. Capillary pericytes regulate cerebral blood flow in health and disease. Nature. 2014;508(7494):55–60.

Computed Tomography Indicators of Deranged Intracranial Physiology in Paediatric Traumatic Brain Injury

Adam M.H. Young, Joseph Donnelly, Xiuyun Liu, Mathew R. Guilfoyle, Melvin Carew, Manuel Cabeleira, Danilo Cardim, Matthew R. Garnett, Helen M. Fernandes, Christina Haubrich, Peter Smielewski, Marek Czosnyka, Peter J. Hutchinson, and Shruti Agrawal

Abstract *Objective*: Computed tomography (CT) of the brain can allow rapid assessment of intracranial pathology after traumatic brain injury (TBI). Frequently in paediatric TBI, CT imaging can fail to display the classical features of severe brain injury with raised intracranial pressure. The objective of this study was to determine early CT brain features that influence intracranial or systemic physiological trends following paediatric TBI.

Materials and methods: Thirty-three patients (mean age, 10 years; range, 0.5–16) admitted between 2002 and 2015 were used for the current analysis. Presence of petechial haemorrhages, basal cistern compression, subarachnoid blood, midline shift and extra-axial masses on the initial trauma CT head were assessed. ICP and arterial blood pressure (ABP) were then monitored continuously with an intraparenchymal microtransducer and an indwelling arterial line. Pressure monitors were connected to bedside computers running ICM+ software. Pressure reactivity was determined as the moving correlation between 30, 10-s averages of ABP and ICP (PRx). The mean ICP, ABP, cerebral perfusion pressure (CPP; ABP minus ICP) and PRx were calculated for the whole monitoring period for each patient.

Results: The presence of subarachnoid blood was related to higher ICP, higher ABP and a trend toward higher PRx. Smaller basal cisterns were related to increased ICP ($R = -0.42$, $p = 0.02$), impaired PRx ($R = -0.5$, $p = 0.003$). The presence of an extra-axial mass was associated with deranged PRx (-0.02 vs. 0.41, $p = 0.003$) and a trend toward higher ICP (14 vs. 40, $p = 0.07$). Interestingly the degree of midline shift was not related to ICP or PRx.

Conclusions: The size of the basal cisterns, the presence of subarachnoid blood or an extra-axial mass are all related to disturbed ICP and pressure reactivity in this paediatric TBI cohort. Patients with these features are ideal candidates for invasive multimodal monitoring.

Keywords Imaging · Pediatric · Brain · Injury · Trauma

Introduction

Traumatic brain injury (TBI) is a major contributor to mortality and morbidity worldwide, particularly in children [1]. The management of paediatric brain injury aims to attenuate evolving secondary brain injury that follows the initial mechanical insult. Hypotension, hypoxia, hypoglycaemia, sustained increased intracranial pressure (ICP), seizures and infections are avoided with the aim of maintaining adequate cerebral perfusion and preventing herniation syndromes [2]. A complex mix of these pathologies can lead to increases in ICP and may compromise brain perfusion by reducing cerebral perfusion pressure. Uncontrolled ICP is widely accepted to be closely linked with disability, poor neurological outcome and decreased survival in paediatric TBI patients [3]; as such, effectively monitoring and managing ICP has become a cornerstone of treatment for severe paediatric TBI [3].

Nevertheless, when to institute ICP monitoring in paediatric TBI is not well defined. The evidence base for an internationally accepted published recommendation for ICP monitoring in children with severe TBI was only sufficient to state that ICP monitoring was appropriate, and only at the level of an option. Not enough support exists for a standard or guideline [3].

In clinical practice, the implementation of ICP monitoring is usually dependent on the severity of the injury according to the level of consciousness as measured with the Glasgow Coma Scale (GCS). However, the increased use of early sedation, intubation and ventilation in more severe patients has decreased the value of the full GCS for purposes of classification [3, 4]. As such, a greater reliance has been placed on morphological criteria based on computed tomographic (CT) or magnetic resonance imaging (MRI) investigations.

Conventional classification of TBI with CT findings differentiates between focal and diffuse injuries [5]. Marshall et al. [6], after analysis of the Traumatic Coma Data Bank, proposed a CT classification for grouping patients with TBI according to multiple CT characteristics. This CT classification identifies six different groups of patients with TBI, based on the type and severity of several abnormalities on the CT scan.

It differentiates between patients with and without mass lesions and permits further discrimination of patients with diffuse injuries into four categories, taking into account signs of raised ICP. Since its introduction, this CT classification has become widely accepted for descriptive purposes and is increasingly being used as major predictor of outcome in TBI. Various studies have confirmed the predictive value of the CT classification [7]. Of these signs, the basal cisterns of the midbrain are arguably the most commonly used measure of the degree of brain swelling, being an indicator of the available perimesencephalic space at the tentorial incisura. Often the assumption is made that if the cisterns are not effaced, ICP is unlikely to be significantly elevated, and ICP monitoring may not be required [8]. Problems arise in paediatric TBI, where initial CT scans fails to demonstrate the same devastating levels of injury found in adult patients with similar ICP trends and mechanism of injury [9].

Here in we analyse the patterns of CT abnormality that are linked to deranged patterns of multi-modality monitoring in a group of paediatric TBI patients. In particular, we have focused on the patency of the basal cisterns and depth of mass lesions to give critical volumes that would encourage surgical intervention.

Methods

Patients

The data in this study were collected retrospectively from data records of paediatric severe traumatic brain injury patients admitted to Addenbrookes Hospital Paediatric Intensive Care Unit (PICU) between January 2002 and December 2015. The insertion of an intracranial monitoring device is part of routine clinical practice and, as such, did not require ethical approval. The data are routinely collected for clinical purposes and guide the management of patients. The analysis of data within this study for the purposes of service evaluation was approved by the Cambridge University Hospital NHS Trust, Audit and Service Evaluation Department (Ref. 2143) and did not require ethical approval or patient consent.

Patients were included in this cohort if they had a clinical need for ICP monitoring. Patients were treated according to current paediatric traumatic brain injury guidelines [2], which aim to keep the ICP below 20 mmHg through a stepwise regime including: positioning, sedation, paralysis, osmotic agents, ventriculostomy and induced hypothermia.

Data Acquisition and Analysis

Arterial blood pressure (ABP) was measured and the radial or femoral artery zeroed at the level of heart (Baxter Healthcare, Newbury Park, CA, USA; Sidcup, UK). ICP was measured with an intraparenchymal microsensor in the frontal cortex (Codman ICP Micro- Sensor; Codman & Shurtleff, Raynham, MA, USA). ICP and ABP data were collected at 100 Hz with an analogue-to-digital converter (DT9801; Data Translation, Marlboro, MA, USA) coupled with a laptop computer running ICM+ software (University of Cambridge, Cambridge Enterprise, Cambridge, UK, http://www.neurosurg.cam.ac.uk/icmplus). Pressure reactivity index was calculated as the moving correlation between 10 s averages of ICP and ABP. The patient's ICP, PRx, mean arterial pressure (MAP) and CPP were then averaged over the first 72 h of their intensive care unit stay.

Basal Cistern Measurements

Independently, two investigators (A.Y., R.P.), not involved with data collection and blinded to the patient's condition, measured the basal cisterns on from the initial admission CT head. All CT scans were performed with a basic non-contrast protocol using a 16-slice scanner (Somatom Sensation 16 scanner; Siemens Healthcare, Erlangen, Germany). Each observer scrolled through the CT head slices to visualise the specific imaging cut demonstrating a visual estimation of the greatest width. The image window was configured to the 'brain' view which yielded the basal cisterns in more detail (Hounsfield unit range, 25–40). The image was then magnified and the cisterns were measured using electronic callipers, with a digital viewer (Centricity PACS; General Electric Healthcare, Little Chalfont, UK) (Fig. 1).

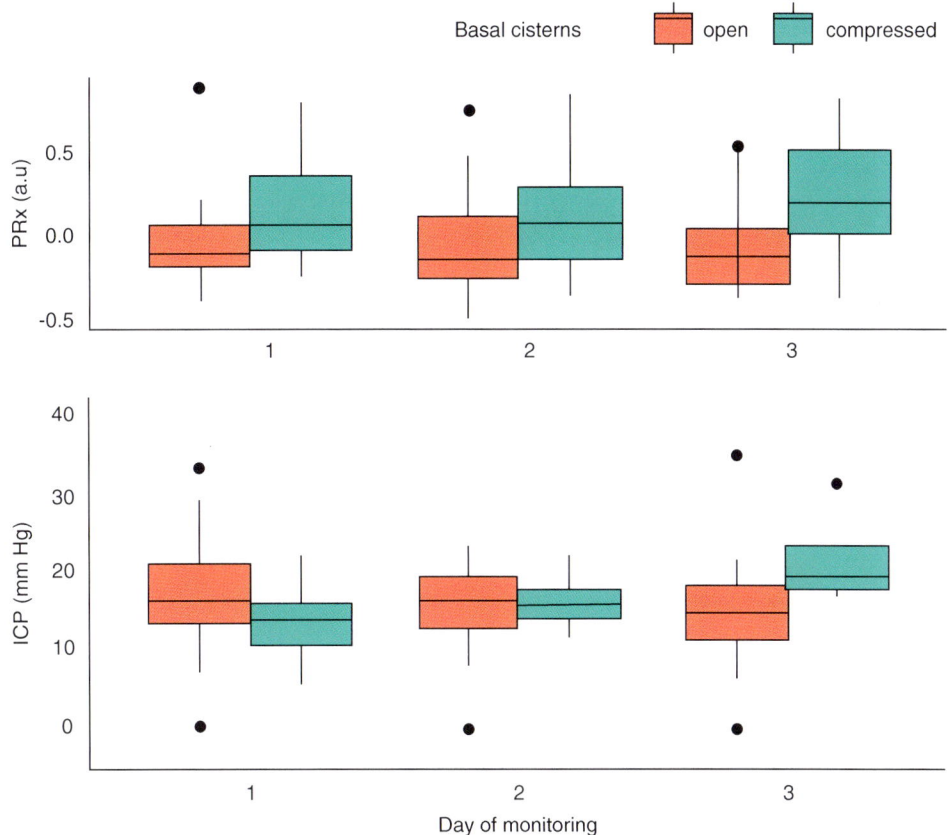

Fig. 1 ICP and PRx in patients with closed versus open cisterns on initial CT. A difference in ICP between open and compressed was observed on day 3 of monitoring ($p = 0.004$)

Statistical Analysis

Mean ICP, PRx, CPP and MAP over the first 3 days of monitoring were calculated. The influence of the presence or absence of pre-hospital factors (hypotension, hypoxia, >1 unreactive pupil. Motor score 3 or less) on subsequent ICP and PRx were tested using a non-parametric Wilcoxon test. All data manipulations and analysis were performed on R language and software environment for statistical computation (version 2.12.1) [10].

Results

The median age was 12 (range, 0.5–15). Of the 39 patients, 36% were female. 23% of patients presented with a low GCS (Motor score 1–4). 5% of patients had bilateral fixed pupils and 13% with a unilateral fixed pupil. Mortality occurred in 18% of patients.

The median ICP was 15.2 (IQR, 12.7–19.2) with a median PRx −0.02 (IQR, −0.18 to 0.14). Baseline CT features included subarachnoid haemorrhage in 31% of patients and midline shift in 63% of patients. Forty-four percent were observed to have a focal lesion in the form of a contusion of an extra-axial haematoma. Fifty-six percent of patients suffered diffuse axonal injury (DAI). Taking a threshold of <2 mm as "compressed basal cisterns", it was observed that on days 1 and 2 of monitoring there was no significant correlation between compression of the basal cisterns and ICP. Only on day 3 of monitoring was there a significant difference in ICP between open basal cisterns (16.2 mmHg) compared to those that were compressed (20.1 mmHg; $p = 0.004$; Fig. 1). With regards to PRx, compressed basal cisterns trended towards impaired PRx; however, this never reach significance. Interestingly, evidence of subarachnoid haemorrhage on CT was associated with raised ICP on days 2 (20.3 mmHg) and 3 (19.8 mmHg) compared to those who did not (14.2 mmHg and 14.9 mmHg) on days 2 and 3 respectively (Fig. 2). Finally, features of midline shift were not associated with deranged ICP or PRx ($p = 0.62$; Fig. 3).

Discussion

In this study, we investigated the relationship between key features of traumatic brain injury on CT and subsequent

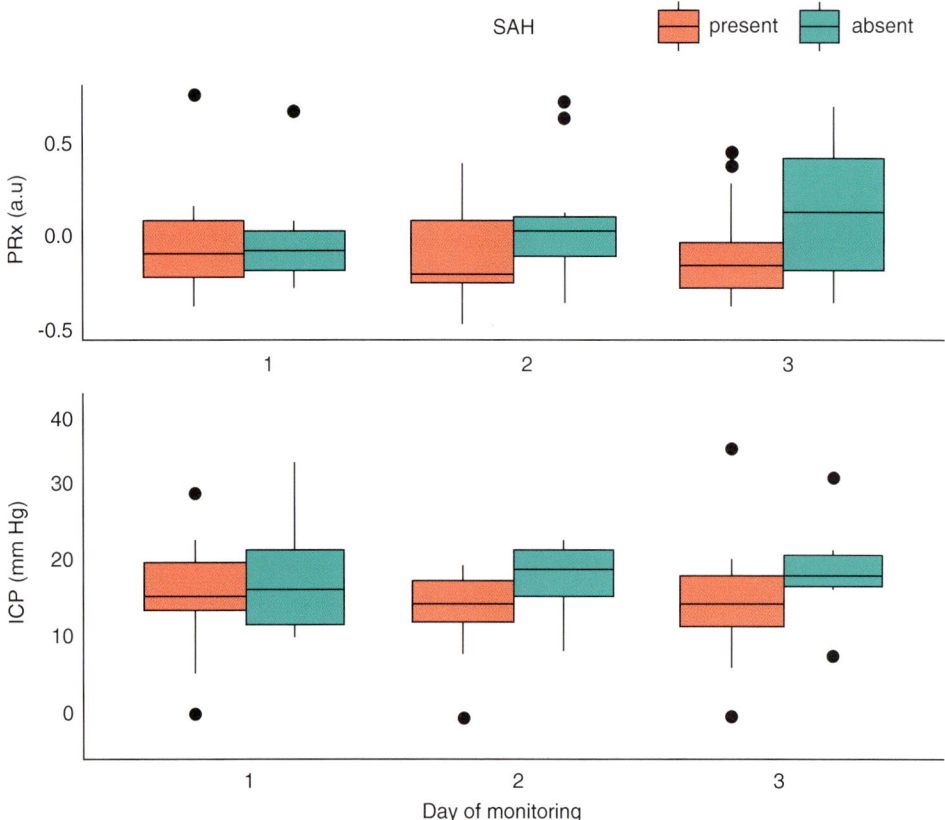

Fig. 2 ICP and PRx in patients with and without subarachnoid haemorrhage on initial CT. The presence of subarachnoid haemorrhage caused significant changes in ICP from day 2 of monitoring ($p = 0.02$) and increased in day 3 ($p = 0.004$)

intracranial physiology after severe traumatic brain injury in children. Children with evidence of severe injury on scan went on to develop higher intracranial pressure. Particularly, evidence of subarachnoid haemorrhage on CT was related to raised ICP but not deranged PRx. Compression of the basal cisterns was linked to increased ICP in these patients; however, unlike adults, complete obliteration of the cisterns was rare. Raised ICP, particularly in days 1 and 2 after injury, was present regardless of the patency of the basal cisterns. This finding replicates that of Kouvarellis et al. [9], who concluded that children with severe TBI frequently may have open basal cisterns on head CT despite increased ICP. Open cisterns should not discourage ICP monitoring.

The relationship between subarachnoid haemorrhage and raised ICP is interesting. It could simply be related to the degree of injury; i.e. a severe injury will be more likely to induced haemorrhage and, as such, raise ICP. However, there is a suspicion that even a subtle occlusion of cerebrospinal fluid drainage could lead to minimal rises in ICP [11].

The lack of correlation between midline shift and ICP or PRx is most likely associated with the fact that extra-axial haematomas that were causing severe shift were evacuated in a timely fashion. Those that were not evacuated were done so on clinical grounds and, as a result, justifiable based on the lack of ICP/PRx derangement.

Implications

Early prediction of raised ICP has the potential to facilitate the management of TBI patients by alerting the clinicians to patients which require more intensive monitoring or perhaps a lower threshold for ICP treatment. However, prediction remains difficult and is usually confined to analysis of high-frequency ICP waveforms. Thus, the current preliminary findings, if confirmed, could enhance existing ICP prediction tools. In addition, the current data potentially indicate that enhanced pre-hospital care may aid in avoiding secondary insults occurring up to 72 h after admission to hospital. Furthermore, the finding of a relationship between subarachnoid haemorrhage and subsequent ICP highlights the need to determine individualised paediatric scoring systems in the analyses between physiological variables and patient outcome.

Limitations

As this current analysis is from quite a small dataset, we cannot exclude that more subtle relationships between CT variables and ICP or PRx may emerge with a larger dataset [12].

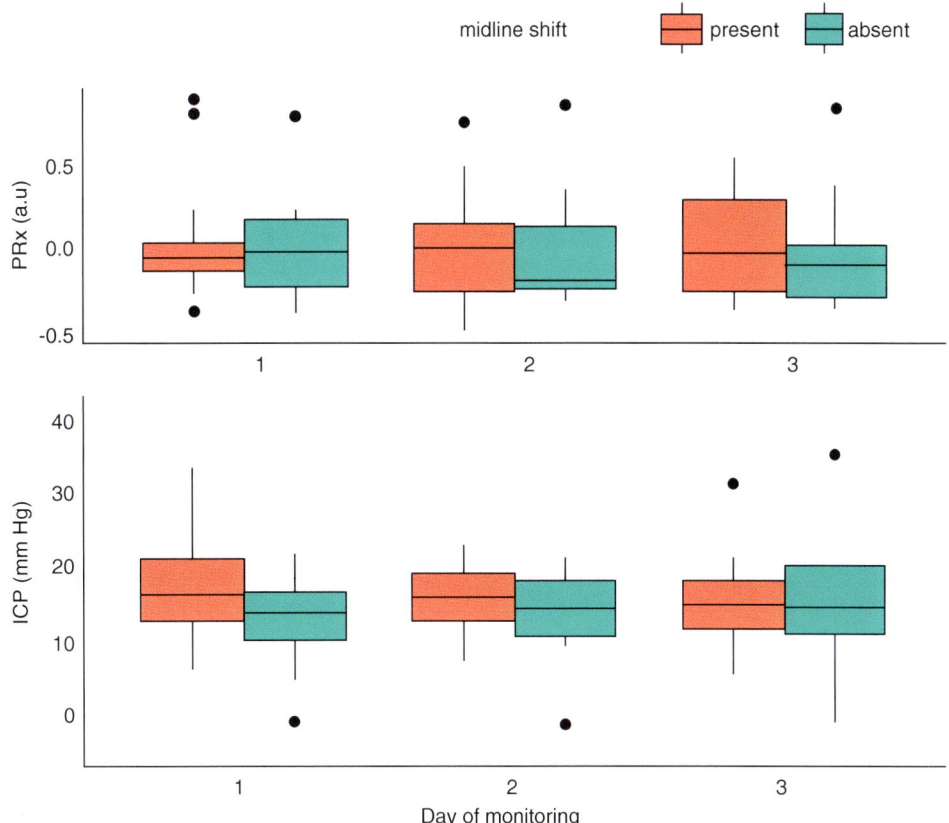

Fig. 3 ICP and PRx in patients with and without mid-line shift on initial CT. The presence of midline shift failed to cause significant differences in ICP or PRx

Conclusion

After severe paediatric TBI, those patients with subarachnoid haemorrhage and compression of the basal cisterns go on to develop higher ICP. It is unusual to have obliterated basal cisterns in children even with deranged ICP.

Conflicts of interest statement We declare that we have no conflict of interest.

References

1. Faul M, Xu L, Wald MM, Coronado VG. Traumatic brain injury in the United States: emergency department visits, hospitalizations, and deaths. Centers for Disease Control and Prevention, National Center for Injury Prevention and Control: Atlanta, GA; 2010.
2. Kochanek PM, Carney N, Adelson PD, et al. Guidelines for the acute medical management of severe traumatic brain injury in infants, children, and adolescents—second edition. Pediatr Crit Care Med. 2012;13(Suppl):S1–82.
3. Adelson PD, Bratton SL, Carney NA, Chesnut RM, du Coudray HE, Goldstein B, Kochanek PM, Miller HC, Partington MD, Selden NR, Warden CW, Wright DW, American Association for Surgery of Trauma, Child Neurology Society, International Society for Pediatric Neurosurgery, International Trauma Anesthesia and Critical Care Society, Society of Critical Care Medicine, World Federation of Pediatric Intensive and Critical Care Societies. Guidelines for the acute medical management of severe traumatic brain injury in infants, children, and adolescents. Chapter 17. Critical pathway for the treatment of established intracranial hypertension in pediatric traumatic brain injury. Pediatr Crit Care Med. 2003;4(3 Suppl):S65–7.
4. Brain Trauma Foundation. Guidelines for the management of severe traumatic brain injury. 3rd edition. J Neurotrauma. 2007;24(Suppl 1):S37–44.
5. Chesnut RM. Computed tomography of the brain: a guide to understanding and interpreting normal and abnormal images in the critically ill patient. Crit Care Nurs Q. 1994;17(1):33–50.5.
6. Marshall LF, Marshall SB, Klauber MR, Van Berkum Clark M, Eisenberg H, Jane JA, Luerssen TG, Marmarou A, Foulkes MA. The diagnosis of head injury requires a classification based on computed axial tomography. J Neurotrauma. 1992;9(Suppl 1):S287–92.
7. Jagannathan J, Okonkwo DO, Yeoh HK, Dumont AS, Saulle D, Haizlip J, Barth JT, Jane JA Sr, Jane JA Jr. Long-term outcomes and prognostic factors in pediatric patients with severe traumatic brain injury and elevated intracranial pressure. J Neurosurg Pediatr. 2008;2(4):240–9.
8. Teasdale E, Cardoso E, Galbraith S, Teasdale G. CT scan in severe diffuse head injury: physiological and clinical correlations. J Neurol Neurosurg Psychiatry. 1984;47(6):600–3.
9. Kouvarellis AJ, Rohlwink UK, Sood V, Van Breda D, Gowen MJ, Figaji AA. The relationship between basal cisterns on CT and time-linked intracranial pressure in paediatric head injury. Childs Nerv Syst. 2011;27(7):1139–44. https://doi.org/10.1007/s00381-011-1464-3. Epub 2011 May 3

10. R Core Team. R: a language and environment for statistical computing. Vienna: R Foundation for Statistical Computing; 2015. http://www.r-project.org/.
11. Noraky J, Verghese GC, Searls DE, Lioutas VA, Sonni S, Thomas A, Heldt T. Noninvasive intracranial pressure determination in patients with subarachnoid hemorrhage. Acta Neurochir Suppl. 2016;122:65–8. https://doi.org/10.1007/978-3-319-22533-3_13.
12. Young AM, Guilfoyle MR, Fernandes H, Garnett MR, Agrawal S, Hutchinson PJ. The application of adult traumatic brain injury models in a pediatric cohort. J Neurosurg Pediatr. 2016;18(5):558–64.

Mean Square Deviation of ICP in Prognosis of Severe TBI Outcomes in Children

Zhanna B. Semenova, V.I. Lukianov, S.V. Meshcheryakov, and L.M. Roshal

Abstract *Objectives*: Prognostic value of intracranial pressure (ICP) is discussed in the recent literature. The aim of our study was to find the parameter that could be representative of ICP variations and might become a good predictor of severe traumatic brain injury (TBI) outcomes in children.

Materials and methods: The study included 81 patients with severe TBI (2004–2014). Inclusion criteria: GCS ≤ 8, age > 3 years old, admission time to our clinic <24 h from the time of injury. Mean daily values of ICP were used as a predictor, Glasgow outcome scale value was used as a grouping variable. Outcomes were assessed 6 months after injury.

Results: Total mortality was 27%. We have entered the indicator "energy ICP" (E^2), which describes the dynamics of the process and energy. E^2 value in the group of survivors was <500 mmHg^2; the probability of accurate forecasting was 91%. Sensitivity, 0.9; specificity; 0.94.

Conclusions: The proposed method is accessible and easy to perform. This method has high specificity in the prediction of severe traumatic brain injury outcome and can be a reliable tool for ICP control.

Keywords Severe brain injury · Decompressive craniectomy · Prognosis · Intracranial hypertension · GOS · Children

Introduction

Scientists and neurosurgeons used to repeat time after time that head injury is one of the most common causes of death and disability in adults and children. However, this problem still remains despite all the latest scientific achievements. Mortality fell markedly, but traumatic brain injury (TBI) outcomes are still unsatisfactory. According to recent studies, the results of severe TBI treatment in different countries remain unsatisfactory in 20–30% of patients [1]. Today, more and more experts in the field of severe TBI treatment speak about the stagnation in results, and it seems that only further development of fundamental science could change the current situation.

However, many unresolved questions exist from a practical point of view. Answers to these questions are directly related to the prognosis of severe TBI in children and adults. The possibility to predict outcome gives us a chance to manage direct care. The understanding of prognosis allows the surgeon not only to confirm the fact of effective or non-effective treatment, but also to choose the optimal evidence-based treatment strategy—in other words, the possibility to control the post-injury process [2–5].

The current conception of primary and secondary brain injury factors determines their effect on the outcome. Intracranial hypertension is considered as one of the most important factors [6–9]. It was shown in 1970s–1980s that intracranial pressure (ICP) monitoring could help to prevent the development of dislocation syndrome and to support adequate cerebral perfusion pressure, oxygenation and brain's metabolism [2, 3, 8, 10]. It is particularly important for the unformed brain of children in case of injury. Such anatomical and physiological aspects as higher intensity of metabolism, increased tendency towards brain oedema and swelling and higher sensitivity to brain hypoxia increase the risk of intracranial hypertension.

No randomised controlled studies have evaluated the effectiveness of ICP monitoring in children with severe TBI and its correlation with treatment outcome. The lack of clear standards for ICP monitoring in children is due to an insufficient data collection process [2].

The aim of our study was to find the parameter that could represent ICP variations and might become a good predictor of severe TBI outcomes in children.

Z.B. Semenova, M.D., Ph.D. (✉) • V.I. Lukianov
S.V. Meshcheryakov L.M. Roshal
Clinical and Research Institute of Emergency Children's Surgery and Trauma, St. Bolshaya Polyanka 22, 119180 Moscow, Russia
e-mail: jseman@mail.ru

Methods and Materials

The study includes 81 patients with severe TBI (2004–2014). Total mortality runs at 27%. Inclusion criteria was a Glasgow Coma Scale (GCS) score ≤8, age >3 years, and admission time to our clinic <24 h from the time of injury. Withdrawal criteria included patients with extracranial complications which resulted in death and age <3 years.

Age ranges from 3 to 17 years. Boys were 67%, girls 33%. Mean GCS was 6 ± 1.5. Combined injury amounted to 67.3%. ICP measurements were performed in accordance with the guidelines. Decompressive craniectomy was made in 22.5% of patients. Patients with GCS 3–4 had mostly unsatisfactory outcome. Good outcomes have been observed in 48% of patients.

All patients were divided into three groups according to outcome: 1— Glasgow Outcome Scale (GOS) 1 (fatal outcome), 2—GOS 2–3 (severe disability), 3—GOS 4–5 (good recovery). Mean daily values of ICP were used as a predictor, GOS value was used as a grouping variable. Outcomes were assessed 6 months after injury.

Software: MS Excel 2003, Statistica version 6, MedCalc version 13.

Results

The initial analysis showed that the prediction could be performed only for two outcome variants—survival and death, but even in this case the probability of correct classification was low and amounted to only 50%. We have developed a new predictor—the mean square deviation as an indicator of process stability. The ICP variation over a certain period of time can be considered as an oscillatory process. It is known that the energy of a contour forms out of the electric field energy and magnetic field energy. During vibrations, the energy of the system transforms from one form to another. The ICP variation (its dynamics and intensity) during a certain time interval can be described in a similar way.

According to classical perception about the oscillatory process, the energy of the process is equal to the sum of the square of the constant component of the average value and the square of the mean-square deviation. For ICP variation this value (E^2) is the sum of the square of the ICP average value and the square of process dispersion:

$$E^2(\text{ICP}) = M(ICP)^2 + \text{STD}(ICP)^2$$

Further analysis of the results showed statistically significant correlation between the ICP variation and outcome: the higher the value of E^2 (ICP), the worse prognosis should be suspected (Fig. 1). A Scheffe test (Table 1) confirmed the statistical significant difference between group 1 and the other groups ($p < 0.05$).

Prognostic threshold of mean daily intracranial pressure amounted to 500 mmHg^2. The risk of unsatisfactory outcome seemed to increase dramatically with higher values of this variable. The E^2 value in the group of survivors was < 500 mmHg^2; the probability of accurate forecasting, 91%. Sensitivity was 0.9, specificity 0.94.

Discussion

Nowadays scientists and practising neurosurgeons are still discussing not only the correlation between ICP values and outcome of TBI, but even the necessity of ICP monitoring, etc. [2, 3, 11]. Current evidence about this correlation is controversial. For example, in a prospective study made by Grinkeviciute et al. [12], 48 children with severe TBI were considered, and according to the study results ICP > 25 mmHg does not affect the outcome. Moreover, over 90% of patients had a satisfactory outcome. It should be recognised that authors used to consider ICP values <20 mmHg or >20 mmHg in most publications about the impact of ICP on TBI outcome. Some authors consider average or maximum value of ICP but state nothing about the duration of hypertension, whereas the prolonged increase of ICP is crucial for the severe TBI outcome. The lack of a unified statistical system is the cornerstone, which leads to confusion in assessing results.

The debate around the effectiveness of decompressive craniectomy drew attention to the threshold values of ICP and the permitted duration of intracranial hypertension again. Anne Vik et al. [13] offered such a thing as a "dose" of intracranial hypertension. They consider the area under the curve (AUC of ICP) as a predictor of outcome.

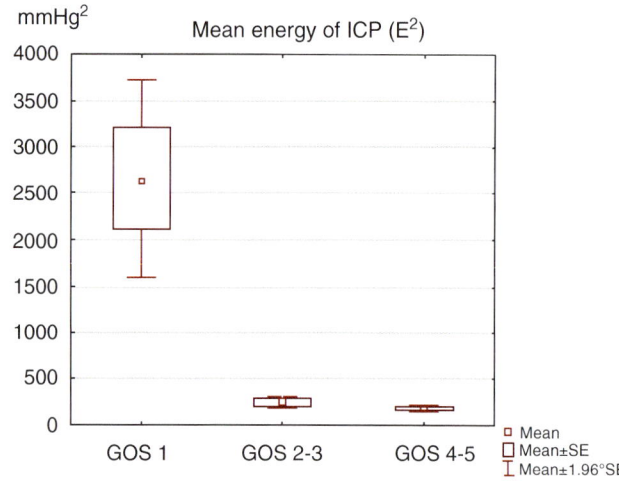

Fig. 1 ICP mean energy

Table 1 Scheffe test

GOS	Variable GOS		
	1	2	3
	M = 2,664.1	M = 2,253.96	M = 191.66
1		0.00	0.00
2	0.00		0.99
3	0.00	0.99	

Marked differences are significant at $p < 0.05$

Kahraman et al. [14] proposed a new predictor—so-called "pressure times time dose"—which reflects the degree and duration of the ICP rise. The authors point at its high predictive value for severe TBI outcome.

The group of Russian authors describes three types of ICP variation in adults during the removal of intracranial haematomas and in the postoperative period (Krylov et al. [4]): type I—decrease of ICP during the operation without a subsequent rise; type II—decrease of ICP during the operation followed by a rise within 2 days after the operation (to values less than 30–35 mmHg; type III—high ICP during the operation with a consequent rise in the postoperative period. The authors have established a correlation between the outcome and the type of ICP variation. Obviously, the type III ICP variation was considered an unsatisfactory outcome predictor.

We found it reasonable to dwell on these publications in detail to show the relevance and importance of ICP variation measurements during a certain time interval. The proposed E^2 parameter is a quantitative indicator that reflects the process oscillation or dispersion objectively. It is easy to register it through the monitor or to extract it from the hardware data registration in a certain period of time. Moreover, the mean square deviation can provide a complete picture of ICP variations, and it can be another tool of stratification during study planning. Of course, such studies are expected to be particularly important for children with TBI.

Conclusion

According to principles of evidence-based medicine, prognosis of the post-injury process course and outcome become increasingly important. The proposed method is accessible and easy to perform in case of ICP monitoring possibility. This method has high specificity (0.94) in the prediction of severe TBI outcome and can be a reliable tool for ICP control, contributing to timely and appropriate clinical decision-making. It is doubtless that a large multi-centre study should be performed in child neurotraumatology centres to collect enough statistically relevant information in this field.

Disclosure The study was approved and supported by the Review Board of Clinical and Research Institute of Emergency Children's Surgery and Trauma, Moscow, Russia.

Conflicts of interest statement We declare that we have no conflict of interest.

References

1. De Silva MJ, Roberts I, Perel P, Edwards P, Kenward MG, Fernandes J, Shakur H, Patel V. Patient outcome after traumatic brain injury in high-, middle- and low-income countries: analysis of data on 8927 patients in 46 countries. Int J Epidemiol. 2009;38:452–8.
2. Kochanek PM, Carney N, Adelson PD, et al. Guidelines for acute medical management of severe traumatic brain injury in infants, children, and adolescents—second edition. Pediatr Crit Care Med. 2012;13(Suppl 1):S1–82.
3. Guidelines for the management of severe traumatic brain injury. J Neurotrauma. 2007;24(Suppl 1):S1–106.
4. Krylov VV, Petrikov SS, Talypov AE, et al. Modern principles of surgery of severe traumatic brain injury. J Emerg Med Care. 2013;4:39–47.
5. Potapov AA, Krylov VV, Lichterman LB, et al. Modern recommendations of the diagnosis and treatment of severe traumatic brain injury. J Voprosy Neurochirurgii. 2006;1:S.3–8.
6. Allen BB, Chiu YL, Gerber LM, Ghajar J, Greenfield JP. Age-specific cerebral perfusion pressure thresholds and survival in children and adolescents with severe traumatic brain injury. Pediatr Crit Care Med. 2014;15(1):62–70.
7. Bruce DA, Alavi A, Bilaniuk L, et al. Diffuse cerebral swelling following head injuries in children: the syndrome of "malignant brain edema". J Neurosurg. 1981;54:170–8.
8. Chambers IR, Tradwell L, Mendelow AD. The cause and incidence of secondary insults in severely head-injured adults and children. Br J Neurosurg. 2000;14:424–31.
9. Miller Ferguson N, Shein SL, Kochanek PM, Luther J, Wisniewski SR, Clark RS, Tyler-Kabara EC, Adelson PD, Bell MJ. Intracranial hypertension and cerebral hypoperfusion in children with severe traumatic brain injury: thresholds and burden in accidental and abusive insults. Pediatr Crit Care Med. 2016;17(5):444–50.
10. Chesnut RM, Marshall LF, Klauber MR, et al. The role of secondary brain injury in determining outcome from severe head injury. J Trauma. 1993;34:216–22.
11. Shafi S, Diaz-Arrastia R, Madden C, Gentilello L. Intracranial pressure monitoring in brain-injured patients is associated with worsening of survival. J Trauma Fed. 2008;64(2):335–40.
12. Grinkeviciute DE, Kevalas R, Matukevicius A, et al. Significance of intracranial pressure and cerebral perfusion in severe pediatric traumatic brain injury. Medicina (Kaunas). 2008;44:119–25.
13. Vik A, Nag T, Fredriclsi OA, Scandsen T, et al. Relationship of "dose" of intracranial hypertension to outcome in severe traumatic injury. J Neurosurg. 2008;109:678–84.
14. Kahraman S, Dutton RP, Hu P, Xiao Y, Aarabi B, Stein DM, Scalea TM. Automated measurement of "pressure times time dose" of intracranial hypertension best predicts outcome after severe traumatic brain injury. J Trauma. 2010;69(1):110–8.

KidsBrainIT: A New Multi-centre, Multi-disciplinary, Multi-national Paediatric Brain Monitoring Collaboration

T. Lo, I. Piper, B. Depreitere, G. Meyfroidt, M. Poca, J. Sahuquillo, T. Durduran, P. Enblad, P. Nilsson, A. Ragauskas, K. Kiening, K. Morris, R. Agbeko, R. Levin, J. Weitz, C. Park, P. Davis, and on Behalf of BrainIT

Abstract *Objectives*: Validated optimal cerebral perfusion pressure (CPP) treatment thresholds in children do not exist. To improve the intensive care unit (ICU) management of the paediatric traumatic brain injury (TBI) population, we are forming a new paediatric multi-centre collaboration to recruit standardised ICU data for running and reporting upon models for assessing autoregulation and optimal CCP (CPPopt).

Materials and methods: We are adapting the adult BrainIT group's approach to develop a new Paediatric Brain Monitoring and Information Technology Group (KidsBrainIT), which will include a repository to store prospectively collected high-resolution physiological, clinical, and outcome data. In the first phase of this project there are 7 UK Paediatric Intensive Care Units, 1 Spanish, 1 Belgium, and 1 Romanian Centre interested in participating. In subsequent phases, we plan to open recruitment to other centres both within Europe, US and abroad. We are collaborating with the Leuven Group and plan to use their LAx (low-frequency autoregulation index), DATACAR (dynamic adaptive target of active cerebral autoregulation), CPPopt and visualisation methodologies. We also plan to use the continuous diffuse optical monitoring and tomography technology developed in Barcelona as an acute surrogate end-point for optimising brain perfusion. This technology allows non-invasive continuous monitoring of deep tissue perfusion and oxygenation in adults but its clinical application in infants and children with TBI has not been studied previously.

Results: We report on the current status of setting up this new collaboration and also on pilot analyses in two centres which are the basis of our rationale for the need for a prospective validation study of CPPopt in children. Specifically, we demonstrated that CPPopt varied with time for each patient during their paediatric intensive care unit (PICU) stay, and the median overall CPPopt levels for children aged 2–6 years, 7–11 years and 12–16 years were 68.83, 68.09, and 72.17 mmHg respectively. Among survivors and patients with favourable outcome (GOS 4 and 5), there were significantly higher proportions with CPP monitoring time within CPPopt ($p = 0.04$ and $p = 0.01$ respectively).

Conclusions: There is a need and an interest in forming a multi-centre PICU collaboration for acquiring data and

on Behalf of BrainIT

T. Lo
Royal Hospital for Sick Children, Edinburgh, UK

I. Piper (✉)
Queen Elizabeth University Hospital, Glasgow, UK
e-mail: ian.piper@brainit.org

B. Depreitere • G. Meyfroidt
Leuven University Hospital, Leuven, Belgium

M. Poca • J. Sahuquillo • T. Durduran
Val D'hebron University Hospital, Barcelona, Spain

P. Enblad • P. Nilsson
Uppsala University Hospital, Uppsala, Sweden

A. Ragauskas
Kaunas University of Technology, Kaunas, Lithuania

K. Kiening
Heidelberg University Hospital, Heidelberg, Germany

K. Morris
Birmingham Children's Hospital, Birmingham, UK

R. Agbeko
Great Northern Children's Hospital, Newcastle Upon Tyne, UK

R. Levin
Royal Hospital for Children, Glasgow, UK

J. Weitz
Oxford Radcliffe Hospitals NHS Foundation Trust, Oxford, UK

C. Park
Alder Hey Childrens NHS Foundation Trust, Liverpool, UK

P. Davis
Nottingham University Hospitals NHS Trust, Nottingham, UK

performing analyses for determining validated CPPopt thresholds in the paediatric TBI population. KidsBrainIT is being formed to meet that need.

Keywords Paediatric brain injury • Neurointensive care • Informatics • BrainIT

Background

Traumatic brain injury (TBI) is the commonest cause of death in children over 1 year of age [1]. It causes significant morbidity, with the majority of survivors suffering from long-term severe disability, such as memory and attention deficits, personality disorders (frontal lobe syndrome) and learning difficulties [2]. The long-term disability socio-economically affects survivors as adults, their carers and their communities [2]. None of the novel experimental TBI therapies tested in the laboratory have translated into effective clinical treatment that improves outcome. The current best therapeutic option to improve paediatric TBI outcome is to optimise physiological support during intensive care management to minimise secondary physiological insults [3] that are known to negatively affect outcome [4–8]. However, therapeutic thresholds for abnormal physiology vary between units [9] and are implemented clinically without validation. To give these patients the best possible recovery, we urgently need clinically relevant and readily translatable research that optimises paediatric brain trauma treatment and reduces inequality between different centres within Britain and worldwide.

Continuous real-time physiological monitoring is a recognised standard in TBI intensive care management. However, unlike many adult neuro-intensive-care units, clinical TBI management, quality improvement and research in the paediatric intensive care unit (PICU) often rely on low-resolution summary measures of these data, such as a single time-point record of an end-of-hour reading. This discards vital information, reduces the fidelity of the data and potentially compromises patient safety, clinical management and outcome [10]. Reasons for wasting these data include difficulty of accessing, organising and using the data from their original sources [10], information overload from the plethora of routine data generated with advances in monitoring technologies [11], variability in clinical documentation methods and quality [10] between different units and countries. To advance paediatric brain trauma care, we urgently need to develop and implement a practical way to systematically capture, analyse and integrate the vital improvement information embedded in the massive amount of routine clinical data generated during patient care [10].

Multi-centre data collection and analysis of such 'big data' have been shown to generate new hypotheses and novel data analysis methods. Examples of such successful informatics initiatives in the adult TBI population include the BrainIT group and more recently the CENTRE-TBI trial. In the paediatric TBI domain, no-one has attempted to set up a similar initiative. Because of the age-related developmental differences in post-TBI physiological responses and outcome, a similar informatics based initiative in paediatrics is much needed to make significant advances in this field. Using prospectively collected high-resolution physiological data from two PICUs, we demonstrated paediatric TBI patients frequently suffered deranged physiology, and the quantitative insult burden was related to worsened outcome [4, 5]. The benefits of using routine high-resolution data generated from clinical care for research is evident from our feasibility study, unfortunately the complexity and burden of such data capture has prevented this from becoming a standard of practice across different PICU. Through close collaboration with adult intensivist colleagues, we know this can be achieved and will improve TBI care and outcome in paediatrics.

The BrainIT group (www.brainit.org) is a multi-centre multi-national data-intensive informatics collaborative clinical and research network that deliver data-derived innovative improvement in adult TBI care, patient safety and outcome. Using innovative analytics [4–8] on the high-quality paediatric TBI 'big-data' in our feasibility study in collaboration with BrainIT, we confirm that current CPP management and raised ICP treatment are sub-optimal. We demonstrated that poor outcome occurs when clinically measured CPP levels fall below the defined critical CPP insult thresholds of any duration [5]. Current CPP treatment thresholds are 'best guess' levels proposed from clinicians' own experience and vary between units [3, 9]. As observed in our feasibility study, although these un-validated CPP treatment thresholds are set higher than the defined critical insult thresholds, TBI patients still have actual CPP recorded below these critical insult thresholds [5]. This highlights the urgent need to have defined and validated cerebrovascular autoregulation-driven optimal CPP target thresholds (CPPopt) for clinical use and a quality improvement feedback mechanism for ensuring adherence to the agreed treatment targets (Fig. 1).

In our feasibility study, we retrospectively calculated CPPopt using the low-frequency autoregulation index (LAx)-CPP plots methodology [2], and then determined the relationship between CPPopt and the patients' clinical global outcome assessed at 6 months after brain trauma [7]. We demonstrated that CPPopt varied with time for each patient during their PICU stay [7]. Among survivors and patients with favourable outcome (GOS 4 and 5), there were significantly higher proportions with CPP monitoring time within CPPopt ($p = 0.04$ and $p = 0.01$ respectively) when considered as a group [7]. Findings from this feasibility study suggest

	Aged 2–6 Yrs	Aged 7–10 Yrs	Aged 11–16 Yrs
Optimal Target Thresholds	?	?	?
Current Un-validated Treatment Thresholds	55 mmHg	60 mmHg	65 mmHg
Critical Insult Thersholds	48 mmHg	54 mmHg	58 mmHg

Fig. 1 The concept of different CPP thresholds (critical insult thresholds vs current unvalidated treatment thresholds vs optimal target thresholds where cerebrovascular autoregulation remains intact)

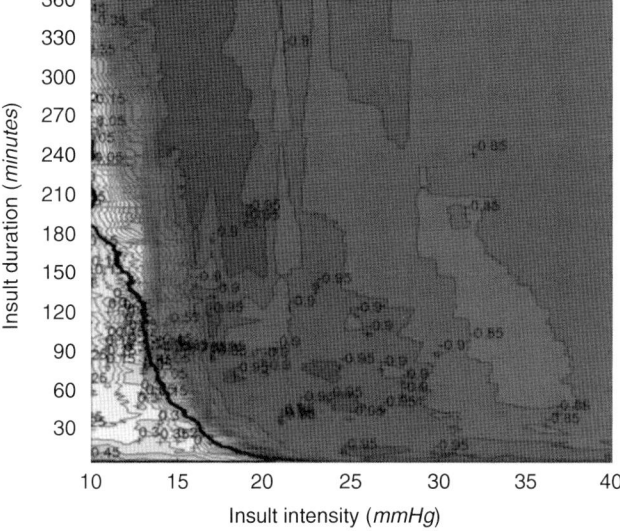

Fig. 2 The ICP dose-response plot for paediatric patients in our feasibility study [8]. It demonstrates that both ICP duration and intensity affect outcome (Area in *red* represents unfavourable outcome.)

that keeping measured CPP within calculated CPPopt may improve global outcome after paediatric TBI.

Our innovative ICP visualisation plots [8] from the feasibility study demonstrate the intuitive concept that episodes of higher ICP can only be tolerated for shorter durations [8] (Fig. 2). This means ICP below the single pre-defined treatment level (for example, 15 mmHg) is not necessarily safe if sustained for longer durations [8]. Thus, to improve outcome, we need to have both cerebral autoregulation derived CPPopt target thresholds and use an ICP dose-response approach that takes into consideration both the duration and magnitude of raised ICP.

Through our feasibility study, we have demonstrated the importance and effectiveness of multi-centre multi-disciplinary multi-national informatics collaborations in deriving and testing clinically relevant hypotheses while addressing the age-maturation challenges we face in managing paediatric brain trauma patients. Translating these research findings may enhance childhood TBI recovery through improving current clinical treatment.

Aims

We, therefore, aim to establish a new multi-centre, multi-disciplinary, multi-national paediatric brain monitoring and information technology group (KidsBrainIT), which uses routinely collected bedside physiological data in 1-min resolutions, and IT (information technology) innovations to improve paediatric traumatic brain injury patients' care, safety and outcome.

In Phase-1, we aim to test two clinically relevant hypotheses derived from our feasibility study: After sustaining TBI, paediatric patients with a longer period of measured CPP maintained within the calculated optimal CPP (CPPopt) range have (1) an improved global clinical outcome, and (2) better tolerance against raised ICP.

Methods

Modelling upon adult BrainIT, we set up a new multi-centre, multi-disciplinary and multi-national paediatric clinical and research group (KidsBrainIT), which was launched at the BrainIT meeting in October 2015. In Phase-1, KidsBrainIT brings together key engineering, technical and scientific staff from adult BrainIT (in Britain, Belgium, and Spain), and also senior clinicians (paediatric intensivists, neurosurgeons and neurologists) from Britain, Belgium, Spain and Romania. The ten contributing centres that have confirmed their commitment to participate in Phase-1 KidsBrainIT include: seven UK PICUs (Edinburgh, Glasgow, Newcastle, Birmingham, Liverpool, Oxford and Nottingham), one Belgian (Leuven), one Spanish (Barcelona) and one Romanian (Iasi) paediatric neuro-surgical/intensive care centres. These key stake-holders, under Dr. Lo and Dr. Piper's leadership, work together to set up and use a central data repository and underlying technical infrastructure to store, analyse and report upon prospectively collected high-resolution physiological, clinical and outcome data.

This is done through a 30-month prospective observational clinical study that forms the Phase-1 KidsBrainIT data-set. Anonymised clinical data are collected using the same pre-designed proforma used in our feasibility study [4–8]. It includes the cause and nature of injury, age, Glasgow Coma Score (GCS) on admission and after acute non-surgical resuscitation, pupillary responses, initial radiological and computerised tomography (CT), operative and other treatment details. Using BrainIT data collection tools, this proforma data is captured electronically and ensures only collection of anonymous data fields. A locally maintained "link database" in each centre is used to enable data-source checking by the contributing unit's local research team should there be any data queries. Each patient's anonymised clinical data are linked to their physiological and outcome data in the KidsBrainIT data-bank using an anonymous study ID.

Routinely measured physiological data in 1-min resolutions are captured from the bedside monitors prospectively. In centres with networked monitors, these data are recorded and stored in the main networked servers (with or without using electronic clinical information systems), where data extraction takes place when the patients are discharged from PICU. For centres without networked monitors (i.e. stand-alone monitors), a mobile data collection unit with ICM+ software installed is connected to the bedside monitor via a serial RS232 connection. This connection allows real-time data storage in 1-min resolutions using the ICM+ software and the data are then exported when the patient is discharged from PICU (Fig. 3). All physiological data are anonymised prior to exporting, and then stored in the KidsBrainIT central data-bank (Fig. 4). The data of the 99 patients from our feasibility study are already stored in the KidsBrainIT central data-bank.

We use this data-set to test clinically relevant hypotheses as described above. We utilise IT analytical innovations developed within BrainIT to calculate CPPopt [6, 7], ICP dose-response [8], quantify physiological insults [4, 5] and determine their relationships to global and functional outcome assessed at 6 and 12 months respectively. We additionally have implemented an open collaborative infrastructure within KidsBrainIT to enable our contributing centres to access the whole data-bank for future hypotheses testing and data sharing with other research groups/institutes in accordance to BrainIT criteria. We plan to expand KidsBrainIT in future phases to include other centres in UK, Europe, North America and beyond. Currently teams in Montreal and Philadelphia have confirmed their interest in joining KidsBrainIT.

In this current report, we described current progress of Phase-1 KidsBrainIT, including the preliminary findings from analyses of the pilot data.

Results

Ten PICUs from four countries confirmed their participation in Phase-1 KidsBrainIT. Site-visits have commenced to ensure successful interface to extract data from bedside monitors prior to KidsBrainIT going live. To-date, we have successfully extracted and anonymised data from bedside monitors in five of the ten centres. Our sample size calculation determines that a sample consisting of 129 patients will provide a 5% significance and 90% power to test our hypothesis; inflating this number by 10% to account for a similar non-

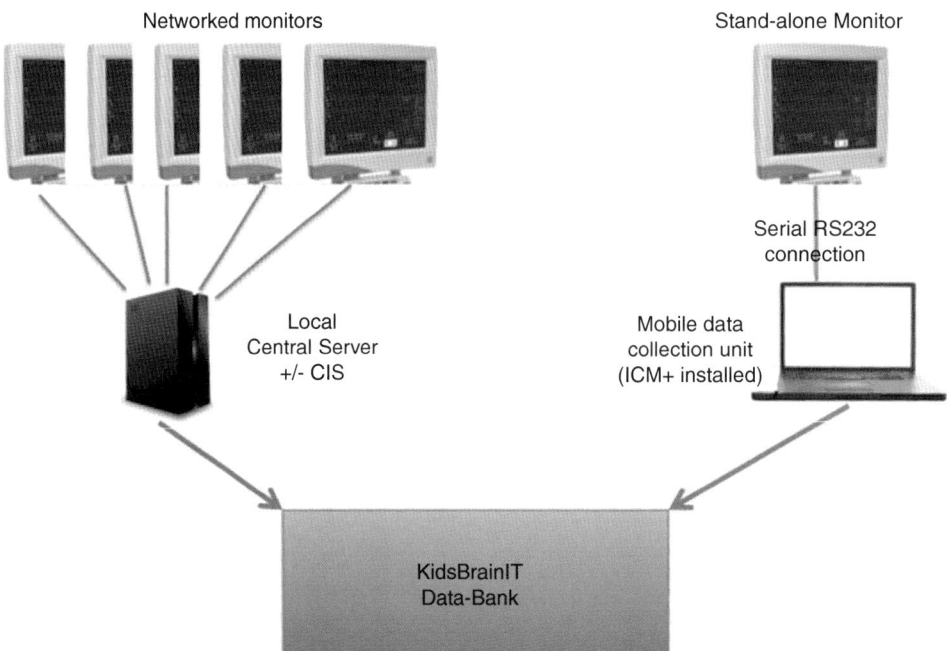

Fig. 3 Data collection and extraction from bedside monitors in units with networked and stand-alone (non-network) monitors. All data are anonymised prior to extraction and archive into the KidsBrainIT data-bank

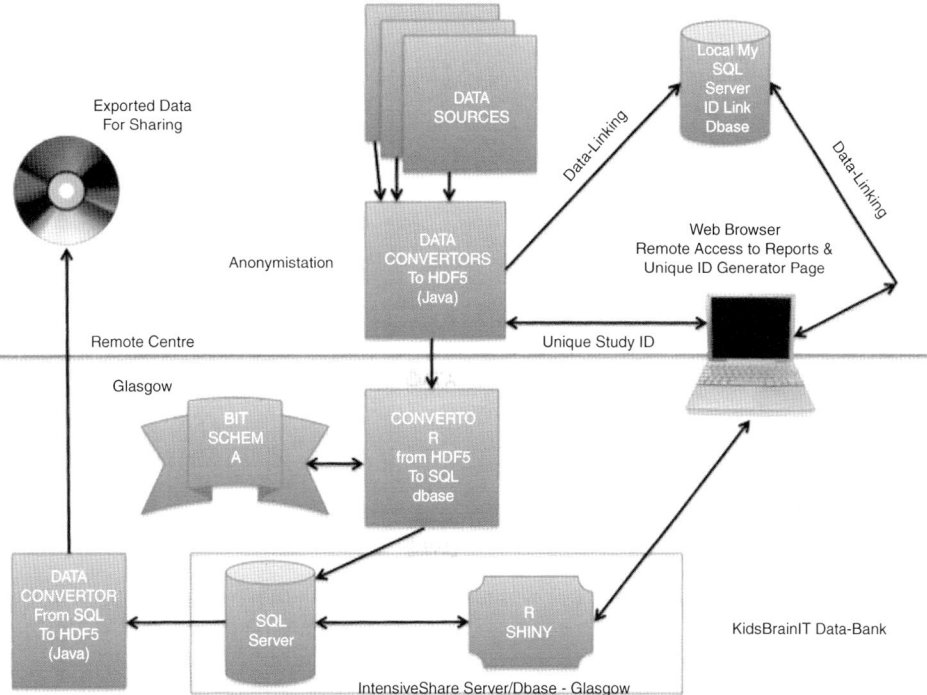

Fig. 4 The anonymisation process used in KidsBrainIT by each contributing unit, and how the data-set may be exported for data sharing in the future with other research groups/institutes

inclusion rate as our feasibility study means that we need to recruit 145 patients in Phase-1 KidsBrainIT. We anticipate we will reach this target number within 18 months of the study period based on the most recent admission data from our contributing units (Fig. 5).

The KidsBrainIT pilot data consisted of 99 critically ill TBI patients aged between 2 and 16 years old (median age was 10.3 years). There were 69 boys and 30 girls. They all sustained accidental brain trauma. Calculated CPPopt varied with time and between patients. Patients with favourable outcome had significantly longer duration of measured CPP within the calculated CPPopt ranges than those with unfavourable outcome ($p < 0.01$). ICP visualisation plot analyses demonstrated that patients with intact cerebral autoregulation was more tolerant of ICP insults than those who had impaired cerebral autoregulation (Fig. 6).

Discussion

In this report, we described the successful establishment of KidsBrainIT, a new multi-centre, multi-disciplinary, multi-national paediatric brain monitoring collaboration. KidsBrainIT is unique and different from other large paediatric TBI trials (including the on-going ADAPT Trial) because it is the first childhood TBI initiative to data-bank continuous prospectively collected physiological data in minute-by-minute resolution from multiple sites in various countries, and to investigate the effect of acute physiological insult quantified using these high-quality clinical and physiological data on outcome. The innovative analytics used in KidsBrainIT are developed within the BrainIT group. Our informatics approach is essential in delivering data-driven improvement in patient care, safety and outcome, and KidsBrainIT is the first such paediatric 'big-data' initiative to have the full support of the highly successful adult BrainIT group. This allows us to address the adult-paediatric divide in TBI management, research and quality improvement, and will bring huge advances to the field.

CPPopt calculation in KidsBrainIT is performed using LAx-CPP plots and DATACAR (dynamic adaptive target of active cerebral autoregulation) methods [6]. These methodologies are those used previously in our feasibility study [7]. We chose to use LAx-CPP plots and DATACAR methodology [6, 7] (developed by the Leuven group within BrainIT) to calculate CPPopt because it only requires routinely measured pressure data in 1-min resolutions extracted from the clinical bedside monitors without the need for costly additional software solutions to capture continuous waveform signals from the bedside monitors at a frequency of at least 60 Hz [6]. The ability to capture high-frequency waveform signals from bedside monitors to calculate optimal CPP using the pressure reactivity index (PRx) method [12] is usually limited to a few research-minded academic centres in the world, making both recruitment and clinical transla-

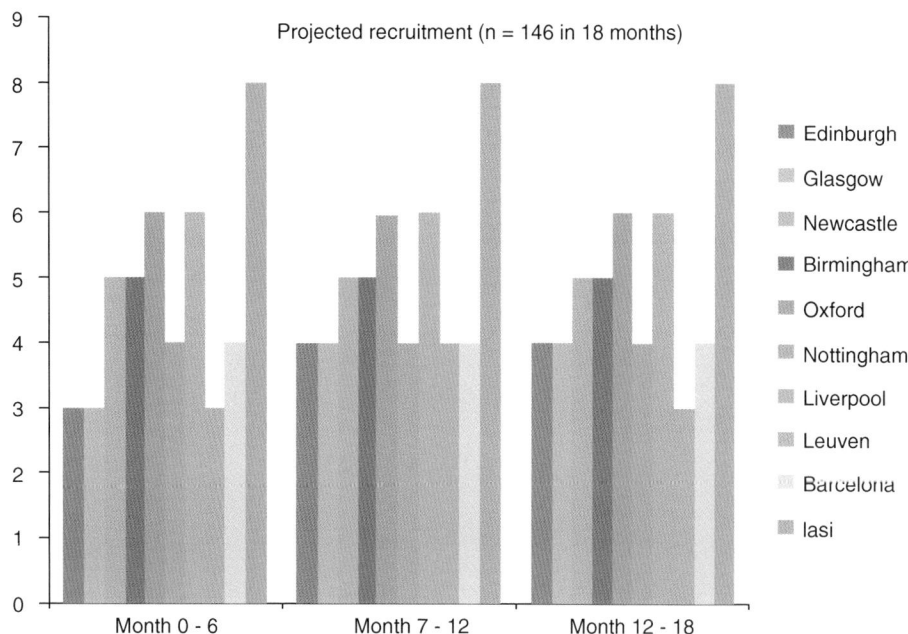

Fig. 5 The projected recruitment from the ten contributing centres within 18 months of the study period

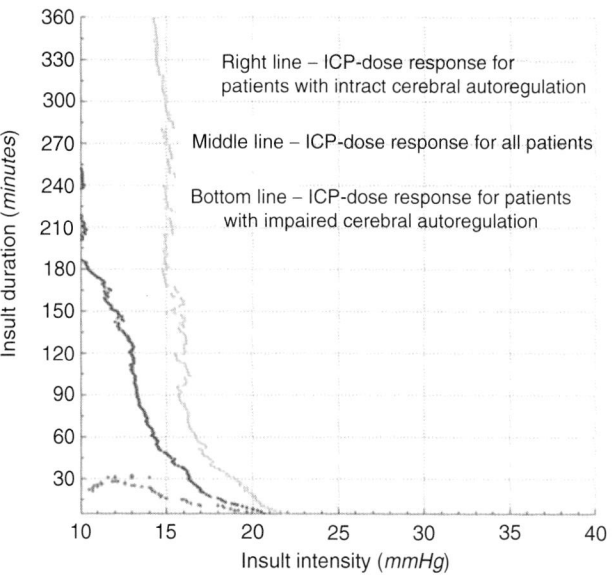

Fig. 6 Patients with intact cerebrovascular autoregulation (*upper line*) are more tolerant of raised ICP insults in our feasibility study [8]. Patients with impaired cerebrovascular autoregulation (*lower line*) had poorer tolerance of raised ICP insults

tion difficult. Thus, our choice of CPPopt calculation using LAx-CPP plots and DATACAR methodology [6, 7] allows KidsBrainIT to theoretically include any PICU across the world that routinely collect minute-by-minute pressure data without requiring costly equipment/software upgrades. Furthermore, findings from our Phase-1 KidsBrainIT study and any treatment target recommendations are directly transferable back to a wider clinical audience because no special equipment or software is required beyond what is currently used for the routine minute-by-minute physiological bedside monitoring. Together with adult BrainIT's expertise in extracting data from a large range of ICU bedside monitors and existing collaborations with monitoring companies, KidsBrainIT plan to expand in future phases to include other centres in the UK, Europe, North America and beyond.

Our colour-coded ICP dose-response visualisation plot (Fig. 2) [8] demonstrates the intuitive concept that episodes of higher ICP can only be tolerated for short durations. Currently, clinical ICP treatment is initiated when ICP exceeds a specific level for a specific duration (for example, many units choose to treat if ICP exceeds 20 mmHg for more than 5 min). There is great variation between different units on the treatment thresholds (both in terms of magnitude and duration) [9]; for example, some units choose to only treat raised ICP if it exceeds 20 mmHg for 15 min, while others will accept ICP values of 25 mmHg lasting less than 5 min. However, these ICP treatment thresholds are based purely on clinicians' own experience rather than evidence-based studies. Our ICP dose-response visualisation plot demonstrates this treatment method is suboptimal because ICP lower than the pre-defined treatment level (for example, 15 mmHg) is not necessarily safe if sustained for longer durations [8]. Thus, developing validated ICP dose-response visualisation plots for paediatric TBI is a much-needed clinical solution to improve current ICP management that may ultimately affect outcome. In our feasibility study, we grouped paediatric patients of all ages in the analyses because of small numbers represented within each age group. But when compared to adults with brain trauma, our paediatric patients had lower tolerance of raised ICP in both magnitude and duration [8]. This indicates tolerance of raised ICP varies with age and different brain maturation or developmental stages. In Phase-1 KidsBrainIT with a larger data-set, we will assess the ICP dose responses in different age bands in addition to as a whole group, so that we may determine the critical ICP dose-response graphs for children of varying ages. These ICP dose-response graphs for children of different ages may be readily translated back to clinical practice to improve patient care at the end of this study.

Conclusion

KidsBrainIT brings clinicians and scientists from multiple centres and different countries together to use high-resolution physiological data and IT innovations to improve TBI patient care and safety.

Conflicts of interest statement We declare that we have no conflict of interest.

References

1. Heron M, Sutton PD, Xu J, Ventura SJ, et al. Annual summary of vital statistics: 2007. Pediatrics. 2010;125(1):4–15.
2. Anderson V, Brown S, Newitt H, Hoile H. Long-term outcome from childhood traumatic brain injury: intellectual ability, personality, and quality of life. Neuropsychology. 2011;25(2):176–84.
3. Kochanek PM, Carney N, Adelson PD, Ashwal S, et al. Guidelines for the acute medical management of severe traumatic brain injury in infants, children, and adolescents (second edition). Pediatr Crit Care Med. 2012;13(Suppl 1):S1–82.
4. Jones PA, Andrews PA, Easton VJ, Minns RA. Traumatic brain injury in childhood: intensive care time series data and outcome. Br J Neurosurg. 2003;17(1):29–39.
5. Chambers IR, Jones PA, Lo TYM, Forsyth RJ, et al. Critical thresholds of intracranial pressure and cerebral perfusion pressure related to age in paediatric head injury. J Neurol Neurosurg Psychiatry. 2006;77(2):234–40.
6. Depreitere B, Güiza F, Van den Berghe G, Schuhmann M, et al. Pressure autoregulation monitoring and cerebral perfusion pressure target recommendation in severe traumatic brain injury patients based on minute-by-minute monitoring data. J Neurosurg. 2014;120(6):1451–7.
7. Güiza F, Meyfroidt G, Lo TYM, Jones PA, et al. Continuous optimal CPP based on minute-by-minute monitoring data: a study on a pediatric population. Acta Neurochir. 2016;122:187–91.
8. Guiza F, Depreitere B, Piper I, Citerio G, et al. Visualizing the pressure and time burden of intracranial hypertension in adult and paediatric traumatic brain injury. Intensive Care Med. 2015;41(6):1067–76.
9. Bell MJ, Adelson PD, Hutchison JS, Kochanek PM, et al. Differences in medical therapy goals for children with severe traumatic brain injury—an international study. Pediatr Crit Care Med. 2013;14(8):811–8.
10. Celi LA, Mark RG, Stone DJ, Montgomery RA. "Big data" in the intensive care unit. Closing the data loop. Am J Respir Crit Care Med. 2013;187(11):1157–60.
11. Jones PA, Minns RA, Lo TY, Andrews PJ, et al. Graphical display of variability and inter-relationships of pressure signals in children with traumatic brain injury. Physiol Meas. 2003;24(1):201–11.
12. Czosnyka M, Smielewski P, Kirkpatrick P, Laing RJ, et al. Continuous assessment of the cerebral vasomotor reactivity in head injury. Neurosurgery. 1997;41(1):11–9.

Increased ICP and Its Cerebral Haemodynamic Sequelae

Joseph Donnelly, Marek Czosnyka, Spencer Harland, Georgios V. Varsos, Danilo Cardim, Chiara Robba, Xiuyun Liu, Philip N. Ainslie, and Peter Smielewski

Abstract *Objectives*: Increased intracranial pressure (ICP) is a pathological feature of many neurological diseases; however, the local and systemic sequelae of raised ICP are incompletely understood. Using an experimental paradigm, we aimed to describe the cerebrovascular consequences of acute increases in ICP.

Materials and methods: We assessed cerebral haemodynamics [mean arterial blood pressure (MAP), ICP, laser Doppler flowmetry (LDF), basilar artery Doppler flow velocity (Fv) and estimated vascular wall tension (WT)] in 27 basilar artery-dependent rabbits during experimental (artificial lumbar CSF infusion) intracranial hypertension. WT was estimated as the difference between critical closing pressure and ICP.

Results: From baseline (~9 mmHg) to moderate increases in ICP (~41 mmHg), cortical LDF decreased (from 100 to 39.1%, $p < 0.001$), while mean global Fv was unchanged (from 47 to 45 cm/s, $p = 0.38$). In addition, MAP increased (from 88.8 to 94.2 mmHg, $p < 0.01$ and WT decreased (from 19.3 to 9.8 mmHg, $p < 0.001$). From moderate to high ICP (~75 mmHg), both global Fv and cortical LDF decreased (Fv, from 45 to 31.3 cm/s, $p < 0.001$; LDF, from 39.1 to 13.3%, $p < 0.001$) while MAP increased further (94.2 to 114.5 mmHg, $p < 0.001$) and estimated WT was unchanged (from 9.7 to 9.6 mmHg, $p = 0.35$).

Conclusion: In this analysis, we demonstrate a cortical vulnerability to increases in ICP and two ICP-dependent cerebro-protective mechanisms: with moderate increases in ICP, WT decreases and MAP increases to buffer cerebral perfusion, while with severe increases of ICP, an increased MAP predominates.

Keywords Intracranial pressure · Cerebral haemodynamics · Autoregulation · Cerebral perfusion pressure

Introduction

Because of the rigid skull encasing the cerebrum, increased intracranial volume from whatever cause can lead to high intracranial pressure (ICP). The consequences of increased ICP are universally harmful and include impaired cerebral blood flow (CBF), electrical activity and metabolism. Therefore, the avoidance of raised ICP is pivotal in the management of many neurological conditions where acute changes in cerebral volume are possible, including traumatic brain injury, subarachnoid haemorrhage or acute hydrocephalus [1].

Increases in ICP lead to a decrease in cerebral perfusion pressure [CPP; calculated as mean arterial pressure (MAP) − ICP] and thus can limit perfusion to the brain [2]. The brain, however, has an intrinsic mechanism to protect itself from injury due to low CPP: cerebral autoregulation [3]. While the haemodynamic response to decreases in MAP have been well described, the response to increases in ICP are less well understood.

In this study, we revisited the question of how raised ICP affects cerebral haemodynamics using a rabbit model of experimental intracranial hypertension. This is a short summary of experimental material, based on our recently published full paper [4].

J. Donnelly · G.V. Varsos · D. Cardim · C. Robba
X. Liu · P. Smielewski
Brain Physics Laboratory, Division of Neurosurgery, Department of Clinical Neurosciences, Cambridge Biomedical Campus, University of Cambridge, Cambridge CB2 0QQ, UK
e-mail: jd634@cam.ac.uk

M. Czosnyka
Institute of Electronic Systems, Warsaw University of Technology, Warsaw, Poland

Brain Physics Laboratory, Division of Neurosurgery, Department of Clinical Neurosciences, Cambridge Biomedical Campus, University of Cambridge, Cambridge CB2 0QQ, UK

S. Harland
Queen Elizabeth Hospital, Birmingham, UK

P.N. Ainslie
University of British Columbia, Kelowna, BC, Canada

Methods

Animals and Ethics

These experiments were carried out in 1995 and 1996 in accordance with the standards provided by the UK Animals Scientific Procedures act of 1986 under a UK Home Office license and with permission from the institutional animal care and use committee at Cambridge University.

Physiological recordings from lumbar CSF infusions in 28 NZ white rabbits (7 female, 21 male; weight, 2.7–3.7 kg) were retrospectively analysed [5]. The experimental procedures for this specific experiment have been described in previous publications [6]. Briefly, ICP was monitored using an intraparenchymal microsensor (Codman and Shurtleff, Raynham, MA, USA), cortical blood flow with a laser Doppler flowmetry probe (Moor Instruments, Axbridge, UK). Basilar artery flow velocity using an 8-MHz Doppler ultrasound probe (PCDop 842;SciMed, Bristol, UK), and arterial blood pressure (ABP) using a catheter in the dorsal aorta (GaelTec, Dunvegan, UK). A lumbar laminectomy facilitated insertion of a catheter for the controlled infusion of artificial cerebrospinal fluid (CSF). The animals were supported in the Sphinx position using a purpose-built head frame with three-point skull fixation. Ventilation was controlled according to arterial PCO_2 via periodic arterial blood gas analyses. All experiments were performed in an animal laboratory at the same time of day.

Importantly these rabbits had their common carotid arteries ligated 2 weeks prior to experimentation so that blood flow to the brain was basilar artery dependent. This made a Doppler assessment of global blood flow possible through the insonation of only the basilar artery.

Protocol

Following 20 min of rest, ICP was artificially increased by infusion of Hartmann's solution into the lumbar CSF space. Infusion rates were initially 0.1 ml/min. ICP increased to reach a plateau of around 40 mmHg after approximately 10 min; thereafter the infusion rate was increased to rates between 0.2 and 2 ml/min to produce severe intracranial hypertension. ICP was increased until the point where diastolic flow velocity approached zero, which corresponded to an ICP of between 60 and 100 mmHg (mean, 75 mmHg) at the termination of the experiment. Rabbits were euthanised with thiopental at the conclusion of the test.

Data Acquisition and Analysis

ABP, ICP, basilar artery flow velocity (Fv) and expired CO_2 signals were recorded digitally at a sampling frequency of 50 Hz. Data were subsequently analysed off-line using custom-built, commercially available data analysis software (ICM+; http://www.neurosurg.cam.ac.uk/icmplus). LDF was expressed as a.u. minus the 'biological zero' as measured in the asystolic rabbit at the conclusion of the experiment. Critical closing pressure (CrCP) was calculated based on an impedance-based methodology as previously described in [7]. Estimated arterial wall tension (WT) was calculated as CrCP − ICP.

Statistical Analyses

Pairwise comparisons of haemodynamic parameters between the three different ICP conditions ("low", "moderate" and "high") were performed using Student's t-test. The alpha-value was set at 0.05 and no corrections were made for multiple comparisons. Of the available 28 experiments, one was excluded from analysis due to an inability to increase ICP above 30 mmHg with CSF infusion, leaving 27 rabbits for the final analysis. Statistical analysis was performed using IBM SPSS version 21.0 software (IBM, Armonk, NY, USA).

Results

A statistical description of monitored parameters is given in Table 1. Increases in MAP were observed between baseline and moderate levels of ICP, and also between moderate and high levels of ICP. As a result of the Cushing vasopressor response, despite an increase in ICP by 35 mmHg between the 'moderate' and 'high' ICP conditions, CPP only decreased by 14 mmHg. Mean flow velocity of the basilar artery was not significantly changed from baseline to moderate ICP, whereas cortical LDF and diastolic flow velocity decreased. End tidal CO_2 remained constant throughout the experiment.

The inter-relationships between changes in ICP, CBF, vascular wall tension, and MAP in all 27 rabbits are shown in Fig. 1. CBF appears well maintained with up to 60 mmHg increases in ICP. This maintenance of CBF was contributed by both decreases in wall tension and increases in MAP. Wall tension progressively decreased with increasing ICP, particularly during early increases in ICP. At the highest levels of ICP, WT started to increase.

Table 1 Haemodynamic consequences of raised intracranial pressure

	Baseline		Moderate ICP			High ICP			
	Mean	SE	Mean	SE	Significance compared to baseline	Mean	SE	Significance compared to baseline	Significance compared to moderate ICP
ICP (mmHg)	9.00	1.51	40.75	2.17	**	75.05	3.65	**	**
MAP (mmHg)	88.84	3.29	94.15	3.21	*	114.54	3.67	**	**
CPP (mmHg)	79.71	3.46	53.08	2.77	**	39.64	2.16	**	**
HR (BPM)	273.27	6.96	262.73	7.64	*	227.21	11.13	**	**
Global Fv mean (cm/s)	47.04	2.99	44.99	2.82		31.33	2.45	**	**
Global Fv diastolic (cm/s)	34.17	2.76	30.49	2.58	*	15.59	1.67	**	**
Global Fv systolic (cm/s)	66.93	3.64	65.51	3.33		50.97	2.66	**	**
WT (mmHg)	19.27	1.84	9.75	1.27	**	9.58	1.36	**	
CrCP (mmHg)	28.42	2.05	50.61	2.12	**	85.09	3.99	**	**
Cortical LDF (%)	100.00	0.00	39.10	29.82	**	13.27	5.19	**	**

ICP intracranial pressure, *MAP* mean arterial pressure, *CPP* cerebral perfusion pressure, *HR* heart rate, *Fv* flow velocity, *WT* wall tension, *CrCP* critical closing pressure, *LDF* laser Doppler flow

* $p < 0.05$
** $p < 0.001$

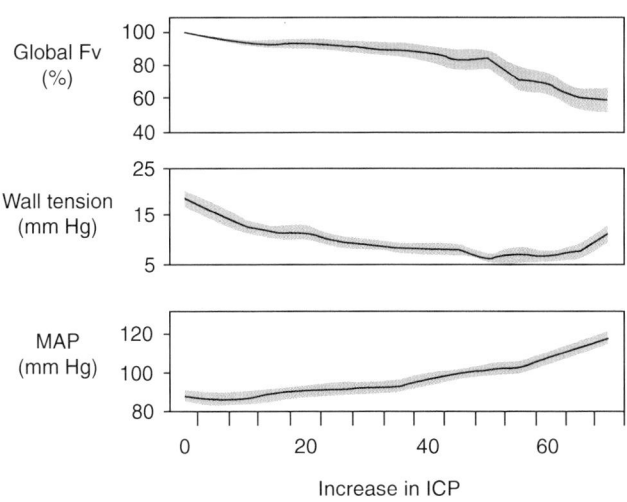

Fig. 1 The haemodynamic response to increased ICP induced by infusion of artificial CSF in NZ rabbits (mean ± standard error, $n = 27$). With moderate increases in ICP, global CBF (basilar artery Fv after common carotid ligation) is maintained through a decrease in vascular wall tension. With more severe increases in ICP (greater than 20-mmHg increase in ICP), a Cushing response-mediated increase in MAP helps to maintain CBF

Discussion

In this experimental investigation, we identified two intrinsic and mechanistically distinct compensatory adaptations to raised ICP: with moderate increases in ICP, CBF is maintained by decreases in vascular wall tension; whereas at higher levels of ICP, cerebral perfusion is protected by the Cushing vasopressor response that maintains CPP. In addition, regional differences in the control of cerebral perfusion were observed, with cortical blood flow being more sensitive to an increase in ICP than global blood flow.

In these experiments, global CBF was maintained until ICP had increased by 55 mmHg above baseline ICP (Fig. 1). This maintenance of CBF seemed to be mediated by a decrease in estimated vascular wall tension (Fig. 1 and Table 1). Estimated wall tension decreased and reached a plateau during ICP increases between 30 and 60 mmHg (Fig. 1 and Table 1). This plateau of vascular wall tension (at around 6–8 mmHg) may represent a condition of maximum vasodilation biologically fixed by the rigid collagen fibres in the tunica adventitia [8]. Further increases in ICP caused a vigorous Cushing response as reflected by reductions in HR and increases in MAP (MAP increasing by >30 mmHg in 13 out of 27 rabbits). However, in contrast to our hypothesis, this hypertensive response was also present with moderate ICP increases (in 12 out of 27 individuals, the hypertensive response was observed with increases of ICP of less than 25 mmHg). This relatively 'early' increase in ICP may indicate that the ICP-induced increases in MAP play a protective role in maintaining perfusion rather than merely signifying irreversible neurological damage. In support of this finding, a similar increase MAP in humans has been observed at even moderate ICP during lumbar CSF infusion studies [9].

Using in vivo global and cortical CBF measurement during dynamic changes in ICP, we demonstrated that cortical blood flow decreased even with moderate increases in ICP, whereas global flow (basilar artery flow velocity) was well maintained until higher levels of ICP (Table 1). A potential explanation for the vulnerability of cortical compared to global CBF could be regional variation in vessel anatomy and compliance or could lie in a differential vascular reactivity of cortical compared with non-cortical brain.

In support of a topographic difference in cerebral vascular reactivity, Horsefield et al. [10] demonstrated using magnetic resonance imaging an intrinsic difference in the autoregulatory efficiency of the grey matter compared to white matter of healthy humans in response to a transient decrease in CPP. Furthermore, in a group of severe TBI patients, Zweifel et al. [11] found there was a higher correlation between CPP and LDF than between CPP and middle cerebral artery Fv. Such cortical sensitivity to high ICP could be a mechanism for diverting blood flow to areas of the brain most crucial for survival: the brainstem nuclei.

Limitations

The current results reflect the cerebral haemodynamic response to raising ICP through the addition of CSF volume. Thus, the observed haemodynamic response may differ somewhat to those observed clinically in the injured, oedematous brain where changes in volume of the intracranial blood, CSF or parenchymal compartments are all common. The current study represents a retrospective analysis and, therefore, some specific details of the surgical procedures (such as the functional integrity of the arterial baroreceptors) cannot be assessed. Application of cortical LDF during an infusion of fluid into the subarachnoid space raises the possibility of LDF probe displacement by the infusion. Finally, bilateral ligation of the common carotid could affect cerebral haemodynamics per se. However, this technique ensured that flow velocity measured at the basilar artery represented a global cerebral perfusion and thus provided a well-controlled model to address our proposed questions.

Conclusions

Decreased vascular wall tension and increased MAP act to protect cerebral perfusion from increases in ICP; however, the relative importance of these mechanisms depends on the prevailing ICP. Furthermore, reductions in cortical blood flow due to increases in ICP may not be detected by global measures of perfusion. Multimodal monitoring including global and local techniques may enhance personalised clinical management in neurocritical disease.

Financial Support for This Project No specific funding for this study.

Conflicts of interest statement ICM+ software (Cambridge Enterprise, Cambridge, UK, http://www.neurosurg.cam.ac.uk/icmplus/) is a multimodal data acquisition and analysis software licensed by the University of Cambridge, Cambridge Enterprise Ltd. P.S. and M.C. have a financial interest in part of the licensing fee. The remaining authors declare no relevant competing financial interests.

References

1. Donnelly J, Budohoski KP, Smielewski P, Czosnyka M. Regulation of the cerebral circulation: bedside assessment and clinical implications. Crit Care. 2016;20:129.
2. Miller JD, Stanek A, Langfitt TW. Concepts of cerebral perfusion pressure and vascular compression during intracranial hypertension. Prog Brain Res. 1972;35:411–32.
3. Lassen N. Cerebral blood flow and oxygen consumption in man. Physiol Rev. 1959;39:183–238.
4. Donnelly J, Czosnyka M, Harland S, Varsos GV, Cardim D, Robba C, Liu X, Ainslie PN, Smielewski P. Cerebral haemodynamics during experimental intracranial hypertension. J Cereb Blood Flow Metab. 2017;37(2):694–705. https://doi.org/10.1177/0271678X16639060.
5. Harland S, Richards HK, Czosnyka M, Piechnik SK, Pickard JD. Dissociation of cerebral autoregulation and CO2 reactivity following carotid occlusion in rabbits. J Cereb Blood Flow Metab. 1999;19:S636.
6. Robba C, Donnelly J, Bertuetti R, Cardim D, Sekhon MS, Aries M, Smielewski P, Richards H, Czosnyka M. Doppler non-invasive monitoring of ICP in an animal model of acute intracranial hypertension. Neurocrit Care. 2015;23:419–26.
7. Varsos GV, Richards H, Kasprowicz M, Budohoski KP, Brady KM, Reinhard M, Avolio A, Smielewski P, Pickard JD, Czosnyka M. Critical closing pressure determined with a model of cerebrovascular impedance. J Cereb Blood Flow Metab. 2013;33:235–43.
8. Dewey RC, Pieper HP, Hunt WE. Experimental cerebral hemodynamics. Vasomotor tone, critical closing pressure, and vascular bed resistance. J Neurosurg. 1974;41:597–606.
9. Varsos GV, Czosnyka M, Smielewski P, Garnett MR, Liu X, Kim D-J, Donnelly J, Adams H, Pickard JD, Czosnyka Z. Cerebral critical closing pressure in hydrocephalus patients undertaking infusion tests. Neurol Res. 2015;37(8):674–82.
10. Horsfield MA, Jara JL, Saeed NP, Panerai RB, Robinson TG. Regional differences in dynamic cerebral autoregulation in the healthy brain assessed by magnetic resonance imaging. PLoS One. 2013;8:e62588.
11. Zweifel C, Czosnyka M, Lavinio A, Castellani G, Kim D-J, Carrera E, Pickard JD, Kirkpatrick PJ, Smielewski P. A comparison study of cerebral autoregulation assessed with transcranial Doppler and cortical laser Doppler flowmetry. Neurol Res. 2010;32:425–8.

What Determines Outcome in Patients That Suffer Raised Intracranial Pressure After Traumatic Brain Injury?

Samuel Patrick Klein and Bart Depreitere

Abstract *Introduction*: Episodes of raised intracranial pressure (ICP) after traumatic brain injury (TBI) are responsible for the majority of secondary brain injury events and thereby strongly affect long-term outcome. However, not all patients with major episodes of raised ICP suffer a poor outcome. The aim of the current analysis was to identify variables contributing to good outcome in patients suffering episodes of high ICP.

Methods: Retrospective analysis of 20 severe TBI patients admitted to the University Hospitals Leuven between 2010 and 2014. All patients had at least one episode of ICP > 30 mmHg for more than 3 min in succession. Outcome was assessed by the extended Glasgow Outcome Scale at 6 months. Partial least squares (PLS) regression was used to derive factors determining outcome. Pressure reactivity index (PRx) was calculated as an index for cerebrovascular autoregulation capacity.

Results: Both outcome groups did not differ for age, Glasgow Coma Score, pupil reactivity, computed tomography Marshall classification, glycaemia, haemoglobin and CRASH and IMPACT scores on admission. Significant differences were found for mean ICP, number of episodes of ICP > 30 mmHg, number and duration of longest PRx episodes. The number of episodes of ICP > 30 mmHg correlated significantly with the number and duration of longest PRx episodes. PLS regression indicates that episodes of impaired autoregulation contributed equally to explaining outcome compared to episodes of raised ICP.

Conclusions: Prolonged episodes of disturbed dynamic cerebral autoregulation contribute to detrimental outcome in patients with increased ICP. Autoregulation seems to have an important protective role in tolerating episodes of raised ICP.

Keywords Intracranial pressure · Outcome · Autoregulation Traumatic brain injury

Introduction

Traumatic brain injury (TBI) can lead to increased intracranial pressure (ICP) as a result of systemic and intracranial events [1]. Raised ICP is associated with poor outcome [2]. However, not all patients with major episodes of raised ICP suffer a poor outcome. CRASH and IMPACT prognostic models have determined baseline predictors for unfavourable outcome such as age, Glasgow Coma Scale score, pupil reactivity, computed tomography abnormalities, haemoglobin and glycaemia, for example [3, 4]. Intact cerebrovascular autoregulation could protect patients suffering raised ICP, maintaining a constant cerebral blood flow despite lower cerebral perfusion pressures (CPPs). The pressure reactivity index (PRx) is considered to be a measure of continuous autoregulation by quantifying the relationship between slow fluctuations in mean arterial blood pressure and ICP [5]. PRx has been shown to be a predictor of clinical outcome [5, 6]. There is evidence that patients with intact cerebrovascular autoregulation benefit more from CPP-oriented therapy, tolerating higher ICPs, and patients with impaired autoregulation benefit more from ICP-lowering therapy [6]. The aim of this analysis is to identify which variables contribute to good outcome in patients suffering episodes of high ICP.

Methods

A retrospective analysis of patients with severe TBI admitted to the University Hospitals Leuven between 2010 and 2014 was performed. Patients with invasive parenchymal ICP monitoring (Codman ICP MicroSensor; Codman & Shurtleff, Raynham, MA, USA) and at least one episode of

S.P. Klein, M.D. (✉) • B. Depreitere, M.D., Ph.D.
Department of Neurosurgery, University Hospitals Leuven, Leuven, Belgium
e-mail: sam.klein@kuleuven.be

ICP >30 mmHg for more than 3 min in succession were included. ICM+ software (Cambridge Enterprise, University of Cambridge, UK) was used for data capture. Outcome was assessed using the extended Glasgow Outcome Scale (GOSE) at 6 months. For bivariate analysis, GOSE was divided in two groups: poor (GOSE 1–4) and good (GOSE 5–8) outcome. Age, Glasgow Coma Scale (GCS), pupillary response, Marshall CT classification, haemoglobin level and glycaemia on admission were determined. CRASH and IMPACT prognostic models were used to calculate the risk of unfavourable outcome at 6 months. For bivariate analysis, differences were compared using a two-tailed Mann-Whitney U test. Dynamic autoregulation was assessed by calculation of the PRx. PRx was calculated as moving Pearson correlation coefficients, using 300-s time windows, between 10-s averages of arterial blood pressure (ABP) and ICP signals. The number of events for ICP and PRx above different thresholds was defined per patient with a duration of 1 min per event. For optimal CPP (CPPopt) calculation, we applied Steiner et al.'s [7] and Aries et al.'s [8] method of plotting CPP and PRx, and fitting a U-shaped curve, with the most negative values of the autoregulation index indicating a 5-mmHg range of optimal CPP from a moving 4-h time window. Statistical analysis was performed using statistical software SPSS 20 (IBM, Armonk, NY, USA) and SmartPLS 3 software (C. M. Ringle, S. Wende, J.-M. Becker, 2015; SmartPLS, Bönningstedt, Germany. Retrieved from http://www.smartpls.com).

Results

Twenty patients were included in the study: 6 female and 14 male. In the good-outcome group, four patients were female and eight male. In the bad-outcome group, two were female and six were male. Table 1 describes the variables analysed and dichotomised for outcome. Significant differences between dichotomised good- and bad-outcome groups were found for mean ICP, number of ICP > 30 mmHg episodes, and number and duration of longest PRx episodes above different thresholds

Table 1 Overview of variables dichotomised for outcome

Variable		Good outcome	Bad outcome	Sign
Age (years)	Mean/median	36/34	57/60	0.27
GCS	Mean/median	8.3/7	10.6/11	0.31
CT Marshall	Mean/median	III/II	III/II	0.80
Glycaemia (mmol/L)	Mean/median	9.8/8.9	8.3/8.3	0.52
Haemoglobin (g/dL)	Mean/median	12.8/13.6	14.2/13.8	0.37
IMPACT 6 months unfavourable outcome (%)	Mean/median	37.8/34	44/40	0.18
CRASH 6 months unfavourable outcome (%)	Mean/median	48.2/45.4	31.2/25.2	0.35
ICP > 30 mmHg number of events (min)	Mean/median	45.9/39	465.2/59	0.05
ICP > 30 mmHg duration longest event (min)	Mean/median	12.4/13	143.6/13	0.20
Mean ICP (mmHg)	Mean (95% Confidence Interval)	39.6 (CI 30.9–41.9)	36.4 (CI 31.9–47.3)	0.03
Mean PRx during ICP > 30 mmHg	Mean (95% Confidence Interval)	0.15 (CI −0.03 to 0.32)	0.32 (CI 0.05–0.6)	0.15
Mean CPP during ICP > 30 mmHg	Mean (95% Confidence Interval)	56.3 (CI 49.9–62.7)	59.3 (CI 46.6–72.0)	0.47
CPPopt mean (mmHg)	Mean (95% Confidence Interval)	73.3 (CI 66.2–80.4)	74.7 (CI 63.0–86.4)	0.80
CPP–CPPopt (mmHg)	Mean (95% Confidence Interval)	−17 (CI −24.6 to −9.4)	−15.4 (CI −19.9 to −10.9)	0.68
PRx > 0.3 number of events	Mean/median	16.6/16	158.4/30	0.03
PRx > 0.3 longest event	Mean/median	6.9/5	15.2/9	0.03
PRx > 0.5 number of events	Mean/median	11.2/8	74.4/29	0.02
PRx > 0.5 longest event	Mean/median	5.5/4	13/9	0.02
PRx > 0.7 number of events	Mean/median	6.8/5	28.6/24	0.01
PRx > 0.7 longest event	Mean/median	2.9/3	9.8/6	0.01
GOSE	Median	7	2	<0.001

Table 2 Spearman's Rho correlation coefficients (p values)

Variable	ICP mean during ICP > 30 mmHg	ICP > 30 number of events during ICP > 30 mmHg	ICP > 30 longest event during ICP > 30 mmHg
PRx mean during ICP > 30 mmHg	0.22 (0.35)	−0.01 (0.96)	0.06 (0.79)
PR > 0.3 number of events during ICP > 30 mmHg	0.42 (0.07)	0.80 (<0.001)	0.71 (<0.001)
PR > 0.3 longest event during ICP > 30 mmHg	0.35 (0.13)	0.66 (<0.001)	0.55 (<0.001)
PR > 0.5 number of events during ICP > 30 mmHg	0.41 (0.07)	0.76 (<0.001)	0.66 (<0.001)
PR > 0.5 longest event during ICP > 30 mmHg	0.25 (0.29)	0.58 (0.01)	0.52 (0.02)
PR > 0.7 number of events during ICP > 30 mmHg	0.41 (0.07)	0.71 (<0.001)	0.57 (0.01)
PR > 0.7 longest event during ICP > 30 mmHg	0.28 (0.22)	0.46 (0.04)	0.41 (0.07)

of 0.3, 0.5 and 0.7. The number and duration of ICP > 30 mmHg episodes correlated significantly with the number and duration of longest PRx episodes above our defined thresholds (Table 2). Due to multicollinearity of the independent variables (correlation of predictors), partial least squares (PLS) regression was performed. Validity for outer loadings was defined using a threshold of >0.7; overall construct validity was good with a Cronbach's alpha value of 0.96 (SD, 0.02). Mean ICP and mean PRx during ICP > 30 mmHg episodes did not reach the predefined validity threshold. Average variance extracted (AVE) by the variables was 0.76 (SD, 0.11). Adjusted model R^2 was 0.31 (SD, 0.16; p = 0.052). PLS regression outer loadings are described in Table 3.

Discussion

This exploratory study investigating factors determining outcome in patients suffering raised episodes of ICP suggests a possible protective role of cerebral autoregulation. Impaired autoregulation was correlated with episodes of raised ICP, and this finding is in agreement with the results of an experimental animal study in piglets by Pesek et al. [9]. Piglets with acute episodes of raised ICP demonstrated loss of autoregulation. Although we found a correlation between impaired autoregulation and episodes of raised ICP, the correlation was not perfect, suggesting autoregulation was not impaired during every episode of raised ICP. The results of our PLS regression indicate that episodes of impaired autoregulation contributed equally to explaining outcome as episodes of raised ICP itself. The number and duration of ICP and impaired autoregulation events were more determining for outcome than mean values of ICP and PRx. This study is limited by the sample size and the exploratory nature of the study, possibly limiting generalisability. The problem of multicollinearity among our variables was present with a moderate-to-high correlation between ICP and impaired autoregulation events. This problem was approached using PLS regression, reducing the effects of multicollinearity but not eliminating them [10].

Table 3 Outer loadings for PLS regression model

Variable	Outer loading	T value	p value
ICP mean during ICP > 30 mmHg	0.64	3.0	0.003
ICP > 30 number of events during ICP > 30 mmHg	0.82	4.2	<0.001
ICP > 30 longest event during ICP > 30 mmHg	0.96	4.8	<0.001
PRx mean during ICP > 30 mmHg	0.57	3.2	<0.001
PR > 0.3 number of events during ICP > 30 mmHg	0.93	5.3	<0.001
PR > 0.3 longest event during ICP > 30 mmHg	0.96	8.1	<0.001
PR > 0.5 number of events during ICP > 30 mmHg	0.93	6.1	<0.001
PR > 0.5 longest event during ICP > 30 mmHg	0.93	9.5	<0.001
PR > 0.7 number of events during ICP > 30 mmHg	0.93	10.1	<0.001
PR > 0.7 longest event during ICP > 30 mmHg	0.96	9.6	<0.001

Conclusions

Prolonged episodes of disturbed dynamic cerebral autoregulation contribute to detrimental outcome in patients with increased ICP. Autoregulation seems to have an important protective role in tolerating episodes of raised ICP.

Conflicts of interest statement We declare that we have no conflict of interest.

References

1. Stocchetti N, AIR M. Traumatic intracranial hypertension. N Engl J Med. 2014;370:2121–30. Available from: http://www.ncbi.nlm.nih.gov/pubmed/24869722.
2. Güiza F, Depreitere B, Piper I, Citerio G, Chambers I, Jones PA, et al. Visualizing the pressure and time burden of intracranial hypertension in adult and paediatric traumatic brain injury. Intensive Care Med. 2015;41(6):1067–76. Available from: http://link.springer.com/10.1007/s00134-015-3806-1.
3. MRC CRASH Trial Collaborators, Perel P, Arango M, Clayton T, Edwards P, Komolafe E, et al. Predicting outcome after traumatic

brain injury: practical prognostic models based on large cohort of international patients. BMJ. 2008;336:425–9.
4. Steyerberg EW, Mushkudiani N, Perel P, Butcher I, Lu J, McHugh GS, et al. Predicting outcome after traumatic brain injury: development and international validation of prognostic scores based on admission characteristics. PLoS Med. 2008;5:1251–61.
5. Czosnyka M, Smielewski P, Kirkpatrick P, Laing RJ, Menon D, Pickard JD. Continuous assessment of the cerebral vasomotor reactivity in head injury. Neurosurgery. 1997;41:11–7. discussion 17–9. Available from: http://www.ncbi.nlm.nih.gov/pubmed/9218290.
6. Howells T, Elf K, Jones PA, Ronne-Engström E, Piper I, Nilsson P, et al. Pressure reactivity as a guide in the treatment of cerebral perfusion pressure in patients with brain trauma. J Neurosurg. 2005;102:311–7.
7. Steiner LA, Czosnyka M, Piechnik SK, et al. Continuous monitoring of cerebrovascular pressure reactivity allows determination of optimal cerebral perfusion pressure in patients with traumatic brain injury. Crit Care Med. 2002;30:733–8. Available from: http://www.ncbi.nlm.nih.gov/pubmed/11940737.
8. Aries MJH, Czosnyka M, Budohoski KP, Steiner LA, Lavinio A, Kolias AG, et al. Continuous determination of optimal cerebral perfusion pressure in traumatic brain injury. Crit Care Med. 2012;40:2456–63.
9. Pesek M, Kibler K, Easley RB, Mytar J, Rhee C, Andropoulos D, et al. The upper limit of cerebral blood flow autoregulation is decreased with elevations in intracranial pressure. Neurosurgery. 2014;75:163–9.
10. Gustafsson A, Johnson MD. Determining attribute importance in a service satisfaction model. J Serv Res. 2004;7:124–41.

Visualisation of the 'Optimal Cerebral Perfusion' Landscape in Severe Traumatic Brain Injury Patients

Ari Ercole, Peter Smielewski, Marcel J.H. Aries, Robin Wesselink, Jan Willem J. Elting, Joseph Donnelly, Marek Czosnyka, and Natasha M. Maurits

Abstract *Objective*: An 'optimal' cerebral perfusion pressure (CPPopt) can be defined as the point on the CPP scale corresponding to the greatest autoregulatory capacity. This can be established by examining the pressure reactivity index PRx–CPP relationship, which is approximately U-shaped but suffers from noise and missing data. In this paper, we present a method for plotting the whole PRx-CPP relationship curve against time in the form of a colour-coded map depicting the 'landscape' of that relationship extending back for several hours and to display this robustly at the bedside.

This is a short version of a full paper recently published in Critical Care Medicine (2016) containing some new insights and details of a novel bedside implementation based on a presentation during Intracranial Pressure 2016 Symposium in Boston.

Methods: Recordings from routine monitoring of traumatic brain injury patients were processed using ICM+. Time-averaged means for arterial blood pressure, intracranial pressure, cerebral perfusion pressure (CPP) and pressure reactivity index (PRx) were calculated and stored with time resolution of 1 min. ICM+ functions have been extended to include not just an algorithm of automatic calculation of CPPopt but also the 'CPPopt landscape' chart.

Results: Examining the 'CPPopt landscape' allows the clinician to differentiate periods where the autoregulatory range is narrow and needs to be targeted from periods when the patient is generally haemodynamically stable, allowing for more relaxed CPP management. This information would not have been conveyed using the original visualisation approaches.

Conclusions: We describe here a natural extension to the concept of autoregulatory assessment, providing the retrospective 'landscape' of the PRx-CPP relationship extending over the past several hours. We have incorporated such visualisation techniques online in ICM+. The proposed visualisation may facilitate clinical evaluation and use of autoregulation-guided therapy.

Keywords Cerebral perfusion pressure · Pressure reactivity PRx · Traumatic brain injury · Optimal CPP

Introduction

'Optimal cerebral perfusion pressure' (CPPopt) has been defined as a pressure value corresponding to the point on the CPP autoregulation characteristic where the autoregulation [as measured by the pressure reactivity index (PRx)] is the strongest [1]. The concept of using CPPopt as an individual target in treating patients with severe brain injury has recently attracted a lot of attention, particularly after the introduction of a continuous measure of CPPopt [2]. However, a single CPPopt value does not fully reflect the character of the PRx-CPP relationship, nor does it capture

A. Ercole, M.B., B.Chir., Ph.D. (✉)
Division of Anaesthesia, Addenbrooke's Hospital, University of Cambridge, Cambridge, UK
e-mail: ae105@cam.ac.uk

P. Smielewski, Ph.D. • J. Donnelly, M.B.Ch.B.
M. Czosnyka, Ph.D.
Brain Physics Group, Department of Clinical Neurosciences, Addenbrooke's Hospital, University of Cambridge, Cambridge, UK

M.J.H. Aries, M.D., Ph.D.
Brain Physics Group, Department of Clinical Neurosciences, Addenbrooke's Hospital, University of Cambridge, Cambridge, UK

Department of Intensive Care, University Medical Centre Groningen, University of Groningen, Groningen, The Netherlands

R. Wesselink, M.B.Ch.B.
Department of Intensive Care, University Medical Centre Groningen, University of Groningen, Groningen, The Netherlands

Department of Technical Medicine, University of Twente, Enschede, The Netherlands

J.W.J. Elting, M.D., Ph.D. • N.M. Maurits, Ph.D.
Department of Neurology, University Medical Centre Groningen, University of Groningen, Groningen, The Netherlands

its dynamic nature, even when plotted as a trend over time. What is more, the CPPopt trends tend to be noisy and may often contain many gaps where the PRx-CPP curves cannot be robustly determined. This represents a barrier to evaluating autoregulation-guided CPP therapy in clinical practice. The objective of this project was to find a way of improving the CPPopt methodology by introducing a new visualisation method that may provide insight into the complete characteristics of the CPP-PRx relationship and its temporal evolution. We have demonstrated that this can be presented at the bedside in real time.

Material and Methods

Monitoring data from patients with severe traumatic brain injury (TBI) admitted to the neurocritical care unit at Addenbrooke's Hospital, Cambridge, were collected using ICM+ software. Patients were managed according to published protocolised TBI guidelines [3]. Patients were sedated, intubated and ventilated. Interventions were aimed at keeping ICP <20 mmHg and CPP >55 mmHg. CPPopt-guided therapy did not form part of the local management algorithm.

Arterial blood pressure (ABP) was monitored invasively using a pressure monitoring kit (Baxter Healthcare, Westlake Village, CA, USA; Sidcup, UK) in the radial artery and zeroed at the level of the heart. An intraparenchymal probe (Codman & Shurtleff, Raynham, MA, USA or Camino Laboratories, San Diego, CA, USA) was used in order to monitor intracranial pressure (ICP). Digital ABP and ICP waveforms were collected from GE Solar monitors at their full available resolution of 120 Hz using ICM+® software (Cambridge Enterprise, Cambridge, UK; http://www.neurosurg.cam.ac.uk/icmplus/). Patient monitoring was approved by the local Ethics Committee (REC97/291) and informed consent was not required for the re-processing of anonymous data. All the analyses on the recorded raw waveforms were performed over 60-s sliding windows using the same software.

Time-averaged means for ABP, ICP, CPP (ABP minus ICP), and PRx (a running correlation coefficient between 10-s averages of ABP and ICP signals) were calculated and stored with time resolution of 1 min. PRx-CPP curves and the corresponding CPPopt values were calculated every minute, with a calculation data buffer of 4 h. The sequential PRx-CPP curves were then used to create a colour-coded map of PRx-CPP relationship evolution over time (Fig. 1). The time (horizontal) axis represents the position of the moving window for CPPopt calculation, the vertical axis represents the scale of CPP, while PRx values are coded, with red representing completely impaired autoregulation

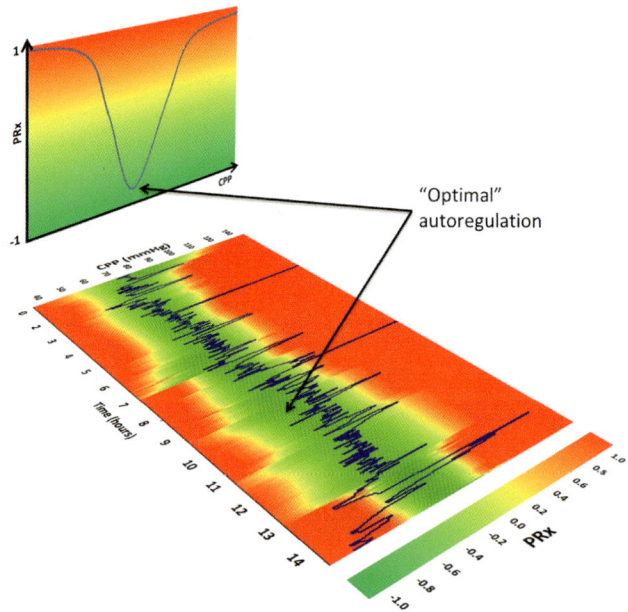

Fig. 1 The concept of CPPopt landscape. The vertical PRx-CPP colour gradient represents the colour-mapping scheme for PRx values. The *blue line* drawn on that colour map denotes the trajectory of the CPPopt curve fitted at that time point, and is coded in the PRx-CPP landscape map (*horizontal*), according to the colours it covers in the colour gradient (*vertical*)

(PRx = 1), green representing fully engaged autoregulation (PRx = −1), with the failing autoregulation zone of PRx 0.1–0.3 coded as yellow. The coding was adapted from the original colour-coding scheme of PRx that has been used in ICM+ for the past decade. The CPPopt landscape chart was fully implemented in ICM+ for bedside display alongside traditional plots of ICP, CPP and PRx.

Results

The new CPPopt visualisation method seems to highlight features that would not have been apparent using the traditional approach. Figure 2 shows an example of recording taken from one patient, with ICP, ABP, CPP, PRx trends plotted together with the CPPopt landscape chart at the bottom. The *light-green* homogeneous areas denote periods where CPPopt calculations were unavailable. The *blue line* represents the trend of CPP values. For clarity, the CPPopt trend was not plotted as it is indicated in the chart anyway by the midpoint of the *green/yellow zone*. By observing the extent of the *green zone*, one can assess the autoregulatory range at any given point of time, while the saturation level of the *green* colour in the centre of that range gives a feedback on the strength of autoregulation there. In the presented example, the patient started off with a relatively wide autoregulatory range centred at about 65 mmHg, and then went through

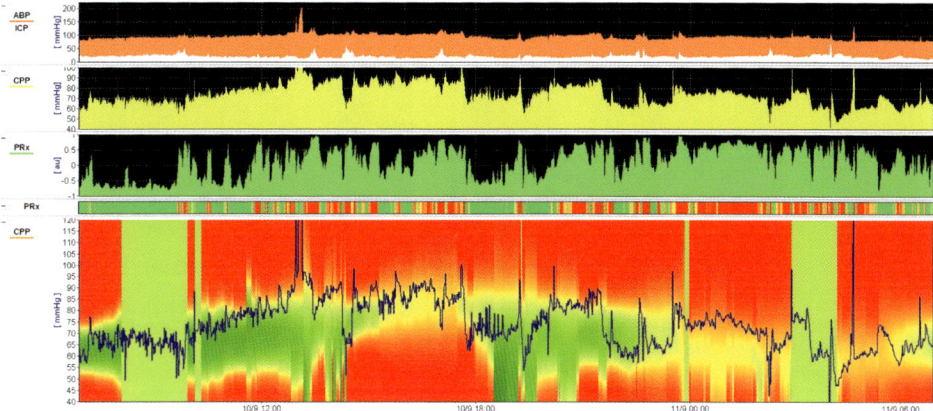

Fig. 2 Example of a recording, available at the bedside, showing the CPPopt landscape alongside the trends of ABP, ICP, CPP and PRx

a phase when that range has substantially narrowed and shifted towards higher CPP values.

Discussion

Individualising targets for management of TBI patients is currently at the forefront of new management policy making efforts in neurocritical care. Whilst the CPPopt concept is still to be prospectively evaluated, it is physiologically attractive. A necessary future evaluation and implementation is impossible, however, unless the data can be presented in a format that is sufficiently robust that the clinician can reliably interpret them at the bedside. Continuous monitoring of cerebral autoregulation using real-time analysis of waveforms of ABP and ICP, via the PRx, has made it possible to relate its dynamically changing state to the corresponding value of cerebral perfusion pressure, thus revealing a relationship between the two. Furthermore, the character of that relationship, which is generally U-shaped, is well suited for using it as the means of arriving at a value of CPP that maximises the autoregulatory capacity (i.e. minimising PRx). However, due to limited spontaneous CPP variability, the errors inherent in the assessment of autoregulation using PRx and other external factors, that relationship is often unclear. This may make the trend of calculated CPPopt values appear noisy, with numerous gaps where the curve was undeterminable. Moreover, efforts to make the automatic calculations of CPPopt more stable and with higher yield of valid values that are currently under way may go a long way in inspiring confidence in this approach, but they still fail to deliver a complete picture of the autoregulatory capacity. This is of particular importance in severe brain trauma management, where the pathological processes often develop rapidly, making cerebral autoregulation a rather fragile defence mechanism. It is not uncommon for the cerebral autoregulation curve to be temporarily shifted towards higher cerebral perfusion pressures or for the autoregulatory plateau to be severely shortened or abolished altogether in a state of total vasoplegia. Additionally, contemporary management of brain trauma patients is multifaceted, requiring constant adjustments of treatment to provide a delicate balance between different target priorities. Incorporating a rigid, even individualised, target for CPP management may not therefore be the best or safest approach of using this promising CPPopt methodology.

On the other hand, giving the clinician an opportunity to examine the whole 'CPPopt landscape' allows one not only to assess the CPPopt trend but also the breadth of the autoregulatory range and its progression over time. Such an approach would allow differentiation of periods where the autoregulatory range is narrow, making careful control important, from periods when the patient is generally cerebrovascularly stable, allowing for more relaxed CPP management and thus prioritising other needs. This information would not have been conveyed using the original visualisation approaches; the trend is for automatically calculated CPPopt or a single optimal CPP curve chart. One could argue that a set of charts showing the optimal CPP, the value of PRx at the optimal CPP point and the CPP range corresponding to intact autoregulation would be sufficient, and perhaps easier to read. Whether or not this is true will have to be investigated further but intuitively the colour-coded, two-dimensional representation of the CPP-PRx relationship contains a lot more information in a relatively simple, compact form and thus may perhaps appeal to clinicians more than a multitude of related charts.

Clearly, this new approach to the CPPopt concept still needs to undergo a more thorough scrutiny, but perhaps a combination of the landscape chart and the more traditional CPPopt trend—possibly with improved automatic calculation algorithms—may provide the ultimate robust, comprehensive and easily digestible information on the patient's dynamically changing state of cerebral autoregulation and offer clearer suggestions for individualised cerebral perfusion pressure targets.

Conclusions

What we describe here is an extension of the concept of autoregulatory assessment, providing the full retrospective 'landscape' of PRx-CPP relationship extending over the past several hours in such a way that it can be presented at the bedside. Although further technical improvements and a test of functionality are needed, the proposed visualisation, while addressing some of the problems of the CPPopt methodology, may improve individual CPP management methods based on the status of cerebral autoregulation, current and past.

Acknowledgements The authors wish to express gratitude to the staff of Neurocritical Care Unit, Addenbrooke's Hospital, Cambridge, UK, for their help and support with the ICM+ brain monitoring project.

Disclosure: ICM+® is a software licensed by Cambridge Enterprise Ltd., Cambridge, UK; P.S. and M.C. have financial interest in a part of the licensing fee.

Conflicts of interest statement We declare that we have no conflict of interest.

References

1. Steiner LA, Czosnyka M, Piechnik SK, Smielewski P, Chatfield D, Menon DK, Pickard JD. Continuous monitoring of cerebrovascular pressure reactivity allows determination of optimal cerebral perfusion pressure in patients with traumatic brain injury. Crit Care Med. 2002;30(4):733–8.
2. Aries MJ, Czosnyka M, Budohoski KP, Steiner LA, Lavinio A, Kolias AG, Hutchinson PJ, Brady KM, Menon DK, Pickard JD, Smielewski P. Continuous determination of optimal cerebral perfusion pressure in traumatic brain injury. Crit Care Med. 2012;40(8):2456–63.
3. Menon DK. Cerebral protection in severe brain injury: physiological determinants of outcome and their optimisation. Br Med Bull. 1999;55(1):226–58.

Is There a Relationship Between Optimal Cerebral Perfusion Pressure-Guided Management and PaO$_2$/FiO$_2$ Ratio After Severe Traumatic Brain Injury?

M. Moreira, D. Fernandes, E. Pereira, E. Monteiro, R. Pascoa, and C. Dias

Abstract *Objective*: Severe traumatic brain injury (TBI) management has been associated with adult respiratory distress syndrome (ARDS) in previous literature. We aimed to investigate the relationships between optimal CPP-guided management, ventilation parameters over time and outcome after severe TBI.

Materials and methods: We performed retrospective analysis of recorded data from 38 patients admitted to the NCCU after severe TBI, managed with optimal cerebral perfusion pressure (CPPopt)-guided therapy, calculated using pressure reactivity index (PRx). All patients were sedated and ventilated with lung protective criteria (Peep > 5, tidal volume 6–8 ml/kg and airway pressure < 30 cmH$_2$O).

Results: Daily mean CPPopt varied between a minimum of 84 mmHg and a maximum of 91 mmHg with an all period mean value of 88 mmHg. The mean value for the difference between CPP and CPPopt was −1.9 mmHg. Daily mean P/F ratio decreased and varied between 253 and 387 with an all-period mean of 294 mmHg. During the 10 days of recording data, five patients (13%) developed criteria of severe ARDS, but only two patients died due to severe ARDS (5%). PaO$_2$/FiO$_2$ (P/F) ratio did not correlate with CPPopt, but showed a strong correlation with tidal volume ($p = 0.000$) and driving pressure ($p = 0.000$).

Conclusions: Although CPPopt-guided therapy may induce a decrease in P/F ratio over time during the first 10 days, we could not find an association with worst outcome, which may be influenced by lung protective ventilation strategies and preservation of cerebral autoregulation.

Keywords Traumatic brain injury · ARDS · Pressure reactivity index · Optimal cerebral perfusion pressure · Driving pressure

M. Moreira • D. Fernandes • E. Pereira • E. Monteiro • C. Dias (✉)
Neurocritical Care Unit, Centro Hospitalar São João,
Porto, Portugal
e-mail: celeste.dias@med.up.pt

R. Pascoa
LAQV/REQUIMTE, Faculty of Pharmacy, University of Porto,
Porto, Portugal

Introduction

The management of cerebral perfusion pressure (CPP) after traumatic brain injury (TBI) is still one of the most controversial topics of neurocritical care [1]. Pulmonary oedema and severe adult respiratory distress syndrome (ARDS) [2] have been reported as independently associated with a higher risk of death in patients with severe TBI [3–6]. Amongst other causes, several authors showed that high cerebral perfusion pressure (CPP) reduced the incidence of secondary ischaemic events to the brain, but increased the incidence of ARDS and global worse outcome [3–5, 7]. The management of patients with ARDS comprises fluid restriction, lung-protective ventilation strategies with high positive end-expiratory pressure (Peep) and permissive hypercapnia [8, 9], which may raise the intracranial pressure (ICP) and decrease CPP. Currently, insufficient data support a level I or IIA recommendation on CPP thresholds for patients with severe TBI [10]. CPP values higher than 70 mmHg were associated with elevated risk for respiratory complications and worse outcome, whereas values of CPP less than 60 mmHg were associated with cerebral ischaemia and hypoxia [11–13]. Moreover, it has been suggested that CPP tailored to individual patients, based on evaluation of autoregulation, is related to favourable outcome [14–17]. The pressure reactivity index (PRx) is a reliable method to continuously evaluate autoregulation at the bedside [18, 19] and to estimate optimal CPP (CPPopt). The aim of this study was to investigate the relationships between CPPopt-guided therapy and ventilation parameters during management of severe TBI.

Methods

Retrospective analysis of recorded data from 38 patients admitted to the Neurocritical Care Unit (NCCU) at Hospital São João, Porto, Portugal, after severe TBI managed with CPPopt-guided therapy, calculated using PRx.

Exclusion criteria included age less than 18 years old and pregnancy. The local research ethics committee approved the protocol and anonymised data collection, and written informed consent was obtained.

The patients were managed according to the Neurocritical Care Unit management protocol previously published [15]. Brain monitoring data (ICP, CPP, CPPopt and PRx), blood gas analysis and respiratory data [PaO_2/FiO_2 (P/F) ratio, tidal volume, Peep and driving pressure] were daily collected during the first 10 days. During the period of recording data, ARDS criteria were applied according to the Berlin definition [2]. Patients were sedated and ventilated with lung protective criteria (Peep > 5, tidal volume 6–8 ml/kg and airway pressure < 30 cmH$_2$O).

The analyses were performed using commercial IBM software SPSS 20. Data were expressed as mean values and standard deviation (mean ± SD). Normal distribution was established with Shapiro–Wilk test. We used Spearman correlation analysis for mean values, and non-parametric Kruskal–Wallis test was used to investigate statistical relationships between the studied variables. Partial least squares discriminant analyses (PLS-DA) was also applied to find fundamental relations between variables. Tests were considered statistically significant for p values < 0.05.

Results

A total of 38 adult patients with TBI (34 males, 89.5%) with mean age 47.3 ± 20 years old, with local median GCS 7 (IQR 4–9) and SAPSII 43.5 ± 9.9 were analysed. Daily mean CPP and CPPopt varied respectively between a minimum of 81 mmHg, 84 mmHg and a maximum of 87 mmHg, 91 mmHg with an all-period mean value of 85 mmHg, 88 mmHg (Table 1). The mean value for the difference between CPP and CPPopt was −1.9 mmHg. Daily mean P/F ratio decreased and varied between 253 and 387 with an all-period mean of 294 mmHg (Fig. 1). According to the Berlin definition and during the 10 days of recording data, seven patients (18%) developed criteria of severe ARDS, 12 patients of moderate ARDS (32%) and 14 patients had no ARDS (37%). Hospital mortality rate was 18% but only two patients died due to severe ARDS. P/F ratio did not correlate with CPP or CPPopt (Fig. 2), but showed a strong correlation with tidal volume ($p = 0.000$) and driving pressure ($p = 0.000$). We found no correlation between CPP or CPPopt

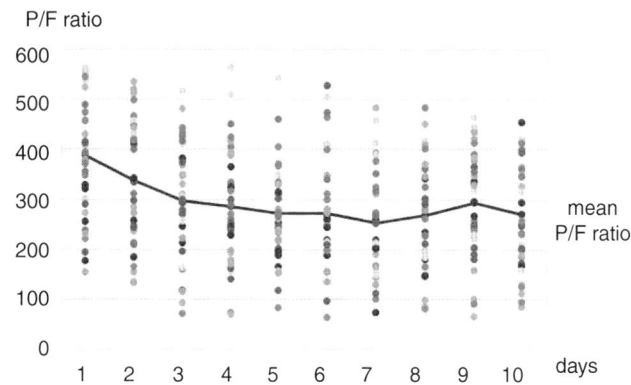

Fig. 1 P/F ratio [daily oxygen arterial pressure (PaO$_2$) and fraction of inspired oxygen (FiO$_2$) ratio] for 38 patients with severe TBI during 10 consecutive days since Neurocritical Care Unit admission

Table 1 Demographic, cerebral and pulmonary data of the 38 patients admitted to the Neurocritical Care Unit with traumatic brain injury (TBI) regarding ARDS (adult respiratory distress syndrome) classification

	No ARDS (mean ± SD)	Mild to moderate ARDS (mean ± SD)	Severe ARDS (mean ± SD)
n	14 (37%)	12 (32%)	7 (18%)
Age (anos)	48 ± 22	50 ± 20	38 ± 14
SAPS II	32 ± 17	42 ± 10	42 ± 8
GCS	8 ± 3	7 ± 3	6 ± 2
Marshall head-CT	4 ± 2	4 ± 2	3 ± 1
ICP (mmHg)	10 ± 4	12 ± 5	17 ± 5
PRx	0.06 ± 0.25	0.11 ± 0.25	0.13 ± 0.15
CPP (mmHg)	81 ± 5	80 ± 9	83 ± 6
CPPopt (mmHg)	82 ± 10	84 ± 10	86 ± 8
CPP − CPPopt (mmHg)	0.2 ± 7	−2 ± 7	−3 ± 6
P/F ratio	471 ± 88	332 ± 113	150 ± 33
Peep (cmH$_2$O)	6 ± 1	6 ± 1	6 ± 1
ΔP = Ppl − Peep (cmH$_2$O)	15 ± 3	14 ± 5	21 ± 2

SAPS II simplified acute physiology score II, *GCS* Glasgow Coma Score, *head-CT* head computed tomography, *ICP* intracranial pressure, *CPP* cerebral perfusion pressure, *CPPopt* optimal CPP, *CPP − CPPopt* difference between CPP and CPPopt, *P/F ratio* PaO$_2$/FiO$_2$ ratio, ΔP = Ppl − Peep difference between plateau pressure and end-expiratory pressure

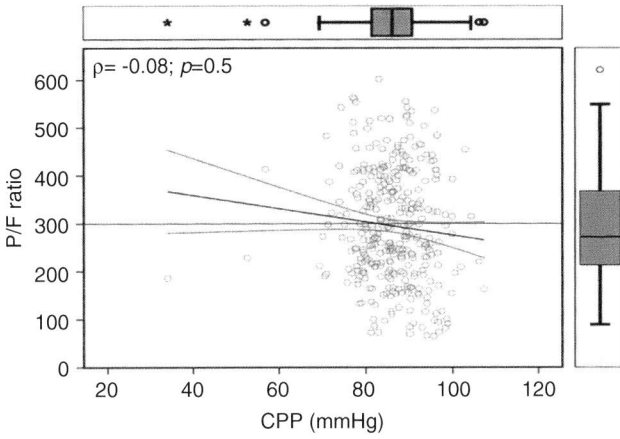

Fig. 2 Correlation between mean cerebral perfusion pressure (CPP) and mean daily P/F ratio [oxygen arterial pressure (PaO$_2$) and fraction of inspired oxygen (FiO$_2$) ratio] for 38 patients with severe TBI during 10 consecutive days and since Neurocritical Care Unit admission ($\rho = -0.08$; $p = 0.5$)

and P/F ratio, tidal volume and driving pressure for different outcomes. By applying PLS-DA model for the P/F ratio, we were able to correctly predict around 90% of the patients with a P/F ratio episode lower than 100 mmHg. The most important variables to the model were FiO$_2$ and Peep and neither CPP nor CPPopt were significantly involved.

Discussion

The desired target for TBI management is the minimum level of CPP that provides adequate blood flow for an injured brain without systemic detrimental effects, namely ARDS [20]. Recently, Aries et al. [16] demonstrated that individualised CPP by bedside evaluation of cerebrovascular reactivity index (PRx) and definition of CPPopt is feasible and seems to be associated with favourable outcome. Our TBI management protocol is autoregulation-guided (CPPopt) based on continuous evaluation of cerebrovascular reactivity (PRx) (Fig. 3). Accordingly, we aimed to study the relationship between this management protocol and the evaluation of development of ARDS. Actually, our mean CPP values are slightly higher than Brain Trauma Foundation recommendations (82 mmHg compared to 60 mmHg), even taking into consideration that patients are treated with 30° head-up elevation and CPP is continuously calculated with ABP transducer located at heart level. Although P/F ratio decreased along the 10-day observation period and seven patients developed severe ARDS, only two died due to this cause. Indeed, we could find no correlation between real CPP values and with P/F ratio, tidal volume and driving pressure for different outcomes. This may be explained by the lung protective ventilation strategy [9], associated with small difference between CPP and CPPopt that preserves cerebral

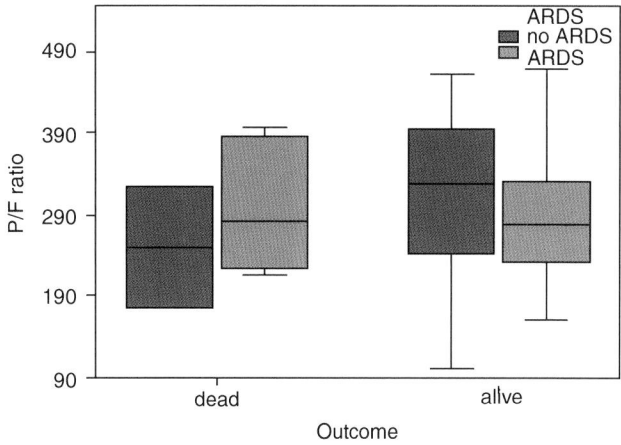
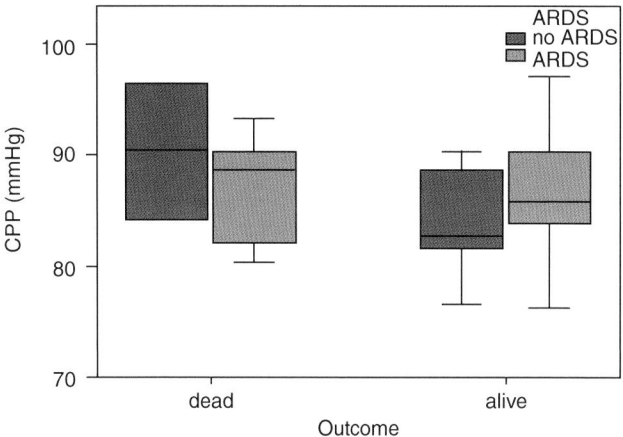

Fig. 3 Box-Plot of P/F ratio [oxygen arterial pressure (PaO$_2$) and fraction of inspired oxygen (FiO$_2$) ratio] and CPP (cerebral perfusion pressure) distributions for different outcomes (dead and alive)

blood flow and avoids overall hyperaemia. Moreover, the patients with severe ARDS had the highest difference between CPP and CPPopt (−3 ± 6 mmHg) and the highest driving pressure [21].

TBI patients managed at averaged real CPP close to CPPopt and with low pulmonary driving pressure seem to be protected from lung complications related to high CPP.

However, the small sample of patients enrolled in this study warrants further evaluation.

Conclusion

Although CPPopt-guided therapy may induce a decrease in P/F ratio over time during the first 10 days, we could not find an association with ARDS or worst outcome, which may be influenced by lung protective ventilation strategies and preservation of cerebral autoregulation.

Conflicts of interest statement We declare that we have no conflict of interest.

References

1. Robertson CS. Management of cerebral perfusion pressure after traumatic brain injury. Anesthesiology. 2001;95(6):1513–7.
2. Ferguson ND, et al. The Berlin definition of ARDS: an expanded rationale, justification, and supplementary material. Intensive Care Med. 2012;38(10):1573–82.
3. Aisiku IP, et al. The incidence of ARDS and associated mortality in severe TBI using the Berlin definition. J Trauma Acute Care Surg. 2016;80(2):308–12.
4. Contant CF, et al. Adult respiratory distress syndrome: a complication of induced hypertension after severe head injury. J Neurosurg. 2001;95(4):560–8.
5. Mackersie RC, et al. Pulmonary extravascular fluid accumulation following intracranial injury. J Trauma. 1983;23(11):968–75.
6. Mascia L, et al. Extracranial complications in patients with acute brain injury: a post-hoc analysis of the SOAP study. Intensive Care Med. 2008;34(4):720–7.
7. Hoesch RE, et al. Acute lung injury in critical neurological illness. Crit Care Med. 2012;40(2):587–93.
8. Ware LB, Matthay MA. The acute respiratory distress syndrome. N Engl J Med. 2000;342(18):1334–49.
9. Amato MB, et al. Effect of a protective-ventilation strategy on mortality in the acute respiratory distress syndrome. N Engl J Med. 1998;338(6):347–54.
10. Carney N, et al. Guidelines for the management of severe traumatic brain injury, fourth edition. Neurosurgery. 2017;80(1):6–15.
11. Robertson C, et al. Prevention of secondary ischemic insults after severe head injury. Crit Care Med. 1999;27:2086–95.
12. Allen BB, et al. Age-specific cerebral perfusion pressure thresholds and survival in children and adolescents with severe traumatic brain injury. Pediatr Crit Care Med. 2014;15(1):62–70.
13. Chang JJ, et al. Physiologic and functional outcome correlates of brain tissue hypoxia in traumatic brain injury. Crit Care Med. 2009;37(1):283–90.
14. Steiner LA, et al. Continuous monitoring of cerebrovascular pressure reactivity allows determination of optimal cerebral perfusion pressure in patients with traumatic brain injury. Crit Care Med. 2002;30(4):733–8.
15. Dias C, et al. Optimal cerebral perfusion pressure management at bedside: a single-center pilot study. Neurocrit Care. 2015;23(1):92–102.
16. Aries MJ, et al. Continuous determination of optimal cerebral perfusion pressure in traumatic brain injury. Crit Care Med. 2012;40(8):2456–63.
17. Le Roux P, et al. Consensus summary statement of the International Multidisciplinary Consensus Conference on Multimodality Monitoring in Neurocritical Care: a statement for healthcare professionals from the Neurocritical Care Society and the European Society of Intensive Care Medicine. Intensive Care Med. 2014;40(9):1189–209.
18. Lang EW, et al. Cerebral vasomotor reactivity testing in head injury: the link between pressure and flow. J Neurol Neurosurg Psychiatry. 2003;74(8):1053–9.
19. Steiner LA, et al. Cerebrovascular pressure reactivity is related to global cerebral oxygen metabolism after head injury. J Neurol Neurosurg Psychiatry. 2003;74(6):765–70.
20. Johnson U, et al. Should the neurointensive care management of traumatic brain injury patients be individualized according to autoregulation status and injury subtype? Neurocrit Care. 2014;21(2):259–65.
21. Amato MB, et al. Driving pressure and survival in the acute respiratory distress syndrome. N Engl J Med. 2015;372(8):747–55.

Cognitive Outcomes of Patients with Traumatic Bifrontal Contusions

George Kwok Chu Wong, Karine Ngai, Wai Sang Poon, Vera Zhi Yuan Zheng, and Carlos Yu

Abstract *Objectives*: We aimed to investigate the prevalence and pattern of cognitive dysfunction in patients with traumatic bifrontal contusions and their association with functional outcome.

Materials and methods: We prospectively recruited patients with bifrontal contusions in a regional neurosurgical center in Hong Kong over a 2-year period. Functional outcome was assessed by modified Rankin Scale (mRS), and cognitive outcomes were assessed by Mini-Mental State Examination (MMSE), Montreal Cognitive Assessment (MoCA), and a comprehensive neuropsychological battery.

Results: We recruited 34 patients with traumatic bifrontal contusions over a 2-year period. Nine (26%) patients had craniotomy for evacuation of left or right frontal contusions. Functional outcome using mRS was significantly correlated with cognitive outcomes using MMSE or MoCA. The effect of cognitive outcome using MMSE or MoCA persisted after adjustments of age, sex, admission Glasgow Coma Scale, and surgery. In patients who completed the comprehensive neuropsychological assessments, cognitive impairment in at least one of the neuropsychological tests was noted in 73% of them.

Conclusions: Cognitive dysfunction had a significant impact on functional outcome, and treatment strategy should be developed to minimize them.

Keywords Traumatic brain injury · Cerebral contusions Cognition · Outcome

---

G.K.C. Wong, M.D. (✉)
Division of Neurosurgery, Department of Surgery, Prince of Wales Hospital, The Chinese University of Hong Kong, Shatin, NT, Hong Kong, China

Department of Surgery, Prince of Wales Hospital, Shatin, NT, Hong Kong, China
e-mail: georgewong@surgury.cuhk.edu.hk

K. Ngai • W.S. Poon • V.Z.Y. Zheng • C. Yu
Division of Neurosurgery, Department of Surgery, Prince of Wales Hospital, The Chinese University of Hong Kong, Shatin, NT, Hong Kong, China

Introduction

Traumatic brain injury (TBI) is still associated with significant mortality and morbidity and drives the development of neurosurgery services in Hong Kong [1–3]. In previous analyses, the pattern of cerebral contusions had prognostic implications [4]. Of 464 patients with head injuries, traumatic intracerebral hematoma was significantly associated with inpatient mortality and 1-year unfavorable outcome after adjusting for age, sex, post-resuscitation Glasgow Coma Scale (GCS) score, and presence of acute subdural hematoma. A total of 114 patients had traumatic intracerebral hematomas and were included for further analysis. The mean age was 49, the male-to-female ratio was 2:1, and the median GCS score at admission was 12. Logistic regression analysis showed that age and GCS score/GCS motor component score were significant factors for inpatient mortality, 1-year mortality, and 1-year outcome. There was an association between temporal hematomas and inpatient mortality, subdural hematomas and inpatient mortality, and bilateral hematomas and unfavorable 1-year outcome. In patients with severe head injury, a traumatic hematoma more than 50 ml was associated with higher inpatient mortality. In addition to age and GCS score, the computed tomography patterns of bilateral hematomas, temporal hematomas, and associated subdural hematomas were suggestive of poor outcome or mortality.

We further postulated that cognitive dysfunction is a major determinant of poor functional outcome in patients with traumatic bifrontal contusions. In this study, we aimed to investigate the prevalence and pattern of cognitive dysfunction in patients with traumatic bifrontal contusions and their associated functional outcome.

Materials and Methods

We prospectively recruited patients with bifrontal contusions in a regional neurosurgical center in Hong Kong over a 2-year period. The study was approved by the Joint NTEC-CUHK (New Territories East Cluster-Chinese University of Hong Kong) Clinical Research Ethics Committee. The study conformed to the Declaration of Helsinki, and written informed consent was obtained from all of the participants or their next of kin. Functional outcome was assessed by modified Rankin Scale (mRS), and cognitive outcomes were assessed by Mini-Mental State Examination (MMSE), Montreal Cognitive Assessment (MoCA), and a comprehensive neuropsychological battery [5].

Montreal Cognitive Assessment

The MoCA is a one-page, 30-point test that usually takes 15 min or less to administer and includes six subtests: visuospatial/executive functions, naming, attention, abstraction, recall and orientation. One point is added for participants with less than 12 years of education. We had reported the application of the Hong Kong version of MoCA in aneurysmal subarachnoid hemorrhage and neurosurgical patients following traumatic and spontaneous intracerebral hemorrhage [6–10].

Mini-Mental State Examination Chinese (Cantonese) Version

The MMSE comprises seven sections (naming, orientation, registration, attention and calculation, recall, praxia, and language). Its maximum total score is 30, and the test can usually be completed in 10 min or less.

The battery of cognitive assessments used in this study was previously applied in a local Chinese population [5]. Its selection was based on (1) its efficacy in previous cognitive studies in local Chinese patients and standard cognitive tests validated in a Cantonese-speaking population, and (2) its balanced range of tests covering verbal and visuospatial memory, attention and working memory, executive functions, psychomotor speed and language. This battery included the following.

Verbal Memory Domain
1. Hong Kong List Learning Test (HKLLT)
Visuospatial Skill and Memory Domain
1. The Rey Osterrieth Complex Figure Test
Attention and Working Memory Domain
1. The verbal and visual digit span forward and backward tests from the Chinese Wechsler Memory Scale-Third Edition
Executive Function and Psychomotor Speed Domain
1. Symbol-Digit Modalities Test
2. Color Trails Test (CTT)
3. Animal fluency
Language Domain
1. Modified Boston Naming Test (mBNT)

Cognitive domain scores were computed by averaging the z scores of the respective test measures derived from established age- and education-matched norms. A cognitive domain deficit was defined as a cognitive domain z score < -1.65 (below the fifth percentile).

Statistical Analyses

Data were analyzed using SPSS for Windows, version 20.0 (SPSS, Chicago, IL, USA). Correlations were assessed by Kendall's tau-b coefficients. Multivariate statistical analyses were performed with multiple logistic regressions using the Enter method. Univariate statistical analyses were performed using contingency analysis (Pearson chi-square test and Fisher exact test) for categorical data. Statistical significance was taken as a two-tailed p value of 0.05 or less.

Results

We recruited 34 patients with traumatic bifrontal contusions over a 2-year period. Nine (26%) patients had craniotomy for evacuation of left or right frontal contusions. Thirty-one (91%) were male and age was 52 ± 16 years.

Functional outcome using mRS was significantly correlated with cognitive outcomes using MMSE or MoCA. The effect of cognitive outcome using MMSE or MoCA persisted after adjustments of age, sex, admission Glasgow Coma Scale, and surgery.

Fourteen patients completed the comprehensive neuropsychological assessments. 36% had verbal memory domain deficit, 36% had executive function and psychomotor speed domain deficit, 18% had visuospatial skill and memory domain deficit, 23% had working memory and attention domain deficit, and 29% had language domain deficit. Unfavorable outcome was significantly associated with language domain deficit, visuospatial skill and memory domain deficit, and working memory and attention domain deficit.

Discussion

We found that cognitive dysfunction was associated with functional outcome measured in mRS. Whether these outcomes were similarly related to the severity of TBI or cognitive dysfunction posed obstacles to activity of daily living remained to be further evaluated. Various cognitive domains, rather than one to two domains, were being affected in patients after traumatic bifrontal contusions.

Concerning possible adjunct to surgical and neurointensive treatment, there has recently been interest in using mesenchymal stem cells (MSCs) in the treatment of TBI [11]. Experimental study suggested that MSCs have the ability to modulate inflammation-associated immune cells and cytokines in TBI-induced cerebral inflammatory responses [12]. In another study, the investigators determined that the CXC chemokine receptor 4 (CXCR4)-SDF1α (stromal cell-derived factor 1α) axis in engineered MSCs serves not only to attract MSC migration to TBI but also to activate the Akt kinase signaling pathway in MSCs to promote paracrine secretion of cytokines and growth factors [13]. The relative abundance of harvest sources of MSCs such as from adipose tissue also makes them particularly appealing. Recently, numerous studies have investigated the effects of infusion of MSCs into animal models of TBI [11]. The results have shown significant improvement in the motor function of the damaged brain tissues.

There were several limitations in our current study. Firstly, the study did not examine how cognitive dysfunction interfered with different tasks of activity of daily living. Secondly, quality of life and neuropsychiatric assessments were not included. Thirdly, the sample size did not allow meaningful evaluation of the effect of surgical evacuation of hematoma with or without primary or secondary decompressive craniectomy. Fourthly, we did not have serial assessments in these patients to see the pattern of cognitive dysfunction at different time points and how these dysfunctions evolved over time.

Our work is important as it provides an understanding of the cognitive dysfunction after traumatic bifrontal contusions. These data suggest that comprehensive neuropsychological battery is necessary for a complete evaluation of cognitive dysfunction in patients with traumatic bifrontal contusions.

Conclusions

Cognitive dysfunction was common after TBI with bifrontal contusion and had a significant impact on functional outcome. Treatment strategy should be developed to minimize them.

Funding This work was supported by Research and Training Fund of the Division of Neurosurgery of the Chinese University of Hong Kong.

Disclosure: None.

Conflicts of interest statement We declare that we have no conflict of interest.

References

1. Wong GK, Graham CA, Ng E, Yeung JH, Rainer TH, Poon WS. Neurological outcomes of neurosurgical operations for multiple trauma elderly patients in Hong Kong. J Emerg Trauma Shock. 2011;4:346–50. https://doi.org/10.4103/0974-2700.83861.
2. Wong GK, Yeung JH, Graham CA, Zhu XL, Rainer TH, Poon WS. Neurological outcome in patients with traumatic brain injury and its relationship with computed tomography patterns of traumatic subarachnoid hemorrhage. J Neurosurg. 2011;114:1510–5. https://doi.org/10.3171/2011.1.JNS101102.
3. Wong GK, Teoh J, Yeung J, Chan E, Siu E, Woo P, Rainer T, Poon WS. Outcomes of traumatic brain injury in Hong Kong: validation with the TRISS, CRASH, and IMPACT models. J Clin Neurosci. 2013;20:1693–6. https://doi.org/10.1016/j.jocn.2012.12.032.
4. Wong GK, Tang BY, Yeung JH, Collins G, Rainer T, Ng SC, Poon WS. Traumatic intracerebral haemorrhage: is the CT pattern related to outcome? Br J Neurosurg. 2009;23:601–5. https://doi.org/10.3109/02688690902948184.
5. Wong GK, Lam SW, Wong A, Ngai K, Poon WS, Mok V. Comparison of montreal cognitive assessment and mini-mental state examination in evaluating cognitive domain deficit following aneurysmal subarachnoid haemorrhage. PLoS One. 2013;8:e59946. https://doi.org/10.1371/journal.pone.0059946.
6. Wong GK, Ngai K, Lam SW, Wong A, Mok V, Poon WS. Validity of the Montreal Cognitive Assessment for traumatic brain injury patients with intracranial haemorrhage. Brain Inj. 2013;27:394–8. https://doi.org/10.3109/02699052.2012.750746.
7. Wong GK, Lam S, Ngai K, Wong A, Mok V, Poon WS, Cognitive Dysfunction after Aneurysmal Subarachnoid Haemorrhage Investigators. Evaluation of cognitive impairment by the Montreal cognitive assessment in patients with aneurysmal subarachnoid haemorrhage: prevalence, risk factors and correlations with 3 month outcomes. J Neurol Neurosurg Psychiatry. 2012;83:1112–7. https://doi.org/10.1136/jnnp-2012-302217.
8. Wong GK, Lam SW, Wong A, Lai M, Siu D, Poon WS, Mok V. MoCA-assessed cognitive function and excellent outcome after aneurysmal subarachnoid hemorrhage at 1 year. Eur J Neurol. 2014;21:725–30. https://doi.org/10.1111/ene.12363.
9. Wong GK, Lam SW, Wong A, Mok V, Siu D, Ngai K, Poon WS. Early MoCA-assessed cognitive impairment after aneurysmal subarachnoid hemorrhage and relationship to 1-year functional outcome. Transl Stroke Res. 2014;5:286–91. https://doi.org/10.1007/s12975-013-0284-z.
10. Wong GK, Wong R, Poon WS. Cognitive outcomes and activity of daily living for neurosurgical patients with intrinsic brain lesions: a one-year prevalence study. Hong Kong J Occup Ther. 2011;21:27–32.
11. Hasan A, Deeb G, Rahal R, Atwi K, Mondello S, Marei HE, Gali A, Sleiman E. Mesenchymal stem cells in the treatment of traumatic brain injury. Front Neurol. 2017;8:28. https://doi.org/10.3389/fneur.2017.00028.
12. Zhang R, Liu Y, Yan K, Chen L, Chen XR, Li P, Chen FF, Jiang XD. Anti-inflammatory and immunomodulatory mechanisms of mesenchymal stem cell transplantation in experimental traumatic brain injury. J Neuroinflammation. 2013;10:106. https://doi.org/10.1186/1742-2094-10-106.
13. Wang Z, Wang Y, Wang Z, Gutkind JS, Wang Z, Wang F, Lu J, Niu G, Teng G, Chen X. Engineered mesenchymal stem cells with enhanced tropism and paracrine secretion of cytokines and growth factors to treat traumatic brain injury. Stem Cells. 2015;33:456–67. https://doi.org/10.1002/stem.1878.

Brain Monitoring Technology

Non-invasive Intracranial Pressure Assessment in Brain Injured Patients Using Ultrasound-Based Methods

Chiara Robba, Danilo Cardim, Tamara Tajsic, Justine Pietersen, Michael Bulman, Frank Rasulo, Rita Bertuetti, Joseph Donnelly, Liu Xiuyun, Zofia Czosnyka, Manuel Cabeleira, Peter Smielewski, Basil Matta, Alessandro Bertuccio, and Marek Czosnyka

Abstract *Background*: Non-invasive measurement of intracranial pressure (ICP) can be invaluable in the management of critically ill patients. Invasive measurement of ICP remains the "gold standard" and should be performed when clinical indications are met, but it is invasive and brings some risks. In this project, we aim to validate the non-invasive ICP (nICP) assessment models based on arterious and venous transcranial Doppler ultrasonography (TCD) and optic nerve sheath diameter (ONSD).

Methods: We included brain injured patients requiring invasive ICP monitoring (intraparenchymal or intraventricular). We assessed the concordance between ICP measured non-invasively with arterious [flow velocity diastolic formula (ICP_{FVd}) and pulsatility index (PI)], venous TCD (vPI) and ICP derived from ONSD ($nICP_{ONSD}$) compared to invasive ICP measurement.

Results: Linear regression showed a positive relationship between nICP and ICP for all the methods, except PIv. ICP_{ONSD} showed the strongest correlation with invasive ICP ($r = 0.61$) compared to the other methods (ICP_{FVd}, $r = 0.26$, p value = 0.0015; PI, $r = 0.19$, p value = 0.02, vPI, $r = 0.056$, p value = 0.510). The ability to predict intracranial hypertension was highest for ICP_{ONSD} (AUC = 0.91; 95% CI, 0.85–0.97 at ICP > 20 mmHg), with a sensitivity and specificity of 85%, followed by ICP_{FVd} (AUC = 0.67; 95% CI, 0.54–0.79).

Conclusions: Our results demonstrate that among the non-invasive methods studied, ONSD showed the best accuracy in the detection of ICP.

Keywords Brain ultrasound · Intracranial pressure · Transcranial doppler · Optic nerve sheath diameter

Introduction

Elevated intracranial pressure (ICP) is an important cause of secondary brain injury and may be associated with a poor outcome [1]. Clinical signs of elevated ICP, such as headache, altered level of consciousness and vomiting, are considered to be non-specific and unreliable predictors of brain damage [2]. The "gold standard" for continuous ICP monitoring is an intraventricular catheter connected to an external pressure transducer [3]. However, the procedure is invasive, and it is at times complicated by infection, haemorrhage, malfunction, obstruction and malpositioning of the catheter [4, 5]. Therefore, non-invasive measurement of ICP (nICP) can be invaluable in the management of critically ill patients [6]. This project is focused on comparing and refining methods for nICP assessment based on arterial and venous transcranial Doppler ultrasonography (TCD) and optic nerve sheath diameter (ONSD) ultrasonography.

C. Robba, M.D. (✉) · T. Tajsic · B. Matta
Neurosciences Critical Care Unit, Addenbrooke's Hospital, University of Cambridge, Cambridge, UK
e-mail: kiarobba@gmail.com

D. Cardim · J. Donnelly · L. Xiuyun · Z. Czosnyka · M. Cabeleira
P. Smielewski · M. Czosnyka
Brain Physics Laboratory, Division of Neurosurgery, Department of Clinical Neurosciences, University of Cambridge, Cambridge, UK

J. Pietersen · M. Bulman
Department of Anaesthesia, Addenbrooke's Hospital, University of Cambridge, Cambridge, UK

F. Rasulo · R. Bertuetti
Neurocritical Care Unit, Department of Anaesthesia, Intensive Care and Emergency Medicine, Spedali Civili, Brescia, Italy

A. Bertuccio
Division of Neurosurgery, S. George's Hospital, London, UK

Methods

This single-centre non-invasive clinical trial was approved by the institutional ethics committee and written informed consent was obtained from all participants' next of kin. Patients admitted to the Neurocritical Care Unit, Addenbrookes Hospital, Cambridge, UK, for intracranial diseases (including traumatic brain injury, subarachnoid haemorrhage and stroke) that necessitate monitoring of ICP with continuous intraparenchymal or intraventricular monitoring were enrolled in this study.

Inclusion criteria were age >18 and necessary ICP monitoring in situ (intraparenchimal or intraventricular). Exclusion criteria were a history of optic nerve lesion or previous optic nerve trauma, cerebral venous thrombosis, skull base fracture with cerebral spinal fluid leakage, inaccessible ultrasound window and the absence of informed consent.

ONSD ultrasound measurements were performed and recorded twice a day from day 1 to day 5 of admission, and in the case of high dynamics of ICP (like plateau waves) on event. Doppler velocity in the middle cerebral artery (MCA) and venous TCD on the straight sinus (SS) was simultaneously measured in all the patients.

ONSD was measured 3 mm behind the retina [7]. A single investigator used a 7.5-MHz linear ultrasound probe oriented perpendicularly in the vertical plane and at around 30° in the horizontal plane on the closed eyelids of both eyes of supine subjects. Ultrasound gel was applied to the outside of each eyelid and recordings made in the axial and longitudinal planes of the widest diameter visible. Measurements were performed in the transverse and sagittal planes of both eyes, and the final ONSD value was calculated by averaging four measured values.

Arterious TCD was performed on the MCA through the temporal window. TCD measurements were conducted trans-temporally using a traditional 2-MHz transducer as previously described [7].

Venous TCD was performed on the SS through an occipital and transforaminal bone window at a depth of 50–80 mm for flow directed towards the probe, as described by Schoser et al. [8].

Pulsatility index (PI) was calculated according to Gosling's method [9]: [PI = (FVs – FVd)/FVm]. FVd based non-invasive ICP (ICP_{FVd}) was derived from the work of Czosnyka et al. [10], in which the authors describe a method for non-invasive estimation of cerebral perfusion pressure (nCPP) in traumatic brain-injured patients:

$$nCPP = ABPm \cdot (FVd / FVm) + 14$$

Non-invasive ICP was estimated as the difference between inflow (ABPm) and non-invasive cerebral perfusion pressure:

$$ICP_{FVd}(mmHg) = ABPm - nCPP$$

PI-derived non-invasive ICP from the SS (vPI) was calculated as [8]:

$$PI = (maximalBFV - minimal\ BFV) / mean\ BFV$$

The value of ONSD-derived ICP was calculated according to our preliminary unpublished results, from the regression plot in a cohort of 23 neurocritical care patients, where invasive ICP was compared with ONSD ultrasound measurements:

$$nICP_{ONSD} = (ONSD - 3.7242) / 0.128$$

Results

A total of 22 patients were included in this study, with a total of 110 measurements. The characteristics of the patients are shown in Table 1. Median value of ICP was 10 (IQR = 17–5.0).

Results from linear regression showed a positive relationship between ICP and nICP calculated with ICP_{ONSD}, ICP_{FVd} and PI, but not for vPI (Fig. 1). ICP_{ONSD} showed the strongest correlation with invasive ICP ($r = 0.61$) compared to the other methods (ICP_{FVd}: $r = 0.26$, p value = 0.001; PI: $r = 0.19$, p value = 0.02; vPI: $r = 0.056$, p value = 0.51). Results from the receiver operator characteristic (ROC) curve analysis are shown in Fig. 2.

The ability to predict intracranial hypertension (threshold 20 mmHg) was highest for ICP_{ONSD} (AUC = 0.91; 95% CI, 0.85–0.97 at ICP > 20 mmHg), with a sensitivity and specificity of 85%, followed by ICP_{FVd} (AUC = 0.67; 95% CI, 0.54–0.79).

Discussion

According to our results, ONSD showed the best accuracy to assess non-invasively ICP when compared with TCD-based methods. To our knowledge, this is the first study comparing ONSD ultrasonography with different (arterious or venous) TCD methods. Non-invasive ICP is a poorly developed tech-

Table 1 Characteristics of the patients

Total number of patients	22
Sex (M/F)	10/12
Age (mean SD) years	62 ± 15.3
Weight (mean SD) kg	78 ± 5.2
Height (mean SD) cm	172 ± 13.4
Comorbidities	4 hypertension 3 diabetes 3 COPD
Reason for admission (n)	Isolated traumatic brain injury $n = 8$ Polytrauma $n = 7$ aSAH $n = 7$
GCS at admission	7 ± 3.2
Complications	Infection $n = 7$

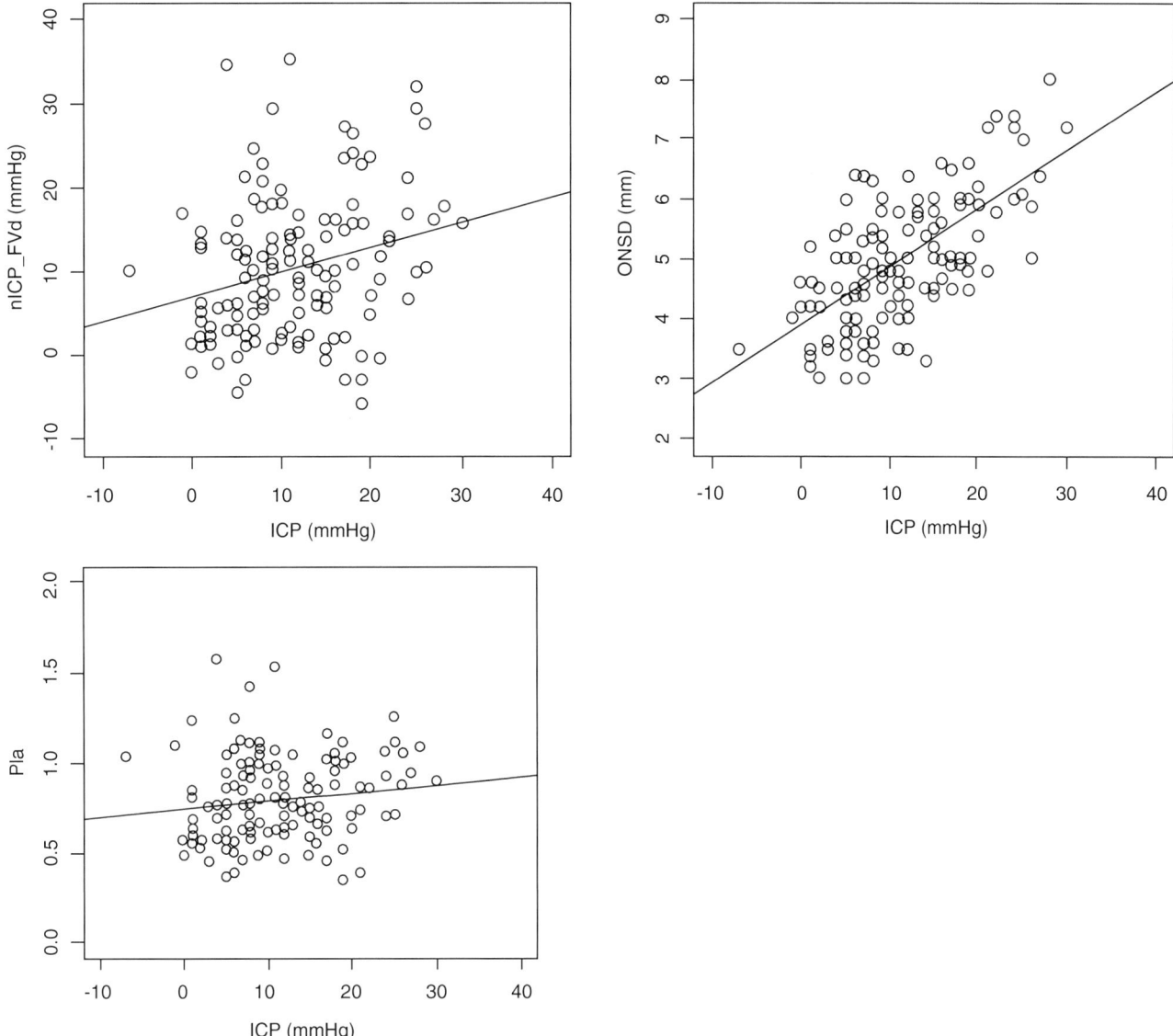

Fig. 1 Scatter plots averaged measured ICP versus ICP_{FVd} (*upper left panel*) ICP_{ONSD} (*upper right panel*) and vPI (*lower panel*)

nique, and several attempts have been made in order to find an accurate method to estimate ICP, but so far none of these can substitute the invasive gold standard [6].

The optic nerve sheath (ONS) is continuous with dura mater; as such, the space within the sheath is continuous with the cranial subarachnoid space. When ICP increases, the pressure in the ONS increases linearly, which distends the ONS. Several studies have directly correlated ONSD measurements on ultrasound with ICP measured invasively [6]. The cut-off value for normal ONSD, measured 3 mm posterior to the globe, ranges from 5.2 to 5.9 mm. The sensitivity is 74–95% and the specificity is 74–100% to identify ICP >20 mmHg [11, 12].

TCD is a non-invasive, safe and bedside tool, and it has been used for multiple applications, including detection of changes in cerebral blood flow, vasospasm and circulatory arrest [13]. The non-invasive evaluation of ICP using TCD has also been studied. TCD generates a velocity–time waveform of cerebral blood flow from which the peak systolic (PSV) and end-diastolic (EDV) flow rates can be measured.

The Gosling pulsatility index (PI) has been for many years the most commonly used formula, but many studies have demonstrated that PI value cannot determine the corresponding ICP with an acceptable clinical precision [13, 14]. Similarly, different formulas and mathematical approaches have been proposed for ICP and CPP estimation [10]. Schmidt et al. [15] proposed a new non-PI-related formula for estimation of CPP and therefore ICP based on FVd, which proved that the absolute difference between real CPP and nCPP so calculated was less than 10 mmHg in 89% of measurements

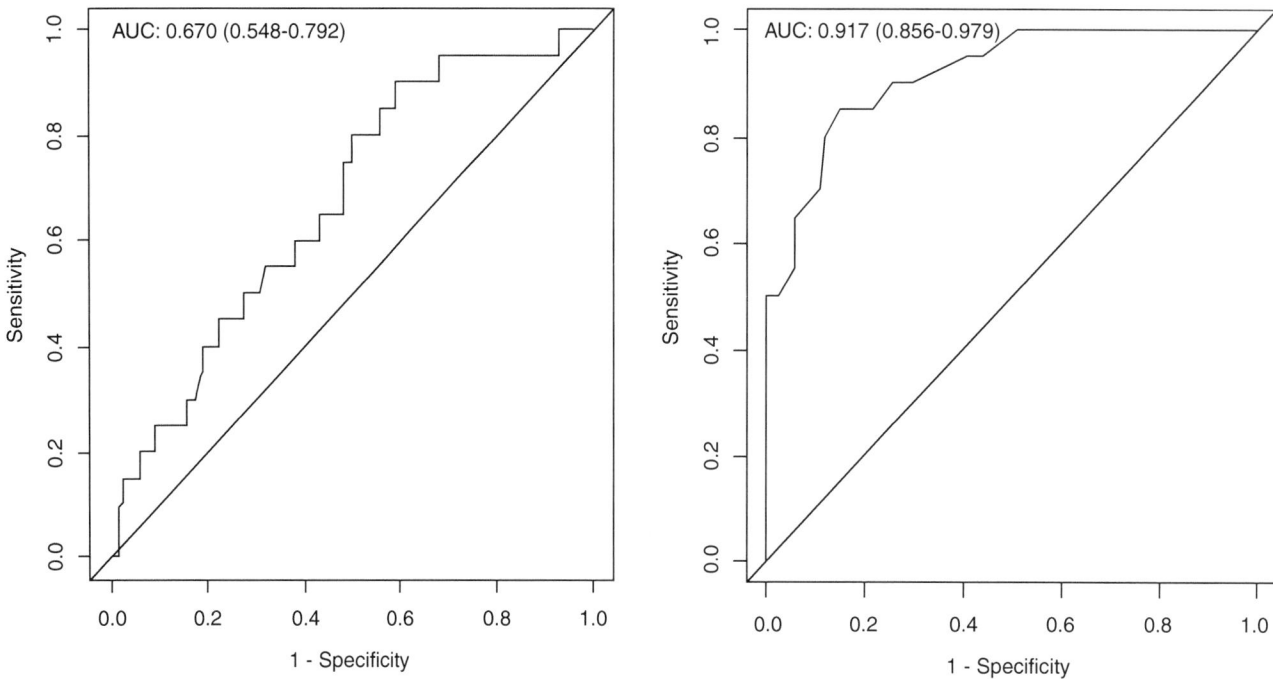

Fig. 2 Univariate ROC curve analysis of the different non-invasive parameters. On the *left panel*, univariate ROC analysis taking in account the use of ICP_{FVd}; in the *right panel*, it takes in account the ICP_{ONSD} method

and less than 13 mmHg in 92% of measurements in their study. The same group of authors, in another study [10], reinforced the results of the above-mentioned study (correlation between and CPP and measured CPP was $r = 0.73$; $p < 0.0001$). Venous TCD ultrasonography is an evolving technique [8]. Within a closed skull, cerebral compliance depends secondarily on the compressibility of the low-pressure venous or capacitance segment of the vascular bed. This venous capacitance segment encompasses 70% of the complete cerebral vascular volume. With progressive increases in ICP, venous blood flow is impaired (venous congestion) before secondary arterial blood flow came to stasis. These venous changes were observed at approximately 50 mmHg of ICP. The main study in this field has been conducted by Schoser et al. [8], who performed venous TCD on 30 control volunteers and 25 patients with raised ICP. Venous bloodflow velocities (BFVs) in the basal vein of Rosenthal showed, within a certain range, a linear relationship between mean ICP and maximal venous BFV ($r = 0.645$; $p < 0.002$). Moreover, a linear relationship was found for maximal venous BFVs in the SS and mean ICP ($r = 0.928$; $p < 0.0003$) [8].

Conclusions

Non-invasive estimation of ICP is a developing field. The ideal non-invasive ICP monitoring method should be safe, low cost, easily available, suitable for emergency settings and accurate. At present, none of these methods seem to be reliable and accurate enough to substitute the invasive ICP measurement. However, ONSD ultrasonography is a simple repeatable, bedside tool, widely used and, among the methods described here, it seems to have highest accuracy in the detection of ICP.

Conflicts of interest statement DC is supported by a Cambridge Commonwealth European and International Trust Scholarship. JD is supported by a Woolf Fisher Trust Scholarship. XL is supported by a Gates Cambridge Trust Scholarship. BC is supported by a CNPQ Scholarship (Research Project 203792/2014-9). MC and DC are partially supported by NIHR Brain Injury Healthcare Technology Co-operative, Cambridge. For the remaining authors nothing was declared.

References

1. Marmarou A, Anderson RL, Ward JD, Young HF, Marmarou A. Impact of ICP instability and hypotension on outcome in patients with severe head trauma. J Neurosurg. 1991;75:S59–66.
2. Tayal VS, Neulander M, Norton HJ, Foster T, Saunders T, Blaivas M. Emergency department sonographic measurement of optic nerve sheath diameter to detect findings of increased intracranial pressure in adult head injury patients. Ann Emerg Med. 2007;49:508–14.
3. Online TBI guidelines 2010. Available at www.braintrauma.org/coma/guidelines. Accessed May 14.
4. Holloway KL, Barnes T, Choi S, Bullock R, Marshall LF, Eisenberg HM, et al. Ventriculostomy infections: the effect of monitoring duration and catheter exchange in 584 patients. J Neurosurg. 1996;85:419–24.

5. Hoefnagel D, Dammers R, Ter Laak-Poort MP, Avezaat CJ. Risk factors for infections related to external ventricular drainage. Acta Neurochir. 2008;150:209–14.
6. Robba C, Bacigaluppi S, Cardim D, Donnelly J, Bertuccio A, Czosnyka M. Non-invasive assessment of intracranial pressure. Acta Neurol Scand. 2016;134(1):4–21. https://doi.org/10.1111/ane.12527. Epub 2015 Oct 30.
7. Robba C, Bragazzi NL, Bertuccio A, Cardim D, Donnelly J, Sekhon M, Lavinio A, Duane D, Burnstein R, Matta B, Bacigaluppi S, Lattuada M, Czosnyka M. Effects of prone position and positive end-expiratory pressure on noninvasive estimators of ICP: a pilot study. J Neurosurg. 1999;91(5):744–9.
8. Schoser BG, Riemenschneider N, Hansen HC. The impact of raised intracranial pressure on cerebral venous hemodynamics: a prospective venous transcranial Doppler ultrasonography study. J Neurosurg. 1999;91(5):744–9.
9. Gosling RG, King DH. Arterial assessment by Doppler-shift ultrasound. Proc R Soc Med. 1974;67:447–9.
10. Czosnyka M, Matta BF, Smielewski P, Kirkpatrick PJ, Pickard JD. Cerebral perfusion pressure in head-injured patients: a non-invasive assessment using transcranial Doppler ultrasonography. J Neurosurg. 1998;88:802–8.
11. Rajajee V, Vanaman M, Fletcher JJ, et al. Optic nerve ultrasound for the detection of raised intracranial pressure. Neurocrit Care. 2011;15:506–15.
12. Moretti R, Pizzi B, Cassini F, et al. Reliability of optic nerve ultrasound for the evaluation of patients with spontaneous intracranial hemorrhage. Neurocrit Care. 2009;11:406–10.
13. Zweifel C, Czosnyka M, Carrera E, et al. Reliability of the Blood Flow Velocity Pulsatility Index for assessment of intracranial and cerebral perfusion pressures in head injured patients. Neurosurgery. 2012;71:237–9.
14. Bellner J, Romner B, Reinstrup P, et al. Transcranial Doppler sonography pulsatility index (PI) reflects intracranial pressure (ICP). Surg Neurol. 2004;62:45–51.
15. Schmidt EA, Czosnyka M, Gooskens I, Piechnik SK, Matta BF, Whitfield PC, Pickard JD. Preliminary experience of the estimation of cerebral perfusion pressure using transcranial Doppler ultrasonography. J Neurol Neurosurg Psychiatry. 2001;70:198–204.

Analysis of a Minimally Invasive Intracranial Pressure Signals During Infusion at the Subarachnoid Spinal Space of Pigs

G. Frigieri, R.A.P. Andrade, C.C. Wang, D. Spavieri Jr., L. Lopes, R. Brunelli, D.A. Cardim, R.M.M. Verzola, and S. Mascarenhas

Abstract *Objective*: We developed a new minimally invasive method for intracranial pressure monitoring (ICPMI). The objective of this project is to verify the similarities between the ICPMI and the invasive method (ICPInv), for different components of the intracranial pressure signal—namely, the mean value (trend) as well as its pulsatile component.

Materials and methods: A 9 kg anesthetized pig was used for simultaneous ICP monitoring with both methods. ICP was increased by performing ten infusions of 6 ml 0.9% saline into the spinal subarachnoid space, using a catheter implanted in the lumbar region. For correlation analysis, the signals were decomposed into two components—trend and pulsatile signals. Pearson correlation coefficient was calculated between ICPInv and ICPMI.

Results: During the infusions, the correlation between the pulsatile components of the signals was above 0.5 for most of the time. The signal trends showed a good agreement (correlation above 0.5) for most of the time during infusions.

Conclusions: The ICPMI signal trends showed a good linear agreement with the signal obtained invasively. Based on the waveform analysis of the pulsatile component of ICP, our results indicate the possibility of using the minimally invasive method for assessing the neuroclinical state of the patient.

Keywords Intracranial pressure · Minimally invasive · ICP waveform · Spinal infusion

Introduction

Intracranial pressure (ICP) is a relevant parameter for the management of many neuropathologies [1]. Current procedures to access ICP are invasive and subject to risks of brain damage and infections. Increased ICP is commonly seen is traumatic brain injury, where the need to know this parameter overcomes the risks associated with its assessment. The possibility to evaluate ICP non-invasively would be valuable in several brain disorders, as it could lead to a better management of the patient in a broader variety of clinical conditions [2–5].

We present in this work the application of a minimally invasive ICP method (ICPMI) based on mechanical extensometers in an experimental model of intracranial hypertension. ICPMI basically consists of a strain gauge (mechanical extensometer) attached to the parietal region laterally to the sagittal suture. The sensor is able to detect small skull deformations resulting from changes in ICP. At the current state of development, this method does not yield pressure values calibrated in millimetres of mercury, but provides continuous information about the ICP waveform and changes in time.

The objective of this study was to verify the similarities between the ICPMI and the invasive method (ICPInv) for different components of the ICP signal—namely, the mean value (trend) and its pulsatile component.

G. Frigieri (✉) · R.A.P. Andrade · C.C. Wang · D. Spavieri Jr.
Braincare, São Carlos, SP, Brazil
e-mail: g.frigieri@gmail.com

L. Lopes
Faculdade de Medicina de Ribeirão Preto, University of São Paulo, Ribeirão Preto, SP, Brazil

R. Brunelli · S. Mascarenhas
Braincare, São Carlos, SP, Brazil

Instituto de Física de São Carlos, Universidade de São Paulo, São Carlos, SP, Brazil

D.A. Cardim
Division of Neurosurgery, Department of Clinical Neurosciences, Brain Physics Laboratory, Cambridge, UK

R.M.M. Verzola
Department of Biological Sciences and Health, Federal University of São Carlos, São Carlos, SP, Brazil

Materials and Methods

Experimental Protocol

A 9 kg anesthetized pig ($n = 1$) was used for simultaneous ICP monitoring with ICPMI and ICPInv methods. The ICPMI (Braincare, São Carlos, Brazil) sensor was glued on the parietal bone. The ICPInv (Codman & Shurtleff) micro transducer was inserted into the brain parenchyma, in the contralateral side of ICPMI (Fig. 1). Both sensors were plugged to the device Braincare CR15. All procedures were approved by the local Ethics Committee (CEEA/FMRP: 014/2013). ICP was increased by performing ten 6 ml infusions of 0.9% saline into the spinal subarachnoid space, using a catheter implanted in the lumbar region. The ICP signals were recorded using the ICP monitor BC Research 1.5 (Braincare), Braincare BCR software v.1.2 and the data were analysed using the Braincare Analytics System.

Data Analysis

To perform the correlation analysis, the signals were decomposed into two components—trend and pulsatile signals. The trend signal was defined as the mean value of the signal envelope, obtained from the interpolation (cubic spline) [6] of the local minima and maxima. To avoid possible drift influences in ICPMI signal, we linearly interpolated the signal before the start of each infusion and subtracted this linear trend from the signals before, during and after each corresponding infusion.

Linear correlation coefficient (Pearson) was calculated between ICP and minimally invasive ICP within temporal windows of 60s, with an overlapping of 50s. We considered correlations above 0.5 as significant. The analysis was performed using custom programs written in Python language, using the libraries Scipy [7], Matplotlib [8] and Scikit-learn [9].

Results

During the infusions, the correlation between the pulsatile components of the signals was above 0.5 for most of the time. The signal trends showed a good agreement (correlation above 0.5) for most of the time during infusions. Figure 2 shows comparisons between minimally invasive and invasive ICP monitoring methods for the first and last infusion procedures, respectively.

Discussion

In this work, skull deformations could be associated with changes in ICPInv using ICPMI. Nevertheless, the calibration in absolute values (mmHg) for the minimally invasive ICP measurement still needs to be developed.

Our findings suggest that the minimally invasive method can be safely used as a simple and cost-effective alternative tool for ICP monitoring. Translated to clinical practice, the ICPMI could be applied where ICP monitoring has been limited due to the risks associated with the invasive procedures.

A potential limitation of this study is associated with the insertion of the needle into the spinal canal without externalizing the animal spine; thus, adequate control of the dural puncture was not feasible and leakage of saline possibly

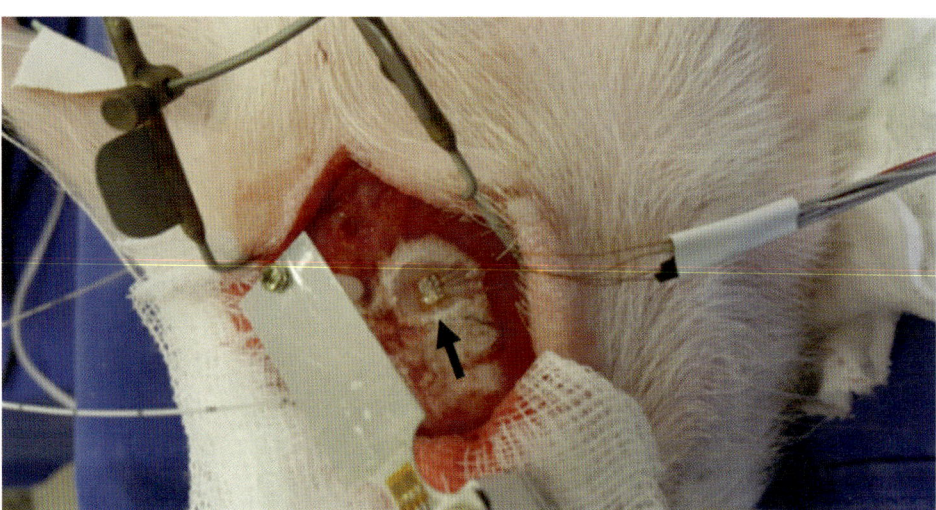

Fig. 1 The minimally invasive sensor placed on the parietal region of the pig skull (*black arrow*)

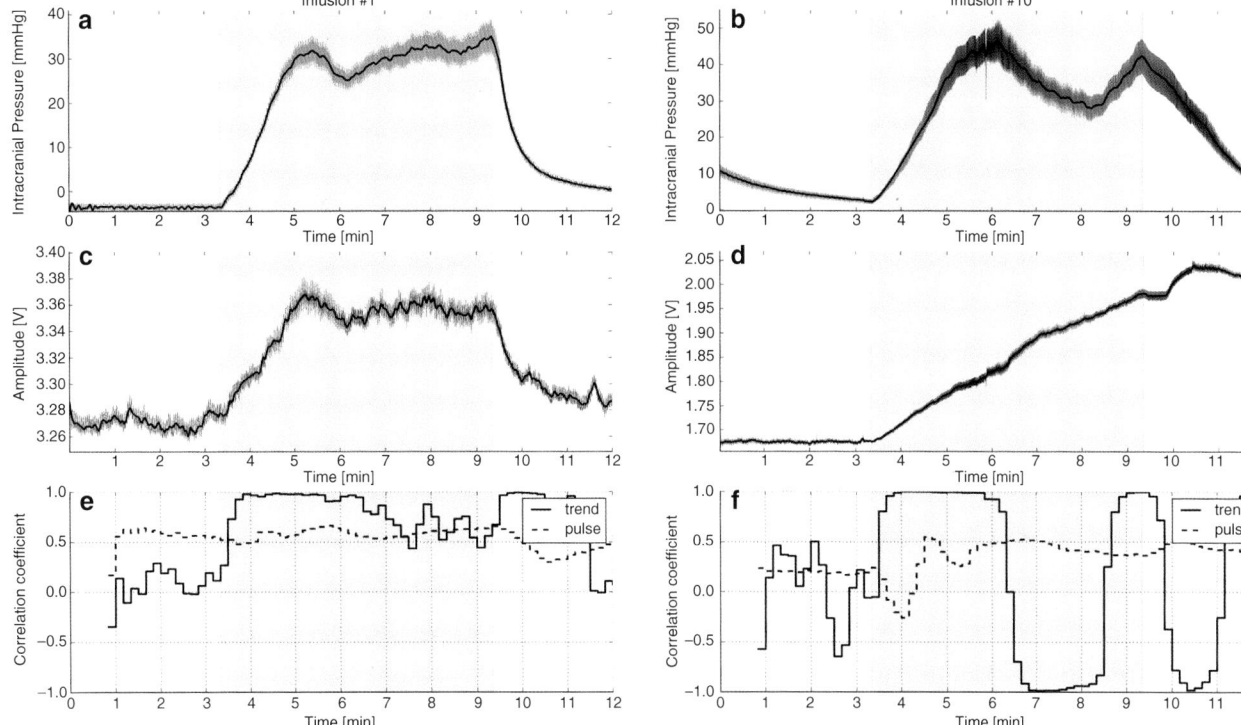

Fig. 2 Comparison between minimally invasive and invasive ICP recording methods. (**a, b**) Invasive ICP recording. (**c, d**) Non-invasive ICP recording. (**e, f**) Linear correlations between trend (*continuous*) and pulsatile (*dashed*) components of the recordings, for the first infusion of the experiment. The *green shadow* represents the period in which the infusion was performed

occurred after reaching a certain pressure threshold. The occurrence of a plateau phase for both methods indicates the moment when the pressure caused the balance between the volume of fluid infused and the fluid leaking through the lumbar puncture. The drift presented by the ICPMI sensor signal is mainly caused by the variation in temperature over the extensometer is subjected. This may have caused a mismatch in the correlation coefficients, as ICPInv is less influenced by temperature once it is in contact with the brain parenchyma.

Conclusions

The ICPMI signal trends showed a good linear agreement with the signal obtained invasively, despite occasional drifts caused by temperature variations or other sources of interference that might influence the minimally invasive sensor's performance. Based on the waveform analysis of the pulsatile component of ICP, our results indicate the possibility of using the minimally invasive method for monitoring changes of ICP.

Conflicts of interest statement We declare that we have no conflict of interest.

References

1. Andrews PD, Citerio G. Intracranial pressure. Intensive Care Med. 2004;30:1730–3. Available from: http://link.springer.com/10.1007/s00134-004-2376-4.
2. Kashif FM, Verghese GC, Novak V, Czosnyka M, Heldt T. Model-based noninvasive estimation of intracranial pressure from cerebral blood flow velocity and arterial pressure. Sci Transl Med. 2012;4:129ra44. Available from: http://stm.sciencemag.org/cgi/doi/10.1126/scitranslmed.3003249.
3. Barone DG, Czosnyka M. Brain Monitoring: do we need a hole? An update on invasive and noninvasive brain monitoring modalities. Sci World J. 2014;2014:1–6. Available from: http://www.hindawi.com/journals/tswj/2014/795762/.
4. Padayachy LC. Non-invasive intracranial pressure assessment. .Child's Nerv Syst. 2016;1–11. Available from: https://doi.org/10.1007/s00381-016-3159-2.
5. Ferreira MCPD. Multimodal brain monitoring and evaluation of cerebrovascular reactivity after severe head injury. Porto: University of Porto; 2015.
6. Press WH, Teukolsky SA, Vetterling WT, Flannery BP. Numerical recipes. 3rd ed. Cambridge: Cambridge University Press; 2007.
7. Jones E, Oliphant T, Peterson P. Scipy: open source scientific tools for Python. 2001. Available from: http://www.scipy.org/.
8. Hunter JD. Matplotlib: a 2D graphics environment. Comput Sci Eng. 2007;9:90–5.
9. Pedregosa F, Varoquaux G, Gramfort A, Michel V, Thirion B, Grisel O, et al. Scikit-learn: machine learning in Python. J Mach Learn Res. 2011;12:2825–30.

Comparison of Different Calibration Methods in a Non-invasive ICP Assessment Model

Bernhard Schmidt, Danilo Cardim, Marco Weinhold, Stefan Streif, Damian D. McLeod, Marek Czosnyka, and Jürgen Klingelhöfer

Abstract *Objective*: Previously we described the method of continuous intracranial pressure (ICP) estimation using arterial blood pressure (ABP) and cerebral blood flow velocity (CBFV). The model was constructed using reference patient data. Various individual calibration strategies were used in the current attempt to improve the accuracy of this non-invasive ICP (nICP) assessment tool.

Materials and methods: Forty-one patients (mean, 52 years; range, 18–77 years) with severe brain injuries were studied. CBFV in the middle cerebral artery (MCA), ABP and invasively assessed ICP were simultaneously recorded for 1 h. Recording was repeated at days 2, 4 and 7. In the first recording, invasively assessed ICP was recorded to calibrate the nICP procedure by means of either a constant shift of nICP (snICP), a constant shift of nICP/ABP ratio (anICP) or by including this recording for a model reconstruction (cnICP). At follow-up days, the calibrated nICP procedures were applied and the results compared to the original nICP.

Results: In 76 follow-up recordings, the mean differences (Bias), the SD and the mean absolute differences (ΔICP) between ICP and the nICP methods were (in mmHg): nICP, −5.6 ± 5.72, 6.5; snICP, +0.7 ± 6.98, 5.5, n.s.; anICP, +1.0 ± 7.22, 5.6, n.s.; cnICP, −3.4 ± 5.68, 5.4, $p < 0.001$. In patients with craniotomy ($n = 19$), the nICP was generally higher than ICP. This overestimation could be reduced by cnICP calibration, but not completely avoided.

Discussion: Constant shift calibrations (snICP, anICP) decrease the Bias to ICP, but increase SD and, therefore, increase the 95% confidence interval (CI = 2 × SD). This calibration method cannot be recommended. Compared to nICP, the cnICP method reduced the Bias and slightly reduced SD, and showed significantly decreased ΔICP. Compared to snICP and anICP, the Bias was higher. This effect was probably caused by the patients with craniotomy.

Conclusion: The cnICP calibration method using initial recordings for model reconstruction showed the best results.

Keywords Intracranial pressure · Cerebral blood flow · Transcranial Doppler ultrasonography · Arterial blood pressure

Introduction

Transcranial Doppler ultrasonography (TCD) has been used for many years to estimate intracranial pressure (ICP) [1–5]. We previously introduced a mathematical model in which TCD assessed cerebral blood flow velocity (CBFV) in the middle cerebral artery (MCA) and arterial blood pressure (ABP) signals were used to generate a continuous non-invasive assessment of ICP (nICP) [6]. A database of data from reference patients, consisting of CBFV, ABP and invasively measured ICP, was used as teaching data to derive the algorithm for nICP assessment. The accuracy of the nICP assessment procedure relies on the general validity of this algorithm. Although the nICP assessment method has been validated in many patients in various clinical studies [7, 8], differing errors of this method suggested individual deviations from the general algorithm. The aim of this study was to investigate how a temporarily implanted ICP probe in a patient could be used for an individual adaptation of the nICP assessment algorithm, that is, an individual calibration of the nICP procedure. Such a

B. Schmidt (✉) · M. Weinhold · J. Klingelhöfer
Department of Neurology, Medical Centre Chemnitz, Chemnitz, Germany
e-mail: B.Schmidt@skc.de

D. Cardim · M. Czosnyka
Brain Physics Lab, Academic Neurosurgical Unit, Addenbrooke's Hospital, Cambridge, UK

S. Streif
Laboratory for Automatic Control and System Dynamics, Technische Universität Chemnitz, Chemnitz, Germany

D.D. McLeod
School of Biomedical Sciences & Pharmacy, The University of Newcastle, Callaghan, NSW, Australia

scenario seems to fit clinical needs for further ICP follow-up after a period of initial direct monitoring. Furthermore, we investigated which type of calibration—of three conceived calibration methods—was the most suitable.

Materials and Methods

Patient Population

Recorded signal data from 41 consecutive patients with severe cerebral diseases (age, 18–77 years; mean age, 52 ± 17 years; 28 men/13 women) who underwent multimodal monitoring between 2005 and 2009 were analysed. Patients were treated in the Neurocritical Care Unit of the Medical Centre Chemnitz. They suffered either from traumatic brain injury (TBI; $n = 20$) with subarachnoid haemorrhages ($n = 7$), intracerebral haemorrhages ($n = 4$) and intracranial hematoma ($n = 11$), or from non-traumatic diseases ($n = 21$), i.e. aneurysmal subarachnoid haemorrhages ($n = 4$), spontaneous intracerebral haemorrhages ($n = 10$), MCA infarction ($n = 4$), cerebral venous sinus thrombosis, hypoxic encephalopathy, and encephalitis. In 19 patients, craniotomy was performed before repeated data recording started. All patients were sedated and mechanically ventilated with fixed ventilator settings at every recording time point. Patients' arterial partial pressure of carbon dioxide ($PaCO_2$) ranged from 26 to 49 mmHg.

The study was approved by the Local Ethics Committee. All signal monitoring was part of a clinical routine. The retrospective data analysis did not require individual patient consent.

Monitoring

A two MHz pulsed Doppler device (Multidop-P; DWL, Sipplingen, Germany) was used for assessment of transcranial Doppler (TCD) signal. The envelope curve of CBFV in the MCA was continuously monitored in the hemisphere ipsilateral to the brain lesion in most cases. TCD signals were recorded during stable periods free from nursing. ABP was measured with a standard manometer line inserted into the radial artery. ICP was measured using either implanted intraparenchymal or intraventricular microsensor catheters (Raumedic, Helmbrechts, Germany).

Computer-assisted Recording

Personal computers fitted with data acquisition systems (Daq 112B; Iotech, Cleveland, OH, USA) and software developed in-house were used for recording and analysing TCD, ABP and ICP signals and for calculation of nICP (see below). For each recording time point, signals were assessed over a 60-min period with a sampling frequency of 25 Hz. If possible, recording was repeated at days 2, 4, and 7. The day 1 recording of each patient was taken to calibrate the nICP assessment procedure while the follow-up recordings were used for its validation. In total, 130 recordings of 41 patients were acquired.

Non-invasive ICP Assessment

The non-invasive ICP is the result of a signal transformation [so-called Dirac Impulse Response (DIR) [9]] of the ABP signal. This transformation (DIR ABP → ICP) is not constant but changes in time. During nICP assessment, the DIR ABP → ICP is controlled and continuously updated by parameters (so-called TCD-characteristics) derived from measured CBFV and ABP signals (Fig. 1b) [6]. The TCD characteristics are recalculated in 10-s intervals. They substantially consist of coefficients of a DIR ABP → CBFV and additional ICP related parameters, such as pulsatility index (Fig. 1a). The model assumes linear relationship between TCD characteristics and the coefficients of the DIR ABP → ICP. This relationship has

Fig. 1 Procedure of non-invasive ICP assessment. (**a**) Generation of nICP procedure. Signal data of 197 reference patients with severe brain injuries was used to assess the relationship between TCD characteristics (**tcd**, parameters calculated from CBFV and ABP) and DIR ABP → ICP (linear transformation of ABP into ICP signal, calculated from ABP and invasively assessed ICP) by means of multiple regression analyses. The relationship was described in terms of nICP matrix (**A, B**). (**b**) Calculation of nICP. From measured CBFV and ABP the TCD characteristics are derived and multiplied with the formerly calculated nICP matrix (**A, B**) (**tcd → A × tcd + B**). This results in the DIR ABP → nICP function (= estimation of the correct DIR ABP → ICP), which transforms the ABP signal into nICP. (**c**) Points of possible calibration. Calibration may be performed at different points in the flow diagram, by either adjusting the nICP matrix (**A, B**), or the DIR ABP → nICP, or by adjusting the calculated nICP signal itself. (**d**) Calibration 1. Day-1 recording data of a patient is added to the reference signal data and the nICP procedure is re-generated. This yields the new nICP matrix (**A^, B^**), adjusted to the individual features of this patient. (**e**) Calibration 2. The difference of ratios ICP/ABP − nICP/ABP is averaged over Day-1 recording of a patient, resulting in **w'**. Assuming that this difference remains approximately constant on subsequent days, calibrated nICP in this patient is achieved by adding the product **w'** × meanABP, (mean =10 s mean), to the (standard) nICP. This product should then provide an approximation of the current difference between ICP and nICP. .(**f**) Calibration 3. The mean difference $K = ICP − nICP$ of the day-1 recording is calculated. Assuming that the difference ICP − nICP remains approximately constant, the constant K is added to the calculated nICP on subsequent days to result in the calibrated snICP signal. (*DIR* Dirac impulse response, *TCD* transcranial Doppler)

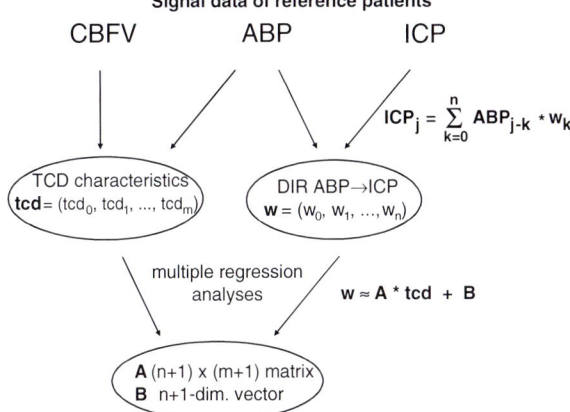
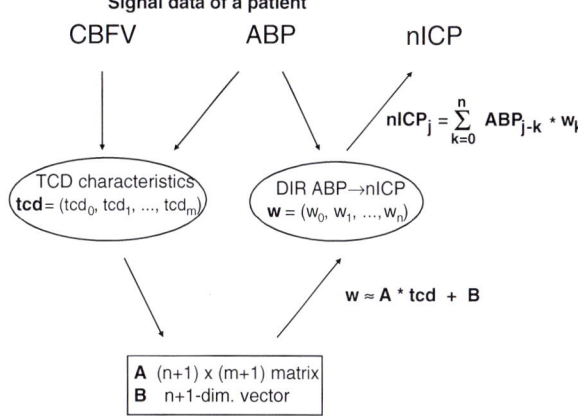
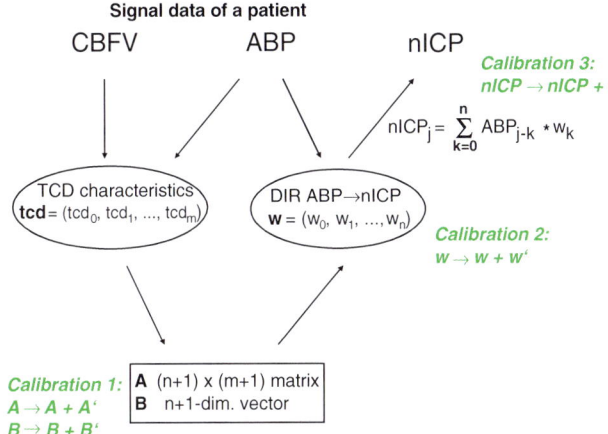
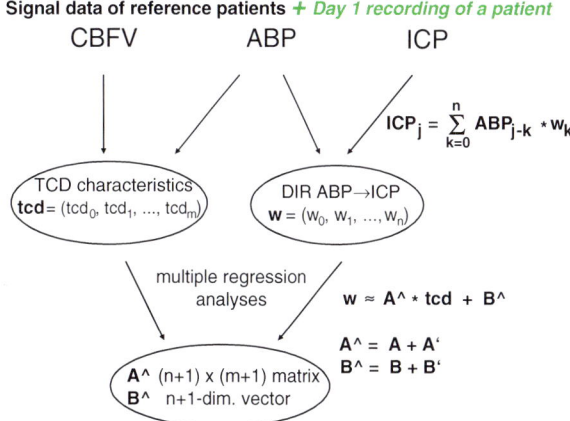
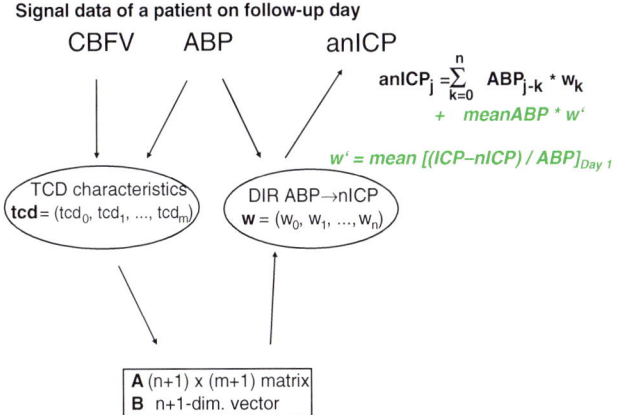
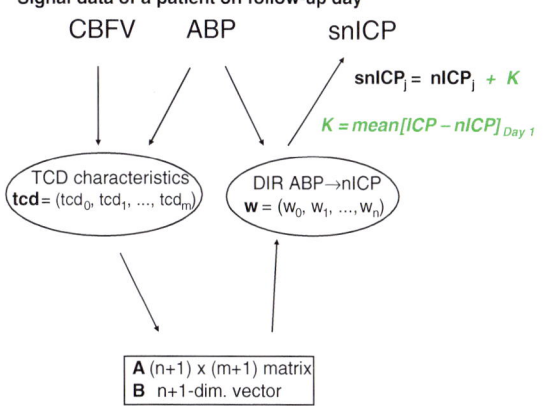

been computed by means of multiple regression analyses on data recordings of CBFV, ABP and (invasively assessed) ICP from a group of 197 reference patients with TBI ($n = 170$) or non-traumatic brain injuries, and it has been expressed in terms of matrix **A** and vector **B** [so-called nICP matrix (**A**, **B**)] (Fig. 1a). The reference patients have been treated earlier in Addenbrooke's Hospital (140) and Medical Centre Chemnitz. None of these patients were part of the study group.

Calibration Methods

If applied to a certain patient, calibration of the nICP procedure means adaptation to the individual characteristics of this patient in order to improve accuracy of ICP estimation. Calibration of the nICP assessment procedure may be achieved by an appropriate adjustment of either the nICP matrix [calibration 1 (Cal1)], the DIR ABP → ICP function [calibration 2 (Cal2)], or the calculated nICP itself [calibration 3 (Cal3)] (Fig. 1c). For Cal1 (Fig. 1d), the data of the day-1 recording of the patient is added to the reference patients' data. Then, multiple regression is reprocessed using this extended data, resulting in the modified nICP matrix ($A^\wedge$, $B^\wedge$). On subsequent days, ($A^\wedge$, $B^\wedge$) is used to calculate the calibrated cnICP signal. For Cal2 (Fig. 1e), the mean ratio $w' =$ mean of the (ICP − nICP)/ABP ratio of the day-1 recording is calculated. On subsequent days, w' is multiplied by the mean ABP (10-s average, recalculated every 10 s) and added to the calculated nICP to result in the calibrated anICP signal. For Cal3 (Fig. 1f), the mean difference $K =$ ICP − nICP of the day-1 recording is calculated. On subsequent days, the constant K is added to the calculated nICP to result in the calibrated snICP signal.

Results

In 2 of 41 patients, follow-up data could not be assessed because of patient death. In 39 patients, 76 follow-up recordings were performed (in nine patients, one follow-up recording; in 23 patients, two in seven patients, three). In these recordings, invasively assessed ICP ranged from 0.1 to 22.1 mmHg, the average ± standard deviation (SD) being 15.3 ± 17.2 mmHg. The mean differences (Bias), its SD and the mean absolute differences (ΔICP) between ICP and the nICP methods were: −5.6 ± 5.72 mmHg and 6.5 mmHg (standard nICP assessment); for cnICP (Cal1), −3.4 ± 5.68 mmHg and 5.4 mmHg ($p < 0.001$); for anICP (Cal2), +1.0 ± 7.22 mmHg and 5.6 mmHg; in the case of snICP (Cal3), +0.7 ± 6.98 mmHg and 5.5 mmHg. ΔICP in cnICP (5.4 mmHg) was significantly lower than ΔICP in nICP (6.5 mmHg) ($p < 0.001$; Wilcoxon test), while ΔICP in both anICP and snICP did not differ from ΔICP in nICP. The 95% confidence intervals (CI) of (ICP − nICP), calculated as the intervals (mean − 2 × SD, mean + 2 × SD), had half-lengths of 11.44, 11.36, 14.44 and 13.96 mmHg in standard, Cal1, Cal2 and Cal3 methods (Fig. 2).

Discussion

Different measures have been used in the past to assess the accuracy of calculated non-invasive ICP in patient populations [10]. Due to this fact, the results of these studies are difficult to compare. However, in recent work there had been a common tendency to assess the mean of the difference (ICP − nICP) together with its standard deviation in the test-population [11]. The mean (ICP − nICP) might be interpreted as the systematic error of nICP compared to invasive ICP reference in the tested population. This explains why mean (ICP − nICP) is also called Bias. The SD of (ICP − nICP) is a measure of the fluctuation of (ICP − nICP) around the Bias and is interpreted as the random error of the method [12]. Moreover, if the differences in ICP − nICP are normally distributed—which is usually true but should be verified—the SD is directly proportional to the size of the 95% CI of the nICP method.

However, both Bias and SD add to the deviation between invasive and non-invasively assessed ICP. In order to quantify this deviation, the authors used the mean of absolute difference ICP − nICP (ΔICP) and its 95th percentile as additional parameters. Both parameters do not need the assumption of a normal distribution.

The calibration methods Cal2 and Cal3 use constant shifts of the nICP (ICP − nICP, Cal3) and the ratio nICP/ABP [(ICP − nICP)/ABP, Cal2] in day 1 recordings to adjust the nICP assessment to the particular patient. By construction of these shifts, both anICP (Cal2) and snICP (Cal2) equals—on average—ICP in each of the day-1 recordings. Therefore, if applied to the day-1 recordings, both methods have a zero Bias. The follow-up recordings, however, belong to the same patient population. Therefore, a systematic error of nICP assessment in the follow-up day recordings should be similar to the systematic error in day-1 recordings. This consideration might explain the Bias of almost zero in methods Cal2 and Cal3.

However, a drawback of these methods was the observed increased SD. Different nICP shifts in different patients may create an inter-patient deviation of (ICP − nICP) which adds to the initial SD. This might be the reason for the increased SD of (ICP − nICP) of both the Cal2 and Cal3 methods. The idea of the Cal1 method was to integrate the individual haemodynamic peculiarities of the patient to the general model. This method is more "in the spirit" of the underlying data-based model than the other two calibrations. Compared to

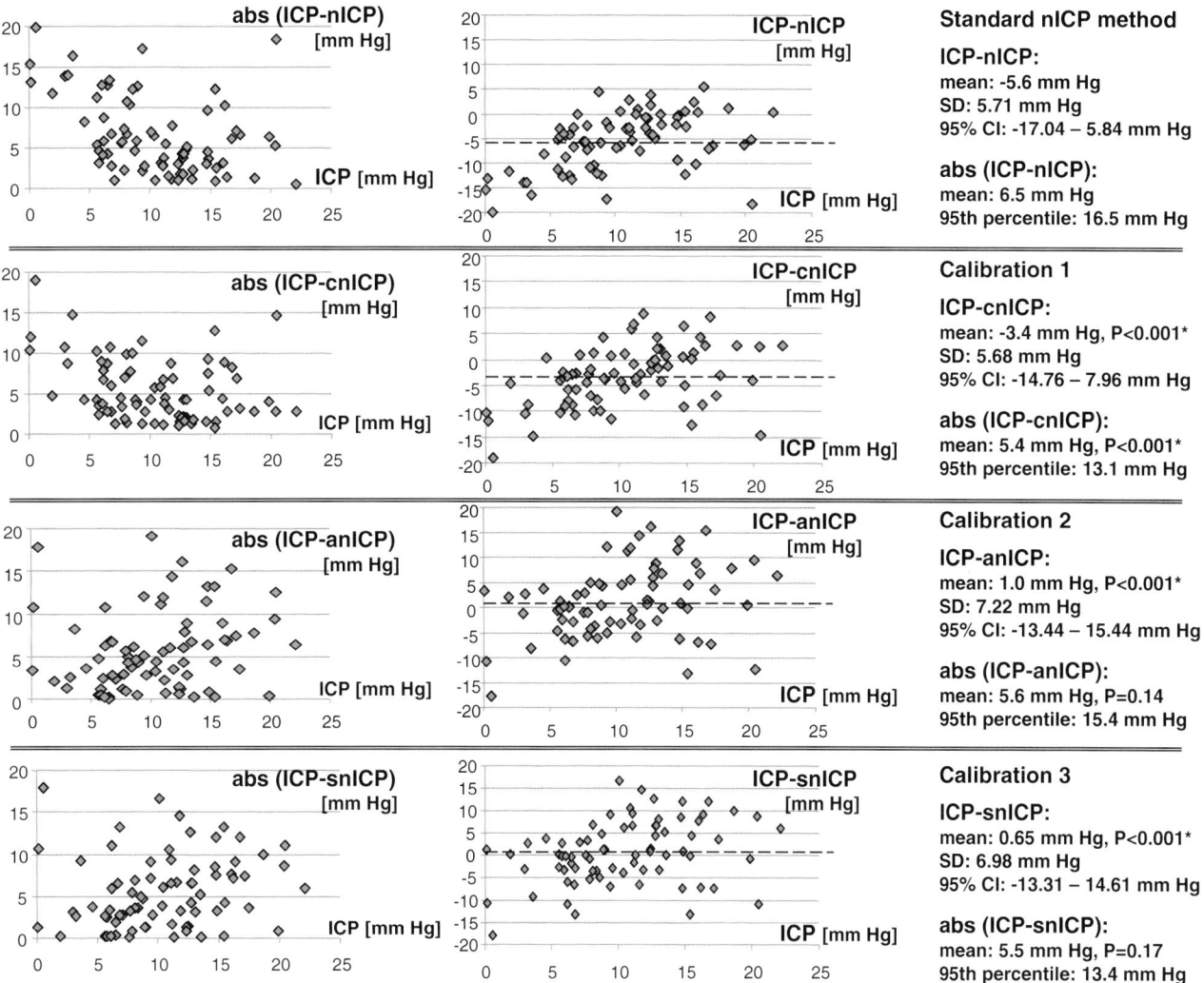

Fig. 2 Comparisons of standard nICP method and three calibration methods with ICP probe results. The figure shows scatter plots of absolute differences (*left*) as well as signed differences (*middle*) between ICP and nICP versus ICP in 76 recordings of 39 patients (all values in mmHg). Parameters describing the similarity between nICP and ICP are shown on the *right side*. The standard nICP assessment method showed a Bias [= mean (ICP − nICP)] of −5.6 mmHg with SD of 5.71 mmHg. ΔICP [= mean abs(ICP − nICP)] was 6.5 mmHg. In calibrations 2 and 3, the Bias could be reduced to almost zero ($p < 0.001$; *t*-test), while SD increased to 7 mmHg. ΔICP did not decrease significantly ($p > 0.1$; Wilcoxon test). In calibration 1, the Bias was reduced to −3.4 mmHg ($p < 0.001$; *t*-test). The SD was slightly lower than in the standard method, ΔICP was significantly lower ($p < 0.001$; Wilcoxon test), and its 95th percentile was the lowest of all methods

the standard nICP method, the Bias of cnICP assessment was reduced by 40%, while the SD decreased marginally. Overall, the deviation between ICP and nICP assessed in terms of ΔICP and its corresponding 95th percentile was lower in Cal1 than in both Cal2 and Cal3 methods.

Limitations

The Cal1 method used a combination of training and testing datasets for the construction of the nICP procedure. The training data should prevent a possible overfitting of the model and keep the model generally applicable. The test patient data (day 1 only) should specialise the model for application to the test patient. A balance between both datasets had to be found for both stability and improved individual accuracy. Although the process of Cal1 might look complicated if compared to Cal3, it may be easily automated using the day 1 recording as input data of specific Cal1 software.

Nineteen patients with craniotomy ($n = 19$) were part of the population studied, but none of the 197 reference patients used earlier for model construction underwent craniotomy. This might explain the strong Bias of nICP (−5.6 mmHg) compared to former studies (Bias = −1.3 mmHg) [13]. On the other hand, the objective of this study was to assess the power of the calibration methods to adapt to the individually differing features of patients.

Conclusions

The studied calibration methods were able to reduce the systematic error, but none of them did reduce the random error of nICP assessment. Cal2 and Cal3 almost completely abolished the Bias of nICP assessment, but increased its SD. Therefore, neither of these methods can be recommended. Cal1 reduced the Bias without increasing the SD. Therefore, the Cal1 method showed a moderate benefit and may be applied for nICP assessment after removal of the ICP probe.

Conflicts of interest statement The procedure of non-invasive ICP assessment is distributed as a plug-in for ICM+ monitoring software. B.S., J.K. and M.C. have financial interest in the fee. ICM+ is licensed by Cambridge Enterprise Ltd., UK. M.C. has financial interest in a fraction of the fee.

References

1. Klingelhöfer J, Conrad B, Benecke R, Sander D, Markakis E. Evaluation of intracranial pressure from transcranial Doppler studies in cerebral disease. J Neurol. 1988;235:159–62.
2. Aaslid R, Lundar T, Lindegaard KF, Nornes H. Estimation of cerebral perfusion pressure from arterial blood pressure and transcranial Doppler recordings. In: Miller JD, Teasdale GM, Rowan JO, Galbraith SL, Mendelow AD, editors. Intracranial pressure VI. New York: Springer; 1993. p. 226–9.
3. Czosnyka M, Matta BF, Smielewski P, Kirkpatrick P, Pickard JD. Cerebral perfusion pressure in head-injured patients: a noninvasive assessment using transcranial Doppler ultrasonography. J Neurosurg. 1998;88(5):802–8.
4. Kashif FM, Verghese GC, Novak V, Czosnyka M, Heldt T. Model-based noninvasive estimation of intracranial pressure from cerebral blood flow velocity and arterial pressure. Sci Transl Med. 2012;4(129):129ra44.
5. Varsos GV, Kolias AG, Smielewski P, Brady KM, Varsos VG, Hutchinson PJ, et al. A noninvasive estimation of cerebral perfusion pressure using critical closing pressure. J Neurosurg. 2015;123:638–48.
6. Schmidt B, Klingelhöfer J, Schwarze JJ, Sander D, Wittich I. Noninvasive prediction of intracranial pressure curves using transcranial ultrasonography and blood pressure curves. Stroke. 1997;28:2465–72.
7. Schmidt B, Czosnyka M, Schwarze JJ, Sander D, Gerstner W, Lumenta CB, Klingelhöfer J. Evaluation of a method for noninvasive intracranial pressure assessment during infusion studies in patients with hydrocephalus. J Neurosurg. 2000;92:793–800.
8. Schmidt B, Czosnyka M, Raabe A, Yahya H, Schwarze JJ, Sackerer D, Sander D, Klingelhöfer J. Adaptive non-invasive assessment of cerebral autoregulation and ICP. Stroke. 2003;34:84–9.
9. Marmarelis P, Marmarelis V. Analysis of physiological systems. New York: Plenum Press; 1978.
10. Cardim D, Robba C, Bohdanowicz M, Donnelly J, Cabella B, Liu X, et al. Non-invasive monitoring of intracranial pressure using transcranial Doppler ultrasonography: is it possible? Neurocrit Care. 2016;25(3):473–91. https://doi.org/10.1007/s12028-016-0258-6.
11. Cardim D, Robba C, Donnelly J, Bohdanowicz M, Schmidt B, Damian M, et al. Prospective study on non-invasive assessment of ICP in head injured patients: comparison of four methods. J Neurotrauma. 2016;33:1–11.
12. Krakauskaite S, Petkus V, Bartusis L, Zakelis R, Chomskis R, Preiksaitis A, et al. Accuracy, precision, sensitivity, and specificity of noninvasive ICP absolute value measurements. In: Ang BT, editor . Intracranial pressure and brain monitoring XV. Acta Neurochir Suppl; 2016;122:317–321.
13. Schmidt B, Czosnyka M, Smielewski P, Plontke R, Schwarze JJ, Klingelhöfer J, et al. Noninvasive assessment of ICP: evaluation of new TBI data. In: Ang B-T, editor. Intracranial pressure and brain monitoring XV. Acta Neurochir Suppl. 2016;122:69–73.

An Embedded Device for Real-Time Noninvasive Intracranial Pressure Estimation

Jonathan M. Matthews, Andrea Fanelli, and Thomas Heldt

Abstract *Objective*: The monitoring of intracranial pressure (ICP) is indicated for diagnosing and guiding therapy in many neurological conditions. Current monitoring methods, however, are highly invasive, limiting their use to the most critically ill patients only. Our goal is to develop and test an embedded device that performs all necessary mathematical operations in real-time for noninvasive ICP (nICP) estimation based on a previously developed model-based approach that uses cerebral blood flow velocity (CBFV) and arterial blood pressure (ABP) waveforms.

Materials and methods: The nICP estimation algorithm along with the required preprocessing steps were implemented on an NXP LPC4337 microcontroller unit (MCU). A prototype device using the MCU was also developed, complete with display, recording functionality, and peripheral interfaces for ABP and CBFV monitoring hardware.

Results: The device produces an estimate of mean ICP once per minute and performs the necessary computations in 410 ms, on average. Real-time nICP estimates differed from the original batch-mode MATLAB implementation of the estimation algorithm by 0.63 mmHg (root-mean-square error).

Conclusions: We have demonstrated that real-time nICP estimation is possible on a microprocessor platform, which offers the advantages of low cost, small size, and product modularity over a general-purpose computer. These attributes take a step toward the goal of real-time nICP estimation at the patient's bedside in a variety of clinical settings.

Keywords Intracranial pressure · Microcontroller · Biomedical device · Model-based estimation · Embedded system

Introduction

Intracranial pressure (ICP) is the hydrostatic pressure of cerebrospinal fluid (CSF). Elevated ICP can be extremely dangerous, as cerebral blood flow might become restricted and brain tissue may be compressed and shifted (herniation); elevated ICP often occurs due to space-filling lesions such as brain tumors, cerebral edema, hydrocephalus, or intracranial hemorrhage [1]. Monitoring ICP in patients suffering from such conditions is therefore imperative for alerting physicians to patient deterioration and the potential need for intervention. Current methods for monitoring ICP are highly invasive, involving the direct placement of a probe into the CSF space or brain tissue and come with inherent risks to the patient that can lead to complications. For this reason, noninvasive methods for estimating ICP are being developed [2].

Kashif *et al*. [3] developed a noninvasive ICP (nICP) estimation algorithm based on a lumped-parameter physiological model of blood flow through the cerebrovascular system. The electric circuit analog model represents the resistance to blood flow of the cerebral vasculature by a resistive element R and the lumped arterial/cerebral tissue elastic properties by a compliance element C. The estimation algorithm uses arterial blood pressure (ABP) and cerebral blood flow velocity (CBFV) waveforms as input to estimate R, C, and nICP. The algorithm was originally developed in MATLAB and runs in batch-mode, acting on windows of patient data after the data have been recorded and archived.

This paper presents a microcontroller-based implementation (Fig. 1) that uses the algorithm developed by Kashif *et al*. [3] to estimate nICP from ABP and CBFV signals acquired in real-time. ICP estimates are generated once every 60 s. The

---

J.M. Matthews, M.Eng. • T. Heldt, Ph.D. (✉)
Department of Electrical Engineering and Computer Science, Massachusetts Institute of Technology, Cambridge, MA, USA

Institute for Medical Engineering and Science, Massachusetts Institute of Technology, Cambridge, MA, USA
e-mail: thomas@mit.edu

A. Fanelli, Ph.D.
Institute for Medical Engineering and Science, Massachusetts Institute of Technology, Cambridge, MA, USA

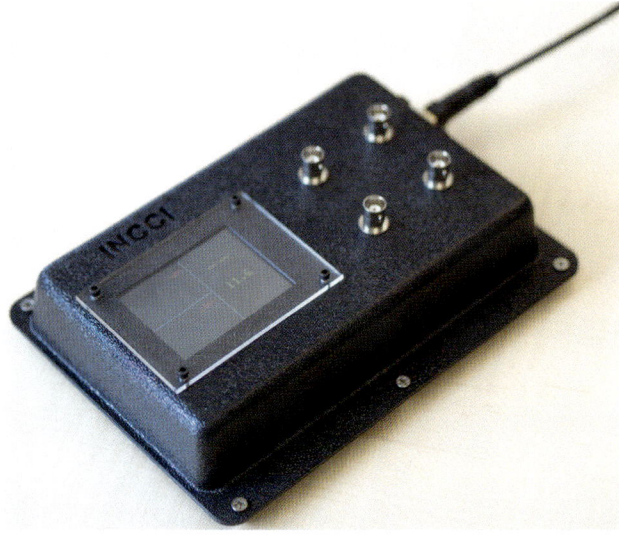

Fig. 1 The assembled device prototype for real-time noninvasive ICP estimation

device was also designed to connect to the analog outputs from standard noninvasive ABP and CBFV measurement hardware. ICP estimates, as well as the ABP and CBFV signals, are displayed on a liquid-crystal display (LCD) screen on the front panel and are also saved to a Secure Digital (SD) card within the device.

Materials and Methods

Core Tool Selection

The algorithm was implemented on an NXP LPC4337 microcontroller unit (MCU) [4], which was selected for its large SRAM capacity, processor speed, and available peripherals. C++ was selected as the implementation language for the device, and several open-source libraries (from the LPCOpen collection [5]) were used for controlling the LPC4337 hardware, such as setting the system control unit (SCU) and GPIO registers to select digital pin functionality.

Strategy for Real-Time Estimation

In the development of the prototype device, we first had to modify the original batch-mode implementation to allow for real-time estimation. To achieve this task, the real-time implementation is broken down into three stages. First, 60 s of CBFV and ABP data are recorded and stored in a local buffer. Second, the onset times of each ABP wavelet are determined [6]. Lastly, the onset times and recorded signals are passed to the model-based estimation procedure, which is also implemented on the embedded device. This three-stage process is repeated on successive data windows to produce a new estimate of nICP every 60 s.

Porting to C++

The MATLAB Coder tool [7] was used to port the original batch-mode MATLAB implementation of the ICP estimation algorithm to C++. The tool supports nearly all of the MATLAB language and produces C and C++ source code. However, the generated code is not optimized for a microcontroller implementation where memory is scarce. The C++ implementations of the heartbeat onset detection and ICP estimation algorithms required 1.8 MB and 348 kB of RAM, respectively, which far exceeded the available 136 kB of SRAM on the MCU. For this reason, a major step in the device implementation process was to reduce the memory usage of the ported algorithm.

To fit the code into the MCU memory, we manually optimized memory usage by addressing several major inefficiencies. The greatest inefficiency in the MATLAB-generated C++ code was that allocated memory was rarely reused. The implementation allocated temporary workspace data to new memory even when memory allocated earlier was no longer being used. We solved this issue by manually changing the C++ files to reuse workspace memory whenever possible. Additionally, the array sizes were unnecessarily large for our real-time estimation approach. For our optimized implementation, we assume that the maximum number of heartbeats possible in the 60-s window is (somewhat arbitrarily) 250 beats. The implementation ignores any heartbeats in excess of 250, and an estimate will be produced for the window containing the initial 250 beats. Further optimizations included using single-precision floating-point variables instead of double-precision variables and performing operations in a manner that reuses memory wherever possible, albeit at the cost of speed.

In the final implementation, the MCU SRAM is spread out over five separate memory locations in block sizes of 40 kB, 32 kB, 32 kB, 16 kB, and 16 kB, which created another memory-related implementation challenge. Some of the allocated arrays in the algorithm were over 30 kB large but could not span more than one SRAM block. To address this issue, we developed a software interface to provide virtual contiguous memory access to the separate memory blocks, allowing for tight packing of allocated space and for large arrays to be accessible even when spanning two or even three RAM blocks.

Peripherals

A Spencer ST[3] transcranial Doppler (TCD) ultrasound system [8] and Nexfin noninvasive cardiovascular monitor [9] recorded the CBFV and ABP, respectively. The analog outputs of both devices were connected to the two analog input ports implemented in our system. Analog waveforms were digitized through the analog-to-digital converters built into the LPC4337, and sampled at 250 samples/s.

An Adafruit 2.8″ thin-film-transistor (TFT) LCD [10] displayed the most recent nICP estimate. To lighten the computational load on the LPC4337, we used an Arduino Nano to control the LCD and display the ABP and CBFV waveforms as well as the estimated ICP.

Results

The device was tested on ABP and CBFV data from two sources: pre-recorded clinical data and real-time data from a human subject. In the first trial dataset, a pre-recorded 17-min clinical record of radial artery ABP and CBFV data was streamed to the device to simulate a real-time recording. In the second dataset, 20 min of ABP and CBFV data were collected from a volunteer subject using the Spencer TCD and Nexfin monitors, streamed in real-time to the device, and saved to the SD card along with the computed nICP estimates. The subject was sitting quietly in a chair for the duration of the measurement.

The real-time estimation approach was compared to the original batch-mode implementation of the estimation algorithm by running both methods on the same data. The real-time nICP estimates differed from the batch-mode estimates by a root-mean-square error (RMSE) of 0.63 mmHg and a mean-absolute-percentage error (MAPE) of 2.87% in the clinical record (Fig. 2) and by a RMSE of 3.03 mmHg and a MAPE of 4.93% in the 20-min trial. The total runtime of the real-time nICP estimation procedure was 52 ms/data window, on average, on a computer with a 2.5 GHz processor. The estimation on the embedded device took 410 ms/data window, on average, which represents a fraction of a cardiac cycle.

Discussion

In this paper, we present the development of an embedded device for estimating ICP through the real-time implementation of Kashif et al.'s algorithm [3]. The nICP estimates produced by the real-time implementation on the device are comparable to those produced by the original batch-mode implementation in MATLAB. Moreover, the device can be directly connected to a Nexfin monitor and to a TCD system and receive analog data from their respective analog outputs. The nICP estimates are displayed on an LCD screen and saved on a microSD card. This system represents a working proof-of-concept that allows continuous estimation of ICP in real time.

Our results show that the real-time nICP estimates differed from the original batch-mode MATLAB implementation of the algorithm by 0.63 mmHg. This discrepancy is negligible in the clinical context of ICP measurement and is largely due to the difference in estimation windows. In the batch-mode algorithm, a 60-beat window is slid across the archived dataset, advancing the data window one heartbeat at a time. In the real-time algorithm, 60 s of data were collected and then processed to produce a single nICP estimate. The remaining discrepancy is attributed to the heartbeat onset detection algorithm, which is run on the entire dataset at once in the batch-mode implementation but is run once per 60-s window in the real-time implementation. Overall, however, the magnitude of the discrepancies between the batch-

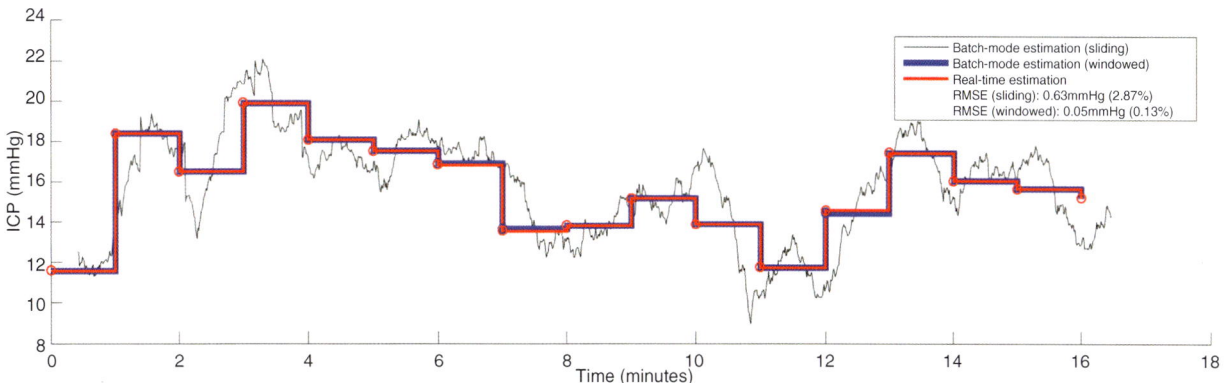

Fig. 2 Comparison of ICP estimates produced by the sliding-window and non-overlapping batch-mode implementation to those produced by the real-time implementation on the MCU

mode implementation of the nICP algorithm and the real-time implementation on the embedded device is clinically irrelevant, as it is a fraction of a millimeter of mercury.

Conclusions

This paper presents a real-time implementation of the Kashif algorithm for continuous and noninvasive estimation of ICP. The device has been developed by: (1) porting the Kashif algorithm to a microprocessor platform and optimizing its performance for real-time ABP and CBFV waveform acquisition; (2) developing an embedded device prototype, complete with peripheral interfaces for connection to existing TCD and ABP monitoring hardware, and display and recording functionality for clinical use and post-acquisition analysis; and (3) verifying that a real-time windowed approach performs comparable to the batch-mode MATLAB implementation of the Kashif algorithm. These contributions take a clear step toward the goal of real-time noninvasive ICP estimation at the patient's bedside in a variety of clinical settings.

Conflicts of interest statement We declare that we have no conflict of interest.

References

1. Steiner LA, Andrews PJ. Monitoring the injured brain: ICP and CBF. Br J Anaesth. 2006;97(1):26–38.
2. Popovic D, Khoo M, Lee S. Noninvasive monitoring of intracranial pressure. Recent Pat Biomed Eng. 2009;2:165–79.
3. Kashif FM, Verghese GC, Novak V, Czosnyka M, Heldt T. Model-based noninvasive estimation of intracranial pressure from cerebral blood flow velocity and arterial pressure. SSci Transl Med. 2012;4(129):129–44.
4. NXP Semiconductor. LPC435x/3x/2x/1x product data sheet. http://www.nxp.com/documents/data_sheet/LPC435X_3X_2X_1X.pdf. May 2016.
5. NXP Semiconductor. LPCOpen libraries and examples. http://www.nxp.com/products/microcontrollers-and-processors/arm-processors/lpc-mcus/software-tools/lpcopen-libraries-and-examples:LPC-OPEN-LIBRARIES. Feb 2017.
6. Zong W, Heldt T, Moody GB, Mark RG. An open-source algorithm to detect onset of arterial blood pressure pulses. Comput Cardio. 2003;30:259–62.
7. MathWorks. MATLAB coder. https://www.mathworks.com/products/matlab-coder.html. Feb 2017.
8. Spencer Technologies. ST^3 transcranial ultrasound system. https://www.spencertechnologies.com. Feb 2017.
9. BMEYE. BMEYE monitor series: continuous, non-invasive cardiovascular monitoring. http://medaval.ie/wp-content/uploads/device-specs/BMEYE-Nexfin-Specs.pdf. Feb 2017.
10. Adafruit. 2.8" TFT LCD with touchscreen breakout board w/ MicroSD socket - ILI9341. https://www.adafruit.com/product/1770. Feb 2017.

Transcranial Bioimpedance Measurement as a Non-invasive Estimate of Intracranial Pressure

Christopher Hawthorne, Martin Shaw, Ian Piper, Laura Moss, and John Kinsella

Abstract *Objectives*: We have previously demonstrated a relationship between transcranial bioimpedance (TCB) measurements and intracranial pressure (ICP) in an animal model of raised ICP. The primary objective of this study was to explore the relationship between non-invasive bioelectrical impedance measurements of the brain and skull and ICP in traumatic brain injury (TBI) patients.

Materials and methods: Included patients were adults admitted to the Neurological Intensive Care Unit with TBI and undergoing invasive ICP monitoring as part of their routine clinical care. Multi-frequency TCB measurements were performed hourly through bi-temporal electrodes. The bioimpedance parameters of Z_c (impedance at the characteristic frequency) and R_0 (resistance to a direct current) were then modelled against ICP using unadjusted and adjusted linear models.

Results: One hundred and sixty-eight TCB measurements were available from ten study participants. Using an unadjusted linear modelling approach, there was no significant relationship between measured ICP and Z_c or R_0. The most significant relationship between ICP and TCB parameters was found by adjusting for multiple patient specific variables and using Z_c and R_0 normalised per patient ($p < 0.0001$, $r^2 = 0.32$).

Conclusions: These pilot results confirm some degree of relationship between TCB parameters and invasively measured ICP. The magnitude of this relationship is small and, on the basis of the current study, TCB is unlikely to provide a clinically useful estimate of ICP in patients admitted with TBI.

Keywords Neurological Intensive Care · Traumatic brain injury · Intracranial pressure · Bioimpedance · Mathematical modelling

Introduction

Background

The Brain Trauma Foundation recommends management of patients with severe traumatic brain injury (TBI) using information from intracranial pressure (ICP) to reduce in-hospital and 2-week post-injury mortality [1]. ICP is typically measured using invasive pressure monitors that are associated with specific complications and can generally only be inserted in specialist centres. To provide ICP monitoring to a wider clinical population, multiple attempts have been made to develop a non-invasive technique. Transcranial bioimpedance (TCB) measurement was considered to be a potential approach to non-invasive ICP monitoring.

Fundamentals of Bioelectrical Impedance

Bioimpedance is the ability of biological tissue to impede electric current. Techniques are available to measure bioimpedance from all or part of the body using cutaneous electrodes in a process known as bioelectrical impedance analysis (BIA) [2].

C. Hawthorne (✉)
Department of Neuroanaesthesia, Institute of Neurological Sciences, Queen Elizabeth University Hospital, Glasgow, UK
e-mail: cwhawthorne@doctors.org.uk

M. Shaw • L. Moss
Department of Clinical Physics, NHS Greater Glasgow and Clyde, Glasgow, UK

Academic Unit of Anaesthesia, Pain and Critical Care Medicine, University of Glasgow, Glasgow, UK

I. Piper
Department of Clinical Physics, NHS Greater Glasgow and Clyde, Glasgow, UK

J. Kinsella
Academic Unit of Anaesthesia, Pain and Critical Care Medicine, University of Glasgow, Glasgow, UK

Bioimpedance is the vector sum of capacitive resistance (or reactance) and resistive resistance (simply called resistance). Electric current of low frequency tends to be conducted through the extracellular space when the cell membrane acts as an insulator, whereas electric current of high frequency is conducted through both the extra- and intracellular spaces. The equation relating the different factors is

$$Z = R + iX_c \quad (1)$$

where Z is overall impedance, R is resistance and iX_c is reactance. The magnitude of bioimpedance can be calculated by

$$|Z| = \left(R^2 + iX_c^2\right)^{\frac{1}{2}} \quad (2)$$

Bioimpedance measured using devices capable of delivering a broad band of frequencies (typically around 1–1000 kHz) is known as bioelectrical spectroscopy. Under these circumstances it is possible to plot the reactance and resistance measurements made at each frequency to construct a Cole-Cole plot [3] (Fig. 1).

Bioimpedance Measurements of the Brain

Application of bioimpedance measurements to the human brain is not a new development. Indeed, rheoencephalography (REG), or electrical impedance measurement of brain circulation, has been investigated for several decades without transitioning into clinical practice [4]. Several more recent studies have investigated intermittent measures of bioimpedance in brain pathologies ranging from ischaemic and haemorrhagic stroke to intracerebral tumours and hydrocephalus [5–7].

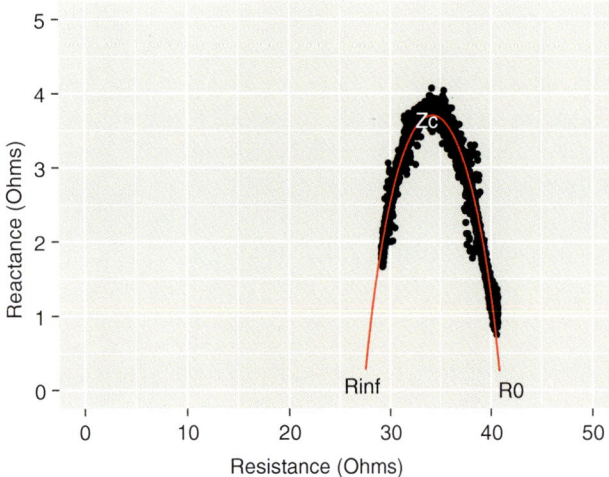

Fig. 1 An example of a fitted Cole-Cole curve from TCB data, where R_0 represents resistance measured with a direct current, R_{inf} the resistance measured with an infinitely high frequency alternating current and Z_c the impedance measured at maximum reactance

TCB as a Non-invasive Estimate of ICP

We postulated that TCB measurements made across the skull would provide an estimate of ICP in traumatic brain injury patients. Bioimpedance measurements are affected by both intracellular swelling and the size of the extracellular space. These factors are also known to affect cerebral compliance. There is a well-defined exponential relationship between ICP and intracranial compliance; there may also be a definable relationship between ICP and transcranial bioimpedance. In support of this approach, there is experimental evidence in a neonatal piglet model of brain tissue hypoxia and in a sheep model of raised ICP, showing that TCB parameters correlate well with ICP [8, 9]. Therefore, the primary objective of this study was to explore the relationship between TCB measurements and ICP in TBI patients.

Materials and Methods

Study Population and Data Collection

Ethical approval was granted for the study by Scotland A Research Ethics Committee (Reference Number: 11/AL/0320). Study participants were prospectively recruited from patients admitted to the Neurological Intensive Care Unit at the Institute of Neurological Sciences. Included patients were over 16 years of age, admitted with a traumatic brain injury and undergoing invasive ICP monitoring as part of their routine clinical care.

TCB measurements were performed using the Impedimed SFB7 Bio-impedance Spectroscopy Unit (ImpediMed, Pinkenba, Queensland, Australia). The device is a single channel BIA unit that acquires 256 separate measurements between 4 and 1000 kHz. The cutaneous electrodes were placed in a bi-temporal configuration and measurements made hourly. At each measurement time point, the device was programmed to perform 40 separate TCB recordings over 1 min.

Data Preprocessing

All data processing and analysis was performed using RStudio Version 0.98.1102 running R Version 3.1.2 [10]. TCB data was downloaded from the SFB7 device and Cole-Cole plots fitted to extract a summary measure for Z_c and R_0 at each measurement point. Waveform resolution ICP recordings were downloaded from the patient monitoring system using iXtrends software [11] and a median ICP for the 5 min around each TCB measurement calculated.

Statistical Modelling and Analysis

Attempts were made to model ICP using both absolute and normalised values of Z_c and R_0. In the animal studies referred to above, Z_c had an inverse relationship with ICP, while R_0 had a direct relationship. An unadjusted linear modelling approach was first taken to confirm some degree of relationship between TCB and ICP.

An adjusted linear modelling approach was subsequently taken to explore which patient specific variables could be used to further define the relationship between ICP and Z_c or R_0. Each of the patient variables of gender, age, weight and height, along with computed tomography (CT)-derived measurements of soft tissue swelling and brain diameter, as well as whole body bioimpedance measurement and temperature, were included in linear models. Patient variables that did not significantly contribute to the model were sequentially removed. The simplified model was then compared against the original using analysis of deviance testing to confirm that they were not significantly different.

The final modelling approach was to use the Akaike information criterion (AIC) in backward stepwise regression to select the models with the best balance of goodness of fit and low complexity.

Results

Patient Demographics

One hundred and sixty-eight TCB measurements were available from ten patients admitted with TBI. There was one female patient and the median age was 51 (29–61) years. The primary diagnosis was subdural haematoma, extradural haematoma or contusions in three cases each, with a single case of diffuse axonal injury.

Unadjusted Linear Models

ICP was first plotted against measured Z_c and R_0 to allow visual inspection for any obvious relationship (Fig. 2). Using an unadjusted linear modelling approach, there was no significant relationship between measured ICP and Z_c or R_0. When Z_c and R_0 values were normalised for each patient, there was a significant relationship between ICP and normalised Z_c ($p < 0.001$), a significant inverse relationship between the log of ICP and normalised Z_c ($p < 0.01$) and a significant relationship between ICP and normalised R_0 ($p < 0.001$). The adjusted r^2 value for each of these relation-

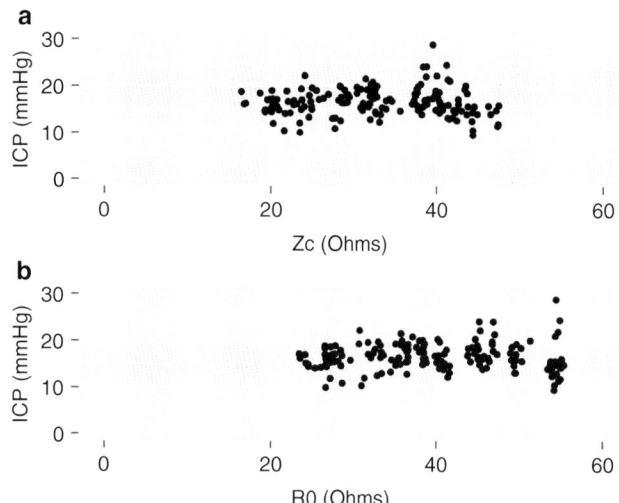

Fig. 2 Plot of ICP against measured Z_c (**a**) and R_0 (**b**) for the entire study population

ships was small (0.09, 0.06 and 0.18 respectively). Attempts were therefore made to explore the relationship between ICP and TCB parameters by adjusting the linear models for patient-specific variables.

Adjusted Linear Models

Using measured TCB parameters, the simplified adjusted model with the greatest r^2 value was:

$$\mathrm{ICP} = a_1 R_0 + a_2 G + a_3 W + a_4 H + a_5 \mathrm{BD} + a_6 \mathrm{WBZ}_c + b \quad (3)$$

where G = gender, W = weight, H = height, BD = brain diameter and WBZc = whole body bioimpedance ($p < 0.0001$, $r^2 = 0.19$, estimates in Table 1).

The simplified adjusted model with the greatest r^2 value using normalised bioimpedance measurements was:

$$\mathrm{ICP} = a_1 \exp\left(\frac{1}{Z_{\mathrm{norm}}}\right) + a_2 R_{\mathrm{norm}} + a_3 G + a_4 \mathrm{ST} + a_5 T + a_6 \mathrm{WBZ}_{\mathrm{norm}} + b \quad (4)$$

where ST = soft tissue thickness and T = temperature ($p < 0.0001$, $r^2 = 0.32$, estimates in Table 2).

Backward Stepwise Regression

The models selected and their r^2 values calculated using a backward stepwise regression approach were essentially the same as those selected in using the adjusted linear modelling approach (Eqs. 3 and 4).

Table 1 Estimates for model shown in Eq. 1

	Estimate	Standard error	p value
a_1	0.20	0.04	<0.0001
a_2	−5.68	0.92	<0.0001
a_3	0.08	0.03	<0.05
a_4	0.28	0.06	<0.0001
a_5	−0.41	0.12	<0.001
a_6	−0.02	0.004	<0.0001
b	15.03	10.10	0.14

Table 2 Estimates for model shown in Eq. 2

	Estimate	Standard error	p value
a_1	2.92	0.94	<0.01
a_2	9.60	1.77	<0.0001
a_3	−3.81	0.80	<0.0001
a_4	0.13	0.03	<0.0001
a_5	0.90	0.31	<0.01
a_6	12.12	5.02	<0.05
b	−48.50	13.17	<0.001

Discussion

TCB has been considered for the early detection of multiple brain pathologies [5–7]. Based on the known relationship between bioimpedance and the volume of the intracellular and extracellular spaces, we investigated the potential use of TCB as an estimate of ICP in TBI. Previously published animal experiments have shown a direct relationship between the TCB parameter of R_0 and ICP [8] and an indirect relationship between Z_c and the log of ICP [9].

In this study, we used a number of linear modelling approaches to explore the relationship between TCB and ICP. Using unadjusted linear models, we were unable to demonstrate any significant relationship between the measured values of either Z_c or R_0 and ICP. When TCB variables were normalised per patient (as was done in the previous animal studies), there was a small but significant relationship. When we accounted for a number of patient-specific variables in both adjusted linear models and backward stepwise regression, the relationship between TCB parameters and ICP was more statistically significant but not likely to be of clinically significant value.

Limitations of this study included the relatively small number of patients with an associated small number of extreme ICP values. Even allowing for this concern, however, within each individual patient's results there was no clear trending of TCB values with ICP. It could be argued that TBI patients were not the best patient population to explore the relationship between TCB and ICP. From a practical point of view, the associated soft tissue injuries made cutaneous electrode contact difficult. In addition, the very mixed nature of the underlying pathological processes is likely to have complicated the modelling task.

Conclusion

These pilot results confirm some degree of relationship between TCB parameters and invasively measured ICP. The magnitude of this relationship is small and, on the basis of the current study, TCB is unlikely to provide a clinically useful estimate of ICP in patients admitted with TBI.

Acknowledgements This study was funded by the Association of Anaesthetists of Great Britain and Ireland/Anaesthesia via the National Institute of Academic Anaesthesia (WKR0-2011-0039).

Conflicts of interest statement We declare that we have no conflict of interest.

References

1. Carney N, Totten AM, O'Reilly C, Ullman JS, Hawryluk GW, Bell MJ, et al. Guidelines for the management of severe traumatic brain injury, fourth edition. Neurosurgery. 2017;80(1):6–15.
2. Kyle UG, Bosaeus I, De Lorenzo AD, Deurenberg P, Elia M, Gomez JM, et al. Bioelectrical impedance analysis—part I: review of principles and methods. Clin Nutr. 2004;23(5):1226–43.
3. Cole KS, Cole RH. Dispersion and absorption in dielectrics I. Alternating current characteristics. J Chem Phys. 1941;9(4):341–51.
4. Bodo M. Studies in rheoencephalography (REG). J Electr Bioimp. 2010;1:18–40.
5. Grasso G, Alafaci C, Passalacqua M, Morabito A, Buemi M, Salpietro FM, et al. Assessment of human brain water content by cerebral bioelectrical impedance analysis: a new technique and its application to cerebral pathological conditions. Neurosurgery. 2002;50(5):1064–72. discussion 72-4
6. Liu LX, Dong WW, Wang J, Wu Q, He W, Jia YJ. The role of noninvasive monitoring of cerebral electrical impedance in stroke. Acta Neurochir Suppl. 2005;95:137–40.
7. Seoane F, Reza Atefi S, Tomner J, Kostulas K, Lindecrantz K. Electrical bioimpedance spectroscopy on acute unilateral stroke patients: initial observations regarding differences between sides. Biomed Res Int. 2015;2015:12.
8. Lingwood BE, Dunster KR, Colditz PB, Ward LC. Noninvasive measurement of cerebral bioimpedance for detection of cerebral edema in the neonatal piglet. Brain Res. 2002;945(1):97–105.
9. Shaw M, Piper I, Campbell P, McKeown C, Britton J, Oommen K, et al. Investigation of the relationship between transcranial impedance and intracranial pressure. Acta Neurochir Suppl. 2012;114:61–5.
10. R Core Team. R: a language and environment for statistical computing. Vienna: R Foundation for Statistical Computing; 2014.
11. ixellence GmbH. ixTrends. Germany; 2011.

Pulsed Electromagnetic Field (PEMF) Mitigates High Intracranial Pressure (ICP) Induced Microvascular Shunting (MVS) in Rats

Denis E. Bragin, Olga A. Bragina, Sean Hagberg, and Edwin M. Nemoto

Abstract *Objective*: High-frequency pulsed electromagnetic field (PEMF) stimulation is an emerging noninvasive therapy that we have shown increases cerebral blood flow (CBF) and tissue oxygenation in the healthy rat brain. In this work, we tested the effect of PEMF on the brain at high intracranial pressure (ICP). We previously showed that high ICP in rats caused a transition from capillary (CAP) to non-nutritive microvascular shunt (MVS) flow, tissue hypoxia and increased blood brain barrier (BBB) permeability.

Methods: Using *in vivo* two-photon laser scanning microscopy (2PLSM) over the rat parietal cortex, and studied the effects of PEMF on microvascular blood flow velocity, tissue oxygenation (NADH autofluorescence), BBB permeability and neuronal necrosis during 4 h of elevated ICP to 30 mmHg.

Results: PEMF significantly dilated arterioles, increased capillary blood flow velocity and reduced MVS/capillary ratio compared to sham-treated animals. These effects led to a significant decrease in tissue hypoxia, BBB degradation and neuronal necrosis.

Conclusions: PEMF attenuates high ICP-induced pathological microcirculatory changes, tissue hypoxia, BBB degradation and neuronal necrosis.

Keywords Cerebral blood flow · High intracranial pressure · Microvascular shunts · Pulsed electromagnetic field · Rats

D.E. Bragin, Ph.D. (✉) • O.A. Bragina • S. Hagberg
E.M. Nemoto
Department of Neurosurgery, University of New Mexico School of Medicine, Albuquerque, NM, USA
e-mail: dbragin@salud.unm.edu

Introduction

High intracranial pressure (ICP) is a serious consequence of severe brain injury that often leads to cerebral ischemia, cerebral edema, tissue compression, herniation, restriction of blood supply to the entire brain, and, finally, brain death. Current treatment paradigms for high ICP are initiated in tiers, each focused on reducing ICP to prevent secondary injury without clinically proven neuroprotective strategies. High-frequency pulsed electromagnetic field (PEMF) stimulation is an emerging noninvasive therapy that induces small electrical currents in tissue. PEMF has an anti-inflammatory effect in the traumatized brain and has been suggested as an adjunctive treatment in brain disorders [1]. We recently demonstrated that PEMF exposure in the healthy rat brain induces vasodilation, increases microvascular blood flow velocity and tissue oxygenation [2]. In previous works we also showed – to our knowledge for the first time – that high ICP in a rat brain induces a transition from low-velocity capillary flow to high velocity non-nutritive microvascular shunt flow (MVS) resulting in tissue hypoxia, brain edema, blood brain barrier damage and neuronal death [3, 4]. Here, we determined whether PEMF could mitigate pathological consequences caused by non-nutritive MVS flow induced by high ICP.

Materials and Methods

The institutional animal care and use committee of the University of New Mexico Health Sciences Center approved the protocol for these studies, which were conducted according to the National Institutes of Health Guide for the Care and Use of Laboratory Animals. Most of the procedures used in this study have been previously described [2, 3].

Experimental Paradigm

Using *in vivo* two-photon laser scanning microscopy (2PLSM) over the rat parietal cortex, we studied the effects of PEMF on microvascular red blood cell flow velocity visualized by serum labeled with tetra-methylrhodamine dextran (TMR), tissue oxygenation (NADH autofluorescence), BBB permeability (TMR extravasation) and neuronal necrosis (i.v. propidium iodide) during 4 h of elevated ICP. ICP and arterial pressure, rectal and cranial temperatures, blood gases and electrolytes were monitored. After baseline imaging at normal ICP (10 mmHg), rats were subjected to high ICP (30 mmHg) by raising an artificial cerebrospinal fluid reservoir connected to a catheter in the cisterna magna. At ICP of 30 mmHg, PEMF was applied for 30 min using the SofPulse device and imaging continuously performed for up to 4 h after the treatment (ten rats). The PEMF signal was a 27.12-MHz carrier modulated by a 3-ms burst repeating at 5 Hz. The signal amplitude was adjusted to provide 6 ± 1 V/m within the rat brain. Controls were treated with sham PEMF (ten rats).

Surgery

Acclimated Sprague–Dawley male rats (Harlan Laboratories, Indianapolis, IN, USA), weighing between 300 and 350 g, were intubated and mechanically ventilated on 2% isoflurane/30% oxygen/70% nitrous oxide. Rectal and temporal muscle temperature thermistors were inserted. Femoral venous and arterial catheters were inserted for injections, arterial pressure monitoring, and blood sampling. A catheter was inserted into the cisterna magna for ICP monitoring and manipulation. For imaging, a craniotomy 5 mm in diameter was made over the left parietal cortex, filled with 2% agarose/saline, and sealed with a cover glass.

Microscopy

An Olympus BX51WI upright microscope and a water-immersion LUMPlan FL/IR 20×/0.50 W objective were used. Excitation (740 nm) was provided by a Prairie View Ultima multiphoton laser scan unit powered by a Millennia Prime 10-W diode laser source pumping a Tsunami Ti: sapphire laser (Spectra-Physics, Mountain View, CA, USA). Blood plasma was labeled by i.v. injection of tetramethylrhodamine isothiocyanate dextran (155 kDa) in physiological saline (5% w/v). All microvessels in an imaging volume (500 × 500 × 300 μm) were scanned at each study point, measuring the diameter and blood flow velocity in each vessel (3–20 μm diameter). Tetramethylrhodamine fluorescence was band pass filtered at 560–600 nm and NADH autofluorescence at 425–475 nm. Imaging data processing and analysis were carried out using the NIH ImageJ processing package.

Statistical Analyses

Statistical analyses were carried out using Student's *t*-test or the Kolmogorov–Smirnov test where appropriate. Differences between groups were determined using two-way analysis of variance (ANOVA) for multiple comparisons and post hoc testing using the Mann–Whitney *U* test. The statistical significance level was set at $p < 0.05$. Data are presented as mean ± SEM.

Results

As in our previous studies, increased ICP to 30 mmHg in the sham-stimulated group caused a redistribution of blood flow from normal capillary flow to MVS flow with an increase in the MVS/CAP ratio from 0.43 ± 0.04 to 0.94 ± 0.08, $p < 0.001$ from baseline (Fig. 1b). The flow velocities of red blood cells in capillaries decreased to $74.2 \pm 13.8\%$, $p < 0.05$ from baseline (Fig. 1a). Pathological changes in cerebral microcirculation led to reduction of tissue oxygenation as reflected by increase in NADH autofluorescence to $129.1 \pm 11.2\%$, $p < 0.01$ from baseline, and BBB damage as reflected by increase of perivascular fluorescence due TMR extravasation to $158.2 \pm 16.3\%$, $p < 0.001$ (Fig. 1c). At the end of monitoring, 4 h after ICP increase, $26.1 \pm 6.2\%$ of neurons died by necrotic mechanism, as reflected by propidium iodide fluorescence in neuronal nuclei, $p < 0.001$ (Fig. 1c); i.v. injected propidium iodide becomes fluorescent after binding to nucleic acids, but as a cell-membrane-impermeable molecule, it labels only necrotic cells with damaged membranes [5].

PEMF treatment dilated arterioles by $4.5 \pm 3.2\%$, $p < 0.05$ from the sham-treated group. The increased blood volume perfused through arterioles elevated blood flow velocities in capillaries to $86.8 \pm 13.2\%$, $p < 0.05$ (Fig. 1a). As a result, MVS/CAP ratio was lower than in the sham-treated group (0.78 ± 0.06, $p < 0.05$, Fig. 1b). These were associated with decreased tissue hypoxia as reflected by a lower NADH autofluorescence ($118.3 \pm 8.4\%$, $p < 0.05$) and decreased BBB permeability as reflected by reduced dye extravasation ($121.1 \pm 14.2\%$, $p < 0.01$c). PEMF reduced neuronal necrosis to $15.2 \pm 3.6\%$, $p < 0.05$ compared with the sham-treated group (Fig. 1c).

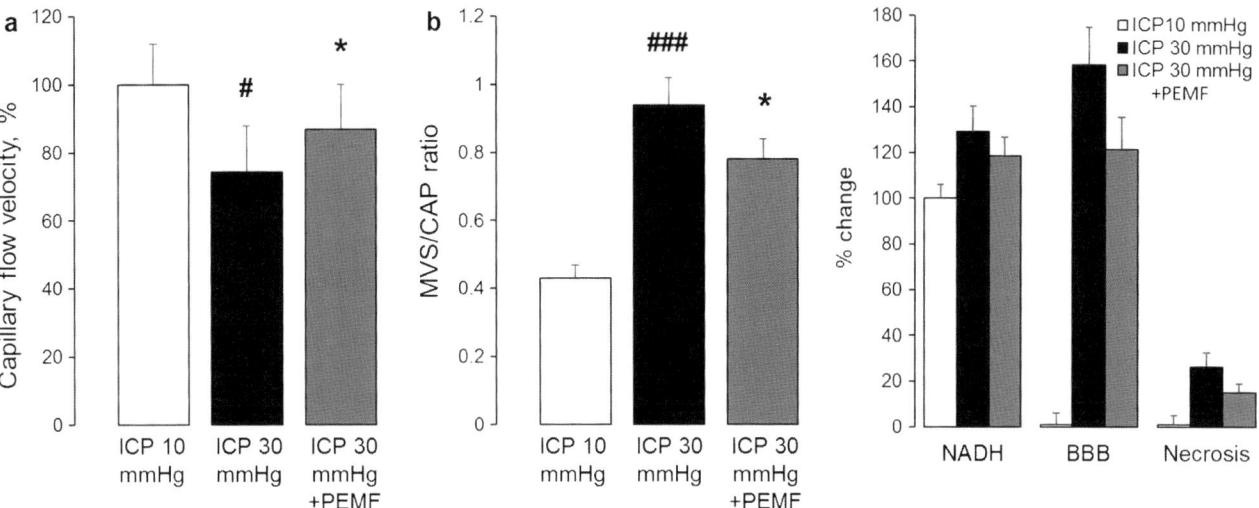

Fig. 1 High-frequency pulsed electromagnetic field stimulation enhances capillary flow velocity (**a**), reduces microvascular shunt/capillary flow ratio (**b**), and attenuates tissue hypoxia, blood brain barrier damage and necrosis of neurons caused by 4 h of intracranial hypertension (ICP = 30 mmHg). Data are presented as mean ± SEM, n = 10 rats per group, $^\#p < 0.05$, $^{\#\#}p < 0.01$, $^{\#\#\#}p < 0.001$ from a baseline of ICP = 10 mmHg, $*p < 0.05$, $**p < 0.01$ from sham-treated group

Discussion

Our results show that PEMF reduces tissue hypoxia, BBB degradation and neuronal necrosis at high ICP by increasing cerebral microvascular perfusion via reducing MVS flow, increasing flow through capillaries as a result of dilatation of arterioles, which we have shown occurs by a nitric oxide-dependent mechanism [1].

Conclusion

PEMF attenuates high ICP-induced pathological microcirculatory changes, tissue hypoxia, BBB degradation and neuronal necrosis and has potential as an effective therapy for high ICP.

Acknowledgments This work was supported by Rio Grande Neurosciences, National Institutes for Health P20GM109089, and RMSE No 12.1223.2017/AP. We thank Anthony Gravagne from the Department of Physics and Astronomy, University of New Mexico, for designing and manufacturing the non-magnetic plastic stereotactic head frame for imaging.

Conflicts of interest statement We declare that we have no conflict of interest.

References

1. Rasouli J, Lekhraj R, White NM, Flamm ES, Pilla AA, Strauch B, Casper D. Attenuation of interleukin-1beta by pulsed electromagnetic fields after traumatic brain injury. Neurosci Lett. 2012;519(1):4–8.
2. Bragin DE, Statom GL, Hagberg S, Nemoto EM. Increases in microvascular perfusion and tissue oxygenation via pulsed electromagnetic fields in the healthy rat brain. J Neurosurg. 2015;122(5):1239–47.
3. Bragin DE, Bush RC, Müller WS, Nemoto EM. High intracranial pressure effects on cerebral cortical microvascular flow in rats. J Neurotrauma. 2011;28(5):775–85.
4. Dai X, Bragina O, Zhang T, Yang Y, Rao GR, Bragin DE, Statom G, Nemoto EM. High intracranial pressure induced injury in the healthy rat brain. Crit Care Med. 2016;44(8):e633–8.
5. Fumagalli S, Coles JA, Ejlerskov P, Ortolano F, Bushell TJ, Brewer JM, De Simoni MG, Dever G, Garside P, Maffia P, Carswell HV. In vivo real-time multiphoton imaging of T lymphocytes in the mouse brain after experimental stroke. Stroke. 2011;42(5):1429–36.

Volumetric Ophthalmic Ultrasound for Inflight Monitoring of Visual Impairment and Intracranial Pressure

Aaron Dentinger, Michael MacDonald, Douglas Ebert, Kathleen Garcia, and Ashot Sargsyan

Abstract *Objective*: The objective is enhanced ophthalmic ultrasound imaging to monitor ocular structure and intracranial dynamics changes related to visual impairment and intracranial pressure (ICP) induced by microgravity. The goals are to improve the ease of use and reduce operator variability by automatically rendering improved views of the anatomy and deriving new metrics of the morphology and dynamics.

Materials and methods: A prototype three-dimensional (3-D) probe was integrated onto a portable ultrasound scanner. Image analysis algorithms were developed to automatically detect the ocular anatomy and simultaneously render views of the optic nerve with improved sheath definition. Curvature metrics were calculated from 3-D retinal surfaces to quantify posterior globe flattening, and tissue velocity waveforms of the optic nerve were analyzed to assess intracranial dynamics.

Results: New 3-D structural measurements were evaluated in a head-down tilt study. The response of optic nerve sheath and globe flattening metrics were quantified in 11 healthy volunteers from baseline to moderately elevated ICP. The optic nerve measurements showed good correlation with existing two-dimensional (2-D) methods and an acute response to increased ICP, while globe flattening did not show an acute response. The tissue velocities were evaluated in a porcine model from baseline to significantly elevated ICP and correlated with invasive ICP readings in four animals.

Conclusions: Volumetric ophthalmic imaging was demonstrated on a portable ultrasound system and structural measurements validated with existing methods. New 3-D structural measurements and dynamic measurements were evaluated during *in vivo* studies. Further investigations are needed to evaluate improvements in performance for non-experts and application to clinically relevant conditions.

Keywords Volumetric (3-D) ultrasound · Intracranial pressure · NASA · Ultrasound image analysis · Optic nerve sheath diameter · Ocular globe flattening · Intracranial dynamics

Introduction

Astronauts have recently experienced visual changes during missions, with inflight and post-flight examinations revealing ocular structural changes [1], and several crew members have exhibited mild elevation in cerebrospinal fluid (CSF) opening pressure. These changes are believed to be the result of systemic and extraocular processes including elevated intracranial pressure (ICP). Further research is needed to understand the role ICP plays in, and to identify countermeasures to, visual impairment resulting from chronic exposure to microgravity.

Direct methods for monitoring ICP clinically are invasive and complicated, making them impractical for routine use in space medicine. Emerging non-invasive technologies are being evaluated that meet the size, mass, and power requirements for space. Several imaging modalities are currently used operationally and for research on the International Space Station (ISS) to monitor ocular health [1]. Fundoscopy and optical coherence tomography allow examination of the retina and choroid for evidence of disc edema, choroidal folds, and cotton-wool spots. Ultrasound allows examination of deeper structures for evidence of optic nerve sheath distension and globe flattening. Ophthalmic ultrasound has been used on the ISS for several years to allow crew members to perform inflight measurements with ground guidance [2], including routine optic nerve sheath diameter (ONSD) measurements for assessing ICP [3].

A. Dentinger (✉) · M. MacDonald
GE Global Research, Niskayuna, NY, USA
e-mail: dentinge@ge.com

D. Ebert · K. Garcia · A. Sargsyan
Wyle Science, Technology and Engineering Gr, Houston, TX, USA

Three-dimensional (3-D) ultrasound and automatic image analysis have the potential to improve the ease of use and accuracy of ocular ultrasound for non-experts and provide operator-independent volumetric imaging of the full ocular anatomy with minimal crew time and ground guidance. For long-duration missions beyond low-earth orbit, operator independence and autonomous operation become essential. Ground-based assessment of ICP at the point of care share similar challenges and can benefit from these innovations.

Materials and Methods

A prototype mechanical 3-D ultrasound probe was integrated on the ISS portable ultrasound platform (GE Vivid q; GE Healthcare, Milwaukee, WI). The prototype probe had a small footprint with a 20-mm width in 2-D imaging mode and operated at transmission frequencies between 8 and 12 MHz for ocular imaging through a closed eyelid. A custom external motor control unit was fabricated to enable 3-D imaging with the ISS platform by sweeping the linear ultrasound transducer array in the prototype 3-D probe through an angle of 60°. The 3-D acquisition hardware is shown in Fig. 1.

The ultrasound image sequences from the swept acquisitions were saved as DICOM files and exported for off-line 3-D reconstruction and analysis. Image analysis algorithms were developed to automatically detect ocular anatomy from the 3-D ultrasound data corresponding to the retinal-vitreous boundary and optic nerve centerline [4, 5]. These anatomical landmarks were then used to simultaneously generate multi-planar reconstructions (MPRs) of standard longitudinal views of the optic nerve in both axial and sagittal orienta-

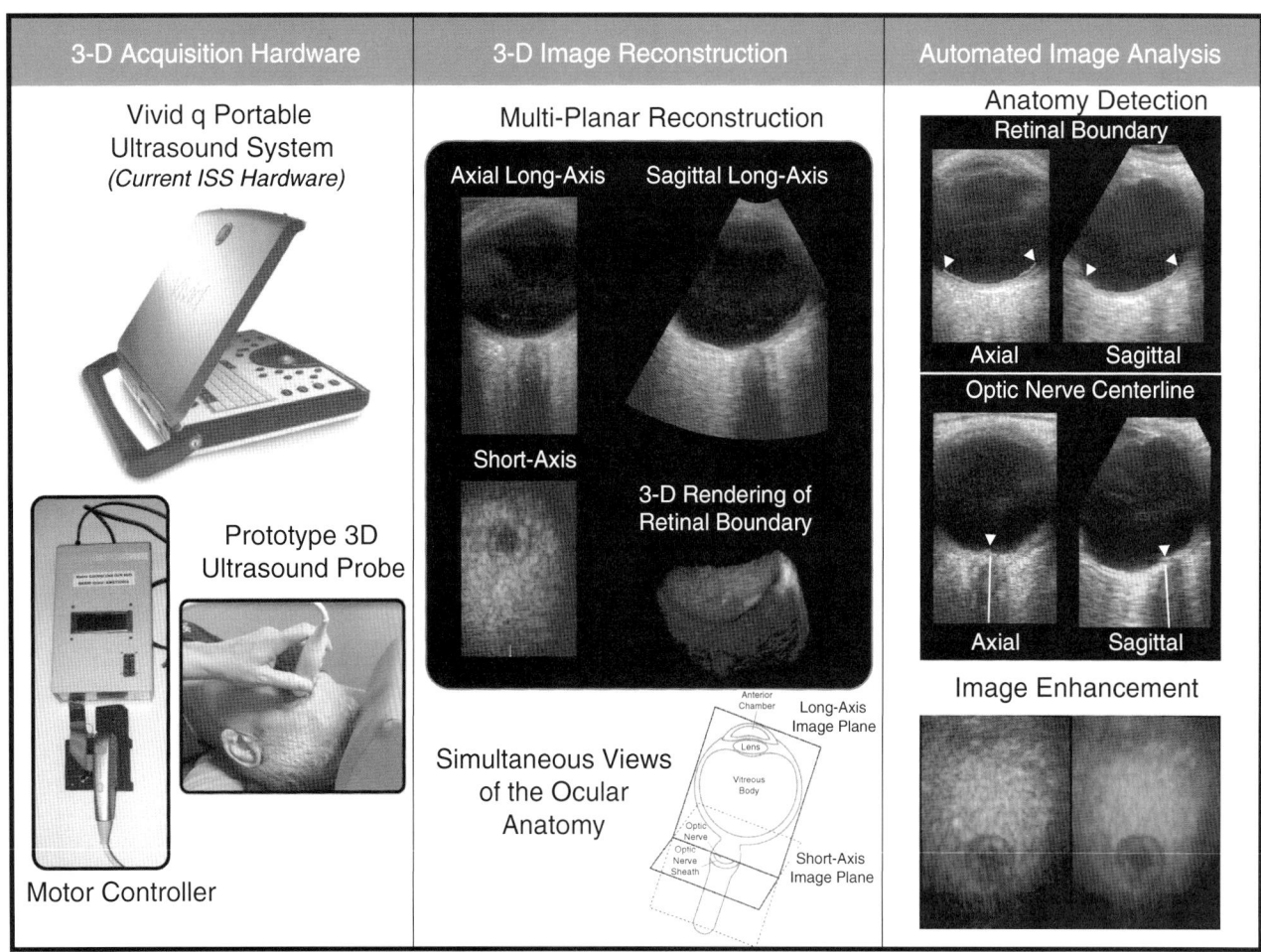

Fig. 1 Three-dimensional ophthalmic ultrasound imaging components: *3-D Acquisition Hardware* including a portable ultrasound system, prototype 3-D probe, and motor control unit; *Multi-planar Reconstruction* of ocular anatomy in long-axis and short-axis views simultaneously; *Automated Image Analysis* to segment retinal boundary (indicated by *white triangles*), detect optic nerve centerline (indicated by *white triangles*), and enhance image contrast from 3-D ultrasound data

tions, as well as new cross-sectional views. Volume contrast imaging techniques were used to enhance the MPRs and improve the contrast of the optic nerve sheath. Examples of the optic nerve views rendered from a single 3-D data set are shown in Fig. 1, along with the results of the image analysis and enhancement.

Several quantitative structural measures were extracted from the 3-D ultrasound data. First, the MPRs were converted to new DICOM files, allowing manual measurements by a reviewer on a clinical review workstation (GE EchoPAC; GE Healthcare, Milwaukee, WI). This included traditional caliper measurements of the optic nerve diameter (OND) and ONSD in long-axis views, as well as the optic nerve area in short-axis views. Secondly, a new 3-D measure of globe flattening was developed through analysis of the retinal boundary. An ellipsoid was fit to a subset of retinal surface points as an indication of the average morphology of the posterior globe, and a single quantitative metric calculated from the mean curvature (average of the minimum and maximum curvature) at the point of intersection of the optic nerve.

Since the optic nerve is surrounded by CSF, the motion of the optic nerve has the potential to provide information about the intracranial dynamics. Due to the fixed volume of the skull, the pulsatility in the arterial blood flow is transferred to the brain, including the CSF, with increased intracranial pulsatility attributed to reduced intracranial compliance [6]. Ultrasound tissue Doppler imaging was used to detect small movement of the tissue around the optic nerve in response to pulsating arterial blood flow. The raw ultrasound data were acquired in a long-axis optic nerve view and the tissue velocity in regions lateral and anterior to the optic nerve were averaged. Temporal waveforms of the average velocity over several cardiac cycles were analyzed and the amplitude of the periodic component at the heart rate was estimated.

The 3-D acquisition, image analysis, and metrics were evaluated via *in vivo* human and animal studies. The first study utilized head-down tilt (HDT) at several angles to induce mild increases in the ICP from hydrostatic pressure changes. Both 2-D and 3-D ophthalmic ultrasound data were collected bilaterally on 11 healthy volunteers at five body postures (seated, supine, 6°, 15°, and 30° HDT) with a 5-min baseline seated period prior to and 5-min equilibrium period after each new body position. The human subjects study was conducted under approval from NASA's Institutional Review Board, and informed consent was obtained from each subject prior to data collection.

In the second study, five adult Yorkshire pigs were anesthetized, intubated, and ventilated. The ICP was increased by infusing normal saline through an intra-parenchymal infusion catheter and ICP adjusted by the height of a saline fluid column. The ICP was increased from a baseline state (10 mmHg) to a significantly elevated state (40 mmHg) and back to baseline. ECG, arterial blood pressure, and ICP through a burr hole were continuously monitored throughout the experiments. Three-dimensional and tissue Doppler ultrasound were acquired bilaterally at each ICP level. The animal study was conducted under approval from the Institutional Animal Care and Use Committee at the University of Texas Medical Branch.

Results

The 3-D acquisition and reconstruction were validated by comparison to current 2-D imaging techniques used for inflight examination on the ISS. The new 3-D ultrasound acquisition showed a high correlation ($r = 0.94$) with the 2-D acquisitions for OND and ONSD measurements taken in both the axial and sagittal planes on healthy volunteers.

The results of the ONSD and globe flattening measurements (mean ± standard error) for the HDT study with healthy volunteers are shown in the bar graphs in Fig. 2. The response for the group showed the expected non-linear increase in ONSD with HDT angle, while the individual responses shown by the line plots in Fig. 2 highlighted significant individual variations. The mean curvature plotted in Fig. 2 is proportional to the reciprocal of the radius of curvature; thus, a decrease in curvature corresponds to increased flattening of the retinal surface. For the acute HDT study, no significant change was observed in globe flattening.

The results of the tissue Doppler measurements for the elevated ICP animal study are shown in Fig. 2. The amplitude of the periodic tissue motion increased and then decreased with ICP. The trends in the physiological data for one animal are also shown in Fig. 2. The physiological plots correspond to the pulse pressure in the arterial blood pressure (ABP) and the ICP along with the respiratory variation of the mean pressures. The ABP pulse pressure remains nearly constant with ICP, while the ICP pulse pressure increased with ICP. The respiratory variation increased and then decreased for both ABP and ICP.

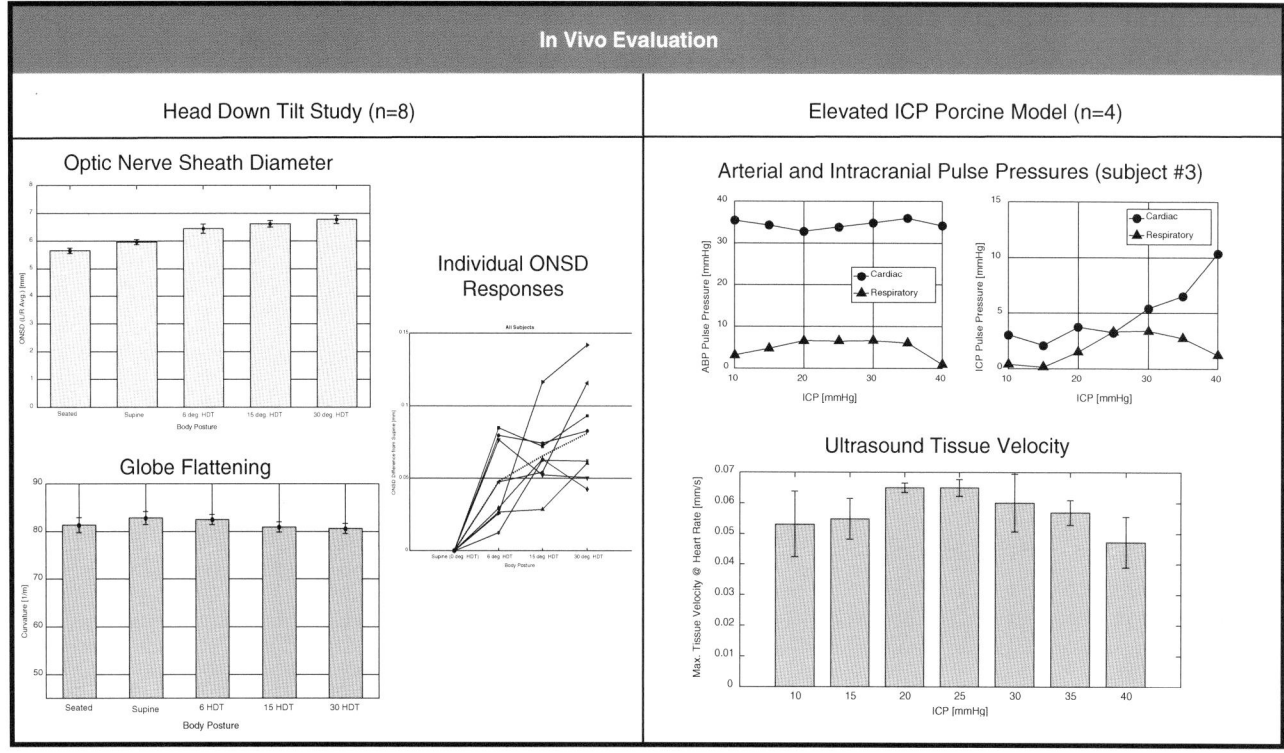

Fig. 2 *In vivo* evaluation of 3-D ultrasound acquisition and image analysis algorithms including optic nerve sheath diameter and globe curvature measurements during a head-down tilt (HDT) subject study in healthy volunteers and ultrasound tissue velocity measurements during an elevated ICP animal study with comparison to arterial blood pressure and ICP pulse pressures

Discussion

Volumetric ultrasound has the potential to improve the ease of use of ultrasound for ONSD measurements by reducing scan times and operator dependence and allowing image findings, like those from other modalities [1], to be acquired inflight and at the point-of-care. Automatic post-processing of the 3-D data has the potential to improve the accuracy of ONSD measurements for novice and experienced reviewers by improving image quality and increasing confidence by providing multiple views.

Although the ONSD response to acutely elevated ICP was readily observable, individual variation in the response to ICP still proves to be a challenge for conversion of the ONSD measurements to an absolute pressure without individualized calibration. Although globe flattening changes were not seen in the acute HDT experiment, 3-D retinal curvature still has the potential to provide quantitative and objective measures independent of probe position but will require further testing in a chronic study. Additional local curvature, as reported by Alperin et al. [7], can also be extracted from analysis of the retinal boundary to further characterize structural changes.

Tissue Doppler and the periodic motion correlated with heart rate for intracranial dynamics assessment is an intriguing new measure provided by ultrasound that requires additional research to understand both the source of the pulsatile motion and explained the relationship to absolute ICP, ICP pulse pressure, and intracranial compliance.

One potential clinical application is non-invasive ICP assessment of traumatic brain injury patients, such as for identifying primary injuries or preventing secondary injuries. Volume scanning with a portable ultrasound system provides the opportunity for frequent, point-of-care assessment of ocular changes, eliminating the need to transport patients to an imaging suite for scanning by an expert sonographer and allowing triage of patients in a timely fashion.

Conclusion

Volumetric and tissue Doppler ultrasound provides additional information to enhance point-of-care assessment of elevated ICP through analysis of ocular structures and dynamics. The 3-D information enables multiple longitudinal views and new cross-sectional views of the optic nerve anatomy to be generated from a single 3-D ultrasound acquisition. Additionally, 3-D image processing allows the contrast between the optic nerve sheath and surrounding orbital fat to be enhanced without apparent loss of the spatial resolution and new quantitative 3-D structural metrics of the optic nerve sheath and posterior globe curvature to be extracted. Lastly, ultrasound Doppler techniques applied to the tissue near the optic nerve and head demonstrated the ability to detect small periodic displacements of the tissue at the heart rate and the variation in the amplitude of these signals with ICP were quantified in a porcine model.

Acknowledgement This work was supported by a grant from the National Space Biomedical Research Institute (NSBRI) through NASA NCC 9-58.

Conflicts of interest statement We declare that we have no conflict of interest.

References

1. Mader TH, Gibson CR, Pass AF, Kramer LA, Lee AG. Optic disc edema, globe flattening, choroidal folds, and hyperopic shifts observed in astronauts after long-duration space flight. Ophthalmology. 2011;118(10):2058–69.
2. Chiao L, Sharipov S, Sargsyan AE, Melton S, Hamilton DR, McFarlin K, Dulchavsky SA. Ocular examination for trauma; clinical ultrasound aboard the International Space Station. J Trauma. 2005;58:885–9.
3. Soldatos T, Chatzimichail K, Papathanasiou M, Gouliamos A. Optic nerve sonography: a new window for the noninvasive evaluation of intracranial pressure in brain injury. Emerg Med J. 2009;26:630–4.
4. Frangi AF, Niessen WJ, Vincken KL, Viergever MA. Multiscale vessel enhancement filtering. MICCAI'98. 1998;1496:130–7.
5. Dalvi R, Hacihaliloglua I, Abugharbieh R. 3D ultrasound volume stitching using phase symmetry and Harris corner detection for orthopaedic applications. SPIE Med Imaging. 2010;7623.
6. Wagshul ME, Eide PK, Madsen JR. The pulsating brain: a review of experimental and clinical studies of intracranial pulsatility. Fluids Barriers CNS. 2011;8(5):1–23.
7. Alperin N, Bagci AM, Lam BL, Sklar E. Automated quantitation of the posterior scleral flattening and optic nerve protrusion by MRI in idiopathic intracranial hypertension. AJNR Am J Neuroradiol. 2013;34:2354–9.

Does the Variability of Evoked Tympanic Membrane Displacement Data (V_m) Increase as the Magnitude of the Pulse Amplitude Increases?

Sammy J. Sharif, Cherith M. Campbell-Bell, Diederik O. Bulters, Robert J. Marchbanks, and Anthony A. Birch

Abstract *Objectives*: Evoked tympanic membrane displacement (TMD) measurements, quantified by V_m, record small volume changes in the ear canal following stimulation of the acoustic reflex. V_m shows a correlation with intracranial pressure (ICP) and has been proposed as an option to non-invasively measure ICP. The spontaneous pulsing of the tympanic membrane, driven by the cardiovascular pulse, may contaminate the recordings and contribute to high measurement variability in some subjects. This study hypothesised that the larger the spontaneous vascular pulse, the larger the variability in V_m.

Materials and methods: Spontaneous and evoked TMD data from each ear in the sitting and supine position were recorded from 100 healthy volunteers using the MMS-14 CCFP analyser. ECG was also recorded to identify each heartbeat. Using bespoke software written in Matlab, spontaneous data were analysed to produce average pulse amplitude (PA) waveforms and evoked data were analysed to calculate average V_m and its standard deviation. Averaged spontaneous PA was plotted against V_m variability and Pearson's correlation coefficient was calculated to test for a significant linear relationship.

Results: There was a strong positive correlation between PA and V_m variability in all conditions: left sitting, $r = 0.758$; left supine, $r = 0.665$; right sitting, $r = 0.755$; right supine, $r = 0.513$. All were significant at $p < 0.001$.

Conclusion: This study shows that large V_m variability is associated with a large spontaneous vascular pulse. This suggests that efforts to reduce vascular pulsing from recordings, either by a subtraction technique during post-processing or ECG-gating of the evoking stimulus, may improve reliability of the V_m measurement.

Keywords Tympanic membrane displacement · V_m · Non-invasive · Vascular pulse · Intracranial pressure

S.J. Sharif
University of Southampton, Hampshire, UK

C.M. Campbell-Bell, Ph.D. • A.A. Birch, Ph.D. (✉)
Neurological Physics, Department of Medical Physics and Bioengineering, University Hospital Southampton National Health Service Foundation Trust, Southampton, UK
e-mail: Tony.Birch@uhs.nhs.uk

D.O. Bulters, F.R.C.S. (S.N.)
Department of Neurosurgery, University Hospital Southampton National Health Service Foundation Trust, Southampton, UK

R.J. Marchbanks, Ph.D.
Neurological Physics, Department of Medical Physics and Bioengineering, University Hospital Southampton National Health Service Foundation Trust, Southampton, UK

Marchbanks Measurements Systems Ltd., Hampshire, UK

Introduction

Measurement of intracranial pressure (ICP) has a vital role in the monitoring, diagnosis and treatment of patients with elevated ICP [1]. Clinically, ICP is measured either through lumbar puncture or by inserting an intracranial catheter [1, 2]. These methods are invasive and have associated complications, such as infection and haemorrhage [2]. Tympanic membrane displacement (TMD) is a non-invasive option [3] that utilises the anatomical connection provided by the cochlear aqueduct (CA) between the perilymph of the scala tympani in the cochlea and the cerebrospinal fluid (CSF) within the subarachnoid space [3, 4].

TMD measures air volume changes in the ear canal caused by movements of the tympanic membrane (TM) [3]. Evoked measurements record TMD during the acoustic reflex (AR); defined as stapedius muscle contraction in response to a loud sound stimulus [3]. When the stapedius contracts, the stapes is pulled medially, the ossicles are compressed and the TM is displaced from its initial position [5]. The position of the oval window of the cochlea, upon which the stapes footplate rests, is influenced by the perilymphatic pressure within the scala tympani [4, 5]. If the CA is patent, then perilymphatic pressure is equal to CSF pressure, which is estimated by measuring the amplitude and direction of the TMD response [4, 5].

Evoked TMD responses are quantified in terms of V_m [4], defined as the mean volume displacement between the point of maximum inward displacement (V_i) and stimulus offset. This is shown in Fig. 1, where A represents V_i (−20.8 nL in this example) and B represents the value at the time of stimulus offset (0.3 s, 278 nL). The mean volume displacement between A and B represents V_m, calculated here as 152 nL.

Spontaneous TMD measures the volume changes in the ear canal induced by the pulsing of the TM, influenced by the cardiovascular pulse and respiration [3]. The spontaneous TMD response is quantified in terms of pulse amplitude and is believed to represent the pulsing of ICP [3].

Evoked TMD is used to provide an estimate of baseline ICP, whether it is low, high or normal [5, 6]. Due to individual variability in evoked TMD measurements, comparisons of V_m values between healthy individuals and patients may be difficult. A larger vascular pulse may lead to more variability in V_m measurements [7], and therefore this study investigated the correlation between the vascular pulse amplitude and variability in V_m. A strong correlation would suggest that developing a method to reduce the influence of the vascular pulse on evoked TMD recordings would be worthwhile.

Materials and Methods

Data Collection

Data from 100 healthy adult participants, including 59 women and 41 men, aged 20–80 (mean age 43.6 years) was extracted from an ongoing study aiming to quantify reference intervals for TMD values in the healthy population. This study was approved by a NHS research ethics committee.

Participants were carefully screened to rule out any otological and neurological pathology by means of otoscopy, tympanometry, AR threshold (ART) testing and a health screen questionnaire. For tympanometry, inclusion criteria consisted of a middle ear pressure between −50 daPa and +50 daPa and a middle ear compliance of between 0.3 ml and 1.5 ml. Maximum ART for inclusion was 95 dB. Sound stimuli were presented at +20 dB above ART or +15 dB above ART for ARTs of 95 dB.

The MMS-14 (Marchbanks Measurement Systems) Cerebral and Cochlear Fluid Pressure (CCFP) Analyser was used to measure spontaneous and evoked TMD data for each participant, in each ear (if possible), both sitting and supine. A three-lead ECG was recorded during the measurements to give timing information for each heartbeat. All signals were recorded at 250 Hz using ICM+ software [8].

Each participant had at least five runs of spontaneous TMD data, 20 s in duration, recorded in each condition. Two sets of ten evoked TMD recordings in each condition were also recorded. Each evoked measurement was obtained by recording the response of the TM to a 1 kHz tone of 0.3 s duration over a 1 s window.

Calculating Pulse Amplitude and V_m Variability

To determine the spontaneous pulse amplitude, each 20 s run of TMD data was analysed using bespoke software written in Matlab [9]. The ECG waveform was used to identify the time of each heartbeat, and the corresponding TMD pulse amplitude was determined as the maximum-minimum TMD value. PA was then calculated as the mean of all recorded pulses. This was determined for each participant, in each ear and in each position. V_m was measured for each of the 20 individual evoked TMD recordings and the V_m variability recorded as the standard deviation of these in each condition.

Statistical Analysis

To assess whether V_m variability increases as PA increases, Pearson's correlation coefficient was calculated to test for a significant linear relationship between mean PA and V_m variability in each condition. All statistical tests were performed using IBM SPSS Statistics version 22 [10].

Results

There was a strong positive correlation between PA and V_m variability in all conditions, as shown in Fig. 2, demonstrating that as PA increases, V_m variability also increases. Table 1

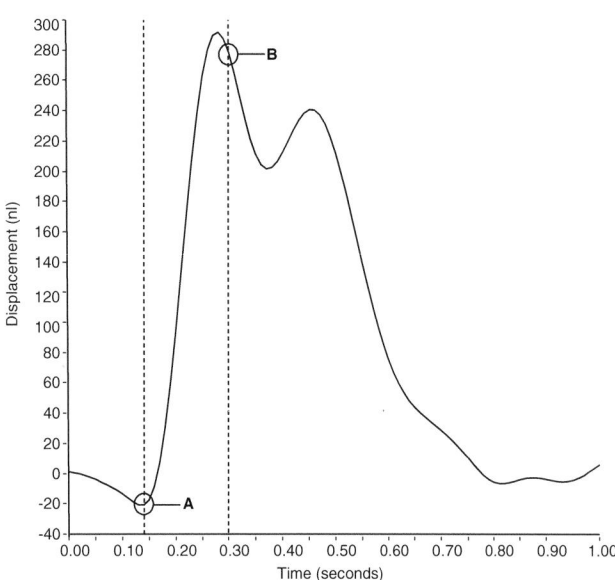

Fig. 1 Showing how V_m is calculated from an evoked TMD waveform

shows the statistical results of the correlations, as well as mean PA and standard deviation (SD) for V_m.

Discussion

Baseline ICP can be estimated from the evoked TMD response; however, the continuous spontaneous pulsing of the TM, driven predominantly by the cardiovascular pulse, might contaminate the recording. This study has shown that the larger the vascular pulse, as measured from the spontaneous TMD waveform, the larger the observed variability in the evoked TMD response (V_m). This suggests that efforts to reduce the artefact introduced by the vascular pulse will improve V_m variability and give a more reliable measure of V_m. One possible method for achieving this could be to use a post-processing vascular subtraction technique, which would involve subtracting the average PA template from

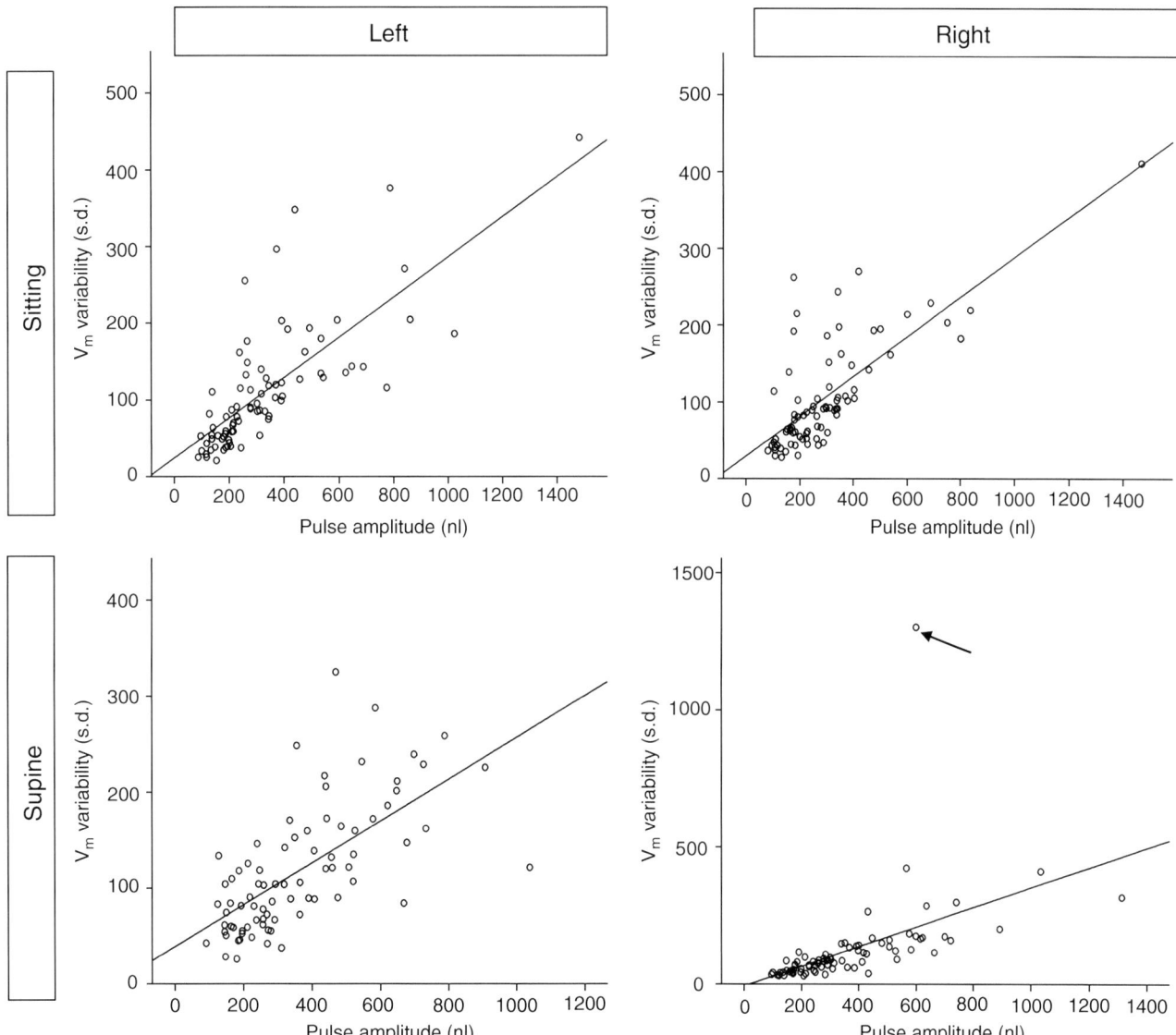

Fig. 2 Pearson's correlation graph for mean PA vs V_m variability (SD) for the 80 participants with left ear sitting, left ear supine, right ear sitting and right ear supine data respectively. The *arrowed data* point in the right supine graph identifies an outlier, discussed later

Table 1 Results from correlation analysis between averaged spontaneous PA and V_m variability for each of the four conditions

	Pearson correlation coefficient (r)	Bootstrap CI	p	Mean PA (nL)	Mean V_m SD
Left sitting	0.758	0.585, 0.880	<0.001	335.456	111.961
Right sitting	0.755	0.529, 0.890	<0.001	295.461	105.703
Left supine	0.665	0.531, 0.796	<0.001	362.451	117.840
Right supine	0.513	0.426, 0.879	<0.001	361.215	123.028

the evoked TMD waveform. Another technique could be ECG-gating of the evoking stimulus, whereby the MMS-14 CCFP analyser would only initiate a sound stimulus when the heart is detected to be in diastole. However, this method would be more complicated and time-consuming.

The influence of respiration on spontaneous TMD was not accounted for in this study; however, the respiratory wave may also influence the variability of the reflex response [3]. Given that it is both lower in frequency and generally of smaller amplitude than the vascular pulse (in healthy participants), we would expect the respiratory wave to produce a lower level of artefact onto TMD recordings [3]. Nonetheless, retrospective analysis of one participant's data showed that the spontaneous TMD waveform was dominated by the respiratory wave. This may help to explain why this particular participant's V_m variability was much larger than would be predicted from their cardiovascular PA (indicated by the *arrow* in Fig. 2). Further investigation of the effect of respiration on TMD recordings is needed and should include differences in respiratory wave PA with posture.

Conclusion

This study has shown that as the amplitude of the vascular pulse increases, the variability in evoked TMD measurements (V_m) also increases. Therefore, efforts to reduce the influence of the vascular pulse on evoked recordings are likely to make TMD a more reliable non-invasive measure of ICP.

Acknowledgements This study was funded by Innovate UK and supported by the NIHR/Wellcome Trust Southampton Clinical Research Facility.

Conflicts of interest statement Dr Robert Marchbanks is the Managing Director of Marchbanks Measurement Systems Ltd, a spin-out company from the University of Southampton (UK) and manufacture of the MMS-14 CCFP Analyser used in this study.

References

1. Hawthorne C, Piper I. Monitoring of intracranial pressure in patients with traumatic brain injury. Front Neurol. 2014;5:121. https://doi.org/10.3389/fneur.2014.00121.
2. Ellenby MS, Tegtmeyer K, Lai S, Braner DAV. Lumbar puncture. N Engl J Med. 2006;355(13):e12. https://doi.org/10.1056/NEJMvcm054952.
3. Shulman A, Goldstein B, Marchbanks RJ. The tympanic membrane displacement test and tinnitus: preliminary report on clinical observations, applications, and implications. Int Tinnitus J. 2012;17(1):80–93.
4. Silverman CA, Linstrom CJ. How to measure cerebrospinal fluid pressure invasively and noninvasively. J Glaucoma. 2013;22(Suppl 5):S26–8. https://doi.org/10.1097/IJG.0b013e3182934a6a.
5. Shimbles S, Dodd C, Banister K, Mendelow AD, Chambers IR. Clinical comparison of tympanic membrane displacement with invasive ICP measurements. Acta Neurochir Suppl. 2005;95:197–9.
6. Samuel M, Burge DM, Marchbanks RJ. Quantitative assessment of intracranial pressure by the tympanic membrane displacement audiometric technique in children with shunted hydrocephalus. Eur J Pediatr Surg. 1998;8(04):200–7. https://doi.org/10.1055/s-2008-1071154.
7. Marchbanks R. A study of tympanic membrane displacement. Ph.D. Thesis. Bristol: Brunel University; 1980.
8. Smielewski P, Czosnyka M. ICM+, Version 8. Department of Clinical Neurosciences: University of Cambridge; 2014.
9. MATLAB. Version R2012b. Natick, MA: The Mathworks Inc.; 2012.
10. IBM, Corp. IBM SPSS Statistics for Windows, Version 22.0. Armonk, NY: IBM Corp.; 2013.

Analysis of a Non-invasive Intracranial Pressure Monitoring Method in Patients with Traumatic Brain Injury

G. Frigieri, R.A.P. Andrade, C. Dias, D.L. Spavieri Jr., R. Brunelli, D.A. Cardim, C.C. Wang, R.M.M. Verzola, and S. Mascarenhas

Abstract *Objective*: We aimed to compare the invasive (iICP) and a non-invasive intracranial pressure (nICP) monitoring methods in patients with traumatic brain injury, based on the similarities of the signals' power spectral densities.

Materials and methods: We recorded the intracranial pressure of seven patients with traumatic brain injury admitted to Hospital São João, Portugal, using two different methods: a standard intraparenchymal (iICP) and a new nICP method based on mechanical extensometers. The similarity between the two monitoring signals was inferred from the Euclidean distance between the non-linear projection in a lower dimensional space (ISOMAP) of the windowed power spectral densities of the respective signals. About 337 h of acquisitions were used out of a total of 608 h. The only data exclusion criterion was the absence of any of the signals of interest.

Results: The averaged distance between iICP and nICP, and between arterial blood pressure (ABP) and nICP projections in the embedded space are statistically different for all seven patients analysed (Mann-Whitney U, $p < 0.05$).

Conclusions: The similarity between the iICP and nICP monitoring methods was higher than the similarity between the nICP and the recordings of the radial ABP for all seven patients. Despite the possible differences between the shape of the ABP waveform at radial and parietal arteries, the results indicate—based on the similarities of iICP and nICP as functions of time—that the nICP method can be applied as an alternative method for ICP monitoring.

Keywords Non-invasive · Intracranial pressure · Arterial blood pressure · Dimensionality reduction · Fourier transform

Introduction

Intracranial pressure (ICP) is usually monitored via the insertion of a catheter and pressure transducer into the subdural, epidural, subarachnoid, intraventricular or intraparenchymal spaces [1]. Potential disadvantages of these methods are the risk of bleeding and infection, calibration problems and obstructions, operation restricted to a neurosurgical environment and high associated cost. In view of these downsides, there have been several initiatives to develop non-invasive methods to continuously monitor ICP [2–5]. We present here the application of a new non-invasive ICP (nICP) monitoring method based on mechanical extensometers.

The new non-invasive monitoring method consists of a strain gauge (mechanical extensometer) fixed on a mechanical device that touches the scalp in the parietal region lateral to the sagittal suture. The non-invasive sensor is able to detect small skull deformations resulting from changes in ICP. In the current state of development, this method does not yet yield pressure values calibrated in millimetres of mercury, but can deliver continuous information about the ICP waveform.

The ICP waveform is directly related to cerebral compliance. The cardiac component of ICP typically comprises three peaks: P1, associated with the systolic blood pressure

G. Frigieri (✉) · R.A.P. Andrade · D.L. Spavieri Jr. · C.C. Wang
Braincare, São Carlos, SP, Brazil
e-mail: g.frigieri@gmail.com

C. Dias
Hospital São João, Universidade do Porto, Porto, Portugal

R. Brunelli · S. Mascarenhas
Braincare, São Carlos, SP, Brazil

Instituto de Física de São Carlos, Universidade de São Paulo, São Carlos, SP, Brazil

D.A. Cardim
Brain Physics Laboratory, Division of Neurosurgery, Department of Clinical Neurosciences, University of Cambridge, Cambridge, UK

R.M.M. Verzola
Department of Biological Sciences and Health, Federal University of São Carlos, São Carlos, SP, Brazil

wave transferred by the choroid plexus to the cerebrospinal fluid; P2, associated with the reflection of systolic wave into the parenchymal tissue; P3, related to the closure of the aortic valve. By observing only the relative amplitude of peaks P1, P2 and P3, it is possible to obtain relevant clinical information. For example, an increase of the amplitude of the three peaks indicates an increase of the mean ICP. A reduction in the P1 amplitude suggests loss of cerebral perfusion, and an increase in P2, loss of brain compliance. Fusion of the peaks P1, P2 and P3 associated with a high mean amplitude may indicate that the autoregulation of the cerebrovascular system is not properly functioning [6–10].

In this study, we compare the waveforms of standard invasive ICP (iICP) and nICP in a lower dimensional space constructed based on signals in the frequency domain. Our goal was to verify the similarities between the two ICP waveforms—invasive and non-invasive—and the radial arterial blood pressure (ABP) along all recording time, without having to look at high dimensional signals directly. In a lower dimensional space, we can see when and how the non-invasive method waveform follows the invasive method as a function of time as changes in ICP occurred.

The comparison between invasive and non-invasive ICP waveforms aim to validate the non-invasive method as an alternative to invasive measurements in situations where the waveform can give additional clinical information. We also compared the nICP with arterial ABP waveforms to verify the possible influence of the peripheral circulation into the nICP signal, which is one of the possible limitations of the present method.

Materials and Methods

The non-invasive sensor consists of a support for a sensor bar for the detection of local skull bone deformations, adapted with extensometers. Detection of these deformations is obtained by a cantilever bar modelled by finite elements calculations. To this bar, strain gauges are attached for strain detection. Non-invasive contact with the skull is obtained by adequate pressure directly on the scalp by a pin. Changes in ICP cause deformations in the skull bone detected by the sensor bar. Variations in ICP lead to deformations in the bar, which are captured by the strain sensors. The equipment filters, amplifies and digitalises the signal from the sensor, and sends the data to a computer [11].

We recorded the ICP of seven patients with traumatic brain injury admitted to Hospital São João, Portugal, using two different methods: a standard intraparenchymal microtransducer (Codman & Shurtleff, Raynham, MA, USA) and the non-invasive method (Braincare, São Paulo, Brazil), placed on the parietal region of the patient's scalp using an elastic head band. We also recorded the ABP thorough the radial artery and the partial pressure of carbon dioxide ($PaCO_2$) simultaneously. We analysed approximately 337 h of recordings from a total of 608 h. The only exclusion criterion was the absence of any of the signals of interest. Table 1 presents the patients' demographics and average recording time for each individual.

The similarity between two time-series at a given temporal window was inferred from the Euclidean distance between the non-linear projection in a lower dimensional space of the windowed power spectral densities of the respective signals. We calculated the power spectral density of the signal x using the short-time Fourier transform [12]:

$$\text{STFT}\left[x(n)\right]_m = \sum_{n=-\infty}^{\infty} x[n] w[n-m] e^{-jwn}$$

where $w[k]$ is the Blackman window. We used window length of 10 s, with a sampling frequency of 250 Hz. We then reduced the dimensionality of STFT (250 dimensions) space to two dimensions using a non-linear dimensionality reduction algorithm (ISOMAP) [13], in which the embedding is done in three steps. First, we calculated the Euclidean distances between the power spectral densities (PSD) of the windowed signals. In the second step, we constructed a graph based on the nearest neighbours of the PSDs; in the final step, we performed classical multidimensional scaling using the geodesical distances between nodes on the graph to embed the signal into the lower space. A schematic representation of the data processing pipeline can be seen in Fig. 1. The whole analysis was performed using custom programs written in the python language, using the libraries Scipy [14], Matplotlib [15] and Scikit-learn [16].

Table 1 Overview of the data analysed

Patient	Age	Gender	Pathology	Acquisition time (h)
1	52	F	Spontaneous haemorrhage	282
2	70	M	Brain tumour	97.8
3	65	M	Brain tumour	77.1
4	77	M	Traumatic injury	37.6
5	72	F	Spontaneous haemorrhage	141.1
6	33	F	Spontaneous haemorrhage	68.3
7	56	F	Traumatic injury	141.1

Analysis of a Non-invasive Intracranial Pressure Monitoring Method in Patients with Traumatic Brain Injury

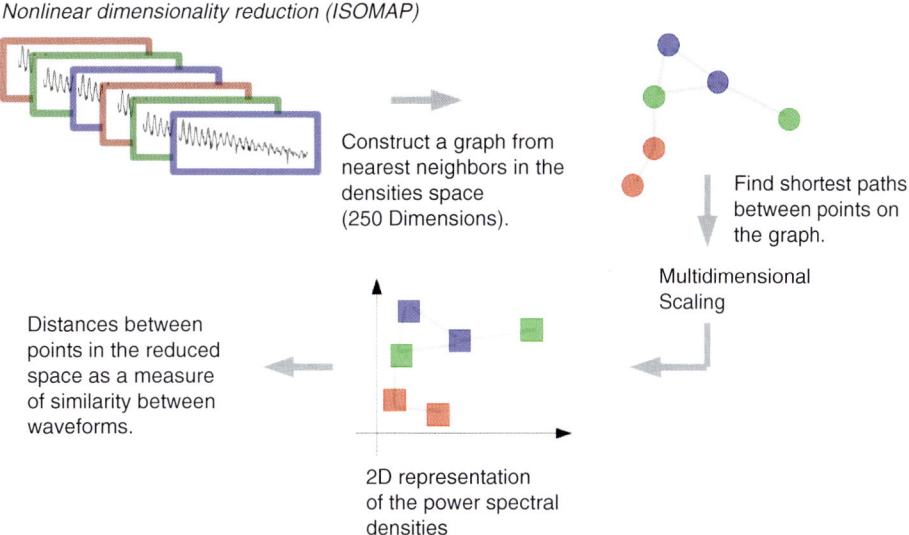

Fig. 1 Schematic representation of the data processing pipeline

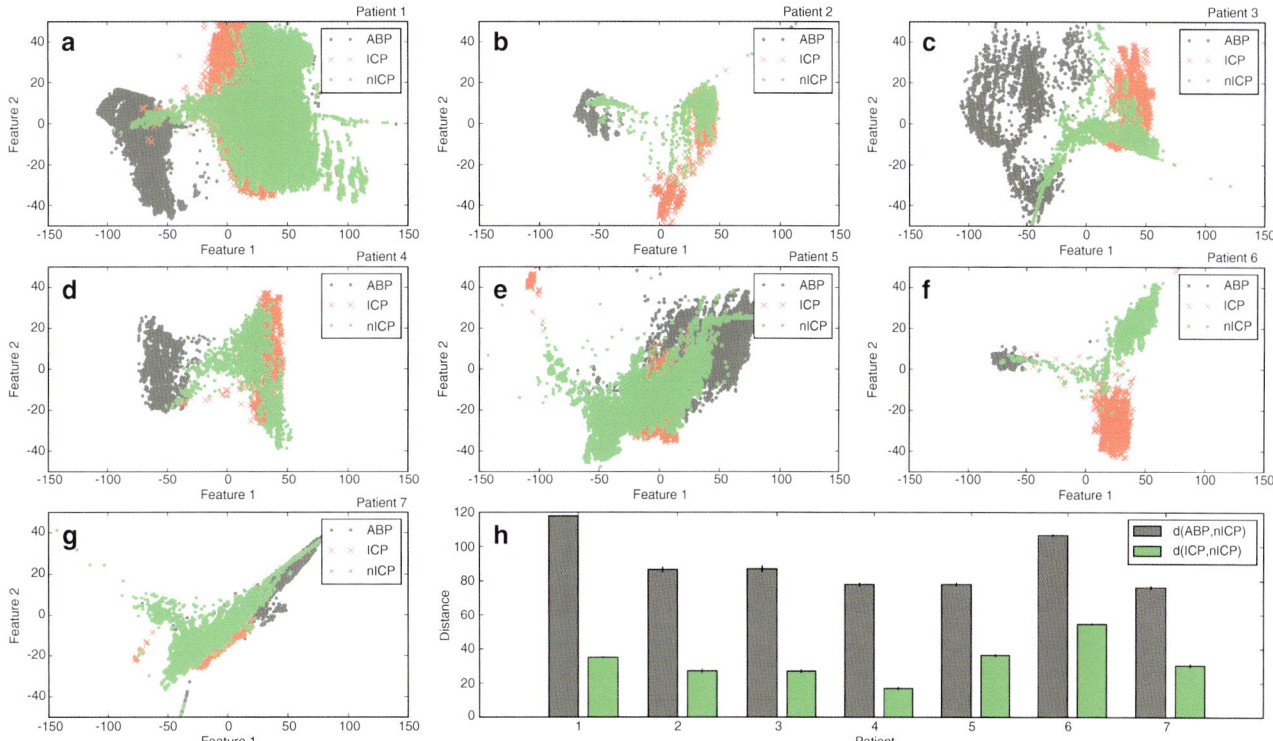

Fig. 2 Projection of the power spectral density into a lower dimensional space for seven patients with traumatic brain injury (**a–g**). (**h**) Average distances for iICP-nICP and ABP-nICP projections for the seven patients. *Errors bars* are non-parametric confidence intervals with $\alpha = 0.05$ and 1000 replications

Results

The ISOMAP projection of the PSD signals of six patients can be observed in the Fig. 2. Each point on the graphs in Fig. 2a–g represents the PSD of a 10-s window of the respective signals embedded into the lower dimensional space. We can qualitatively observe that nICP and iICP points are on average closer than ABP and iICP points for most of the patients. Indeed, the average distances between the respective points confirm that (Fig. 2h, Table 2). The differences between iICP-nICP and ABP-nICP are statistically significant for all seven patients (Mann-Whitney $U, p < 0.05$). A dynamic comparison as a function of time can be seen at the following link (https://youtu.be/dK1XK-4jCkE). The

Table 2 Measure of similarities between iICP, ABP and nICP for seven patients (arbitrary units)

Similarities	Patient ID						
	1	2	3	4	5	6	7
iICP-nICP	35.0	27.2	26.9	16.9	36.3	54.7	30.3
ABP-nICP	117.3	86.6	86.9	77.9	78.1	106.6	76.3

video shows the representation of three signals—iICP (red), nICP (green) and ABP (grey)—for one patient during 24 h. In the upper panel, one can observe the nonlinear projection of the three signals power spectral densities, which are shown in the lower right panel. In the lower left panel, one can see the corresponding morphologies.

Discussion

We did not expect that the waveforms—and respective frequency domain signatures—of the ICP recording methods were identical, because they are recorded at different sites—one inside the parenchyma and other outside the skull. Both waveforms are, however, an indirect result of mechanical waves generated by the blood inflow to the brain and, therefore, should share some similarities. Indeed, we were able to observe a dynamic similarity between the waveforms as ICP changed in time. Given the importance of ICP waveform analysis to monitor the clinical state of the patient, and the similarities between the invasive and non-invasive methods, we suggest that the non-invasive method can be used for monitoring relative changes in ICP despite the absence of absolute values in mmHg.

One possible limitation of the non-invasive method could be the interference of peripheral circulation on the nICP signal. We therefore compared the iICP and nICP waveforms with the radial artery blood pressure waveform, and observed that similarities between nICP and iICP are greater than the similarities between ABP and nICP or ABP and iICP. Nevertheless, such limitation could be minimised if the non-invasive sensor positioning is optimised, i.e. away from major vessels in the parietal region. This could attenuate the potential influence of the peripheral circulation on the nICP waveform, and consequently approximate its pattern to the direct ICP waveform.

Conclusions

The waveform similarity between iICP and nICP methods was greater than the similarity between nICP and radial ABP for all seven patients. Despite the possible differences between the shape of the ABP waveform at radial and parietal arteries, the results indicate—based on the similarities of iICP and nICP as functions of time—that the nICP method can be used as an alternative tool for ICP monitoring in conditions where the knowledge of absolute values might not be essentially relevant.

Acknowledgements Funded by FAPESP, PAHO, CNPq and Ministry of Health of Brazil.

Conflicts of interest statement We declare that we have no conflict of interest.

References

1. Lee KR, Hoff JT. Intracranial pressure. In: Youmans JR, editor. Youmans neurological surgery, vol. 1. 4th ed. Philadelphia: WB Saunders; 1996. p. 491–518.
2. Kashif FM, Verghese GC, Novak V, Czosnyka M, Heldt T. Model-based noninvasive estimation of intracranial pressure from cerebral blood flow velocity and arterial pressure. Sci Transl Med. 2012;4:129ra44.
3. Ragauskas A, Daubaris G, Dziugys a, Azelis V, Gedrimas V. Innovative non-invasive method for absolute intracranial pressure measurement without calibration. Acta Neurochir Suppl. 2005;95:357–61.
4. Barone DG, Czosnyka M. Brain monitoring: do we need a hole? An update on invasive and noninvasive brain monitoring modalities. Sci World J. 2014;2014:1–6.
5. Padayachy LC. Non-invasive intracranial pressure assessment. Childs Nerv Syst. 2016;32:1–11.
6. CJJ A, Van Eijndhoven JH, Wyper DJ. Cerebrospinal fluid pulse pressure and intracranial volume-pressure relationships. J Neurol Neurosurg Psychiatry. 1979;42:687–700.
7. Hashimoto M, Higashi S, Tokuda K, Yamamoto Y, Yamashita J. Changes of intracranial pressure and pulse wave form induced by various mechanical stresses upon intracranial hemodynamics. In: Avezaat CJJ, van Eijndhoven JHM, Maas AIR, Tans JTJ, editors. Intracranial pressure. VIII SE—79. Heidelberg: Springer; 1993. p. 367–71.
8. Ferreira MCPD. Multimodal brain monitoring and evaluation of cerebrovascular reactivity after severe head injury. Porto: University of Porto; 2015.
9. Fan JY, Kirkness C, Vicini P, Burr R, Mitchell P. Intracranial pressure waveform morphology and intracranial adaptive capacity. Am J Crit Care. 2008;17:545–54.
10. Scalzo F, Hamilton R, Hu X. Real-time analysis of intracranial pressure waveform morphology. In: Chen K-S, editor. Adv Top Neurol Disord InTech. 2012;99–128.
11. Cabella B, Vilela GHF, Mascarenhas S, Czosnyka M, Smielewski P, Dias C, Colli BO (2016) Validation of a new noninvasive intracranial pressure monitoring method by direct comparison with an invasive technique. Acta Neurochirurgica. Supplement 2016;122:93–96.
12. Allen J. Short term spectral analysis, synthesis, and modification by discrete Fourier transform. IEEE Trans Acoust Speech Signal Process. 1977;25(3):235–8.
13. Tenenbaum JB, de Silva V, Langford JC. A global geometric framework for nonlinear dimensionality reduction. Science (New York, N.Y.), 290(5500), 2319–23.
14. Jones E, Oliphant T, Peterson P. Scipy: open source scientific tools for Python. 2001. http://www.scipy.org.
15. Hunter JD. Matplotlib: a 2D graphics environment. IEEE Comput Sci Eng. 2007;9:90–5.
16. Pedregosa F, Varoquaux G, Gramfort A, Michel V, Thirion B, Grisel O, et al. Scikit-learn: machine learning in Python. J Mach Learn Res. 2011;12:2825–30.

A Wearable Transcranial Doppler Ultrasound Phased Array System

Sabino J. Pietrangelo, Hae-Seung Lee, and Charles G. Sodini

Abstract *Objective*: Practical deficiencies related to conventional transcranial Doppler (TCD) sonography have restricted its use and applicability. This work seeks to mitigate several such constraints through the development of a wearable, electronically steered TCD velocimetry system, which enables noninvasive measurement of cerebral blood flow velocity (CBFV) for monitoring applications with limited operator interaction.

Materials and Methods: A highly-compact, discrete prototype system was designed and experimentally validated through flow phantom and preliminary human subject testing. The prototype system incorporates a custom two-dimensional transducer array and multi-channel transceiver electronics, thereby facilitating acoustic beamformation via phased array operation. Electronic steering of acoustic energy enables algorithmic system controls to map Doppler power throughout the tissue volume of interest and localize regions of maximal flow. Multi-focal reception permits dynamic vessel position tracking and simultaneous flow velocimetry over the time-course of monitoring.

Results: Experimental flow phantom testing yielded high correlation with concurrent flowmeter recordings across the expected range of physiological flow velocities. Doppler power mapping has been validated in both flow phantom and preliminary human subject testing, resulting in average vessel location mapping times <14 s. Dynamic vessel tracking has been realized in both flow phantom and preliminary human subject testing.

Conclusions: A wearable prototype CBFV measurement system capable of autonomous vessel search and tracking has been presented. Although flow phantom and preliminary human validation show promise, further human subject testing is necessary to compare velocimetry data against existing commercial TCD systems. Additional human subject testing must also verify acceptable vessel search and tracking performance under a variety of subject populations and motion dynamics—such as head movement and ambulation.

Keywords Cerebral blood flow velocity · Transcranial Doppler · Power Doppler · Phased array · Wearable ultrasound

Introduction

Transcranial Doppler (TCD) sonography is a specialized Doppler ultrasound technique that enables the measurement of cerebral blood flow velocity (CBFV) from the basal intracerebral vessels. The use of TCD sonography is highly compelling as a cerebrovascular diagnostic modality because of its safety in prolonged studies, high temporal resolution, and relative portability. Although TCD sonography has been clinically indicated in a variety of neurovascular diagnostic applications [1], general acceptance of conventional TCD methods by the medical community has been impeded by several critical limitations—including the need for a highly-trained TCD operator, operator-dependent measurement results, and severe patient movement restrictions [2].

This work seeks to address these concerns through the development of a wearable TCD system with algorithmic steering capabilities. The wearable prototype form factor alleviates certain movement-related constraints particular to existing cart-based TCD systems, permitting applications requiring extended monitoring (e.g., emboli detection) [3]. Algorithmic vessel location and tracking can further reduce operator dependencies by both expediting and systematizing vessel location and identification procedures and by continuously

S.J. Pietrangelo (✉)
Department of Electrical Engineering and Computer Science, Massachusetts Institute of Technology, Cambridge, MA, USA
e-mail: sabinop@mit.edu; sjpietrangelo@gmail.com

H.-S. Lee • C.G. Sodini
Department of Electrical Engineering and Computer Science, Massachusetts Institute of Technology, Cambridge, MA, USA

updating acoustic focusing to regions of maximal flow, thereby ensuring measurement integrity. Additionally, autonomous operation can potentially lessen patient movement restrictions through a reduction in operator engagement and an increase in motion tolerance. Such capabilities eliminate the need for fine manual transducer adjustment and allow for an expansion of TCD measurement applications.

Materials and Methods

Recent advances in ultrasound electronics have led to substantial decreases in instrumentation dimensions. This work extends such reductions to a wearable form factor by identifying the anatomic, acoustic, and algorithmic constraints relevant to portable TCD sonography [4, 5].

To facilitate development and limit system complexity, this work concentrates on unilateral transtemporal acoustic window (TAW) insonation of the middle cerebral artery (MCA) for velocimetry applications. Of the major cerebral vessels, insonation and spectral Doppler (i.e., non-imaging) identification of the MCA through the TAW is generally the most straightforward due to favorable anatomical structure. The MCA is a high flow velocity, relatively large diameter cerebral vessel with approximately lateral course (i.e., normal to skull surface). TAW insonation of the ipsilateral MCA typically results in moderate insonation depths with modest steering and Doppler angles.

By restricting maximum steering angles and neglecting sonographic imaging requirements, electronic channel and transducer element count remain manageable without significant degradation in system performance. For azimuth and elevation steering angles less than ±17°, the 64 channel prototype device of this work maintains an acoustic focal intensity above the maximum on-axis intensity of an unfocused single element transducer at an equal acoustic output power. Grating lobes are generated by the relatively large transducer element pitch (1.6 mm ≈ 2λ), which produce spatial aliasing that may alter perceived volumetric position and combine backscattering from multiple regions at the same depth. These effects, however, have minimal influence on the accuracy of MCA spectral envelope generation when the MCA is the dominant source of positive volumetric flow at the depth of interest.

The discrete prototype electronic system has dimensions of 16.5 × 14 × 2.5 cm and is worn at the chest. The transducer array is affixed at the temporal region with an adjustable headframe. A block diagram of the discrete prototype system is presented Fig. 1.

Beamforming is achieved on transmit and receive through timing delays at each channel. Delays are discretized to 31 ns, resulting in phase resolution of 22.5° at the 2 MHz carrier frequency and steering angle resolution of approximately 1.5°. Following initialization, the prototype system controls define a coarse volumetric grid over the entire volume of interest and scan each coarse grid location for the specified dwell period (10–20 ms). Each grid location is characterized by the relative Doppler power ratio P_{rel} acquired over the dwell duration:

$$P_{rel}[n] = \frac{\int_0^\pi |X[n,\omega]|^2 d\omega}{\int_\pi^{2\pi} |X[n,\omega]|^2 d\omega}$$

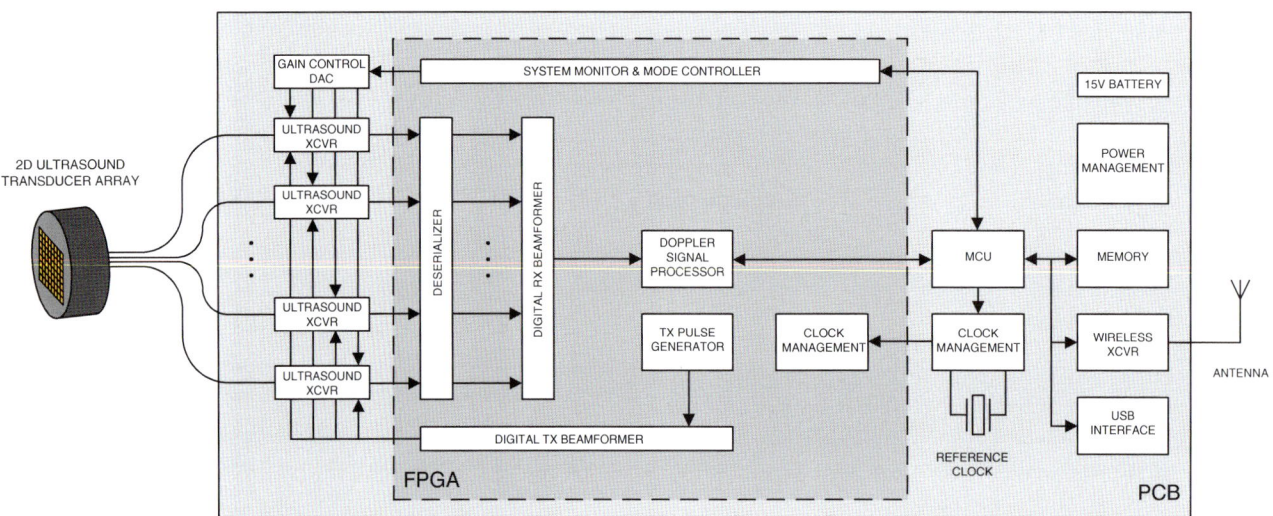

Fig. 1 Discrete prototype hardware block diagram

where $X[n,\lambda]$ is the time-dependent discrete Fourier transform of the baseband receive waveform $x[n]$ after clutter reject filtering, as described in [5, 6]. For unidirectional positive flow, spectral power at positive frequencies ($0 < \omega < \pi$) greatly exceeds spectral power at negative frequencies ($\pi < \omega < 2\pi$), yielding large values of P_{rel} (~5–100). Because a simultaneous ratio of powers is employed, P_{rel} values can be equitably compared without accounting for focal depth, acoustic attenuation and reflection, transducer beam pattern, transmit power level, and tissue backscattering coefficient.

For MCA localization, the search region extent is confined to −15 to +15 mm in both lateral dimensions and 40–65 mm in depth. A pulse repetition rate of 10 kHz with a 192 sample dwell period results in coarse search times of approximately 12 s—including communication overhead. For coarse grid locations yielding a Doppler power ratio above a specified threshold value, a subsampled local grid is defined and the dwell process repeated. The Doppler mapping procedure returns the location corresponding to maximal Doppler power ratio following local subsampling and redundancy checks. Because the MCA is generally the dominant source of positive flow within the search region, the search process nominally infers a suitable focal location for MCA velocimetry.

Vessel tracking is a continuous background process that defines a secondary receive focus. Tracking steers the secondary receive focus at offsets from the common transmit focus and compares the Doppler power ratio of the primary and secondary receive paths. Multiple range gates are added to the secondary receive path to increase effective tracking volume coverage. When the Doppler power ratio in the secondary path exceeds that of the primary velocimetry path for sufficient duration, the common transmit and primary receive focal points are updated. This process allows the system to track relative vessel motion simultaneous to CBFV measurement. Limitations in tracking robustness are highly dependent on both transmit 3 dB beamwidth at the depth of interest (≈2–4 mm) and relative vessel movement dynamics. If vessel tracking fails to maintain sufficient Doppler power ratio, the mapping search process is repeated until a suitable vessel segment is found.

Results

Velocimetry data from the prototype TCD system was validated on a Doppler flow phantom. Accurate flow velocity measurements were achieved over the expected range of physiological CBFV values (25 cm/s to 125 cm/s), yielding a normalized root-mean-square error < 3.0%, with a mean error of −1.7 cm/s and a standard deviation of the error of 2.4 cm/s. Figure 2a presents human subject test data from the vessel search procedure, where Doppler power ratio is measured throughout the search volume. Following Doppler power maximization, the system computes the spectrogram and spectral envelope, as shown in Fig. 2b. Under this procedure, operator interaction is limited to placement of the transducer array at the TAW via palpation; translation and angulation of the transducer array after placement is not required.

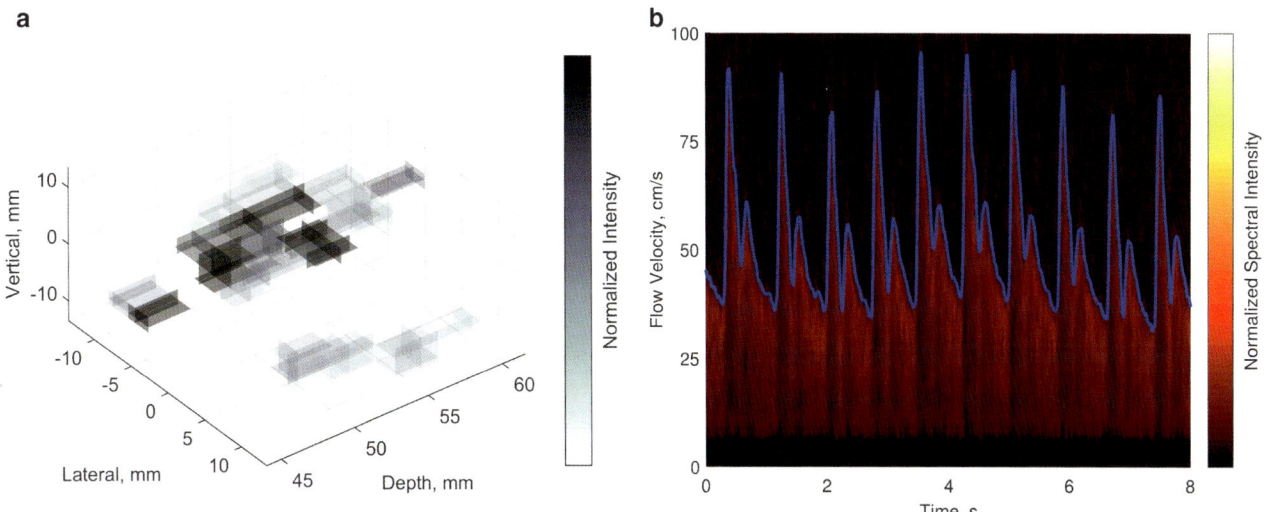

Fig. 2 (a) Spatial variation of transcranial Doppler power ratio via coarse mapping. (b) Transcranial spectrogram at the algorithmically located Doppler power ratio maxima

Discussion

Flow phantom experiments have demonstrated accurate velocimetry operation of the prototype system. Such measurement conditions, however, differ significantly from human subject receive signal levels—due primarily to excessive acoustic attenuation and reflection introduced by cranial bone and minimal erythrocytic backscattering. Results from initial human subject testing are encouraging, but additional human testing is necessary to validate the system across a breadth of subjects and measurement environments.

Doppler mapping techniques have exhibited utility in determining suitable focal locations for flow velocimetry—a tedious manual process under conventional TCD techniques. The codification of vessel search and identification through algorithmic procedures may yield a reduction in inter-operator and intra-operator variability.

Although operator interaction with the TCD sonography system during monitoring may be significantly mitigated through the use of algorithmic control, operator proficiency remains essential in determining TAW location. Improvements in acoustic window detection techniques are needed to further reduce necessary TCD operator qualifications.

Conclusions

Enabling technological advancements and a changing atmosphere toward point-of-care testing and mobile health paradigms has stimulated interest in portable, non-invasive, and highly usable tools for cerebrovascular monitoring and diagnostics. Preliminary human validation demonstrates a compact, wearable, and algorithmically steered TCD system that largely resolves several key shortcomings of established TCD measurement techniques. The successful execution of our current objectives can profoundly alter the standard clinical approach to neurovascular evaluation, especially in applications where the role of non-invasive diagnostics has not yet been clearly established (e.g., extended monitoring, emergency assessment).

Conflicts of interest statement We declare that we have no conflict of interest.

References

1. Sloan MA, Alexandrov AV, et al. Assessment: transcranial Doppler ultrasonography report of the Therapeutics and Technology Assessment Subcommittee of the American Academy of Neurology. Neurology. 2004;62:1468–81.
2. Shen Q, Stuart J, Venkatesh B, Wallace J, Lipman J. Inter observer variability of the transcranial Doppler ultrasound technique: impact of lack of practice on the accuracy of measurement. J Clin Monit Comput. 1999;15:179–84.
3. Mackinnon AD, Aaslid R, Markus HS. Ambulatory transcranial Doppler cerebral embolic signal detection in symptomatic and asymptomatic carotid stenosis. Stroke. 2005;36:1726–30.
4. Mackinnon AD, Aaslid R, Markus HS. Long-term ambulatory monitoring for cerebral emboli using transcranial Doppler ultrasound. Stroke. 2004;35:73–8.
5. Pietrangelo SJ. An electronically steered, wearable transcranial Doppler ultrasound system. S.M. Thesis. Cambridge, MA: Massachusetts Institute of Technology; 2013.
6. Jensen JA. Estimation of blood velocities using ultrasound: a signal processing approach. New York: Cambridge University Press; 1996.

Quantification of Macrocirculation and Microcirculation in Brain Using Ultrasound Perfusion Imaging

Eline J. Vinke, Jens Eyding, Chris de Korte, Cornelis H. Slump, Johannes G. van der Hoeven, and Cornelia W.E. Hoedemaekers

Abstract *Objective*: The aim of this study was to investigate the feasibility of simultaneous visualization of the cerebral macrocirculation and microcirculation, using ultrasound perfusion imaging (UPI). In addition, we studied the sensitivity of this technique for detecting changes in cerebral blood flow (CBF).

Materials and methods: We performed an observational study in ten healthy volunteers. Ultrasound contrast was used for UPI measurements during normoventilation and hyperventilation. For the data analysis of the UPI measurements, an in-house algorithm was used to visualize the DICOM files, calculate parameter images and select regions of interest (ROIs). Next, time intensity curves (TIC) were extracted and perfusion parameters calculated.

Results: Both volume- and velocity-related perfusion parameters were significantly different between the macrocirculation and the parenchymal areas. Hyperventilation-induced decreases in CBF were detectable by UPI in both the macrocirculation and microcirculation, most consistently by the volume-related parameters. The method was safe, with no adverse effects in our population.

Conclusions: Bedside quantification of CBF seems feasible and the technique has a favourable safety profile. Adjustment of current method is required to improve its diagnostic accuracy. Validation studies using a 'gold standard' are needed to determine the added value of UPI in neurocritical care monitoring.

Keywords Contrast enhanced ultrasound · Cerebral blood flow · Ischemia · Acute brain injury · Intensive care

Introduction

Acute brain injury is associated with high morbidity and mortality. Ischemia is an important mediator in the development of (secondary) brain injury. Increasing evidence shows that the microcirculation plays a key role in the pathophysiology of acute brain injury [1, 2]. Currently available monitoring techniques are unable to measure microvascular and macrovascular cerebral blood flow (CBF) simultaneously, require transportation of the patient outside the intensive care unit or are invasive in nature.

Ultrasound perfusion imaging (UPI) is a promising method to measure brain perfusion [3]. Ultrasound contrast agents (UCAs) are used to visualize the cerebral arteries to overcome the low level of acoustic intensity due to the ultrasound absorption of the skull [4]. Hereby, flow velocities and characteristics of the cerebral arteries can be determined as markers of macrocirculation. UCAs can also function as a tracer of microcirculation, that is, perfusion measurements, in a similar way as contrast agents in magnetic resonance imaging or computed tomography perfusion imaging.

The aim of this study was to investigate the feasibility of simultaneous visualization of cerebral macrocirculation and microcirculation using UPI. In addition, we studied the sensitivity of this technique for detecting changes in CBF.

E.J. Vinke · J.G. van der Hoeven · C.W.E. Hoedemaekers, M.D., Ph.D. (✉)
Department of Intensive Care, Radboud University Nijmegen Medical Centre, Nijmegen, The Netherlands
e-mail: Astrid.Hoedemaekers@radboudumc.nl

J. Eyding
Department of Neurology, Universitätsklinikum Knappschaftskrankenhaus, Ruhr University Bochum, Bochum, Germany

C. de Korte
Department of Radiology, Radboud University Nijmegen Medical Centre, Nijmegen, The Netherlands

C.H. Slump
MIRA Institute for Biomedical Technology and Technical Medicine, University of Twente, Enschede, The Netherlands

Methods

Study

We performed an observational study in ten healthy volunteers. All participants gave written informed consent before entering the study. The study was approved by the ethics committee of the Radboud University Medical Centre (NL 52854.091.15) and in accordance with the ethical standards laid down in the 1964 Declaration of Helsinki and its later amendments.

Population

The population comprised ten young healthy volunteers, between 18 and 35 years of age. Subjects were screened by physical examination and electrocardiography. Main exclusion criteria were known hypersensitivity to the active substance(s) or to any of the excipients of SonoVue (Bracco International, Amsterdam, The Netherlands), history, signs or symptoms of cardiovascular, pulmonary or neurological disease, pregnancy and participation in another clinical trial within 3 months prior to the experimental day.

Study Protocol

Duplex and UPI measurements were performed on the subjects during normoventilation and during hyperventilation. The measurements comprised of bilateral duplex measurements of the middle cerebral artery (MCA) blood flow velocity (CBFV), followed by a UPI measurement using the bolus technique. Duplex followed by UPI measurement was performed three times. Intervals between each examination in one volunteer were at least 20 min to allow wash-out of the contrast agent.

Following three baseline measurements, a baseline duplex measurement was performed while on continuous end-tidal CO_2 monitoring. Following baseline duplex measurement, subjects were asked to hyperventilate to reduce end-tidal CO_2 by at least 20%. After the end-tidal CO_2 was reduced sufficiently, a duplex followed by UPI measurement of cerebral blood flow was performed at one side (unilaterally).

Ultrasound Protocol

A Philips iU22 ultrasound system was used, with a 2.5-MHz phased-array S5-1 probe for all duplex and UPI measurements. In the contrast mode, a mechanical index of 1.09 with a gain of 76% was used. UPI was performed in contrast mode after a rapid IV bolus injection of 2.4 ml of a sulphurhexafluoride-dispersion (SonoVue; Bracco International, Amsterdam, The Netherlands), followed by a rapid flush of 10 ml normal saline. An insonation plane was chosen visualizing the MCA and other parts of the circle of Willis to allow simultaneous analysis of the flow in the macrocirculation and parenchyma.

Data Analysis

For the data analysis of the UPI measurements, an in-house algorithm was developed in Matlab (R2014b; The MathWorks, Natick, MA, USA). With this algorithm, the DICOM files were visualized, parameter images were calculated, and regions of interest (ROIs) selected, from which time intensity curves (TIC) were extracted and bolus curves were fitted.

One ROI was selected in the ipsilateral MCA at a depth of 4–5 cm, and three in the parenchyma: region of interest (ROI1) was selected on the contralateral side at a depth of 9–10 cm at the same anterior level as the MCA region. The second parenchyma region (ROI2) was selected at the contralateral side at a depth of 9–10 cm, posterior to ROI1. The final parenchyma region (ROI3) was selected on the ipsilateral side at a depth of 4–5 cm posterior to the ipsilateral MCA region. Curve fitting and calculation of the perfusion parameters from the TIC was performed using the method of least squares with the model function as described by Eyding et al. [5]. Peak intensity (PI) was defined as the maximum amplitude the curve reaches; area under the curve (AUC) was calculated by a summation of all the acoustic intensities starting from the start of the bolus curve; time to peak intensity (T_{PI}) was defined as the time at which the curve reaches its maximum amplitude; time to peak (TTP) was defined as T_{PI} minus the start of the bolus curve.

Statistical Analyses

Statistical analysis was performed using GraphPad Prism version 5.0 (GraphPad Software, La Jolla, CA, USA). Data are presented as mean values with standard deviation or median values with interquartal ranges depending on their distribution. Differences between the perfusion parameters of the macrocirculation were compared to the three different ROIs of the microcirculation using the Friedman test for non-parametric repeated measures. Differences in perfusion parameters in the four ROIs between normoventilation and hyperventilation were analysed using the Wilcoxon signed rank sum test. Linear regression was used to determine the correlation between CBFV in the MCA and perfusion parameters. A p value < 0.05 was considered to indicate statistical significance.

Results

Population

Ten healthy volunteers were included in the study. No adverse events occurred during the study. Due to technical failure, data of the first subject could not be used. Results of the remaining nine subjects are presented.

Normal Cerebral Blood Flow

The blood volume-related parameters PI and AUC were significantly different in the macrocirculation compared to the microcirculation (Fig. 1a, b). The PI in the macrocirculation was 25.4 [24.7–26.3] dB compared to 2.3 [1.5–2.9], 2.4 [2.1–3.4] and 3.2 [1.8–3.8] dB in the microcirculation ($p = 0.0008$); the AUC was 10,195 [9,129–12,699] dB in the macrocirculation and 332 [268–398], 389 [303–651] and 540 [259–722] dB in the microcirculation ($p = 0.0005$).

The velocity-related parameters TPI and TTP were also significantly different in the macrocirculation and microcirculation (Fig. 1c, d). The TPI in the macrocirculation was 13.8 [12.6–14.8] s compared to 18.1 [16.8–19.2] s, 17.8 [17.3–18.1] s and 17.3 [16.5–18.3] s in the microcirculation

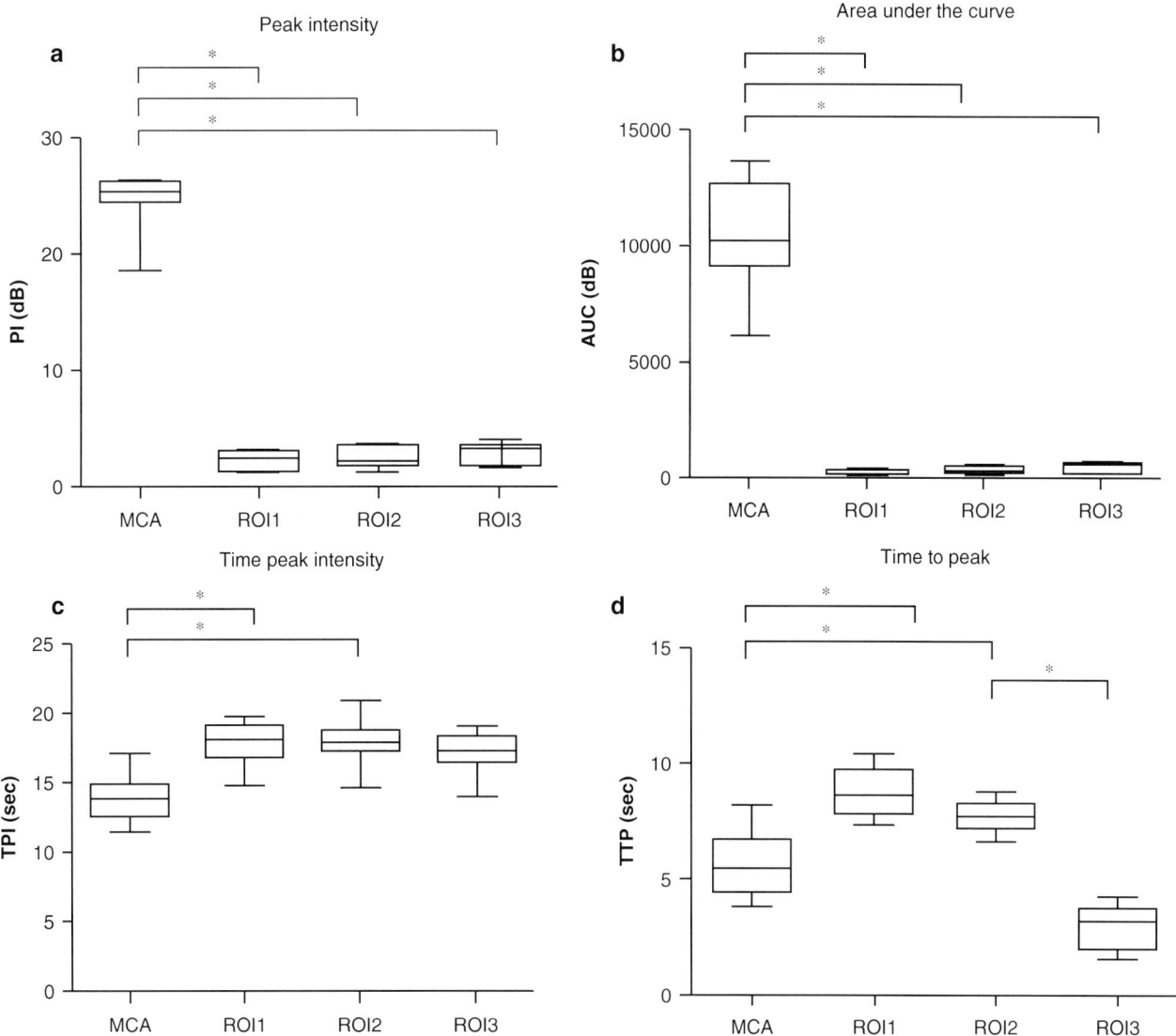

Fig. 1 (a) Perfusion parameter values in the ipsilateral MCA region (MCA), (b) anterior contralateral parenchyma region (ROI1), (c) posterior contralateral parenchyma region (ROI2) and (d) the posterior ipsilateral region (ROI3)

($p < 0.0001$); the TTP was 5.5 [4.4–6.7] s in the macrocirculation and 8.6 [7.8–9.7] s, 7.7 [7.3–8.3] s and 3.2 [2.0–3.8] s in the microcirculation ($p < 0.0001$).

Effects of Hyperventilation on Cerebral Blood Flow

Hyperventilation effectively decreased the end-tidal CO_2 values from 5.4 ± 0.37% to 3.9 ± 0.4% (28.2 ± 7.1% decrease). The mean blood flow velocity in the MCA significantly decreased during hyperventilation from 60.6 ± 7.1 to 49.9 ± 3.4 cm/s ($p = 0.0128$); the peak systolic blood flow velocity decreased from 101.6 ± 13.0 to 90.1 ± 10.5 cm/s ($p = 0.0078$) (data not shown).

The blood volume-related parameter PI in the macrocirculation decreased from 25.4 [24.7–26.3] to 20.2 [12.9–26.0] dB ($p = 0.0547$) and the AUC decreased from 10,195 [9129–12,699] to 4509 [2214–6,299] dB ($p = 0.0039$) during hyperventilation (Fig. 2a, b). Similarly, the PI in the microcirculation decreased significantly from 2.3 [1.5–2.9] to 0.52 [0.35–1.24] ($p = 0.0078$), 2.4 [2.1–3.4] to 0.49 [0.45–1.23] ($p = 0.0078$) and 3.2 [1.8–3.8] to 1.18 [0.82–2.77] dB ($p = 0.0195$). The AUC in the microcirculation decreased during hyperventilation in the ROI1 and ROI2 from 332 [268–398] to 39.0 [28.2–121.6] and 389 [303–651] to 57.7 [26.1–146] dB ($p = 0.0039$ and 0.0078) respectively (Fig. 2e, f). The decrease in ROI3 was not significant.

The velocity-related parameters TPI and TTP did not change significantly in the MCA (Fig. 2c, d). In the microcirculation, TPI decreased significantly in ROI1 and ROI3 from 18.1 [16.8–19.2] to 14.9 [12.1–15.8] ($p = 0.0195$) and from 17.3 [16.5–18.3] to 13.3 [10.6–15.1] s ($p = 0.0117$) (Fig. 2g). Similar results were calculated for the TTP in ROI1 and ROI3 {decrease from 8.6 [7.8–9.7] to 6.4 [5.2–7.8] ($p = 0.017$) and from 3.2 [2.0–3.8] to 1.1 [0.8–2.8] ($p = 0.0195$) s} (Fig. 2h).

Changes in size of the ROIs did not significantly change the results (data not shown). We have correlated changes in CBFV measured by duplex to changes in perfusion parameters derived from the UPI. Mean CBFV in the MCA correlated significantly with perfusion parameters PI and AUC ($p = 0.004$), but not with TTP or TPI (data not shown).

Discussion

Simultaneous (semi-)quantitative analysis of the cerebral macrocirculation and microcirculation seems feasible in healthy volunteers. Both volume- and velocity-related parameters were significantly different between the macrocirculation and the parenchymal areas. Hyperventilation-induced decreases in CBF were detectable by UPI in both the macrocirculation and microcirculation, most consistently by the volume-related parameters. The method was safe, with no adverse effects in our population.

The volume-related parameters PI and AUC were significantly higher in the MCA compared to the parenchyma, due to the increased concentration of microbubbles within the blood vessel. Decrease in CBF resulted in a consistent decrease in most volume-related parameters in both macrocirculation and microcirculation, suggesting that a change in CBF was detectable with UPI. Although the change in perfusion parameters was significant, quantification of CBF was not validated in this (feasibility) experiment. In order to quantify flow using a contrast agent, the contrast intensity must be correlated to the concentration of the contrast agent. Recently, linearity between contrast intensity and the concentration of perflubutane microbubbles was confirmed in an ex vivo phantom study in liver tissue [6]. Similar results were found using galactose-based (first-generation) microbubbles in myocardial tissue [7].

Velocity-dependent parameters were more affected by variation compared to the volume-related parameters. This may be a reflection of variation in administration and the dosage of the microbubbles. Reconstitution of the microbubbles prior to administration, together with variation in the physical and physiological environment, changes the size distribution, stability and concentration of the contrast agents and strongly influences the perfusion parameters [8]. At high doses, especially in the MCA recordings, multiple scattering can occur, with the sound waves scattered by one bubble affecting the oscillation and scattering from its neighbours. In addition, the measurement may become saturated as seen most evidently in the PI measurements in the MCA. This is supported by the fact that the PI in the microcirculation (with lower contrast agent concentrations) decreased significantly. Reduction in microbubble dose may overcome this issue.

This study has a number of limitations. Several velocity and volume parameters failed to detect the change in CBF induced by hyperventilation, most likely as a result of the high variability in the results. High variability of UPI is a key challenge of this technique and the causes of this high variability have not yet been fully understood [9]. UPI is operator dependent, due to differences in microbubble dosing and speed of injection and probe positioning. Imaging parameters and specific equipment settings strongly influence the quantification outcomes. Since all experiments were performed by the same operator, and scanner settings were unchanged during the experiment, variation from these factors was considered to be limited. The variability was highest in ROI3, situated closely to the skull base; bone artefacts may underlie the high variability of parameters in this region.

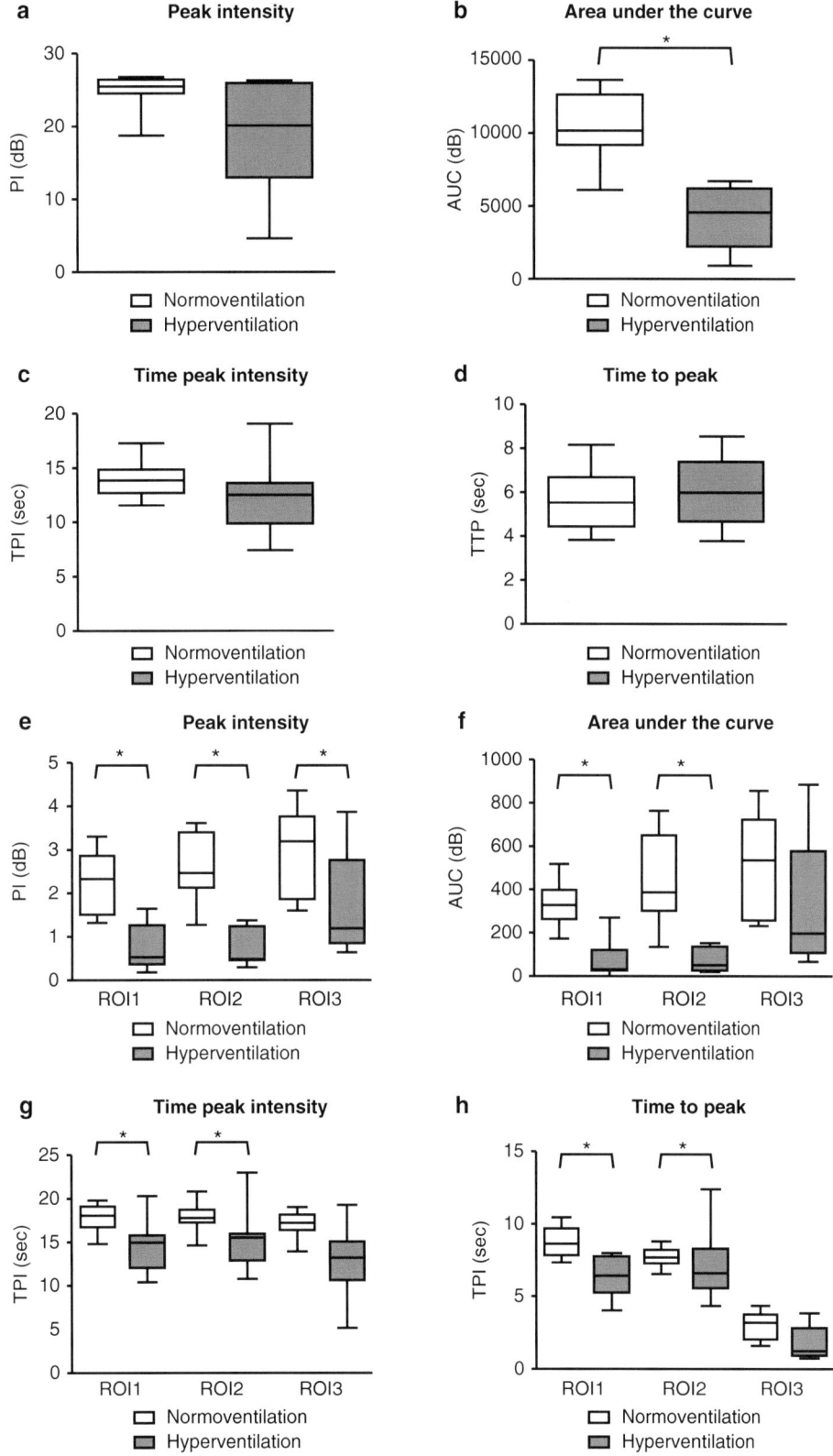

Fig. 2 Perfusion parameter values in the ipsilateral MCA region (MCA) during normoventilation and hyperventilation (a–d) and in the three parenchymal regions (e–h) during normoventilation and hyperventilation

Conclusion

Bedside quantification of CBF seems feasible and the technique has a favourable safety profile. Adjustment of the current method is needed to improve its diagnostic accuracy. Validation studies using a 'gold standard' are needed to determine the exact role of UPI in neurocritical care monitoring.

Conflicts of interest statement We declare that we have no conflict of interest.

References

1. Gursoy-Ozdemir Y, Yemisci M, Dalkara T. Microvascular protection is essential for successful neuroprotection in stroke. J Neurochem. 2012;123(Suppl 2):2–11. https://doi.org/10.1111/j.1471-4159.2012.07938.x.
2. Taccone FS, Su F, Pierrakos C, He X, James S, Dewitte O, Vincent JL, De Backer D. Cerebral microcirculation is impaired during sepsis: an experimental study. Crit Care. 2010;14:R140. https://doi.org/10.1186/cc9205.
3. Meairs S, Kern R. Intracranial perfusion imaging with ultrasound. Front Neurol Neurosci. 2015;36:57–70. https://doi.org/10.1159/000366237.
4. Shpak O, Verweij M, de Jong N, Versluis M. Droplets, bubbles and ultrasound interactions. Adv Exp Med Biol. 2016;880:157–74. https://doi.org/10.1007/978-3-319-22536-4_9.
5. Eyding J, Krogias C, Wilkening W, Meves S, Ermert H, Postert T. Parameters of cerebral perfusion in phase-inversion harmonic imaging (PIHI) ultrasound examinations. Ultrasound Med Biol. 2003;29:1379–85.
6. Ohno N, Miyati T, Yamashita M, Narikawa M. Quantitative assessment of tissue perfusion in hepatocellular carcinoma using perflubutane dynamic contrast-enhanced ultrasonography: a preliminary study. Diagnostics. 2015;5:210–8. https://doi.org/10.3390/diagnostics5020210.
7. Yamada S, Komuro K, Mikami T, Kudo N, Onozuka H, Goto K, Fujii S, Yamamoto K, Kitabatake A. Novel quantitative assessment of myocardial perfusion by harmonic power Doppler imaging during myocardial contrast echocardiography. Heart. 2005;91:183–8. https://doi.org/10.1136/hrt.2004.035857.
8. Seidel G, Algermissen C, Christoph A, Claassen L, Vidal-Langwasser M, Katzer T. Harmonic imaging of the human brain. Visualization of brain perfusion with ultrasound. Stroke. 2000;31:151–4.
9. Tang MX, Mulvana H, Gauthier T, Lim AK, Cosgrove DO, Eckersley RJ, Stride E. Quantitative contrast-enhanced ultrasound imaging: a review of sources of variability. Interface Focu.s. 2011;1:520–39. https://doi.org/10.1098/rsfs.2011.0026.

HDF5-Based Data Format for Archiving Complex Neuro-monitoring Data in Traumatic Brain Injury Patients

Manuel Cabeleira, Ari Ercole, and Peter Smielewski

Abstract *Objectives:* Modern neuro-critical care units generate high volumes of data. These data originate from a multitude of devices in various formats and levels of granularity. We present a new data format intended to store these data in an ordered and homogenous way.

Material and methods: The adopted data format was based on the hierarchical model, HDF5, which is capable of dealing with a mixture of small and very large datasets with equal ease. It is possible to access and manipulate individual data elements directly within a single file, and this is extensible and versatile.

Results: The file structure that was agreed divided the patient data into four different groups: 'Annotations' for clinical events and sporadic observations, 'Numerics' for all the low-frequency data, 'Waves' for all the high-frequency data and 'Summaries' for the trend data and calculated parameters. The addition of attributes to every group and dataset makes the file self-described. More than 200 files have been successfully collected and stored using this format.

Conclusion: The new file format was implemented in ICM+ software and validated as part of a collaboration with participating centres across Europe.

Keywords HDF5 · Multimodal monitoring · Data storage · Data format

Introduction

High volumes of data are generated during a patient's stay in any modern intensive care unit and in neurointensive care in particular. Data come not only from a multitude of bedside monitors [arterial blood pressure (ABP), intracranial pressure (ICP), electrocardiogram (ECG)] but also from lab data, manual measurements/observations and event annotation. With the introduction of electronic medical record systems, these data are captured and archived electronically. Currently, a notable exception to this is the routine storage of high-resolution, full waveform data. These are generally displayed at the bedside but only summary values are archived. Such a situation is problematic for research and clinical care, whereas important clinical information can be extracted from multimodal waveform data.

Despite numerous attempts to address these interoperability issues with unifying medical communication standards, notably the ISO standard IEEE11073 [1], none have managed to truly fulfil the needs for physiological data and thus have not been widely adopted. A number of proprietary formats have emerged, but these all suffer from limitations, making the creation of multi-centre databases difficult. Developing a well-annotated standard for data archiving is of paramount importance to facilitate further advances in computer-supported individualised management of patients.

We propose a prototype format that that can be used as the foundation for the creation of a standard that covers all the needs of modern critical care environment. This format has been implemented for the CENTER-TBI study [2], where it will be used as the main data storage format for high resolution data generated across Europe.

M. Cabeleira (✉)
Brain Physics Lab, Division of Neurosurgery, Department of Clinical Neurosciences, Addenbrooke's Hospital, University of Cambridge, Cambridge, UK

Neurosurgery Unit, Addenbrooke's Hospital, Cambridge, UK
e-mail: mc916@cam.ac.uk

A. Ercole
Division of Anaesthesia, Addenbrooke's Hospital, University of Cambridge, Cambridge, UK

P. Smielewski
Brain Physics Lab, Division of Neurosurgery, Department of Clinical Neurosciences, Addenbrooke's Hospital, University of Cambridge, Cambridge, UK

Materials and Methods

This project builds on the hierarchical model developed by the open source HDF5 file format specification [3]. This file format is already extensively used in other areas of science where extensive amounts of data need to be stored [4–6]. In particular, it has found application as a standard for experimental neuroinformatics [7].

HDF5 is attractive for its flexible format, offering a self-describing hierarchical, tree-like structure capable of holding almost any kind of well-annotated data objects in a single file. To add to its versatility, most of the most widely used scientific tools already provide libraries to handle this type of files (MATLAB, Python, Java, C), with MATLAB even adopting the file format as its primary storage format. An HDF5 file is composed of two main building blocks: Groups and Datasets (Fig. 1). The groups form the tree's stem and branches and are therefore responsible for the hierarchical organisation of the data. Every dataset is a uniform multidimensional array of data objects or elements, represented by one of the predefined simple data types or compound elements composed of a mixture of data types. Groups and datasets can be further annotated with metadata contained in associated 'Attributes'.

HDF5 may be compressed for storage efficiency and the format reduces data access time and facilitates access and extraction of only data subsets.

The following requirements for the file internal structure design were defined:

- Accommodate all data types from bedside monitors at full temporal resolution.
- Each data object fully described by its attributes.
- Accommodation of structured clinical annotation. Provision for metadata.
- Completely self-described.

Results

HDF5 Data File Structure

Our file structure is presented in Fig. 1. The data are divided into different groups (categories) (Table 1). Each group contains a specific data type associated with it and a set of attributes.

Waveform and numeric datasets include one dataset per modality or, in case of composite recordings such as electroencephalograms (EEGs), one group of datasets (individual channels) per modality (see Fig. 1). Each dataset in turn includes a series of uninterrupted (continuous) data streams characterised by its position in the dataset, its actual start time and its sampling frequency detailed in the dataset 'Index Table' attributes (Table 2, Fig. 2). In addition, each of those datasets also has an attribute data quality tracking (Table 2, Fig. 2). Episodic (Table 2) and annotation data (Table 2) contain individual data samples (simple or composite), each with its own time stamp and a quality flag, where relevant.

In addition, the file structure also contains: Summaries, Definitions and Clinical annotations groups as well as two datasets, PatientInfo and Presentation—all of which are described in Tables 1 and 2.

Finally, a set of attributes was chosen for the root group containing the most important metadata describing the dataset.

Data Compression and Performance

Data compression intrinsic to the HDF5 standard is used to minimise overall file size. For time-series datasets (numeric, waveform and electrophysiology), the Scale Offset algorithm

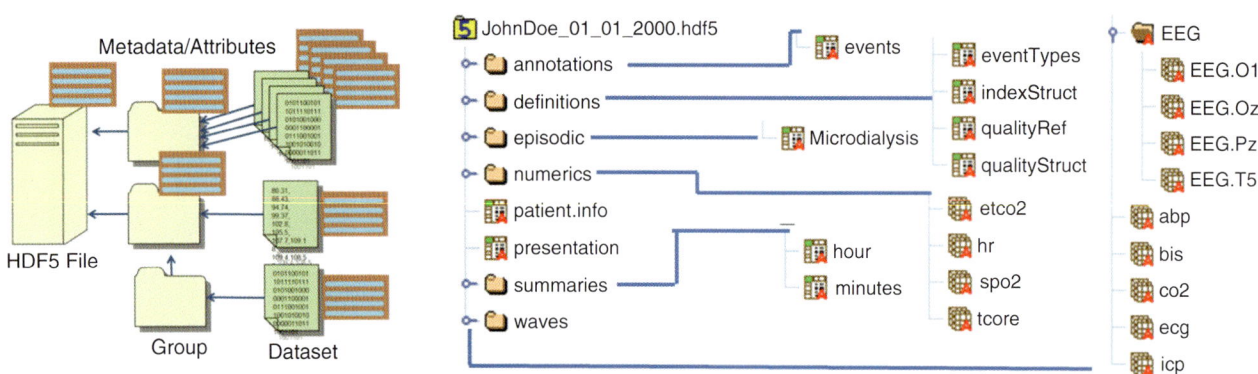

Fig. 1 *Left*: HDF5 hierarchical data storage concept. *Right*: structure of the proposed neurocritical care physiological data file

Table 1 Division of data into logical categories—HDF5 groups

Data type	Modalities	HDF5 dataset type	Attributes	Description
Numerics	• ETCO2 • SPO2 • PBTO2 • HR • Temperature			• For all the low temporal resolution data (sampled ≤ 1 Hz)
Waveforms	• ABP • ICP • ECG • CVP • EEG[a] • ECoG[a]	One-dimensional array of 32-bit float numbers	• Index Table (Composite array) • Quality Table (Composite array) • Units (String) • Location (String) • Metric (String) • Modality (String) • Source (String)	• For high temporal resolution, waveforms
EEG/ECoG (inside waveform group)[a]	• EEG channels			• Group inside the Waveforms used to store EEG data
Summaries	(Processed data) • Minute-by-minute • Hourly	One-dimensional array of a composite type[b]	• Index Table (Composite array) • Column labels (String) • Title (String)	• Group which stores synchronised Excel spread sheet type, time synchronised, representation of the numerics and waveforms datasets, produced by averaging values with granularity of 1 min in one dataset, and 1 h in the other
Episodic	• Microdialysis • Clinical observations		• Columns labels (String) • Title (String) • Textual description (String)	• For irregularly sampled data and manual measurements
Clinical annotations	• Nursery events • Spontaneous notes			• Including datasets with labelled events and textual notes (ex. Nursing events)
Definitions	• eventTypes • indexStruct • qualitied • qualityStruct			• Group containing details, with descriptions, of any complex data formats used for datasets or attributes. The group is also meant to contain physiological variables' and events' labels nomenclature
Patient.info[c]	(Patient Demographics)		• Columns labels (string) • Title (string) • Textual description (string)	• A dataset in the root group that contains name=value pairs of patient demographics, if such patient identifier are to be stored in the files, otherwise may be omitted
Presentation[c]	(Clinical information)			• A dataset in the root group that contains name=value pairs of any auxiliary clinical data fields that are useful to keep together with the physiological data, and which do not de-anonymise the data (example, GCS at admission, type of trauma, etc.)

[a]EEG/ECoG are part of a group that is inside the waveforms group
[b]Composite types are explained in Table 2
[c]Patient.info and presentation are not associated to any group

was used. For the summaries group, the GZip algorithm [8] was used with a power level of 6 for its handling of NAN values (ensuring seamless Excel compatibility). This data compression was shown to be effective (Table 3) and capable of processing an average of 1.7MB HDF5 data per second. Within-file data access time was negligible.

This format has already been used to archive and transfer to a central repository of more than 200 recordings from 22 different centres across Europe. The average file size was 512 MB, containing an average of 7.4 days of data and at least ABP, ICP and ECG full-resolution waveforms.

Table 2 Table describing the composite data types

Composite type	Data arrangement	Descriptions
Summaries	• [*Time-stamp* (64-bit float), *1xN* 32-bit float]	• *Time-stamp*—Excel date time format (number of days since 1/1/1990) • *1xN*—one-dimensional array with one value for each (*N*) variable collected in the file
Episodic	• [*Code* (String), *Time-stamp* (64-bit Float), *Duration* (32-bit Float), *Comment* (String), *Value* (32-bit Float)]	• *Code*—Textual code for the variable/observation being inserted • *Time-stamp*—UNIX format time stamp (milliseconds since 1/1/1970) • *Duration*—Duration of the duration/effect of the variable being inserted (to use only if applicable) • *Comment*—Textual comment on the variable/observation being inserted (to use only if applicable) • *Value*—Numerical value of the variable/observation being inserted (to use only if applicable)
Clinical annotations	• [*Code* (String), *UNIX Time-stamp* (64-bit Float), *Duration* (32-bit Float), *Comment* (String)]	• *Code*—Textual code for the Clinical Annotations being inserted • *Time-stamp*—UNIX format time stamp (milliseconds since 1/1/1970) • *Duration*—Duration of the duration/effect of the Clinical Annotations being inserted (to use only if applicable) • *Comment*—Textual comment on the Clinical Annotations being inserted (to use only if applicable)
Definitions[a]	• [*Name* (String), *Description* (String)] or • [*Value* (32-bit unsigned integer), *Description* (String)]	• *Name*—Name of the element being described • *Description*—Textual description of the element or • *Value*—Numeric code of the element being described • *Description*—Textual description of the element
Index Table	• *Start index* (64-bit integer), *Start time* (64-bit Unsigned integer), *Duration* (64-bit integer), *Sampling frequency* (64-bit float)	• *Start index*—index of the first sample in this continuous data block • *Start time*—modified UNIX format time stamp (microseconds since 1/1/1970) • *Duration*—number of data samples in this data block • *Sampling frequency*—data sampling frequency [Hz]
Quality Table	• [*TimeStamp* (64-bit unsigned integer), *Code* (32-bit unsigned integer)] • [*TimeStamp Code*] • [64-bit unsigned integer 32-bit unsigned integer]	• *Time-Stamp*—UNIX format time stamp (milliseconds since 1/1/1970) • *Code*—(bit) set of quality indicators valid for data starting at this time point until the next quality indicator or until the end of data
Patient.info (Patient demographics) Presentation (Clinical information)	• [*Field* (String), *Value* (String)]	• *Filed*—Textual name of the patient or clinical information • *Value*—Textual value for the field representing the patient name or Clinical information

[a]Depending of the specific needs of the definition table these two composite arrangements can be found

Discussion

The HDF5 data platform proved to be robust, extensible, scalable, self-describing and easy to handle. One important advantage of our format is the capacity for easy manipulation of its contents. In particular, it allows post-creation removal, addition or transformation of datasets. This feature allows supplementing the intensive care unit recordings with external data. Unlike other formats, it is possible to extract subsets of data without parsing the whole file, making handling very large files practical.

The compression ratios observed in this file format were very good compared to others, allowing the creation of lightweight databases and facilitating the overall file handling, yet still retaining excellent performance of the data-archiving process.

Conclusions

The developed format can be used to archive multi-centre data in a homogenous, robust, self-described and accessible way. We propose our format as a prototype for a standard for clinical physiological data from intensive care. The creation of such standard is of paramount importance not only to ease

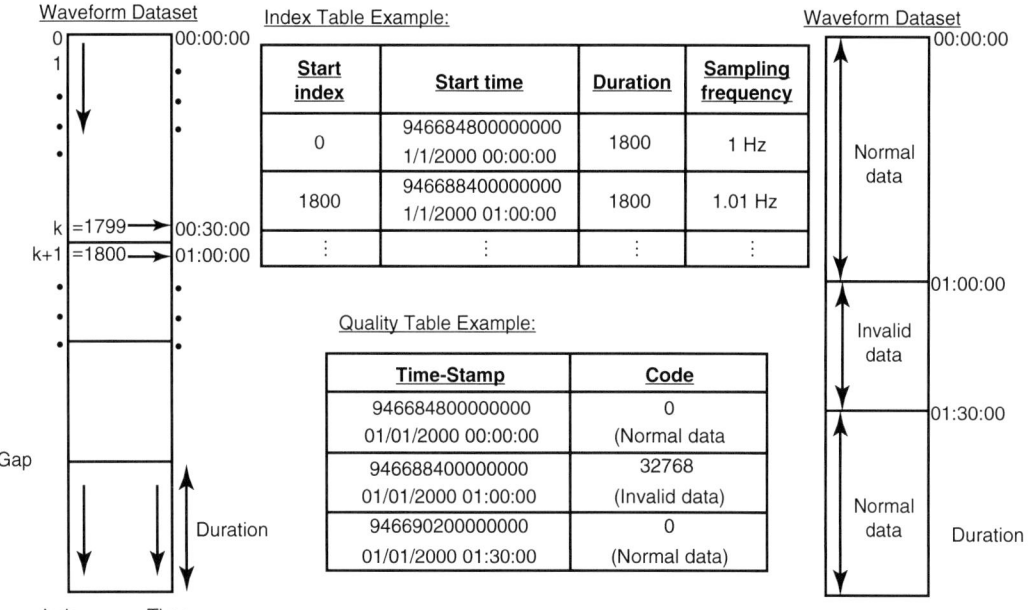

Fig. 2 The concepts of the Index Table (*left*), and the Quality Table (*right*)

Table 3 Achieved compression rates

Original file type	Average compression rates achieved
ICM+ Raw	3.37
LabChart	4.99
Draeger proprietary binary	1.62
Moberg binary	2.8

inter-centre collaborations, but also to simplify planning and execution of future multi-centre studies.

Acknowledgements This work was supported by a European CoER-TBI).

Conflicts of interest statement P. Smielewski and M. Czosnyka have partial financial interest in the licensing of ICM+.

References

1. Franklin DF, Ostler DV. Proposed standard IEEE P1073 Medical Information Bus: medical device to host computer interface network overview and architecture. In: Eighth Annual International Phoenix Conference on Computers and Communications 1989 Conference Proceedings. IEEE Comput Soc Press; [cited 2016 Oct 26]. p. 574–8. Available from: http://ieeexplore.ieee.org/document/37448/.
2. Maas AIR, Menon DK, Steyerberg EW, Citerio G, Lecky F, Manley GT, et al. Collaborative European NeuroTrauma Effectiveness Research in Traumatic Brain Injury (CENTER-TBI): a prospective longitudinal observational study. Neurosurgery [Internet]. 2015 .[cited 2016 Oct 31];76(1):67–80. Available from: http://www.ncbi.nlm.nih.gov/pubmed/25525693.
3. HDF5 file format specification version 3.0. Available from: https://support.hdfgroup.org/HDF5/doc/H5.format.html.
4. Dougherty MT, Folk MJ, Zadok E, Bernstein HJ, Bernstein FC, Eliceiri KW, et al. Unifying biological image formats with HDF5. Commun AMC. 2009;52(10):42–7.
5. Rees N, Billich HR, Koziol Q, Wintersberger E, Götz A, Pourmal E, et al. Developing HDF5 for the Synchrotron Community. 2015;WEPGF063.
6. Rübel O, Prabhat M, Denes P, Conant D, Chang E, Bouchard K. BRAINformat: a data standardization framework for neuroscience data. 2015. bioRxiv.
7. Eglen SJ, Weeks M, Jessop M, Simonotto J, Jackson T, Sernagor E, et al. A data repository and analysis framework for spontaneous neural activity recordings in developing retina. Gigascience. 2014 [cited 2016 Oct 31];3(1):3. Available from: http://gigascience.biomedcentral.com/articles/10.1186/2047-217X-3-3.
8. HDF5 Users Guide. [cited 2017 Feb 28]. Available from: https://support.hdfgroup.org/HDF5/doc/UG/HDF5_Users_Guide.pdf.

Neurocritical Care Informatics

Are Slow Waves of Intracranial Pressure Suppressed by General Anaesthesia?

Despina Afroditi Lalou, Marek Czosnyka, Joseph Donnelly, Andrea Lavinio, John D. Pickard, Matthew Garnett, and Zofia Czosnyka

Abstract *Objectives*: Slow waves of intracranial pressure (ICP) are spontaneous oscillations with a frequency of 0.3–4 cycles/min. They are often associated with pathological conditions, following vasomotor activity in the cranial enclosure. This study quantifies the effects of general anaesthesia (GA) on the magnitude of B-waves compared with natural sleep and the conscious state.

Materials and methods: Four groups of 30 patients each were formed to assess the magnitude of slow waves. Group A and group B consisted of normal pressure hydrocephalus (NPH) patients, each undergoing cerebrospinal fluid (CSF) infusion studies, conscious and under GA respectively. Group C comprised conscious, naturally asleep hydrocephalic patients undergoing overnight ICP monitoring; group D, which included deeply sedated head injury patients monitored in the intensive care unit (ICU), was compared with group C.

Results: The average amplitude for group A patients was higher (0.23 ± 0.10 mmHg) than that of group B (0.15 ± 0.10 mmHg; $p = 0.01$). Overnight magnitude of slow waves was higher in group C (0.20 ± 0.13 mmHg) than in group D (0.11 ± 0.09 mmHg; $p = 0.002$).

Conclusion: Slow waves of ICP are suppressed by GA and deep sedation. When using slow waves in clinical decision-making, it is important to consider the patients' level of consciousness to avoid incorrect therapeutic and management decisions.

Keywords General anesthesia · Slow waves · B-waves Intracranial pressure · Hydrocephalus

Introduction

We previously published the complete version of this paper [1]. Slow waves of intracranial pressure (ICP), also called B-waves, are spontaneous rhythmic oscillations of the ICP within a low frequency bandwidth of 0.3–4 cycles/min. Even though they are mostly associated with hydrocephalus and head injury, they may also be present in healthy individuals [2, 3]. It is widely accepted that they originate from changes in intracranial blood volume, following vasodilation and vasoconstriction [3, 4]. More theories, suggesting that cyclical changes in arterial CO_2 are probably the causative factor in B-waves, have been called into question by findings that showed that artificial ventilation does not affect B-waves [3, 4].

The clinical significance of slow waves is also something that remains unclarified. They have been used as a reliable indicator of decreased brain elasticity and shunt responsiveness in hydrocephalus; the intracranial volume buffering reserve correlates inversely with B-wave amplitude and correlates directly with resistance to cerebrospinal fluid (CSF) outflow (RCSF) [4–6]. In turn, increased B-wave activity correlates with clinical improvement after shunt insertion in normal pressure hydrocephalus (NPH). In head injury patients, the presence of B-waves is associated with a positive outcome, reflecting preserved autoregulation [5, 6].

D.A. Lalou (✉) · M. Czosnyka · J. Donnelly · J.D. Pickard
M. Garnett · Z. Czosnyka
Division of Neurosurgery, Department of Clinical Neuroscience,
Cambridge University Hospital,
Cambridge, UK
e-mail: adl43@cam.ac.uk

A. Lavinio
Neurosciences Critical Care Unit, Department of Anaesthesia,
Cambridge University Hospitals NHS Foundation Trust,
Cambridge, UK

Monitoring of ICP is performed according to indication in a variety of clinical settings ranging from conscious, self-ventilating patients, mechanically ventilated patients under general anaesthesia (GA) and during physiological sleep [6, 7]. Based on previous observations, it has been evident that slow waves recorded in conscious, self-ventilated patients undergoing CSF infusion studies are lessened or absent in patients studied under GA. So far, there are no published data quantifying the influence of GA on vasogenic ICP oscillations. The wealth of data collected in our laboratory over many years allows us to quantify and compare B-wave activity in NPH and head injury patients.

Materials and Methods

The first two groups of patients, group A and group B, consisted of two cohorts of 30 non-shunted patients, each undergoing CSF infusion studies for diagnostic confirmation of suspected NPH [6, 7]. Group A patients were conscious and lying in a recumbent position. Group B patients underwent the procedure under GA; these patients were either unable to tolerate the diagnostic procedure (which may require up to 1 h of monitoring) or assessed preoperatively to confirm the need for shunt insertion within the same surgical session [5–7]. All patients presented with ventriculomegaly and with at least two elements of the Hakim's triad of symptoms (urinary incontinence, shuffling gait and memory loss); gait problems were present in all patients. During the infusion study, anaesthesia was induced using propofol, fentanyl and atracurium or vecuronium [8, 9] and maintained with either propofol target controlled infusion (3–6 mcg/ml) at the effect site alone or combined with remifentanil (0.05–0.2 mcg/kg/min).

Group C and group D consisted of two cohorts of 30 patients each, undergoing overnight ICP monitoring. Group C involved naturally asleep patients being evaluated for or diagnosed with hydrocephalus, with or without a shunt in place [1, 5, 7]. Group D patients had undergone ICP monitoring following severe traumatic brain injury (TBI) [9]. These patients were under deep sedation with propofol and fentanyl or remifentanil, with or without neuromuscular blockade.

Research ethics committee approval was obtained (29 REC 97/291) and all patients had given their informed consent for their digital data to be analysed anonymously.

Data Analysis

The magnitude of slow waves [SLOW] was calculated using spectral analysis of digitised ICP recordings [8, 9]. Artefacts were manually extracted in all groups before analysis. In groups A and B, de-trending of ICP was performed before analysis to minimise the influence of the induced increase in ICP on slow wave activity (Fig. 1).

Baseline ICP, intracranial elasticity [1, 6], RAP (an index of volume compensatory reserve), CSF production and RCSF were assessed in all patients, as previously described [8–10]. Data were analysed using SPSS version 22.0. A one-way ANOVA was used to examine between-group differences in examined parameters. Spearman rank correlation coefficient was used to examine the relationship between descriptors of slow waves and CSF compensatory parameters.

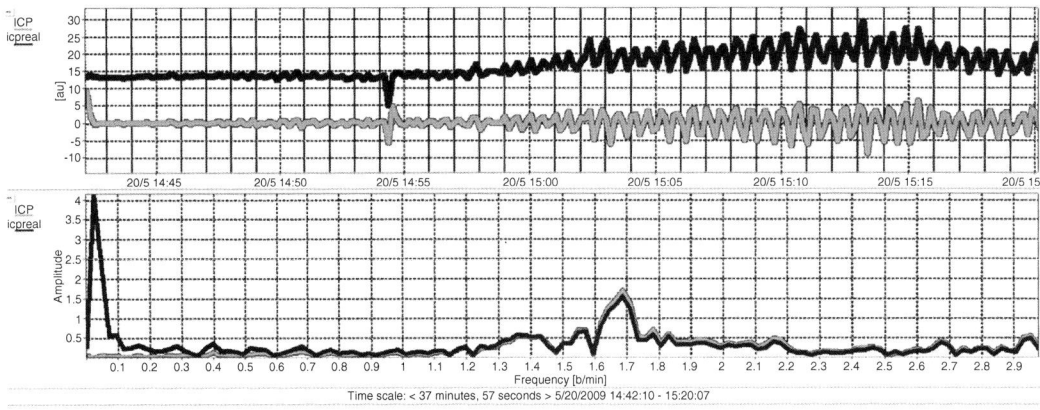

Fig. 1 Spectral analysis of slow waves during infusion study: effect of detrending. *Upper*: difference in the trend between the original intracranial pressure (ICP) recording (darker trend) and the detrended singal (lighter trend). *Lower*: difference between the original spectrum and the spectrum of the detrended ICP starts to minimise from a frequency of around 1.4 cycles/min

Results

Groups A and B included age-matched (73 ± 7 vs 75 ± 8 years) NPH patients undergoing infusion testing, in a conscious state (group A; $n = 30$) and under GA (group B; $n = 30$). Male to female ratio in both groups was approximately 4:3.

Groups C and D included age-matched patients undergoing overnight ICP monitoring for diagnostic investigation of NPH during natural sleep (group C; $n = 30$; age = 23 ± 8) and deeply sedated and mechanically ventilated patients (group D; $n = 30$; age = 29 ± 7 years).

Overall, the average magnitude of slow waves and standard deviations of 10 s-averaged ICP was lower in the GA patients (groups B and D; 0.15 ± 0.10 mmHg; $p = 0.01$ and 0.11 ± 0.09 mmHg; $p = 0.002$, respectively) in comparison with conscious patients (groups A and C; 0.23 ± 0.10 mmHg and 0.20 ± 0.13 mmHg respectively; Fig. 2).

In groups A and B, there was no correlation between compensatory reserve and the volume of slow waves. There was no significant correlation between any measures describing the magnitude of B waves and resistance to CSF outflow or elasticity, both in the GA and conscious patients group. The magnitude of B waves correlated positively with baseline ICP ($R = 0.48$; $p = 0.0067$), but only in conscious patients.

There is a significant difference in the duration of the recording between the first (groups A and B) and the second (groups C and D) cohort, which was the initial purpose of their formation. The duration of the infusion studies was approximately half an hour, therefore different methodology was used for analysis of slow waves. Formally, there is no statistical difference between slow waves in groups A (baseline values, before start of infusion) and C, and between groups B and D ($p > 0.05$).

Discussion

The number by which slow waves are dampened by GA is demonstrated in this study. By quantifying these previously observational findings, a reference for further studies and for clinical interpretation of ICP recordings is provided.

Both the average magnitude of slow waves and standard deviation of mean ICP were significantly lower in patients under GA than in conscious ones, indicating a suppression of ICP dynamics by GA. There were no differences between conscious and sedated patients with regard to baseline ICP, excluding mean ICP as a contributing factor to B-wave suppression [8, 9]. Therefore, lower brain metabolism rate (lower cerebral blood flow [CBF]) mainly accounted for the lower magnitude. Adding to this hypothesis is the fact that CSF production was significantly lower in the GA group [6]. Contrary to what would be expected because of the between-group difference in cerebral arterial blood volume (CaBV), intracranial elasticity did not vary between the two groups [6, 7]. The resistance (R) to the CSF outflow was found to be significantly higher in the GA group (group B). This could be attributed to selection bias, as GA infusion studies involve patients with severe clinical features who are most likely to be candidates for CSF shunting procedures [10].

Regarding the use of anaesthetic drugs, propofol has been widely used for CSF dynamics studies, with known effects [8]. The safety of fentanyl and remifentanil as adjuvants in neuroanaesthesia and neurointensive care is also supported by a large body of evidence [9]. Nonetheless, the current study demonstrates that even propofol-based anaesthesia and sedation are associated with a considerable reduction in the amplitude of vasogenic waves compared with wakefulness or natural sleep [5, 6, 8]. Patients in the TBI group were selected because they did not have significant intracranial

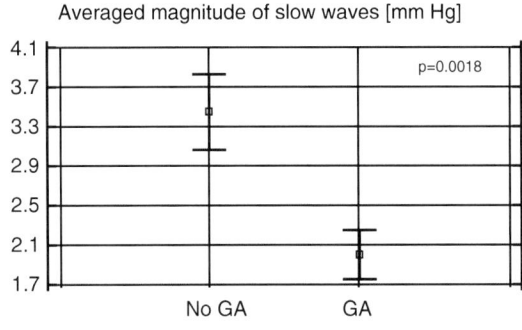

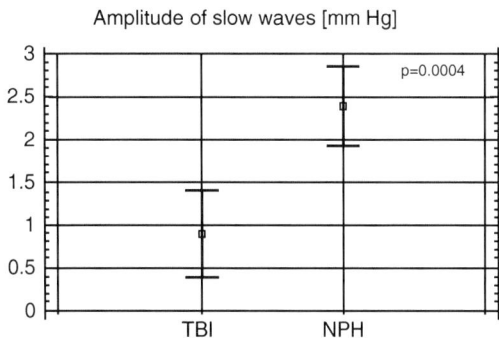

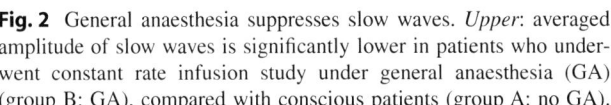

Fig. 2 General anaesthesia suppresses slow waves. *Upper*: averaged amplitude of slow waves is significantly lower in patients who underwent constant rate infusion study under general anaesthesia (GA) (group B: GA), compared with conscious patients (group A: no GA). *Lower*: significantly decreased amplitude of slow waves in deeply sedated traumatic brain injury (TBI) patients (group D), compared with naturally asleep hydrocephalus patients (NPH) (group C: NPH)

hypertension (ICP < 18 mmHg) and their CSF parameters were considered for the first day of their admission [3–5].

Because of the undetermined origin of B-waves, it is hard to conclude that a specific mechanism is responsible for the suppression phenomenon. Arterial $PaCO_2$ fluctuations partly explain the changes in CaBV and ICP, but not the sole cause of the reported amplitude differences [2–4]. It has been shown that GA-induced changes in arterial blood pressure (ABP) do not influence cerebral autoregulation, especially under the well-controlled conditions of the ICU [6, 8].

Quantifying the influence of anaesthesia and deep sedation on B-waves may have clinical relevance om improving the management of hydrocephalic patients; slow waves are often used to predict shunt response and select NPH candidates for surgery [2, 5, 7, 10]. Results of long-term ICP monitoring also vary between conscious and sedated patients. The use of anaesthesia should hence be considered in an effort to prevent the misidentification of potential shunt-responders as non-responders.

Limitations of the Study

Head injury patients may not be absolutely comparable with hydrocephalus patients, even though the main difference in raised ICP was eliminated by selecting subjects with preserved autoregulation. A possible selection bias may be present in group B, with a significantly higher RCSF linked with advanced clinical disease. Although there may be considerable within-group heterogeneity in the anaesthetised and sedated group, there remains a consistent and statistically significant difference in the magnitude of vasogenic waves in patients undergoing infusion studies under GA compared with patients in the awake state. CBF and ABP were not measured in this study.

Finally, the difference in the magnitude may appear quite minimal (0.08 mmHg and 0.09 mmHg during infusion studies and long-term monitoring respectively). However, our aim was to quantify and describe an empirically observed difference statistically and that was achieved in this paper. Using our paper as a reference, it is important to begin considering the practical issues demonstrated by our numerical results.

Further studies need to be performed to confirm these findings and provide a better insight into how to interpret slow-wave analysis derived from anaesthetised patients.

Conflicts of interest statement We declare that we have no conflicts of interest.

References

1. Lalou DA, Czosnyka M, Donnelly J, Lavinio A, Pickard JD, Garnett M, Czosnyka Z. Influence of general anaesthesia on slow waves of intracranial pressure. Neurol Res. 2016;38(7):587–92.
2. Droste DW, Krauss JK. Simultaneous recording of cerebrospinal fluid pressure and middle cerebral artery blood flow velocity in patients with suspected symptomatic normal pressure hydrocephalus. J Neurol Neurosurg Psychiatry. 1993;56:75–792.
3. Lescot T, Naccache L, Bonnet MP, et al. The relationship of intracranial pressure Lundberg waves to electroencephalograph fluctuations in patients with severe head trauma. Acta Neurochir. 2005;147(2):125–9.
4. Lemaire JJ, Khalil T, Cervenansky F, et al. Slow pressure waves in the cranial enclosure. Acta Neurochir. 2002;144(3):243–54.
5. Kasprowicz M, Bergsneider M, Czosnyka M, et al. Association between ICP pulse waveform morphology and ICP B waves. Acta Neurochir Suppl. 2012;114:29–34. https://doi.org/10.1007/978-3-7091-0956-4_6.
6. Weerakkody RA, Czosnyka M, Zweifel C. Slow vasogenic fluctuations of intracranial pressure and cerebral near infrared spectroscopy—an observational study. Acta Neurochir. 2010;152(10):1763–9.
7. Swallow DM, Fellner N, Varsos GV, et al. Repeatability of cerebrospinal fluid constant rate infusion study. Acta Neurol Scand. 2014;130(2):131–8.
8. Girard F, Moumdjian R, Boudreault D, et al. The effect of sedation on intracranial pressure in patients with an intracranial space-occupying lesion: remifentanil versus propofol. Anesth Analg. 2009;109(1):194–8.
9. Fodale V, Schifilliti D, Praticò C, et al. Remifentanil and the brain. Acta Anaesthesiol Scand. 2008;52(3):319–26.
10. Pickard JD, Teasdale G, Matheson M, et al. Intraventricular pressure waves—the best predictive test for shunting in normal pressure hydrocephalus. In: Shulman K, Marmarou A, Miller JD, Becker DP, Hochwold GM, Brock M, editors. Intracranial pressure IV. Berlin: Springer-Verlag; 1980. p. 498–500.

Critical Closing Pressure During a Controlled Increase in Intracranial Pressure

Katarzyna Kaczmarska, Magdalena Kasprowicz, Antoni Grzanka, Wojciech Zabołotny, Peter Smielewski, Despina Afroditi Lalou, Georgios Varsos, Marek Czosnyka, and Zofia Czosnyka

Abstract *Objectives*: The objectives were to compare three methods of estimating critical closing pressure (CrCP) in a scenario of a controlled increase in intracranial pressure (ICP) induced during an infusion test in patients with suspected normal pressure hydrocephalus (NPH).

Methods: We retrospectively analyzed data from 37 NPH patients who underwent infusion tests. Computer recordings of directly measured intracranial pressure (ICP), arterial blood pressure (ABP) and transcranial Doppler cerebral blood flow velocity (CBFV) were used. The CrCP was calculated using three methods: first harmonics ratio of the pulse waveforms of ABP and CBFV ($CrCP_A$) and two methods based on a model of cerebrovascular impedance, as a function of cerebral perfusion pressure ($CrCP_{inv}$), and as a function of ABP ($CrCP_{ninv}$).

Results: There is good agreement among the three methods of CrCP calculation, with correlation coefficients being greater than 0.8 ($p < 0.0001$). For the $CrCP_A$ method, negative values were found for about 20% of all results. Negative values of CrCP were not observed in estimators based on cerebrovascular impedance. During the controlled rise of ICP, all three estimators of CrCP increased significantly ($p < 0.05$). The strongest correlation between ICP and CrCP was found for $CrCP_{inv}$ (median R = 0.41).

Conclusion: Invasive CrCP is most sensitive to variations in ICP and can be used as an indicator of the status of the cerebrovascular system during infusion tests.

Keywords Critical closing pressure · Wall tension Intracranial pressure · Cerebral autoregulation · Infusion test

Introduction

Critical closing pressure (CrCP) is the arterial blood pressure (ABP) threshold, below which small arterial vessels collapse and blood flow ceases. Theoretically, cerebral CrCP is the sum of intracranial pressure (ICP) and vascular wall tension (WT) [1]. With the introduction of transcranial Doppler (TCD) ultrasound, it became possible to assess CrCP non-invasively by comparing the waveforms of cerebral blood flow velocity (CBFV) and ABP. One of the methods, proposed by Aaslid et al. [2] estimates CrCP from the fundamental harmonics of the pulse waveforms of ABP and CBFV. However, these methods may provide an inaccurate estimation of CrCP, as they can produce negative values that cannot be interpreted physiologically [3]. Recently, Varsos et al. proposed a new methodology for CrCP estimation based on a cerebrovascular impedance model [4] as a function of cerebral perfusion

K. Kaczmarska (✉)
Department of Neurosurgery, Mossakowski Medical Research Centre Polish Academy of Sciences, Warsaw, Poland

Institute of Electronic Systems, Warsaw University of Technology, Warsaw, Poland
e-mail: kkaczmarska@imdik.pan.pl

M. Kasprowicz
Department of Biomedical Engineering, Wroclaw University of Technology, Wroclaw, Poland

A. Grzanka · W. Zabołotny
Institute of Electronic Systems, Warsaw University of Technology, Warsaw, Poland

P. Smielewski · D.A. Lalou · G. Varsos · Z. Czosnyka
Division of Neurosurgery, Department of Clinical Neurosciences, Addenbrooke's Hospital, University of Cambridge, Cambridge, UK

M. Czosnyka
Institute of Electronic Systems, Warsaw University of Technology, Warsaw, Poland

Division of Neurosurgery, Department of Clinical Neurosciences, Addenbrooke's Hospital, University of Cambridge, Cambridge, UK

pressure (CPP), ABP, cerebrovascular resistance (CVR), arterial compliance (Ca), and heart rate (HR). An important advantage of this method of CrCP calculation is the fact that it is not providing the non-physiological negative values of pressure, as was the case with Aaslid's method.

In this study, we aim to compare three methods of CrCP estimation in a scenario of a controlled increase in ICP induced by the infusion test. It was previously shown that an increase in CrCP is related to an increase in ICP [5]. However, it is unknown whether and to what extent the non-invasive and invasive methods of CrCP estimation can be used interchangeably in a scenario of a controlled rise in ICP.

Material and Methods

Based on imaging examinations (the median width of the third cerebral ventricle was 13.64 mm, quartile range: 10.15–17.22 mm) and the clinical symptoms of hydrocephalus, patients were admitted to the Hydrocephalus Clinic, Addenbrooke's Hospital, Cambridge, UK, to undergo the infusion test. Tests were performed as a standard clinical procedure. Patients gave their consent and anonymized digital recordings of monitored variables were post-processed as part of a clinical audit. Additional non-invasive TCD monitoring during the test was approved by the Ethics Committee (08/H0306/103).

The inclusion criterion was suspected NPH, requiring an infusion test with simultaneous TCD monitoring. Thirty-seven patients with an entry diagnosis of NPH were studied. The median age of the patients was 57.0 years (quartile range: 37.0–64.0 years).

The cerebrospinal fluid space was accessed by a lumbar puncture. The needle was connected to an infusion pump and to the pressure transducer, from which the signal was transferred to the standard invasive pressure input of a bed-side monitor. After about 10 min of baseline pressure measurement, the infusion was started. The test was performed with a constant-rate infusion. The infusion was continued until a new steady-state ICP (plateau) was reached, or until an ICP safety limit of 40 mmHg was achieved.

Data Acquisition and Analysis

Cerebral blood flow velocity (CBFV) was measured from the middle cerebral artery with a 2-MHz probe and monitored using TCD (Neuroguard, Medasonics, Fremont, CA, USA). Arterial blood pressure was measured non-invasively using a Finapres finger cuff (Ohmeda, Englewood, CO, USA). Raw signals were digitized using an analog–digital converter (DT2814; Data Translation, Marlboro, CA, USA) sampled at a frequency of 50 Hz, recorded by WREC software (Wojciech Zabolotny, Warsaw University of Technology) and re-analyzed using ICM+ software (Cambridge Enterprise, Cambridge, UK, http://www.neurosurg.cam.ac.uk/icmplus/). The amplitudes of the fundamental harmonics of ABP, CBFV and ICP were derived using 10-s discrete Fourier transformations. The HR was assessed as the frequency associated with the first harmonic of ABP. All the calculations were performed over a 10-s window.

The CrCP was determined using the first harmonics ratio of the pulse waveforms of ABP and CBFV according to the following formula [6]:

$$CrCP_A = ABP_{mean} - \frac{Amp_{ABP}}{Amp_{CBFV}} \cdot CBFV_{mean} \quad (1)$$

where: ABP_{mean} – mean value of ABP; Amp_{ABP} and Amp_{CBFV} – amplitudes of the fundamental harmonics of ABP and CBFV respectively.

To calculate a multiparameter model of CrCP it is necessary to estimate CVR and compliance (Ca). CVR represents the resistance of small cerebral arteries and it can be estimated using TCD mean blood flow velocity (CBFV), and mean cerebral perfusion pressure (CPP = meanABP − meanICP):

$$CVR = \frac{meanCPP}{meanCBFV \cdot S_a} \quad (2)$$

The arterial compliance (Ca) represents the change in arterial blood volume in response to a change in arterial pressure and can be estimated as:

$$C_a = \frac{Amp_{CaBV} \cdot S_a}{Amp_{ABP}} \quad (3)$$

In Eqs. 2 and 3, Sa represents the cross-sectional area of the insonated vessel. Obtaining of amplitude of the fundamental harmonic of cerebral arterial blood volume (CaBV) is described in detail in Kim et al. [7].

The $CrCP_{inv}$ is calculated based on the mathematical model of cerebrovascular impedance and expressed by Eq. 4.

$$CrCP_{inv} = ABP - \frac{CPP}{\sqrt{(CVR \cdot C_a \cdot HR \cdot 2\pi)^2 + 1}} \quad (4)$$

In some clinical scenarios, when there is no need or possibility of monitoring ICP, the CrCP can be calculated from Eq. 5 with CPP approximated by ABP:

$$CrCP_{ninv} = ABP \cdot \left(1 - \frac{1}{\sqrt{(CVR_{ninv} \cdot C_a \cdot HR \cdot 2\pi)^2 + 1}}\right) \quad (5)$$

where CVR_{ninv} is CVR calculated from Eq. 2 with CPP approximated by ABP. This a simple modification of formula 4, taking ICP = 0.

Statistical Analysis

To determine whether the data are normally distributed, the Shapiro–Wilk test was used. Non-parametric Wilcoxon test was utilized to examine the significance of a difference in analyzed parameters between the baseline and plateau phase of the test. The significance level of all tests was set at 0.05. Results are presented as median value ± quartile range (QR). Pearson's method was used for the bivariate correlation analysis.

Results

The changes in ICP, ABP, CPP, and CBFV between the baseline and the plateau phase of the test and the calculated variables $CrCP_A$, $CrCP_{inv}$, $CrCP_{ninv}$, WT_A, WT_{inv}, along with ratios of WT and CrCP, are presented in Table 1.

Following the rise in ICP, median CrCP obtained with all three methods significantly increased by 7.78 ± 6.00 mmHg, $p < 0.0001$, for $CrCP_{inv}$, 5.89 ± 4.66 mmHg, $p < 0.0001$ for $CrCP_{ninv}$ and by 9.38 ± 9.87 mmHg, $p = 0.0001$ in the case of $CrCP_A$. However, the values of Aaslid's estimator were lower than impedance methods by 10.80 ± 20.56 mmHg, $p < 0.0001$ in the baseline and by 12.45 ± 16.99 mmHg, $p < 0.0001$ in the plateau phase.

Results obtained using all three methods of CrCP calculation correlated strongly. The strongest correlation was found between $CrCP_{inv}$ and $CrCP_{ninv}$ ($R = 0.9675$, $p < 0.0001$). The associations between $CrCP_A$ and either $CrCP_{inv}$ or $CrCP_{ninv}$ were also significant, but correlation coefficients were weaker ($CrCP_{inv}$ vs $CrCP_A$, $R = 0.8398$, $p < 0.0001$ and $CrCP_{ninv}$ vs $CrCP_A$, $R = 0.8295$, $p < 0.0001$).

The largest discrepancies were seen when the $CrCP_A$ demonstrated negative values.

Correlation analysis among CrCP obtained using three methods and ICP was also performed based on data recorded in each individual patient. The results were highly variable, the strongest correlation being between $CrCP_{inv}$ and ICP ($R = 0.41$; $p < 0.01$). Examples of good and bad correlations are shown in Fig. 1.

In 7 patients (20.6%), the correlation coefficient between ICP and CrCP had a negative value. Negative values of R occurred most often in the case of $CrCP_{ninv}$. In 4 patients the correlation coefficient between ICP and the three estimators of CrCP had negative values.

It was also observed that changes in CrCP from baseline to plateau ICP (ΔCrCP) correlated significantly with changes in ICP (ΔICP) in all three methods: ΔICP and $ΔCrCP_A$, $R = 0.4451$, $p = 0.0075$, ΔICP and $ΔCrCP_{ninv}$, $R = 0.3901$, $p = 0.0205$, ΔICP and $ΔCrCP_{inv}$, $R = 0.4349$, $p = 0.0090$.

Discussion

We have demonstrated a close relationship between the values of CrCP obtained using impedance model-based methods (invasive and non-invasive) and based on Aaslid's equation. CrCP calculation methods correlate relatively well, although non-invasive CrCP expresses changes in ICP to a weaker degree. Moreover, in individual patients, the absolute difference between these estimators was the smallest in the case of $CrCP_{inv}$ and $CrCP_{ninv}$. Correlation between CrCP from Aaslid's equation and invasive/non-invasive CrCP was undoubtedly lower. The existence of negative $CrCP_A$ values caused discrepancies between the methods. $CrCP_A$ was lower than impedance model-based estimators. This was caused by the methodological limitations of Aaslid's formula. During a controlled increase in ICP, the $CrCP_A$ rendered negative values in situations of changes in amplitude and mean values of CBFV and/or ABP. The issue of low and negative values of $CrCP_A$ has been a known drawback in cases such as hyperemia or vasospasm [3, 4]. Therefore physiological interpretation of $CrCP_A$ is sometimes difficult.

Conclusions

There was a significant correlation between the analyzed methods of determining CrCP. All three indices were in agreement, although the best agreement between impedance

Table 1 Median and quartile range of measured and calculated variables from the baseline and plateau level

Parameter	Baseline	Plateau	p value
ICP (mmHg)	6.81 (7.27)	19.76 (11.16)	<0.0001
ABP (mmHg)	95.12 (36.36)	100.40 (33.74)	0.0030
CPP (mmHg)	86.98 (26.59)	81.87 (32.54)	0.0010
CBFV (cm/s)	52.40 (16.80)	50.34 (17.58)	<0.0001
$CrCP_{inv}$ (mmHg)	44.99 (16.11)	52.72 (20.74)	<0.0001
$CrCP_{ninv}$ (mmHg)	44.73 (22.12)	48.90 (24.29)	0.0001
$CrCP_A$ (mmHg)	33.39 (27.86)	38.03 (33.68)	0.0003

ICP intracranial pressure, *ABP* arterial blood pressure, *CPP* cerebral perfusion pressure, *CBFV* cerebral blood flow velocity, *CrCPinv* function of cerebral perfusion pressure, *CrCPninv* function of arterial blood pressure, *CrCPA* ratio of the pulse waveforms of ABP and CBFV

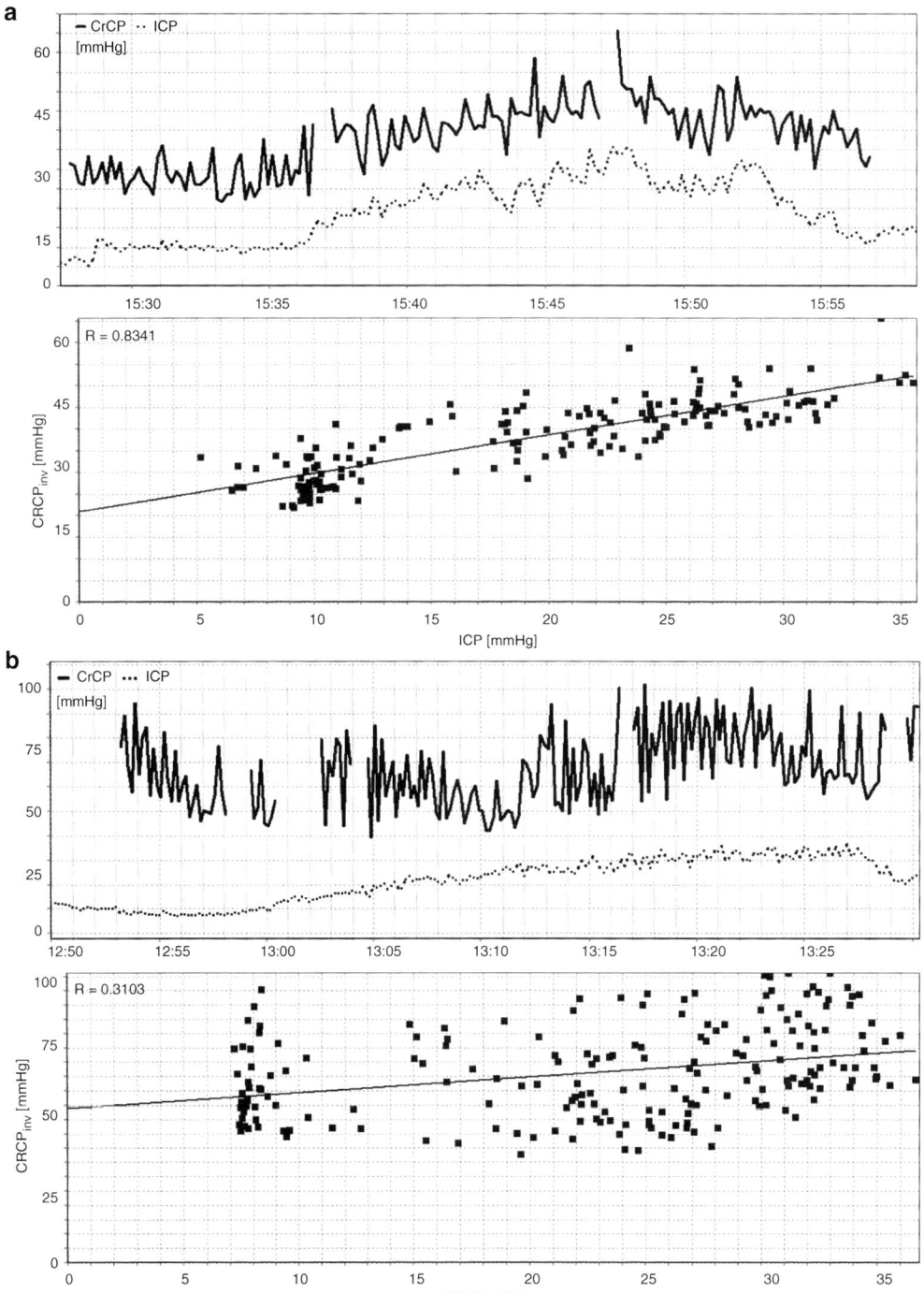

Fig. 1 Example of (**a**) high and (**b**) low correlation between intracranial pressure and critical closing pressure with the corresponding time plots

model-based methods (invasive and non-invasive) were demonstrated.

Acknowledgements This study was partially supported by the statutory fund of Mossakowski Medical Research Centre Polish Academy of Sciences and Institute of Electronic Systems, Warsaw University of Technology. Katarzyna Kaczmarska was also supported by the European Union in the framework of European Social Fund through the Warsaw University of Technology Development Programme.

Conflicts of interest statement ICM+ software is licensed by Cambridge Enterprise Ltd. (UK). M.C. and P.S. have a financial interest in a part of the licensing fee.

References

1. Dewey RC, Pieper HP, Hunt WE. Experimental cerebral hemodynamics. Vasomotor tone, critical closing pressure, and vascular bed resistance. J Neurosurg. 1974;41:597–606.
2. Aaslid R, Lash SR, Bardy GH, Gild WH, Newell DW. Dynamic pressure-flow velocity relationships in the human cerebral circulation. Stroke. 2003;34:1645–9.
3. Puppo C, Camacho J, Varsos GV, Yelicich B, Gómez H, Moraes L, Biestro A, Czosnyka M. Cerebral critical closing pressure: is the multiparameter model better suited to estimate physiology of cerebral hemodynamics? Neurocrit Care. 2016;25:446–54.
4. Varsos GV, Richards H, Kasprowicz M, Budohoski KP, Brady KM, Reinhard M, Avolio M, Smielewski P, Pickard JD, Czosnyka M. Critical closing pressure determined with a model of cerebrovascular impedance. J Cereb Blood Flow Metab. 2012;33:235–43.
5. Varsos GV, Czosnyka M, Smielewski P, Garnett MR, Liu X, Kim DJ, Donnelly J, Adams H, Pickard JD, Czosnyka Z. Cerebral critical closing pressure in hydrocephalus patients undertaking infusion tests. Neurol Res. 2015;37(8):674–82.
6. Michel E, Zernikow B. Goslig's Doppler pulsatility index revisited. Ultrasound Med Biol. 1998;24:597–9.
7. Kim DJ, Kasprowicz M, Carrera E, Castellani G, Zweifel C, Lavinio A, Smielewski P, Sutcliffe MP, Pickard JD, Czosnyka M. The monitoring of relative changes in compartmental compliances of brain. Physiol Meas. 2009;30:647–59.

Effect of Mild Hypocapnia on Critical Closing Pressure and Other Mechanoelastic Parameters of the Cerebrospinal System

Peter Smielewski, Luzius Steiner, Corina Puppo, Karol Budohoski, Georgios V. Varsos, and Marek Czosnyka

Abstract *Objective*: Brain arterial critical closing pressure (CrCP) has been studied in several diseases such as traumatic brain injury (TBI), subarachnoid haemorrhage, hydrocephalus, and in various physiological scenarios: intracranial hypertension, decreased cerebral perfusion pressure, hypercapnia, etc. Little or nothing so far has been demonstrated to characterise change in CrCP during mild hypocapnia.

Method: We retrospectively analysed recordings of intracranial pressure (ICP), arterial blood pressure (ABP) and blood flow velocity from 27 severe TBI patients (mean 39.5 ± 3.4 years, 6 women) in whom a ventilation increase (20% increase in respiratory minute volume) was performed over 50 min as part of a standard clinical CO_2 reactivity test. CrCP was calculated using the Windkessel model of cerebral arterial flow. Arteriolar wall tension (WT) was calculated as a difference between CrCP and ICP. The compartmental compliances arterial (Ca) and cerebrospinal fluid space (Ci) were also evaluated.

Results: During hypocapnia, ICP decreased from 17±6.8 to 13.2±6.6 mmHg ($p < 0.000001$). Wall tension increased from 14.5 ± 9.9 to 21.7±9.1 mmHg ($p < 0.0002$). CrCP, being a sum of WT + ICP, changed significantly from 31.5 ± 11.9 mmHg to 34.9±11.1 mmHg ($p < 0.002$), and the closing margin (ABP-CrCP) remained constant at an average value of 60 mmHg. Ca decreased significantly during hypocapnia by 30% ($p < 0.00001$) and Ci increased by 26% ($p < 0.003$).

Conclusion: During hypocapnia in TBI patients, ICP decreases and WT increases. CrCP increases slightly as the rise in wall tension outweighs the decrease in ICP. The closing margin remained unchanged, suggesting that the risk of hypocapnia-induced ischemia might not be increased.

Keywords Traumatic brain injury · Hypocapnia · Intracranial pressure · Critical closing pressure · Arterial wall tension · Cerebrovascular compliance · Brain monitoring · ICM+

Introduction

Critical closing pressure (CrCP) is the lowest threshold of arterial blood pressure (ABP) below which the cerebral blood flow ceases. The flow cessation happens when the transmural pressure in the cerebral arteries, expressed as the difference between ABP and intracranial pressure (ICP), becomes too low to oppose the tension of the arterial walls leading to collapse of the arteries. Therefore, CrCP is defined as the sum of intracranial pressure (ICP) and the wall tension (WT) pressure. The phenomenon of critical closing pressure in the brain was first described with the appearance of transcranial Doppler (TCD) measurements of blood flow velocity in the middle cerebral artery when the intercept of the regression line through the systolic and diastolic values of flow velocity and arterial blood pressure was studied. Since then, CrCP has been studied in many conditions, including traumatic brain injury, subarachnoid haemorrhage, and hydrocephalus under various haemodynamic conditions such as increased intracranial pressure, decreased cerebral perfusion, and moderate hyper- and hypocapnia.

Moderate hypocapnia has at one point been proposed as a means of controlling elevated intracranial pressure in severe brain trauma patients because of its vasoconstrictive properties, leading to a reduction in cerebral blood volume, and thus ICP. However, subsequent studies showed that despite lowering ICP and improving global brain perfusion, the direct vasoconstriction effect often leads to worsening deficits in local cerebral perfusion in particularly vulnerable regions of the brain. This has led to changes in the management strategies of severe head trauma patients, allowing only for mild hypocapnic treatment to be applied in those patients. However, little is currently known of the effects of such mild hypocapnia on the properties of cerebral arteries.

In this study, we set out to examine what happens to the arterial compliances, the WT and the critical closing pressure in TBI patients with elevated ICP during mild hypocapnic challenges.

Materials and Methods

We retrospectively analysed waveform recordings of ICP, arterial blood pressure (ABP) and TCD blood flow velocity (FV) taken from 27 sedated and ventilated severe TBI patients (mean age 39.5 ± 3.4 years, 6 were women) admitted to the Neurocritical Care Unit at Addenbrooke's Hospital, Cambridge, in whom an increase in ventilation (20% increase in respiratory minute volume) was performed over 50 min as part of a standard clinical CO_2 reactivity test.

ABP was monitored invasively using a pressure monitoring kit (Baxter Healthcare CA, USA; Sidcup, UK) at the radial artery, zeroed at the level of the heart, whereas an intraparenchymal probe (Codman & Shurtleff, MA, USA or Camino Laboratories, CA, USA) was used to monitor ICP. FV was measured from the middle cerebral artery with a 2-MHz probe and monitored with the Doppler Box (DWL Compumedics, Germany) or Neuroguard (Medasonics, Fremont, CA, USA). All the monitoring was performed as part of the standard protocol for the management of traumatic brain injury [1]. Patient monitoring was approved by the local Ethics Committee (REC97/291).

The raw data signals were digitised at a sampling frequency of 50 Hz using an analogue–digital converter (DT9801 and DT9803, Data Translation, Marlboro, MA, USA), and recorded using ICM +® software (Cambridge Enterprise, ltd, Cambridge, UK, http://icmplus.neurosurg.cam.ac.uk). All the analyses on the recorded raw waveforms were performed over 10-s long-sliding windows using the same software ICM+.

Critical closing pressure (CrCP) was calculated using the Windkessel model of cerebral arterial flow [2] according to the following formula:

$$CrCP = ABP - \frac{CPP}{\sqrt{(R_a \cdot C_a \cdot HR \cdot 2\pi)^2 + 1}} \quad [mmHg],$$

where Ra is the composite cerebrovascular resistance estimated as:

$$R_a = \frac{CPP}{FV \cdot S_a} \quad \left[\frac{mmHg \cdot s}{cm^3}\right],$$

Ca is the lumped cerebral arterial compliance estimated as:

$$C_a = \frac{AMP_{CaBV}}{AMP_{ABP}} \quad \left[\frac{cm^3}{mmHg}\right],$$

AMP here denotes the amplitude of the first, Fourier, harmonic of the pulse component of ABP, and CaBV respectively.

CaBV is the cerebral arterial blood volume, which is derived from FV by means of time integration:

$$CaBV(n) = S_a \cdot \sum_{i=1}^{n} (FV(i) - ABP(i)/R_a) \varnothing \quad [cm^3],$$

and finally, HR is the heart rate.

Both Ra and Ca formulae contain unknown factor Sa (directly, or indirectly inside the CaBV formula, as above) used to convert blood flow velocity measurements into blood flow, which cancels out when the product of the two (denoted as time constant τ in the results) is used in the CrCP formula.

Subsequently, vascular wall tension (WT) was estimated as (Dewey et al.): WT = CrCP − ICP, which when using the impedance model becomes:

$$WT = CPP \cdot \left[1 - \frac{1}{\sqrt{(R_a \cdot C_a \cdot HR \cdot 2\pi)^2 + 1}}\right], \quad [mmHg]$$

In addition, the compliance of the cerebrospinal space Ci was also calculated as:

$$C_i = \frac{AMP_{CaBV}}{AMP_{ICP}} \quad \left[\frac{cm^3}{mmHg}\right]$$

The exact derivation of all the above formulae with detailed explanations can be found elsewhere [2, 3].

For statistical analysis of the effects of hypocapnia, mean values of the studied parameters at baseline and during the hypotension period were compared using univariate tests (paired t test).

Results

A representative example of the behaviour of the studied parameters during the 20% increase in the respiratory rate is shown in Fig. 1 and the statistical comparisons of baseline versus hypocapnic period values are given in Table 1. $PaCO_2$, ICP, FV and CrCP decreased significantly, whereas ABP, CPP, Ci, Ra, and WT increased significantly. The other parameters, HR and Ca, did not change. For completeness measures of cerebral blood flow autoregulation, the mean index, Mx, and the pressure reactivity index, PRx, were also added, showing in both cases intact reactivity at both levels of CO_2, with no significant difference between the two levels. Also, the diastolic closing margin (DCM), defined as the difference between the diastolic arterial blood pressure and CrCP, was calculated at both levels, and the difference was found to be non-significant.

Discussion

The increase in ventilation led to a state of mild hypocapnia in all cases. As expected, this produced a decrease in both ICP and TCD blood FV, evidence of induced vasoconstriction. Not surprisingly, the compliance of the CSF space (Ci) increased significantly because of the decrease in the cerebral blood volume. Cerebrovascular time constant τ also increased, despite the opposing behaviour of Ra and Ca. The former increased as a direct effect of the vasoconstriction whereas the latter decreased in individual cases, but as a group statistically not significantly, and in all cases, the change in Ra prevailed over the change in Ca. Similarly, WT and ICP changed in the opposite direction, with WT increasing significantly during the hypocapnia period. In this case, however, those opposite effects were largely balanced out; thus, the resulting critical closing pressure, being the sum of WT and ICP, decreased only a little, though statistically significantly.

What is even more important is that the diastolic closing margin (DCM), which provides a "safety" window for arterial blood pressure before the first ischaemic threshold for the cerebral blood flow is reached during the diastolic phase of the heart cycle, not only did not decrease but even showed a tendency to increase.

It is also worth noting that cerebral autoregulation was not significantly affected by this low degree of hypocapnia. The pressure reactivity index (Prx) showed a general tendency towards a slight improvement, but the mean flow index (Mx) did not change at all.

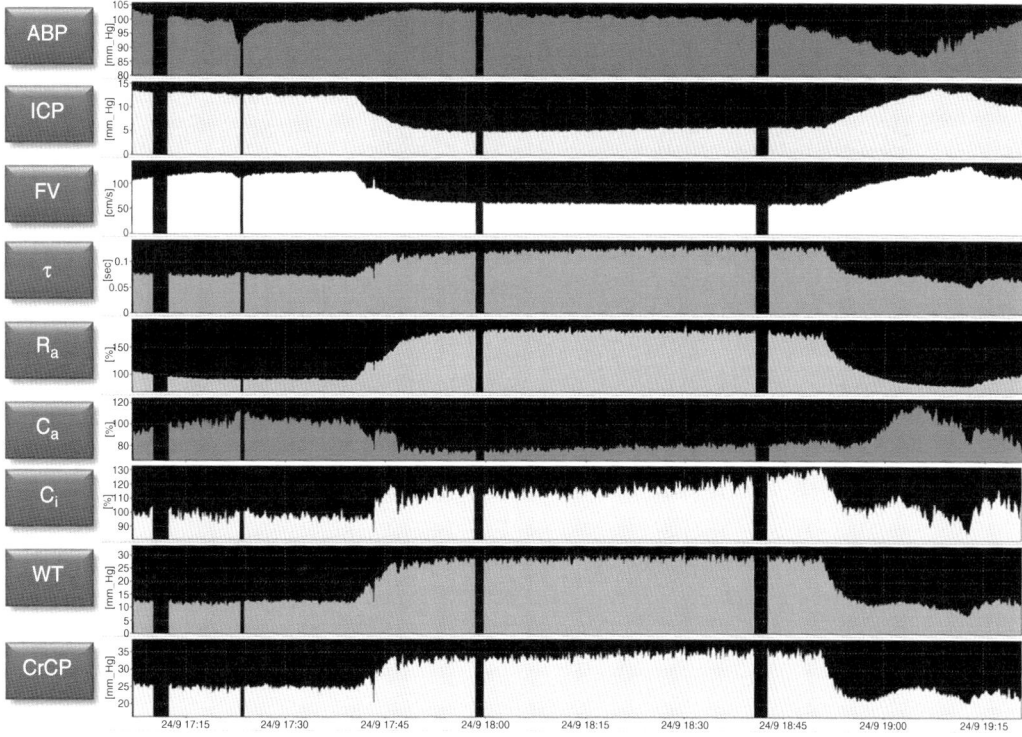

Fig. 1 Typical example of time trends of the haemodynamic parameters studied during one episode of a 20% increase in ventilation-induced mild hypocapnia

Table 1 Mean values (and standard deviations) of all the studied haemodynamic parameters at baseline and during the hypocapnia period

Variable	Unit	Baseline Mean	SD	Hypocapnia Mean	SD	Change	p value
$PaCO_2$	kPa	5.22	0.34	4.89	0.331	Down	0.027
ABP	mmHg	106.24	9.50	109.47	12.05	Up	0.022
ICP	mmHg	19.73	6.80	15.48	6.38	Down	<0.0001
FV	cm/s	113.16	36.22	103.54	30.37	Down	<0.0001
CPP	mmHg	86.50	8.73	94.00	11.76	Up	<0.0001
HR	1/min	69.25	16.31	69.64	15.47		0.474
τ (=Ra·Ca)	s	0.046	0.038	0.058	0.04	Up	<0.0001
CrCP	mmHg	24.20	10.50	22.59	11.21	Down	0.003
WT	mmHg	4.47	7.80	7.12	9.24	Up	<0.0001
Mx		0.056	0.316	0.110	0.254		0.237
PRx		−0.073	0.25	−0.362	0.187		0.372
DCM[a]	mmHg	56.04	8.61	60.15	10.17		0.098
Ca	cm/mmHg	0.053	0.026	0.055	0.025		0.247
Ra	mmHg/(cm/s)	0.877	0.77	1.07	0.83	Up	<0.0001
Ci	cm/mmHg	0.581	0.709	0.987	1.03	Up	<0.0001

[a]Diastolic closing margin (DCM), is defined as ABPdiastolic − CrCP

Of course, these global measures still do not necessarily reflect what happens in local, vulnerable areas of the injured brain. However, the finding that the increase in ventilation induced mild hypocapnia caused a reduction in ICP. There was no evidence of any other accompanying significant haemodynamic consequences, though, which seems to suggest that the use of the mild form of hypocapnia might indeed be a safe option. This is because it is unlikely to produce the adverse effects observed under conditions of pronounced hypocapnia.

Last, the authors would like to accentuate the usefulness of the presented methodology for a more thorough interpretation of the TCD measurements. This sort of analysis providing clinically important additional insights into the cerebral haemodynamics would have not been possible without the support of dedicated real-time analysis software such as ICM+.

Conclusions

During hypocapnia in TBI patients, ICP decreases and WT increases. CrCP increases slightly as the rise in wall tension outweighs the decrease in ICP. Closing margins remained unchanged, suggesting that the risk of hypocapnia-induced ischaemia might be low.

Acknowledgements The authors wish to express gratitude to the staff of Neurocritical Care Unit, Addenbrooke's Hospital, Cambridge, UK, for their help and support with the ICM+ brain monitoring project.

Disclosure: ICM+® is software licensed by Cambridge Enterprise Ltd., UK; P.S. and M.C. have a financial interest in a part of the licensing fee.

Conflicts of interest statement We declare that we have no conflict of interest.

References

1. Menon DK. Cerebral protection in severe brain injury: physiological determinants of outcome and their optimisation. Br Med Bull. 1999;55(1):226–58.
2. Varsos GV, et al. Critical closing pressure determined with a model of cerebrovascular impedance. J Cereb Blood Flow Metab. 2013;33(2):235–43.
3. Kim DJ, Kasprowicz M, Carrera E, et al. The monitoring of relative changes in compartmental compliances of brain. Physiol Meas. 2009;30(7):647–59.

Occurrence of CPPopt Values in Uncorrelated ICP and ABP Time Series

M. Cabeleira, M. Czosnyka, X. Liu, J. Donnelly, and P. Smielewski

Abstract *Objectives*: Optimal cerebral perfusion pressure (CPPopt) is a concept that uses the pressure reactivity (PRx)–CPP relationship over a given period to find a value of CPP at which PRx shows best autoregulation. It has been proposed that this relationship be modelled by a U-shaped curve, where the minimum is interpreted as being the CPP value that corresponds to the strongest autoregulation. Owing to the nature of the calculation and the signals involved in it, the occurrence of CPPopt curves generated by non-physiological variations of intracranial pressure (ICP) and arterial blood pressure (ABP), termed here "false positives", is possible. Such random occurrences would artificially increase the yield of CPPopt values and decrease the reliability of the methodology.

In this work, we studied the probability of the random occurrence of false-positives and we compared the effect of the parameters used for CPPopt calculation on this probability.

Materials and methods: To simulate the occurrence of false-positives, uncorrelated ICP and ABP time series were generated by destroying the relationship between the waves in real recordings. The CPPopt algorithm was then applied to these new series and the number of false-positives was counted for different values of the algorithm's parameters.

Results: The percentage of CPPopt curves generated from uncorrelated data was demonstrated to be 11.5%.

Conclusion: This value can be minimised by tuning some of the calculation parameters, such as increasing the calculation window and increasing the minimum PRx span accepted on the curve.

Keywords Optimal CPP · Pressure reactivity · PRx · ICM+ · Brain trauma · Brain monitoring · Neuro-critical care

Introduction

The rise in computer-assisted patient monitoring in neuro-critical care units has demonstrated the inherent heterogeneity of traumatic brain injury and the importance of developing individualised therapies, tailored for each individual patient to better target this condition.

One of the popular strategies for the management of these patients is careful control of cerebral perfusion pressure (CPP) by following a generalised CPP management protocol, including fixed population-based CPP targets. In recent years, a new technique, intended to individualise CPP targets, has been increasing in popularity amongst the clinical research community [1]. This technique, called optimal CPP (CPPopt), makes use of continuous computerised patient monitoring to access the state of autoregulation of the patient by calculating the well-established pressure reactivity index (PRx) and analysing its relationship to CPP. It has been demonstrated that the PRx–CPP characteristics can be modelled by an approximately U-shaped curve, where the minimum of the curve (lowest average PRx) is associated with a value of CPP corresponding to a point where the cerebral autoregulation is the most active.

Despite the promising nature of the technique, it has received some criticism because the parameters being compared are derived from the same primary variables, arterial blood pressure (ABP) and intracranial pressure (ICP), with PRx being the result of Pearson's correlation of mean values of ABP and ICP and CPP being the difference between the two.

M. Cabeleira (✉)
Division of Neurosurgery, Department of Clinical Neurosciences, Addenbrooke's Hospital, University of Cambridge, Cambridge, UK

Neurosurgery Unit, Addenbrooke's Hospital, Cambridge, UK
e-mail: mc916@cam.ac.uk

M. Czosnyka · X. Liu · J. Donnelly · P. Smielewski
Division of Neurosurgery, Department of Clinical Neurosciences, Addenbrooke's Hospital, University of Cambridge, Cambridge, UK

Therefore, the often-observed U-shaped relationship could simply be statistically favoured.

Another problem that plagues the method is its blindness to nursing-related artefacts that affect the time trends being used for the calculation in non-physiological ways. The effect of these artefacts may be that U-shaped curves are not related to the true underlying physiology, and thus generate false CPP targets. These in turn would lead to the erratic (highly variable) appearance of the CPPopt time trends, thus reducing the clinician's overall confidence in the methodology, or at worst it may misguide management of the patient.

In this project, we have set out to study the alleged favouritism of the algorithm for generating U-shaped curves by calculating CPPopt from uncorrelated, surrogate time trends of ICP and ABP, in which any physiological relationship was destroyed. In addition, influence of the individual parameters of the current algorithm on the rate of appearance of false CPPopt curves was also studied.

Materials and Methods

The CPPopt algorithm implemented in this project follows the method presented in Aries et al. [1] and is summarised in Fig. 1.

Uncorrelated ABP and ICP time series were generated using original data recorded at full waveform resolution using ICM+ software [2] from 280 traumatic brain injury patients admitted to the Neuro-Critical Care Unit, Addenbrooke's Hospital, Cambridge. Patient monitoring was approved by the Ethics Committee (REC97/291). Minute-by-minute values of CPP and PRx were calculated in ICM+ and then further processed in MATLAB.

The inherent correlation of the two time series was destroyed by applying a fast Fourier transform (FFT) to ICP, scrambling its phase and applying the inverse FFT to the result. By using this method, any correlation between the signals was eliminated whilst keeping the signal within physiological ranges and dynamics.

To test the occurrence of stand-alone curves of CPPopt, the following protocol was devised:

1. Randomly pick a chunk of n hours of ICP and ABP from the raw data
2. Destroy the correlation using the method described above
3. Calculate CPP and PRx
4. Calculate a CPPopt curve
5. Save 1 if there is a U-shaped curve present and accepted, 0 otherwise
6. Repeat 10,000 times

This protocol was first applied using the most accepted values for the CPPopt calculation parameters proposed in

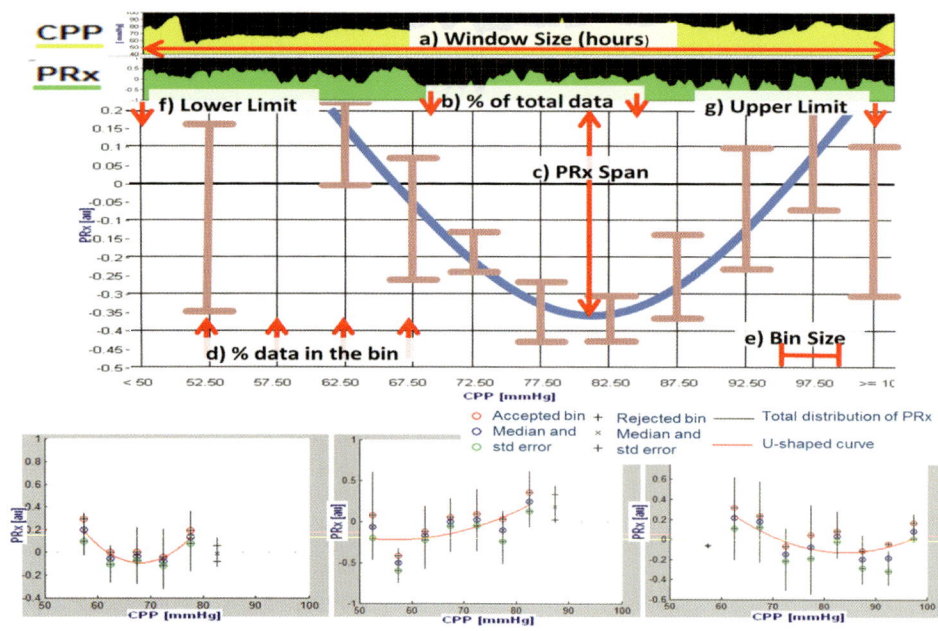

Fig. 1 *Top*: Optimal cerebral perfusion pressure (CPPopt) calculation algorithm. (1) Pressure reactivity (Prx) values from the last n hours (a) are normalised by the Fisher transform and distributed into "bins" of corresponding CPP values. (2) Number of bins calculated using preconfigured lower (f) and upper (g) limit of CPP and the bin width (e). (3) The bins that do not contain a minimum percentage of data (d) stored in them are eliminated (bins < 50 and bins with a centre value of 57.5. (4) Bins with median values of PRx generating rising left edges and falling right edges are also eliminated (bin 52.5). (5) The remaining bins must contain a minimum percentage of total data held (b) for the calculation to proceed. (6) A 2nd order polynomial curve is fitted to the bin mean values. (7) The curve is accepted if it has a positive concavity and if the PRx span (c) is higher than the minimum accepted. *Bottom*: some examples of CPPopt curves generated with noise

Aries et al. [1] (highlighted in Table 1) and then repeated with the parameters adjusted in steps, one at a time (Table 1).

Last, the percentage of occurrence of "false positive" CPPopt curves (i.e. the false yield) in individual patient recordings was also tested using the following protocol:

1. Select a random patient from the pool of 280 recordings
2. Destroy the correlation of ICP and ABP
3. Calculate the CPPopt curves for the whole file in sliding windows of 60 s
   Save 1 if a U-shape curve is present at a given moment, 0 otherwise
4. Calculate the percentage of curves present in the analysed file
5. Repeat 100 times
6. Calculate the average percentage of CPPopt curves of the group of files

To compare the performance of protocol 2 in relation to optimal CPP calculated in real data, the calculations were repeated without the step where correlation is destroyed.

Results

The probability of generating a CPPopt curve from stand-alone uncorrelated curves was 11.5%. Table 1 presents the probabilities of generating CPPopt curves when varying values of the calculation parameters for both protocols and for protocol 2 with real data. The highlighted results were obtained using parameters with the values as recommended in Aries et al. [1]. Examples of accepted U-shaped curves generated with uncorrelated data are presented in Fig. 1.

Discussion

The tests carried out showed that the probability of generating acceptable CPPopt curves from uncorrelated time series (11.5%) is low, but this effect cannot be neglected and measures should be taken to minimise its occurrence.

Table 1 Results of the application of the calculation protocols on the data for each parameter combination tested

Calculation parameter		Value ranges				
(a) Calculation window size	Values range	2	4	8		12
	Protocol 1	16.3	11.7	6.1		3.6
	Protocol 2	17.2 (0–84.7)	11.3 (0–98.2)	5.2 (0–62.9)		3.1 (0–87.9)
	Real CPPopt yield	24.4 (1.3–55.8)	23.5 (0.1–47.1)	22.6 (0–60.1)		23.9 (0–84.4)
(b) Percentage of total data	Values range	40	*50*	60	70	80
	Protocol 1	12.0	11.9	11.3	10.6	9.4
	Protocol 2	11.1 (0–59.3)	10.4 (0–94.1)	9.49 (0–40.4)	8.56 (0–38.8)	9.52 (0–49.7)
	Real CPPopt yield	23.8 (0.1–47.1)	23.5 (0.1–47.1)	22.6 (0.1–47.1)	21.5 (0.0–47.1)	19.9 (0.0–46.9)
(c) Minimum PRx span	Values range	0.1	*0.2*	0.3	0.4	0.5
	Protocol 1	18.5	11.7	5.4	2.0	0.7
	Protocol 2	17.4 (0–76.5)	11.7 (0–53.2)	4.3 (0–21.0)	1.7 (0–25.3)	0.4 (0–4.1)
	Real CPPopt yield	27.3 (8.9–49.2)	23.5 (0.1–47.1)	18.8 (0.0–45.9)	14.5 (0.0–44.5)	9.8 (0.0–34.5)
(d) Percentage of total PRx/Bin	Values range	1	2	3		4
	Protocol 1	19.3	11.8	5.9		3.6
	Protocol 2	17.3 (0–56.6)	10.1 (0–35.3)	5.4 (0–30.7)		2.9 (0–12.8)
	Real CPPopt yield	33.6 (0.2–60.8)	23.5 (0.1–47.1)	13.0 (0.1–26.5)		7.8 (0.0–21.9)
(e) Bin size	Values range	2.5	5		10	
	Protocol 1	12.8	11.8		1.6	
	Protocol 2	10.5 (0–44.5)	11.3 (0–64.7)		9.7 (0–16.0)	
	Real CPPopt yield	25.5 (0.1–56.0)	23.5 (0.1–47.1)		1.3 (0.0–4.7)	
(f) Lower CPP limit and (g) upper CPP limit	Values range	40/120		*50/100*		
	Protocol 1	12.3		11.9		
	Protocol 2	11.1 (0–52.5)		10.7 (0–67.5)		
	Real CPPopt yield	25.8 (1.4–63.1)		23.5 (0.1–47.1)		

PRx pressure reactivity index, *CPP* cerebral perfusion pressure

The discrepancy in yield of CPPopt on recordings from real patients between the result found in Aries et al., (55%) [1], and the result obtained in this study (23.5%) can be explained by the fact that we only considered pure U-shaped curves and not monotonically ascending or descending parts of the curve. Another factor was that the data used here were not "cleaned," meaning that gaps and artefacts were still present at the time of the calculations.

Analysis of the sensitivity of the algorithm's false-positive yield rate to the value of its parameters showed that the total percentage of data (b) in the bins and the CPP limits (f) and (g) do not affect the yield of false-positives. The parameters that seem to have the most preventive effect on the spontaneous calculation of valid CPPopt values are the minimum PRx span (c) and the duration of calculating window (a). Making these parameters stricter will not considerably affect the performance of the algorithm in correlated data, but would decrease the yield of false-positives in the calculations. Increasing the minimum percentage of data in each bin (d) also has a preventive effect on the yield of false-positives, but also considerably affects the yield when using real data. The bin size (e) is the worst parameter to tune because decreasing the size of the bin does not affect the yield and increasing it is more destructive to the yield in real data than in uncorrelated data.

Although visually scrutinising the CPPopt curves generated with uncorrelated data (Fig. 1), the poor quality of fit of the generated curves became immediately evident as the mean values for each bin are very erratic and tend not to follow the U-shaped format. It is also quickly noted that the PRx span is at the minimum in most of the curves and proof of this is the big fall in the percentage of accepted CPPopt curves when using a higher minimum PRx span (1.7% when the minimum span is 0.4).

It is also important not to rely solely on the calculated CPPopt values alone, but to take into consideration the historical values in addition to other related parameters, such as PRx at CPPopt, and their time profile. Visual inspection of the CPPopt charts, and perhaps other forms of CPPopt visualisation, should also help a great deal to discard suspicious curve fitting.

Conclusions

We have shown that it is possible to generate CPPopt curves using uncorrelated data. However, the probability of such false-positives is low, but not negligible and should be taken into account when choosing the parameters for CPPopt calculation. The results also show the importance of annotations in the data that could flag moments when CPPopt calculations might be unreliable.

Acknowledgement The authors wish to express their gratitude to the staff of the Neurocritical Care Unit in Addenbrooke's Hospital, Cambridge, UK, for their help and support for the ICM+ brain monitoring project.

Conflicts of interest statement P. Smielewski and M. Czosnyka have partial financial interest in the licensing of ICM+.

References

1. Aries MJH, Czosnyka M, Budohoski KP, Steiner LA, Lavinio A, Kolias AG, et al. Continuous determination of optimal cerebral perfusion pressure in traumatic brain injury. Crit Care Med [Internet]. 2012;40(8):2456–63. Available from: http://www.ncbi.nlm.nih.gov/pubmed/22622398.
2. Smielewski P, Czosnyka M. Cambridge University: Neurosurgery Unit | About ICM+ [Internet]. Available from: http://www.neurosurg.cam.ac.uk/pages/ICM/about.php.

Simultaneous Transients of Intracranial Pressure and Heart Rate in Traumatic Brain Injury: Methods of Analysis

Giovanna Maria Dimitri, Shruti Agrawal, Adam Young, Joseph Donnelly, Xiuyun Liu, Peter Smielewski, Peter Hutchinson, Marek Czosnyka, Pietro Lio, and Christina Haubrich

Abstract *Objectives*: The detection of increasing intracranial pressure (ICP) is important in preventing secondary brain injuries. Before mean ICP increases critically, transient ICP elevations may be observed. We have observed ICP transients of less than 10 min duration, which occurred simultaneously with transient increases in heart rate (HR). These simultaneous events in HR and ICP suggest a direct interaction or communication between the heart and the brain. Methods: This chapter describes four mathematical methods and their applicability in detecting the above heart–brain cross-talk events during long-term monitoring of ICP. Results: Recurrence plots, cross-correlation function and wavelet analysis confirmed the relationship between ICP and HR time series. Using the peaks detection algorithm with a sliding window approach we found an average of 37 cross-talk events (± SD 39). The number of events detected varied among patients, from 1 to more than 150 events.

Pietro Lio and Christina Haubrich contributed equally to this work.

G.M. Dimitri • P. Lio
Computer Laboratory, University of Cambridge, Cambridge, UK

S. Agrawal
Department of Pediatric Intensive Care, Addenbrooke's Hospital, University of Cambridge, Cambridge, UK

A. Young • P. Hutchinson
Division of Academic Neurosurgery, Department of Clinical Neurosciences, Addenbrooke's Hospital, University of Cambridge, Cambridge, UK

J. Donnelly • X. Liu • P. Smielewski • M. Czosnyka
Brain Physics Laboratory, Division of Neurosurgery, Department of Clinical Neuroscience, Addenbrooke's Hospital, University of Cambridge, Cambridge, UK

C. Haubrich (✉)
Brain Physics Laboratory, Division of Neurosurgery, Department of Clinical Neuroscience, Addenbrooke's Hospital, University of Cambridge, Cambridge, UK

Faculty of Neurology, RWTH Aachen University, Aachen, Germany
e-mail: ch723@cam.ac.uk

Conclusion: Our analysis suggested that the peaks detection algorithm based on a sliding window approach is feasible for detecting simultaneous peaks, e.g. cross-talk events in the ICP and HR signals.

Keywords Intracranial pressure · Heart rate · Cross-talk · Recurrence plots · Wavelet analysis · Peaks detection

Introduction

Intracranial pressure (ICP) after severe brain injuries or similar life-threatening conditions can be continuously monitored [1]. The ICP signal contains useful information for predicting critical conditions such as intracranial hypertension. So far, monitoring approaches are focusing mainly on the relationship between arterial blood pressure and intracranial pressure. There are however, transient elevations of heart rate (HR) and ICP, which occur simultaneously. These transients appear variable in rate and intensity. Our hypothesis, therefore, is that these "cross-talk" events in the HR–ICP relationship can be quantified via methods of complex event processing. There are only a few papers modelling the dynamics of intracranial pressure. Hu et al. for instance, presented an estimation algorithm based on a hidden state estimation approach and nonlinear Kalman filters to estimate unobserved variables in the monitoring data of ICP and cerebral blood flow velocity (CBFV) [2]. Various methods have been applied to investigate the interrelationship between ICP and cardiovascular parameters. Hu et al. also presented ApEN, an algorithm based on the adaptive calculation of approximate entropy, integrated with a causal coherence analysis that is able to exploit the potential interaction between ICP and R wave intervals [3]. The same authors have shown that causal spectral measures and generalised synchronisation measures can be used to extract indices from beat-to-beat mean intracranial pressure measurements and intervals between consecutive normal sinus heart beats (ICP and RR intervals; [4]). To systematically detect simultaneous transients in HR and ICP, e.g., cross-talk events from our initially described observations, we applied different mathematical methodologies to identify the relationships between the two time series. We then implemented a sliding window approach to detect simultaneous HR and ICP peaks (see section "Peaks Detection Algorithm: A Sliding Window Approach"), obtaining promising results.

Monitoring Data

The data in this study were collected prospectively from 27 pediatric TBI patients admitted to Addenbrooke's Hospital, Cambridge, Pediatric Intensive Care Unit (PICU) between August 2012 and December 2014. Consecutive TBI patients with a clinical need for ICP monitoring were included for analysis. The insertion of an intracranial monitoring device is part of routine clinical practice and as such did not require ethical approval. The data are routinely collected for clinical purposes and guide the management of patients. The analysis of data within this study for the purposes of service evaluation was approved by the Cambridge University Hospital NHS Trust, Audit and Service Evaluation Department (Ref: 2143) and did not require ethical approval or patient consent. ABP mean arterial pressure was measured in mmHg, heart rate (HR) in Hz and intracranial pressure (ICP) in mmHg. The data sampling rate was 200 Hz.

Methods

We describe in this section the methods used for performing the analysis of the two time series and to study the behaviour of the ICP with regard to the HR. In the following section we describe the results obtained.

Recurrence Plots

We used recurrence plots (RP) to further analyse nonlinear dynamics simultaneously occurring in ICP and HR time series. The data are visualised through a graph in a square matrix (column and rows represent a pair of times). The elements represent the time points at which a specific state of the dynamical system recurred [5]. In mathematical terms, RP represents the time stamps in which the phase space trajectory of the system under consideration passes through the same area in the phase space [6]. In recurrence plots there are two parameters to be fixed, the so-called d and m: the time delay and the embedding dimension respectively [7]. This is in fact derived from recurrence plots theories and the way in which the time series is represented in the phase space. In particular, the mathematical description comes from Takens' embedding theorem. For details on the theorem please see Takens [8].

Cross-Correlation Function and Wavelet Analysis

In signal theory, cross-correlation represents the similarity between two signals, as a function of the shift or temporal translation applied to one of the two signals [9]. In particular, if g and f are two continuous functions, the cross-correlation is defined as:

$$(f \otimes g)(\tau) = \int_{-\infty}^{\infty} f^*(t) g(t+\tau) dt.$$

where f^* is the complex conjugate of f and τ is the time displacement.

Another methodology we used to understand the behaviour of the system is wavelet analysis. The method is based on the decomposition of a time series into the time–frequency space. This allows us to determine and study the variability of a given time series and its behaviour. In particular, the continuous wavelet transform (CWT) is able to decompose the time series in the time–frequency domain by convolving the time series with a scaled and translated form of the so-called mother wavelet function, a continuous function both in frequency and time domain [10, 11]. The wavelet coherence method determines and visualises areas with a high common power (i.e. high common correlation) between time series [12]. Wavelet coherence analysis is based on the CWT. The CTW given scaling factor $\alpha \in \mathbb{R}^+$ and a value for translation $\beta \in \mathbb{R}$ is defined as:

$$\chi_\omega(\alpha,\beta) = \frac{1}{|\alpha|^{\frac{1}{2}}} \int_{-\infty}^{\infty} x(t) \Psi(t)^* \left(\frac{t-\beta}{\alpha}\right) dt$$

where $\Psi(t)$ is the mother wavelet. $\Psi(t)^*$ is the complex conjugate of the mother wavelet function.

Peaks Detection Algorithm: A Sliding Window Approach

After the relationship between the ICP and HR time series was confirmed, the next step was to implement a peak detection algorithm to systematically collect the ICP-HR cross-talk events from initial observations (as shown in Fig. 1). We

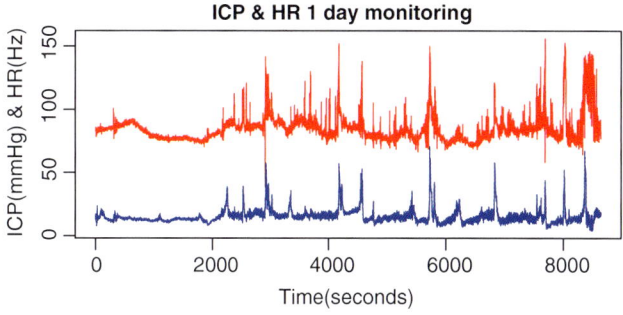

Fig. 1 Plot of the intracranial pressure (ICP; *blue*) and heart rate (HR; *red*) behaviour in a day time span of a patient in our cohort. As we can see, there are multiple cross-talk events happening in the time range considered (some of them are highlighted in *green*). Each time stamp in the x axis is 10 s

first followed the algorithm suggested in Palshikar [13]. Our aim was to find visual correlations between peaks happening in the ICP and in the HR series and to consider the temporal correlation between events. To take into account the fact that both time series originate from biological systems, we implemented a peaks detection algorithm based on a naive sliding window approach. This algorithm works as follows:

1. Consider two time series $X = x_1, x_2, x_3, \ldots, xT$ and $Y = y_1, y_2, y_3, \ldots, yT$ (which in our case are the HR and ICP time series)
2. Consider a window W of length L (in our case we considered a window with a dimension of 10 min)
3. Consider all the simultaneous sub-windows of length (L) in the two time series x and y
4. If the maximum value in the i-th time window considered is at least a 20% increase with regard to the minimum value in this time window, and if after the maximum value, there is a decrease of at least 20%, then a peak is detected.
5. If in both time series such a peak is detected, then a cross-talk event is registered in that particular time window.

Results

As a starting point of our analysis, we first plotted the time series for each patient, to visually explore ICP–HR cross-talk events. Figure 1 is an sample plot of ICP and HR time series monitored from a patient in our cohort. Figure 1 show several simultaneous transients in ICP and HR. The ICP time series is coloured in blue, whereas the HR is red and several peaks appear to take place in the same time window (i.e. cross-talk events). Starting from this visual observation, we further analysed such cross-talk events, using several statistical and time series analysis approaches, such as recurrence plots, cross-correlation function, wavelet analysis and peak detection algorithms.

We used recurrence plots to explore the behaviour of the two time series, as explained in section "Methods". In Fig. 2a, b, the black dots represent recurrent points and the lines parallel to the diagonal line show the determinism of the system. This happens both for the ICP and HR and is coherent with the nature of the two signals. Moreover, the two recurrent plots look quite similar, suggesting our hypothesis of an interaction between the two time series considered. The presence of parallel lines and similarity between the HR and ICP were verified in the plots of 27 patients from the cohort.

We then performed the cross-correlation function between the two time series ICP and HR. Figure 3c exemplifies the correlation between the two time series and provides further support for the hypothesis of an interdependency between the two signals.

In Table 1, we report the Pearson correlation coefficient between the ICP and HR for the 27 patients available.

We then performed wavelet analysis on the ICP and HR time series of 27 patients. Before performing this analysis, we checked for the normality of the two time series considering the Shapiro–Wilk test for normality. As the test showed normality of the data proposed, we performed the wavelet

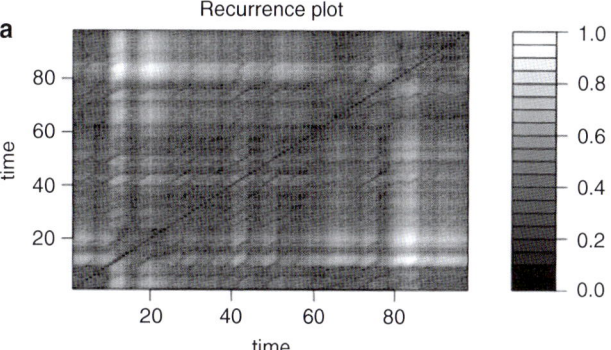

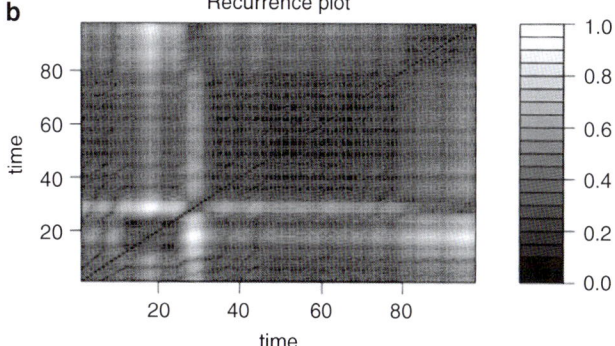

Fig. 2 Recurrence plots for a patient in our cohort for (**a**) ICP and (**b**) HR. The parameters used for the recurrence plots were ($d = 2$ and $m = 3$, where m is the embedding dimension and d is the delay. Those two parameters are needed for setting the time window in which the recurrence of the system is analysed using the recurrence plot method.). See Marwan et al. [5] for details

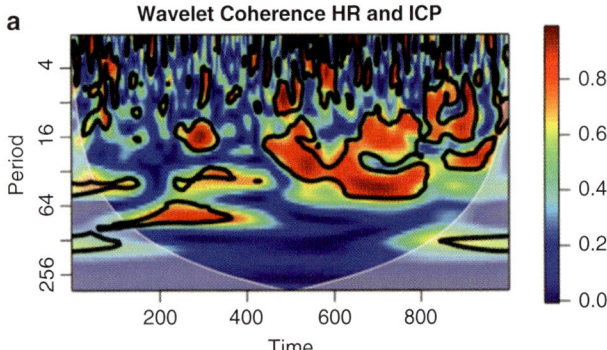

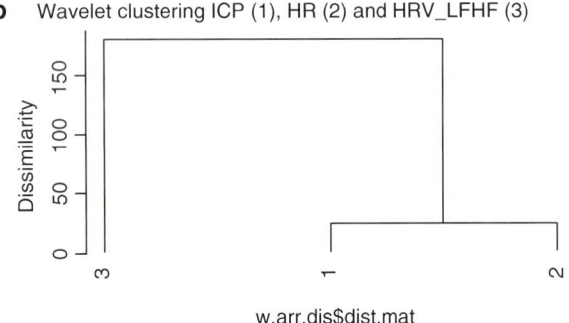

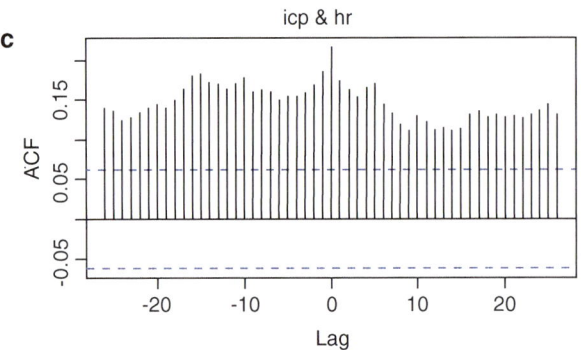

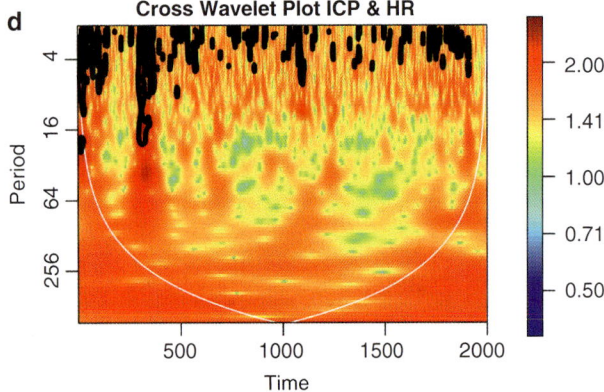

Fig. 3 (**a**) Wavelet coherence; (**b**) wavelet clustering; (**c**) cross-correlation; (**d**) cross-wavelet

two signals show high correlation, and it also tells us in which time instants such a correlation happens. This is particularly useful for our analysis, because we are looking for a correlation in particular time instances (i.e. when peaks occur). Moreover, we performed two additional analyses with wavelets, in particular, wavelet correlations and wavelet clustering. The wavelets showed a high correlation between the ICP and HR, as we can see from Fig. 3a, where the red parts indicate the presence of highly correlated episodes. In the case of clustering, we have so far analysed the wavelet power clustering considering three time series, HR, ICP and HRVLF/HF. As we can see from Fig. 3b, the ICP and HR time series are clustered together (1 and 2 in the tree) and further away from the frequency domain-derived parameter, LF/HF ratio, supporting even further our hypothesis about the similarity between HR and ICP behaviours.

Finally, we applied our sliding window approach to detect cross-talk events between ICP and HR described in section "Peaks Detection Algorithm: A Sliding Window Approach". This enabled us to identify multiple cross-talk events happening in the HR and ICP time series. We found an average of 37 cross-talk events (±SD 39).

The number of events detected varied among patients, from 1 to more than 150 events (Table 2).

Discussion and Conclusions

This analysis was performed with no a priori regard for a possible relationship between HR and ICP. The 27 records of monitored data are consecutive samples of pediatric patients admitted to Addenbrooke's Hospital, Cambridge. We performed a series of correlation analyses and tests to understand the behaviour and the relationship between peaks happening in the ICP and HR. The two parameters were obtained independently one from the other and with no previous assumption regarding the causal relationship or behavioural relationship between the two time series. Recurrence plots, cross-correlation function and wavelet analysis confirmed the relationship between ICP and HR time series. These were performed as part of a preliminary analysis to understand if the two time series correlated and showed similar behaviours.

In a first instance, we applied recurrence plots analysis to study the determinism and behaviour of each individual time series (ICP and HR considered separately). We then introduced wavelet analysis to study the interaction between HR and ICP. Using wavelet coherence and cross wavelets, we were able to understand that correlated behaviours were occurring. We also obtained the Pearson correlation coefficients, which allowed us to evaluate even further the presence of a correlation between the ICP and HR series of each patient. As a next step, we implemented a sliding window peaks detection

coherence between HR and ICP time series, as shown in Fig. 3d. The resulting plot shows particularly interesting characteristics. In fact, it identifies regions (in red) where the

Table 1 Pearson correlation coefficient of the 27 patients between intracranial pressure (ICP) and heart rate (HR)

P1	P2	P3	P4	P5	P6	P7	P8	P9
0.46	−0.1	0.01	−0.50	0.17	−0.02	0.11	0.33	−0.22
P10	P11	P12	P13	P14	P15	P16	P17	P18
−0.01	0.10	0.12	0.31	0.40	0.23	0.04	0.11	0.24
P19	P20	P21	P22	P23	P24	P25	P26	P27
0.24	−0.13	−0.39	0.09	0.47	0.30	−0.6	0.09	−0.32

P patient

Table 2 Number of HR–ICP cross-talk events detected for each patient

P1	P2	P3	P4	P5	P6	P7	P8	P9
17	32	65	20	1	23	22	43	55
P10	P11	P12	P13	P14	P15	P16	P17	P18
67	20	142	27	29	7	35	2	0
P19	P20	P21	P22	P23	P24	P25	P26	P27
1	19	188	55	2	15	0	14	17

algorithm. With this algorithm, we were able to detect the cross-talk events happening in the two time series for each patient. The sliding window peaks detection algorithm detected a significant number of cross-talk-events using the peaks detection algorithm. Using a sliding window approach, we found an average number of simultaneous peaks in HR and ICP. We found an average of 37 cross-talk-events (±SD 39).

The results showed that a peaks extraction method may be a feasible approach for the automated detection of simultaneous peaks in HR and ICP. On the one hand, however, we do not know about a causal relationship between the transient elevations of HR and ICP. Hence, further work will include the analysis of the time series using the Granger causality method, trying to understand the causality of correlations between the ICP and HR time series. When considering the inter-individual variations in the number of cross-talks events, on the other hand, influencing factors such as the pressure–volume reserve or the autonomic nervous activity should be analysed as well. Therefore, we are currently extending our analysis, investigating the relationship between ICP–HR cross-talk events and measures derived from time- and frequency domains.

Conflicts of interest statement We declare that we have no conflicts of interest.

References

1. Hu X, et al. Morphological clustering and analysis of continuous intracranial pressure. IEEE Trans Biomed Eng. 2009;56:696–705.
2. Hu X, et al. Estimation of hidden state variables of the intracranial system using constrained nonlinear Kalman filters. IEEE Trans Biomed Eng. 2007;54:597–610.
3. Hu X, et al. Adaptive computation of approximate entropy and its application in integrative analysis of irregularity of heart rate variability and intracranial pressure signals. Med Eng Phys. 2008;30:631–9.
4. Hu X, et al. Characterization of interdependency between intracranial pressure and heart variability signals: a causal spectral measure and a generalized synchronization measure. IEEE Trans Biomed Eng. 2007;54:1407–17.
5. Marwan N, Romano MC, Thiel M, Kurths J. Recurrence plots for the analysis of complex systems. Phys Rep. 2007;438(5–6):237–329.
6. Eckmann J-P, Oliffson Kamphorst S, David R. Recurrence plots of dynamical systems. Europhys Lett. 1987;4:973.
7. Fabretti A, Ausloos M. Recurrence plot and recurrence quantification analysis techniques for detecting a critical regime. Examples from financial market indices. Int J Mod Phys C. 2005;16(05):671–706.
8. Takens F. Detecting strange attractors in turbulence. Dynamical systems and turbulence, Warwick 1980. Berlin: Springer; 1981. p. 366–81.
9. Kapinchev K, Bradu A, Barnes F, Podoleanu A. GPU implementation of cross-correlation for image generation in real time. ICSPCS 2015. 2015.
10. Tian F, et al. Wavelet coherence analysis of dynamic cerebral autoregulation in neonatal hypoxic-ischemic encephalopathy. Neuroimage Clin. 2016;11:124–32.
11. Mallat SG. A wavelet tour of signal processing. San Diego: Academic Press; 1999.
12. Grinsted A, Moore JC, Jevrejeva S. Application of the cross wavelet transform and wavelet coherence to geophysical time series. Nonlinear Proc Geophys. 2004;11:561–6.
13. Palshikar G. Simple algorithms for peak detection in time-series. Proc. 1st Int. Conf. Advanced Data Analysis, Business Analytics and Intelligence. 2009.

Increasing the Contrast-to-Noise Ratio of MRI Signals for Regional Assessment of Dynamic Cerebral Autoregulation

José L. Jara, Nazia P. Saeed, Ronney B. Panerai, and Thompson G. Robinson

Abstract *Objective*: To devise an appropriate measure of the quality of a magnetic resonance imaging (MRI) signal for the assessment of dynamic cerebral autoregulation, and propose simple strategies to improve its quality.

Materials and methods: Magnetic resonance images of 11 healthy subjects were scanned during a transient decrease in arterial blood pressure (BP). Mean signals were extracted from non-overlapping brain regions for each image. An ad-hoc contrast-to-noise ratio (CNR) was used to evaluate the quality of these regional signals. Global mean signals were obtained by averaging the set of regional signals resulting after applying a Hampel filter and discarding a proportion of the lower quality component signals.

Results: Significant improvements in CNR values of global mean signals were obtained, whilst maintaining significant correlation with the original ones. A Hampel filter with a small moving window and a low rejection threshold combined with a selection of the 50% component signals seems a recommendable option.

Conclusions: This work has demonstrated the possibility of improving the quality of MRI signals acquired during transient drops in BP. This approach needs validation at a voxel level, which could help to consolidate MRI as a technological alternative to the standard techniques for the study of cerebral autoregulation.

J.L. Jara (✉)
Departamento de Ingeniería Informática, Universidad de Santiago de Chile, USACH, Santiago, Chile
e-mail: joseluis.jara@usach.cl

N.P. Saeed
Ageing and Stroke Medicine, Department of Cardiovascular Sciences, University of Leicester, Leicester, UK

R.B. Panerai • T.G. Robinson
Ageing and Stroke Medicine, Department of Cardiovascular Sciences, University of Leicester, Leicester, UK

NIHR Biomedical Research Unit for Cardiovascular Sciences, University of Leicester, Leicester, UK

Keywords Dynamic cerebral autoregulation · Magnetic resonance imaging · Contrast-to-noise ratio · Hampel filter

Introduction

Using magnetic resonance imaging (MRI) as an alternative to the standard transcranial Doppler (TCD) approach to assess dynamic cerebral autoregulation (dCA) is under investigation. The similarity between the time courses of the signal recorded with TCD and the MRI signal was established for healthy subjects in Saeed et al. [1]. A mean map of dCA efficiency for a group of healthy subjects was presented in Horsfield et al. [2]. More recently, the use of hemispheric TCD signals and hemispheric MRI signals to discriminate between healthy and acute ischaemic stroke populations was investigated in Panerai et al. [3]. However, as reported in the most recent study, many time courses were excluded from the analysis, mostly from stroke patients, by a panel of four of the authors who visually inspected the signals on a computer screen, because they presented large artefacts or they did not show the expected temporal pattern, reflecting a sudden drop in arterial blood pressure (BP).

The MRI-based method of evaluating dCA efficiency proposed in Horsfield et al. [2] resembles the functional MRI paradigm (fMRI) of cognitive neuroimaging studies. Both approaches seek variations in the blood-oxygen-level-dependent (BOLD) contrast as a surrogate of changes in cerebral blood flow. Although in fMRI, the goal is to identify an increase in the BOLD signal in response to neuronal activity, the MRI-based dCA evaluation is aimed at detecting a drop in the BOLD signal in response to a slump in BP produced by the sudden release of inflated bilateral thigh cuffs (THCs). In both cases, the change in BOLD signal is rather small and transient, starting a few seconds after the stimulus and returning to baseline level over time.

The signal of an individual voxel in an MRI image can be affected by BOLD fluctuations due to ghost images, blood flow artefacts in the vicinity of large vessels and, in particular, by spontaneous neuronal activity [4, 5]. Similar to the hemispheric MRI signals of Panerai et al. [3], regional indicators for the efficiency of cerebral autoregulation could be obtained from a dCA efficiency map by averaging the values of the hundreds or thousands of voxels that usually comprise the region of interest (ROI). Moreover, recognising and filtering out corrupted voxels in the ROI could yield less noisy regional signals or more accurate regional measures of dCA efficiency.

Two important questions arise from these observations, which are addressed in this study. First, it is necessary to devise a more objective and easily comparable measure of the quality of a signal time course than visual inspection. This measure must be applicable to the hundreds of thousands of voxels in an MRI image and consider that spontaneous fluctuations should be limited, whereas the variation introduced by the THC deflation should be much larger and clear. Second, simple strategies must be proposed to further reduce common artefacts and improve the quality of the MRI signals at both voxel level and regional level.

Materials and Methods

Subjects and Data

Gradient-echo EPI sequences were used to scan the brains of 11 healthy subjects at a rate of 1 Hz. During the initial 3 min, the subjects lay supine in the scanner with filled THCs. Then, a transient decrease in BP was provoked by the sudden deflation of the THCs. The series continued until 240-s images were acquired. After the first run was completed, the THCs were re-inflated and the procedure was repeated twice more during a single session. The protocol is detailed in Saeed et al., Horsfield et al. and Panerai et al. [1–3] and the 33 images considered in this study are the same as those used in Horsfield et al. [2]. The study was approved by the Leicestershire, Northamptonshire and Rutland Research Ethics Committee (REC 09/H0403/25) and all subjects gave written informed consent.

As it would be impossible to hand-inspect for improvements in the quality of the signal of all voxels in a real situation, a more manageable simplification was used: the global mean signal of an image is the result of averaging regional mean signals that result from the applications of 32 masks of non-overlapping brain regions. In this way, a global mean signal can be compared before and after manipulating its 32 component signals, which can also be examined to determine the effect on them of any proposed method.

MRI Signal Quality

Contrast-to-noise ratio (CNR) has been found to be more suitable for fMRI than more traditional measures of signal quality [6, 7], as higher CNR values yield to better identification of the actual stimulus-related fluctuations and it encapsulates all relevant quality factors into a single and intuitive parameter [8]. There are different definitions and methods of estimating CNR, but all of them conceptualise this parameter as the ratio between the amplitude of BOLD fluctuations produced by the stimulus and the variability of the noise over time [7, 8]. The definition used is $CNR = A/\sigma_N$. The estimation begins with the selection of two segments of the signal: the baseline samples b_i are the 10 signal values before the deflation of the THCs, and the response samples r_i correspond to the 10 values between the 3 s and 12 s after the THC deflation, in which the reaction to the stimulus is expected. The variability of the noise in the signal is the standard deviation of the baseline residuals: $\sigma_N = \mathrm{sd}(b_i - \mathrm{mean}(b_i))$, and the amplitude of the response to the stimulus is determined as the difference between the baseline value and the minimum signal value in the response segment: $A = \mathrm{mean}(b_i) - \min(b_i)$. Thus, the clearer the response to the stimulus with regard to the observed noise, the higher the CNR value obtained. It must be noted that negative CNR values are possible when the signal exhibits an increase during the stimulus segment.

Outlier Filtering

The estimation of CNR involves mean and standard deviation values, which are both known to be sensitive to outliers. In addition, artefacts in the form of "narrow spikes" (<3 s) have been reported in the signals under study [2, 3]. Thus, outliers must be dealt with to obtain reliable CNR values.

Filtering and denoising methods for fMRI have been intensely studied. Out of many options [4, 9], the Hampel filter was selected for this study as it is much simpler to compute, it does not require knowledge of the process model, it replaces only outliers, preserving all other information in the signal, and it is often extremely effective in practice [10]. This filter has two parameters: k, the half-size of a moving window $\{s_{-k}, ..., s_0, ..., s_k\}$ to assess the "outlierness" of the centre sample s_0, and the rejection threshold t_0, so that s_0 is replaced by the window's median value when it is greater than t_0 times the median absolute deviation scale of the window [10]. The combinations of several values for the parameters were tested: $k = \{2, 3, ..., 9, 10\}$ and $t_0 = \{2.0, 2.5, 3.0, 3.5, 4.0\}$.

Low CNR Filtering

Low-quality component signals should have low CNR values with regard to the other component signals and they could be discarded when calculating mean signals. This CNR filter was added to the experiments filtering out 1\4, 1\3, 1\2, 2\3 and 3\4 of the component signals with lowest CNR values. Using proportions to discard component signals allows the selection of the weak elements relative to the quality of all component signals, avoiding the need for a fixed threshold and securing a number of component signals to be averaged.

Statistical Analysis

Mean signals of each of the 33 run images were calculated with the resulting component signals for each combination of a Hampel filter and a CNR filter. Resulting mean signals were compared with the original, unfiltered signal using the Spearman correlation coefficient and their statistical significance was tested. CNR values of the unfiltered mean signal and the three best combination of filters were compared using repeated-measures ANOVA and Tukey's post hoc analysis when differences were found. In all cases, differences were considered significant with $p < 0.05$.

Results

Table 1 summarises the results obtained. Every pair of filters evaluated yielded significant increments in the CNR values of global mean signals, producing improvements in 25 to all 33 images, and at the same time maintaining significantly high correlations with the unfiltered version that range from 0.85 to 0.97 approximately.

Discussion

No inflexion point was observed for the effect of CNR filters and the larger the proportion of weak component signals disregarded, the higher the CNR value of the overall signal. Thus, the selection of this proportion is determined by the trade-off between this improvement in CNR values and how much of the original signal is to be preserved. The number of component signals should obviously be taken into consideration as well.

In general, the combination of a Hampel filter with a short moving window (2–3 s) and a low rejection threshold (2.0–2.5) and a selection of the 50% of component signals seems a recommendable option that would yield 3.5–4.0 points increase in overall CNR value maintaining a mean correlation coefficient over 0.9 with the original global mean signals. Figure 1 shows the application of the approach to one particular image.

Table 1 Results of the best three combinations for each proportion of component signals discarded

CNR proportion	Hampel filter		CNR values of the 33 global signals			Correlation with original	
	k	t_0	Improved	Median increase	Mean increase	Median	Mean
25%	3	2.0	27	1.92	2.45	0.97	0.96
	2	2.0	25	1.68	2.26	0.97	0.96
	3	2.5	25	1.63	2.02	0.97	0.97
33%	2	2.0	30	2.32	2.73	0.96	0.94
	3	2.0	29	2.21	3.03	0.96	0.95
	4	2.0	29	2.06	3.02	0.96	0.95
50%	3	2.0	32	2.78	4.01	0.93	0.92
	2	2.0	32	3.16	3.93	0.92	0.91
	2	2.5	32	2.61	3.66	0.93	0.92
67%	3	2.0	33	4.28	5.53	0.90	0.88
	2	2.0	33	4.37	5.51	0.91	0.88
	2	2.5	33	4.28	4.89	0.92	0.89
75%	3	2.0	33	3.19	5.69	0.88	0.86
	2	2.0	33	3.29	5.18	0.87	0.85
	3	2.5	33	2.49	5.14	0.89	0.86

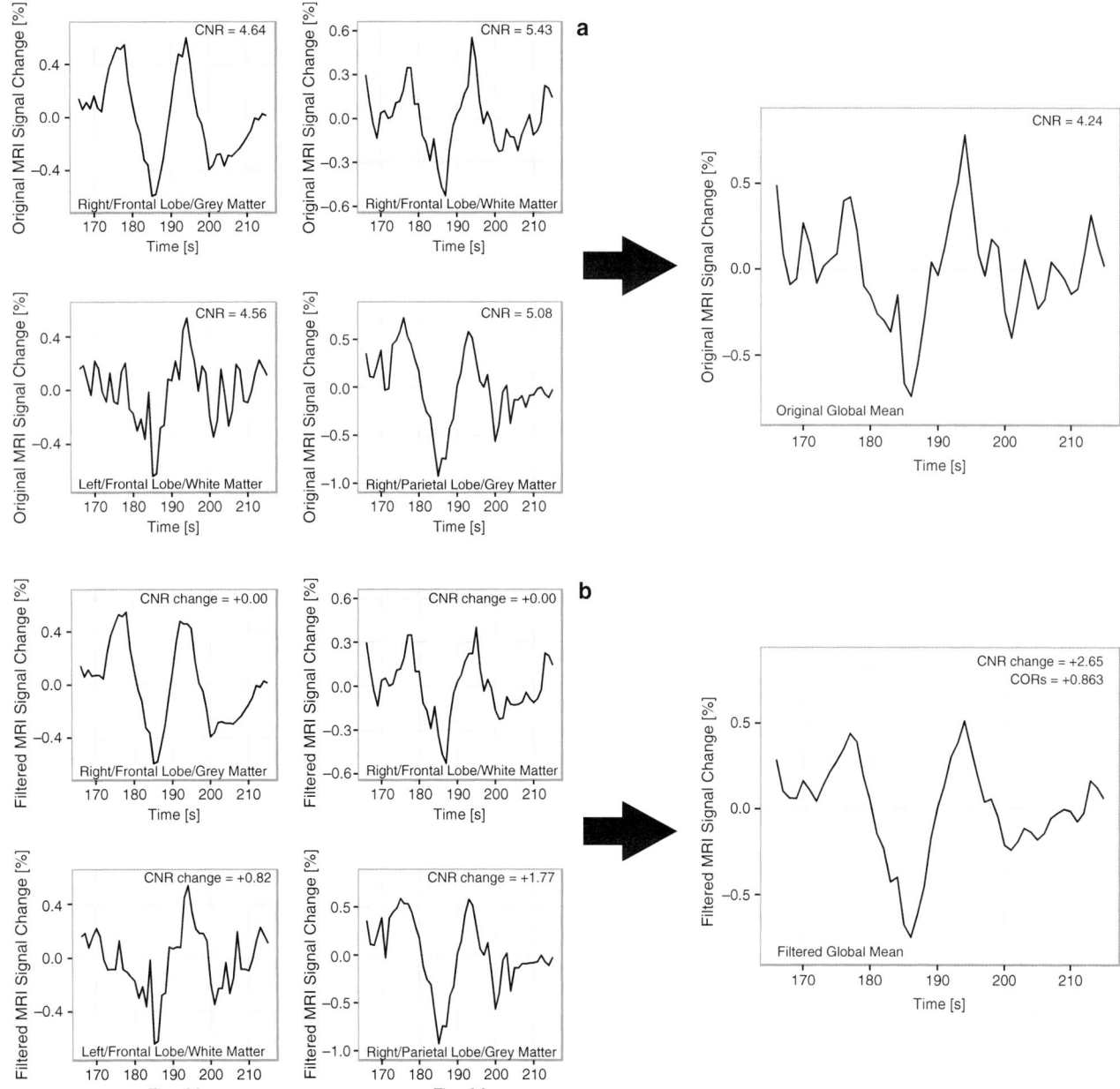

Fig. 1 Examples of original (**a**, *left*) regional MRI signals that compose the (**a**, *right*) global mean MRI signal of a subject. (**b**) The same signals are shown after filtering with the recommended approach. The final global mean MRI signal correlates significantly with the original one ($r_S = 0.863$, $p < 0.001$)

Although future work is needed to validate it, the approach seems scalable to voxel level, as both the Hampel filter and the CNR filter are not computationally expensive. If corrupted voxels can indeed be detected and filtered out, then more reliable measures of dCA efficiency could be obtained from particular regions of the brain, information that could have great potential in guiding the clinical management of diseases such as stroke and traumatic brain injury [2].

Conclusions

This study has demonstrated the possibility of improving the quality of MRI signals, as measured by CNR, with the combination of two simple filtering strategies. This approach could help to consolidate MRI as an alternative to the standard TCD technique for the assessment of dCA, with the clear advantage of obtaining information about regional variations that has been unavailable so far.

Funding Partially funded by DICYT-USACH.

Conflicts of interest statement We declare that we have no conflicts of interest.

References

1. Saeed N, Horsfield M, Panerai R, Mistri A, Robinson T. Measurement of cerebral blood flow responses to the thigh cuff maneuver: a comparison of TCD with a novel MRI method. J Cereb Blood Flow Metab. 2010;31:1302–10.
2. Horsfield M, Jara J, Saeed N, Panerai R, Robinson T. Regional differences in dynamic cerebral autoregulation in the healthy brain assessed by magnetic resonance imaging. PLoS One. 2013;8:e62588.
3. Panerai R, Jara J, Saeed N, Horsfield M, Robinson T. Dynamic cerebral autoregulation following acute ischaemic stroke: comparison of transcranial Doppler and magnetic resonance imaging techniques. J Cereb Blood Flow Metab. 2015. 0271678X15615874.
4. Kruggel F, von Cramon D, Descombes X. Comparison of filtering methods for fMRI datasets. NeuroImage. 1999;10:530–43.
5. Bianciardi M, Fukunaga M, van Gelderen P, Horovitz S, de Zwart J, Shmueli K, Duyn J. Sources of functional magnetic resonance imaging signal fluctuations in the human brain at rest: a 7 T study. Magn Reson Imaging. 2009;27:1019–29.
6. Triantafyllou C, Polimeni J, Wald L. Physiological noise and signal-to-noise ratio in fMRI with multi-channel array coils. NeuroImage. 2011;55:597–606.
7. Welvaert M, Rosseel Y. On the definition of signal-to-noise ratio and contrast-to-noise ratio for fMRI data. PLoS One. 2013;8:e77089.
8. Geissler A, Gartus A, Foki T, Tahamtan A, Beisteiner R, Barth M. Contrast-to-noise ratio (CNR) as a quality parameter in fMRI. J Magn Reson Imaging. 2007;25:1263–70.
9. Liu H, Shah S, Jiang W. On-line outlier detection and data cleaning. Comput Chem Eng. 2004;28:1635–47.
10. Pearson R. Outliers in process modeling and identification. IEEE Trans Control Syst Technol. 2002;10:55–63.

Comparing Models of Spontaneous Variations, Maneuvers and Indexes to Assess Dynamic Cerebral Autoregulation

Max Chacón, Sun-Ho Noh, Jean Landerretche, and José L. Jara

Abstract *Objective*: We analyzed the performance of linear and nonlinear models to assess dynamic cerebral autoregulation (dCA) from spontaneous variations in healthy subjects and compared it with the use of two known maneuvers to abruptly change arterial blood pressure (BP): thigh cuffs and sit-to-stand.

Materials and methods: Cerebral blood flow velocity and BP were measured simultaneously at rest and while the maneuvers were performed in 20 healthy subjects. To analyze the spontaneous variations, we implemented two types of models using support vector machine (SVM): linear and nonlinear finite impulse response models. The classic autoregulation index (ARI) and the more recently proposed model-free ARI (mfARI) were used as measures of dCA. An ANOVA analysis was applied to compare the different methods and the coefficient of variation was calculated to evaluate their variability.

Results: There are differences between indexes, but not between models and maneuvers. The mfARI index with the sit-to-stand maneuver shows the least variability.

Conclusions: Support vector machine modeling of spontaneous variation with the mfARI index could be used for the assessment of dCA as an alternative to maneuvers to introduce large BP fluctuations.

Keywords Dynamic cerebral autoregulation · Spontaneous variations · Thigh cuff maneuver · Sit-to-stand maneuver · Support vector regression · Linear and nonlinear models

M. Chacón • S.-H. Noh • J.L. Jara (✉)
Departamento de Ingeniería Informática, Facultad de Ingeniería, Universidad de Santiago de Chile, Estación Central, Santiago, Chile
e-mail: joseluis.jara@usach.cl

J. Landerretche
Unidad de Neurología, Facultad de Ciencias Médicas, Universidad de Santiago de Chile, Santiago, Chile

Introduction

Dynamic cerebral autoregulation (dCA) is usually assessed by analyzing the cerebral blood flow velocity (CBFV) response signal to a change in arterial blood pressure (BP). There are several maneuvers for producing the BP stimulus, such as the sudden release of bilateral thigh cuffs [1, 2], varying the body posture [3, 4], the Valsalva maneuver, hand grip exercises and others that can induce significant transient changes in BP. However, these maneuvers are hard to implement in routine clinical practice, require patients' cooperation, cause discomfort, increase sympathetic activity or cannot be used in certain pathological conditions. Therefore, dCA should ideally be assessed from the spontaneous BP-CBFV fluctuations of subjects at rest (baseline). For this, it is usual to use a system identification method to capture the relationship between BP and CBFV, and manipulate a parameter or introduce changes in the inputs (i.e., BP) to obtain the response signal (i.e., CBFV), which can then be assess using, for example, the classic autoregulation index (ARI) [5]. Unfortunately, the signal-to-noise relationship in baseline signals has so far proved to be challenging for the adequate assessment of dCA.

The standard system identification method for evaluating dCA with baseline signals is transfer function analysis [6], whose potential has already been established, for example in Panerai et al. [7]. On the other hand, promising new methods that use nonlinear models of dCA have emerged [8, 9], but they have not been sufficiently compared with traditional BP maneuvers.

Materials and Methods

Subjects and Measurement

Twenty healthy subjects were recruited, aged between 21 and 41 years (27.6 ± 5.4), with no history of cardiovascular pathological conditions, hypertension, epilepsy, aneurysms or any other neurological disorder. The study was performed in the Biomedical Informatics Lab of the Departamento de Ingeniería Informática at the Universidad de Santiago de Chile. The study was approved by the university's ethics committee and all subjects gave written informed consent.

After a period of resting, 5-min-long beat-to-beat non-invasive baseline BP and CBFV signals were obtained using a Finometer MIDI Finapres, on the contra-lateral middle finger, and a DWL Doppler Box system with 2 MHz transducers, on the middle cerebral arteries respectively. Both signals were then recorded while the subjects were subjected to thigh cuff maneuvers (as in [10]) and sit-to-stand maneuvers (as in Sorond et al. [11], only the period moving from sitting to standing position was analyzed). Hereafter, these maneuvers for manipulating BP are referred to as the THC and the STAND methods respectively. Signals were directly recorded in a computer, via the analog/digital converter of the Doppler box, for off-line preprocessing that yielded mean BP and CBFV signals re-sampled at 5 Hz using spline interpolation.

Models were built from the baseline signals re-sampled at 2 Hz (see details below) and their step responses were obtained. dCA effectiveness was measured on the CBFV responses in all experimental conditions using classic ARI. In addition, we used a newer autoregulation index that does not make assumptions of linearity, as the classic ARI does [5], namely the model-free ARI (mfARI) [12]. Both indexes range between 0 (no autoregulation) and 9 (most effective autoregulation).

Modeling

Models were built using support vector regression (SVR) [13] with BP as input and CBFV as output. Input time delays were introduced to obtain finite impulse response (FIR) dynamic models. Specifically, we procured linear (LFIR) and nonlinear models (NFIR) using the usual linear kernel and radial basis function kernel respectively. The number of time delays and the model's hyper-parameters (v, C, and, in the case of NFIR, σ) were set empirically by grid search. Twofold cross-validation was applied to select the models with the best test correlations. A smoothed inverted BP step was introduced to each model and the resulting step response was evaluated by an algorithm on how physiologically plausible it looked and scored accordingly. The model with highest test correlation coefficient and highest plausibility score was chosen from each set of baseline signals.

Statistics

Data normality was confirmed using the Shapiro–Wilk statistic. Paired comparisons between LFIR and NFIR models were made using the Student's t test. Intra-subject variability of the four dCA assessment methods (THC, STAND, LFIR, and NFIR) were compared in terms of their standard deviation normalized as a percentage of the mean, that is, their unbiased coefficient of variation (CoV). A global comparison of the four methods and the two autoregulation indexes was obtained with a two-way repeated-measures ANOVA. Tukey's method was used for post-hoc analysis. In all tests, a value $p < 0.05$ was considered significant.

Results

Good baseline recordings were procured for 19 out of the 20 subjects, which allowed valid LFIR and NFIR models to be obtained. Mean ± SD values of the training parameters and goodness-of-fit are shown in Table 1. NFIR models achieved borderline-significantly higher test correlation coefficients ($p = 0.051$).

Figure 1 presents the ANOVA plot of means. No significant interaction was observed ($p = 0.080$[1]) and the factors were then analyzed individually, finding relevant differences between indexes ($p < 0.001$), but not between methods ($p = 0.084$[1]). Post-hoc analysis revealed that only a few combinations of method/index are dissimilar: THC/mfARI vs STAND/ARI, LFIR/ARI and NFIR/ARI ($p = 0.003$, $p = 0.036$, and $p < 0.001$ respectively) and STAND/mfARI vs STAND/ARI and NFIR/ARI ($p = 0.020$ and $p < 0.005$ respectively).

Mean ± SD values of both autoregulation index and CoV are detailed in Table 2. mfARI consistently exhibited the best

Table 1 Statistics for the training hyper-parameters and correlations of selected LFIR and NFIR models

Models	np	C	σ	v	Test CC
LFIR	10 [2–10]	28.5 ± 56.9	–	0.4 ± 0.3	0.67 ± 0.16
NFIR	10 [2–19]	3455.4 ± 4457.2	17.6 ± 13.8	0.5 ± 0.3	0.70 ± 0.13

Mode and range is reported for the number of input time delays (np). Mean ± SD for the other values

CC Pearson's correlation coefficient

---

[1] Corrected using the Greenhouse–Geisser procedure.

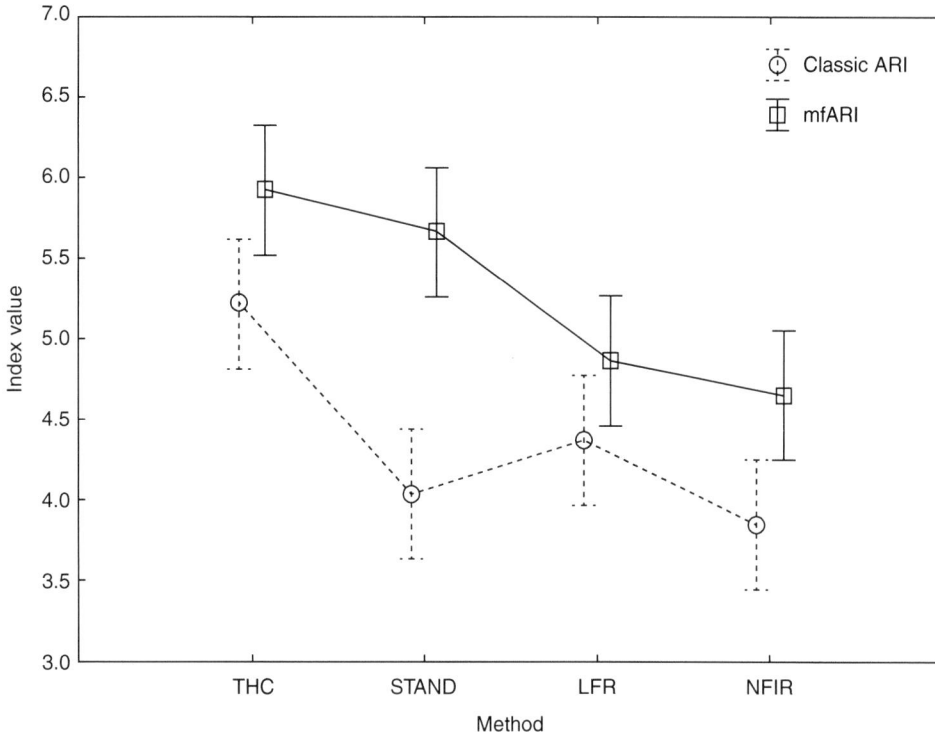

Fig. 1 Two-way ANOVA. Mean autoregulation index values for each method of assessing dynamic cerebral autoregulation (dCA; THC, STAND, LFIR, and NFIR) as measured with the classic ARI (*dashed line*) and mfARI (*solid line*)

Table 2 Autoregulation index mean ± SD values and coefficients of variation (CoV) for each combination of method–index

Autoregulation Index		Method			
		THC	STAND	FIR	NFIR
mfARI	Means ± SD	5.8 ± 1.4	5.7 ± 1.1	4.9 ± 1.5	4.7 ± 2.0
	CoV	23.73%	19.30%	30.61%	42.55%
ARI	Means ± SD	5.2 ± 1.4	4.0 ± 1.4	4.4 ± 2.2	3.8 ± 2.2
	CoV	26.92%	35.00%	50.00%	57.90%

intra-subject variability in every method. STAND/mfARI and NFIR/ARI are the combinations with the lowest and higher variations respectively.

Discussion

Models were successfully acquired with high correlation levels, of around 0.7, between the real CBFV signal and the models' output. It should be noted that multi-step-ahead prediction was applied in the evaluation; thus, the 2.5-min test signal was reproduced using exclusively the input BP signal.

The analysis of variance showed that significant differences were due to the autoregulation index utilized. mfARI achieved significantly higher values than the classic ARI in every method. High index values, on the upper half of the scale 0–9, were expected for the group of subjects studied, as none of them had neurological or cardiovascular problems, confirming the findings in Chacón et al. [12].

Considering measures with mfARI only, although models showed lower values, there was no significant difference between assessment methods ($p > 0.164$). Therefore, using mfARI, the efficiency of the dCA can be equivalently evaluated with signals from two of the most frequently used maneuvers to perturb BP or from spontaneous variations at rest, with the clear advantage of being simpler to perform and applicable to a wider range of patients.

mfARI also exhibited the least variability. Nonetheless, the BP maneuvers obtained lower CoV values than the models, indicating that even though mfARI improved the discriminatory ability of the models, the index could not completely eliminate the intra-subject variability of the latter.

Future studies are necessary. For instance, the age range should be broadened to include older subjects. Also, pathological cases should be considered, to investigate the performance of the proposed method–index pairs so as to recognize impaired dCA. Finally, a reliability study may be of great relevance, but this would require repeated measurements in both baseline and BP maneuver conditions [12].

Conclusion

We have shown that SVR models built from spontaneous BP-CBFV fluctuations of healthy subjects at rest can measure dCA efficiency in a way that is statistically equivalent to two of the most commonly used methods based on maneuvers to produce large BP perturbations. We believe that conducting a reproducibility analysis of the proposed methods is necessary.

Acknowledgements We would like to thank DICYT (project 061119CP) and VRIDEI at Universidad de Santiago de Chile, and the Department of Cardiovascular Sciences, University of Leicester.

Conflicts of interest statement We declare that we have no conflicts of interest.

References

1. Aaslid R, Lindegaard K, Sorteberg W, Nornes H. Cerebral autoregulation dynamics in humans. Stroke. 1989;20:45–52.
2. Hlatky R, Valadka A, Robertson C. Analysis of dynamic autoregulation assessed by the cuff deflation method. Neurocrit Care. 2006;4:127–32.
3. Lipsitz L, Mukai S, Hamner J, Gagnon M, Babikian V. Dynamic regulation of middle cerebral artery blood flow velocity in aging and hypertension. Stroke. 2000;31:1897–903.
4. Claassen J, Levine B, Zhang R. Dynamic cerebral autoregulation during repeated squat-stand maneuvers. J Appl Physiol. 2008;106:153–60.
5. Tiecks F, Lam A, Aaslid R, Newell D. Comparison of static and dynamic cerebral autoregulation measurements. Stroke. 1995;26:1014–9.
6. Claassen J, Meel-van den Abeelen A, Simpson D, Panerai R. Transfer function analysis of dynamic cerebral autoregulation: a white paper from the International Cerebral Autoregulation Research Network. J Cereb Blood Flow Metab. 2016;36:665–80.
7. Panerai R, White R, Markus H, Evans D. Grading of cerebral dynamic autoregulation from spontaneous fluctuations in arterial blood pressure. Stroke. 1998;29:2341–6.
8. Mitsis G, Poulin M, Robbins P, Marmarelis V. Nonlinear modeling of the dynamic effects of arterial pressure and CO_2 variations on cerebral blood flow in healthy humans. IEEE Trans Biomed Eng. 2004;51:1932–43.
9. Chacón M, Araya C, Panerai R. Non-linear multivariate modeling of cerebral hemodynamics with autoregressive support vector machines. Med Eng Phys. 2011;33:180–7.
10. Mahony P, Panerai R, Deverson S, Hayes P, Evans D. Assessment of the thigh cuff technique for measurement of dynamic cerebral autoregulation. Stroke. 2000;31:476–80.
11. Sorond F, Serrador J, Jones R, Shaffer M, Lipsitz L. The sit-to-stand technique for the measurement of dynamic cerebral autoregulation. Ultrasound Med Biol. 2009;35:21–9.
12. Chacón M, Jara J, Panerai R. A new model-free index of dynamic cerebral blood flow autoregulation. PLoS One. 2014;9:e108281.
13. Schölkopf B, Smola A, Williamson R, Bartlett P. New support vector algorithms. Neural Comput. 2000;12:1207–45.

ICP and Antihypertensive Drugs

Charlotte Rouzaud-Laborde, Pierre Lafitte, Laurent Balardy, Zofia Czosnyka, and Eric A. Schmidt

Abstract *Objectives*: Arterial hypertension is among the leading risks for mortality. This burden requires in hypertensive patients the use of single, double or more antihypertensive drugs. The relationship between intracranial pressure (ICP) and arterial blood pressure is complex and still under debate. The impact of antihypertensive drugs on ICP is unknown. We wanted to understand whether the use of antihypertensive drugs has a significant influence on ICP and cerebrospinal fluid (CSF)/brain related parameters.

Materials and methods: In a cohort of 95 patients with suspected normal pressure hydrocephalus, we prospectively collected drug details according to the Anatomical Therapeutic Chemical (ATC) classification. Lumbar infusion studies were performed. Using ICM+ software, we calculated at baseline and plateau ICP and pulse amplitude, resistance to CSF outflow, elastance, and pressure in the sagittal sinus and CSF production rate. We studied the influence of the administration of 1, 2, 3 or more antihypertensive drugs on ICP-derived parameters. We compared the data using Student's and Mann–Whitney tests or Chi-squared and Fisher's exact test.

Results: Elastance is significantly higher in patients with at least one antihypertensive drug compared with patients without medication. On the contrary, pressure volume index (PVI) is significantly decreased in patients with antihypertensive drugs compared with patients not on these medications. However, the number of antihypertensive drugs does not seem to influence other ICP parameters.

Conclusions: Patients on antihypertensive drugs seem to have a stiffer brain than those not on them.

Keywords Antihypertensive drugs · Hypertension · Elastance · PVI · PSS

Introduction

The interaction between intracranial pressure (ICP) and arterial blood pressure (ABP) is complex and still ill-understood. Hypertension, i.e., high ABP, has no symptoms, but if not treated it can damage the kidneys, heart, and brain, with an increased risk of renal failure, myocardial infarction, and stroke. In that respect, hypertension is among the leading risks for mortality. Hence, lowering ABP reduces the risk, in particular, of stroke. Hence, antihypertensive drugs must influence directly or indirectly not only brain biomechanical characteristics but also ICP.

This burden of hypertension requires the use of one, two or more antihypertensive drugs. These drugs are classified by the Anatomical Therapeutic Chemical (ATC) system. This is an international system [1] that defines a drug as part of different groups according to the organ or system on which they act and their therapeutic, pharmacological, and chemical properties. Drugs are classified in groups at five different levels. The drugs are divided into 14 main groups (the first level, which is an alphabetic letter), with pharmacological/therapeutic subgroups (second level). The third and fourth levels are used to identify pharmacological subgroups when that is considered more appropriate than therapeutic or chemical subgroups. Examples of the main groups: A alimentary tract and nutrition, B blood and blood forming organs, C cardiovascular system, D dermatologicals, etc.… With regard to antihypertensive drugs, the most

C. Rouzaud-Laborde (✉) · P. Lafitte
Department of Pharmacy, University Hospital Toulouse, Toulouse, France
e-mail: laborde.c@chu-toulouse.fr; charlotte.laborde@yahoo.fr

L. Balardy
Department of Geriatry, University Hospital Toulouse, Toulouse, France

Z. Czosnyka
Brain Physics Lab, Academic Neurosurgery, University of Cambridge, Cambridge, UK

E.A. Schmidt
Department of Neurosurgery, University Hospital Toulouse, Toulouse, France

common medications are angiotensin-converting enzyme (ATC C09A), angiotensin-2 receptor blockers (ATC C09C), calcium channel blockers (ATC C08), diuretics (ATC C03), and beta-blockers (ATC C07).

We hypothesize that the use of one or several antihypertensive drugs might influence ICP and brain biomechanical characteristics.

Materials and Methods

Study Population

Our analysis was carried out in a prospective cohort of 95 patients with suspected normal pressure hydrocephalus. We collected drug details according to the ATC classification. Thus, we classified patients according to the number of antihypertensive drugs they take to compare the potential effects of these treatments on ICP and brain characteristics.

Infusion Studies

Lumbar infusion studies were performed for every patient [2]. Using ICM+ software we analyzed nine parameters of cerebral hydrodynamics: baseline and plateau ICP, baseline and plateau of pulse amplitude, resistance to CSF outflow and an estimation of elastance, pressure volume index (PVI), pressure in the sagittal sinus (PSS), and CSF production rate.

Statistical Analysis

We studied the influence of antihypertensive drugs on the mean value of all nine parameters. For our statistical analysis, we made two comparisons. The first one was between patients with 0–2 antihypertensive drugs and patients with 3 or 4 antihypertensive drugs. The second one was between patients without treatment and patients with at least one antihypertensive drug. Quantitative values were compared using Student's test or Mann–Whitney test and qualitative values were compared using Chi-squared test or Fisher's exact test.

Results

Characteristics of the population are detailed in Table 1. Comparative overview shows that the two subpopulations have similar characteristics according to age, gender, and mean arterial blood pressure. Parameters of 84 patients with 0, 1 or 2 antihypertensive drugs were compared with param-

Table 1 Subpopulation characteristics

		0 to 2 AHT drugs	3 to 4 AHT drug	p	No AHT drug	At least 1 AHT drug	p
Average age (years)		74.45	75	0.75	74.52	74.5	0.99
Gender	Male	42	9	0.095	19	32	0.14
	Female	42	2		23	21	
Mean arterial blood pressure (mmHG)		114	108	0.18	112	114	0.55

AHT antihypertensive

Table 2 Antihypertensive (*AHT*) drug influence on intracranial pressure (*ICP*) parameters

	0 to 2 AHT drugs	3 to 4 AHT drugs	p value	No AHT drug	At least 1 AHT drug	p value
	Mean ± SEM			Mean ± SEM		
ICP baseline (mmHg)	10.35 ± 0.3	10.78 ± 1.2	0.65	10.19 ± 0.5	10.3 ± 0.5	0.81
ICP plateau (mmHg)	28.7 ± 0.8	31.9 ± 1.9	0.25	29.5 ± 1.2	28.1 ± 1.1	0.36
AMP basal (mmHg)	0.96 ± 0.05	0.8 ± 0.12	0.52	0.95 ± 0.08	0.93 ± 0.06	0.84
AMP plateau (mmHg)	4 ± 0.2	4.6 ± 0.6	0.37	4.2 ± 0.3	3.9 ± 0.2	0.49
Resistance to CSF (mmHg × min/mL)	17.5 ± 1.3	19.1 ± 3.5	0.44	18.4 ± 1.8	15.6 ± 1.5	0.25
Elastance (1/mL)	0.22 ± 0.02	0.27 ± 0.06	0.36	0.16 ± 0.01	0.26 ± 0.03	0.001
PVI (mL)	15.2 ± 0.8	13.2 ± 2.4	0.46	17.8 ± 0.9	13.24 ± 1	0.021
PSS (mmHg)	1.3 ± 0.9	4.3 ± 1.9	0.31	2.42 ± 1.5	4.3 ± 0.8	<0.0001
CSF production rate (mL/min)	0.77 ± 0.2	0.53 ± 0.22	0.14	1.1 ± 0.3	0.49 ± 0.07	0.054

AMP amplitude, *PVI* pressure volume index, *PSS* pressure in the sagittal sinus, *CSF* cerebrospinal fluid

eters of 11 patients with 3 or 4 antihypertensive drugs. The number of antihypertensive drugs does not seem to be associated with ICP parameters (Table 2, left panel).

However, the presence of at least one antihypertensive drug is significantly associated with an increased estimation of brain elastance compared with patients not taking antihypertensive drugs (0.16 ± 0.01 vs 0.26 ± 0.003, $p = 0.0017$). Unsurprisingly, the PVI parameter is significantly decreased in the same group (13.24 ± 1 vs 17.8 ± 0.9, $p = 0.021$).

The PSS is significantly increased in patients with at least one antihypertensive drug compared with those not taking antihypertensive drugs (2.42 ± 1.5 vs 4.3 ± 0.8, $p < 0.0001$ respectively).

Conclusion

Our study reveals that brain stiffness is associated with the use of antihypertensive drugs through elastance, PVI, and PSS markers. Arterial stiffness is emerging as an important risk marker for pathological brain aging and dementia through its associations with cerebral small vessel disease, stroke, β-amyloid deposition, brain atrophy, and cognitive impairment [3]. Indeed, arterial stiffness provides an important link between systemic hypertension and dementia, because it serves as the driving force behind the effects of hypertension on the microvasculature of the brain. Brain stiffness probably provides an indirect expression of arterial stiffness. One hypothesis could be that the use of antihypertensive drugs is probably an indirect marker of an altered microcirculation. Our data reinforce the concept that vascular diseases participate in brain alteration. We plan to further explore the influence of other drugs on ICP and CSF/brain biomechanics.

Conflicts of interest statement We declare that we have no conflicts of interest.

References

1. Word Health Organization. WHOCC – structure and principles. Collaboration Centre for Drug Statistics Methodology. 2011 [accessed 8 Nov 2016]. http://www.whocc.no/atc/structure_and_principles/.
2. Czosnyka M, Czosnyka Z, Momjian S, Pickard JD. Cerebrospinal fluid dynamics. Physiol Meas. 2004;25:R1–27. PII: S0967-3334(04)70217-8.
3. Hughes TM, Craft S, Lopez OL. Review of the potential role of arterial stiffness in the pathogenesis of Alzheimer's disease. Neurodegener Dis Manag. 2015;5(2):121–35.

ICP: From Correlation to Causation

Eric A. Schmidt, Olivier Maarek, Jérôme Despres, Manon Verdier, and Laurent Risser

Abstract Intracranial pressure (ICP) is a complex modality in the sense that it largely interconnects various systemic and intra-cranial variables such as cerebral blood flow and volume, cerebrospinal fluid flow and absoption, craniospinal container. In this context, although empirical correlation is an interesting tool for establishing relations between pairs of observed variables, it may be limited to establishing causation relations. For instance, if variables X and Y are mainly influenced by variable Z, their correlation is strong, but does not mean that X has a causation relation with Y or vice versa. In this work, we explore the use of the statistical concept of partial correlation to ICP and other derived measures to apprehend the interplay between correlation and causation.

Keywords ICP · Correlation · Causation · Complex data analysis

Introduction

Post hoc ergo propter hoc; after this, therefore because of this. This Latin sophism is a logical fallacy, often shortened to post hoc fallacy, that states "since event Y follows event X, event Y must be caused by event X."

Causation and correlation are two statistical concepts that are often mixed up, although they are fundamentally different.

Correlation quantifies how the observed (empirical) fluctuations of one variable X are related to the observed fluctuations of another variable Y in a group of patients, or more generally in a dataset. Two correlation measurements are often distinguished: Pearson's correlation, which measures whether the variables are linearly related, and Spearman's correlation, which measures whether the variables are similarly ranked (e.g., if an observation of X is one of the smallest in one patient, observation of Y is also one of the smallest in the same patient). In both cases, correlation directly quantifies the observed relations among paired variables in a dataset.

Causation is a more abstract concept meaning that variable X has a direct influence on variable Y. If variables X and Y present no or little correlation, they are unlikely to have a causation relation, at least in the experimental context of the dataset considered. If X and Y present a high correlation level (close to -1 or 1), they also do not necessarily present a causation relation for one main reason: both of them could be mainly influenced by another variable Z; thus, fluctuations of Y could not be influenced by variations of X, although they show strong correlation.

It is clear that such complex relations occur in intracranial pressure (ICP): various systemic and intracranial variables such as cerebral blood flow or volume, cerebrospinal fluid flow and absoption, craniospinal container are known to be interconnected. In this context, we explore the use of partial correlation for ICP data obtained in a group of 70 patients. Indeed, partial correlation makes it possible to remove the influence of a variable Z when computing the correlation between X and Y by considering linear relations between these variables. If more than three variables are observed in a dataset, which is the case for us, high partial correlations between X and Y by removing the influence of all other variables Z_i therefore appears to be an appealing tool for establishing causation relations.

E.A. Schmidt (✉)
Department of Neurosurgery, University Hospital, Toulouse, France

INSERM1214—ToNIC, Toulouse NeuroImaging Center, Toulouse, France
e-mail: schmidt.e@chu-toulouse.fr

O. Maarek · J. Despres
Department of Neurosurgery, University Hospital, Toulouse, France

M. Verdier · L. Risser
Institut de Mathématiques de Toulouse (UMR5219), Université de Toulouse; CNRS, UPS IMT, F-31062, Toulouse Cedex 9, France

Materials and Methods

Nine intracranial biomechanical variables have been measured prospectively in a group of 70 patients: ICP baseline, ICP plateau, pulse amplitude (AMP) baseline, AMP plateau, static, and dynamic resistance to CSF outflow (RCSF), estimation of CSF production rate, pressure in the sagittal sinus (PSS), and elastance.

Histograms of these different variables in the group of subjects under consideration clearly present heterogeneous distributions of values. This can be an issue when comparing the variables using Pearson-based correlations, which we will use in this work. Linear relations are indeed tested between the compared variables. To tackle this issue, we therefore consider the ranks of the different variables in our group of subjects instead of their raw values. The ranks of all variables are then distributed following a single uniform distribution and linear relations between the variables make more sense. Note that an alternative strategy would have been to project each variable distribution to a single uniform law by minimizing Wasserstein distances [1]. Ranks of the value (r) lead to more homogeneous distributions in practice and were therefore preferred.

Measures of correlation between two variables range from -1 to $+1$ inclusive, where $+1$ is total positive correlation, 0 is no correlation, and -1 is total negative correlation. For a sufficiently large number of subjects, which is reasonable here, the p values also indicate whether the correlations are significant. A classic threshold for the p values is 0.05. In the context of our work, we use partial correlation to measure extending Pearson's correlation. We use the ranks of our data and not their values. This allows to mimic Spearman's correlation, which we empirically verified on our data.

Pearson's partial correlation measures the strength of a linear relationship between two variables, X and Y, while removing the effect of another variable Z by assuming linear relations. If there is an influence of Z in X and Y, the following hypotheses are made:

$$X \approx X_{woZ} + \beta_1 Z$$
$$Y \approx Y_{woZ} + \beta_2 Z$$

where X_{woZ} and Y_{woZ} are X and Y without the influence of Z respectively. The scalars $\beta 1$ and $\beta 2$ are optimal coefficients for removing the influence of Z in X and Y. Partial correlation between X and Y relative to Z is then Pearson's correlation between $XwoZ$ and $YwoZ$. Mathematical details about how to compute X_{woZ}, Y_{woZ}, $\beta 1$ and $\beta 2$ can be found in references [1–3] and MATLAB, R or Python routines for this purpose can be easily found on the internet.

As mentioned earlier, we measured nine properties related to ICP in a group of 70 patients. When studying the relation between two of these variables, it appeared interesting to remove the influence of each of the remaining variables. Removing the influence of a variable can also make some correlation measures stronger, as the residuals only express the influence of these variables. Note that it is also technically possible to remove the influence of all remaining variables at once. However, we prefer to remove the influence of single variables to make explanations of the results straightforward and to limit fitness approximation issues (overfitting with too much of a parameter on complex data).

Results

Figure 1a displays Pearson's correlation coefficient among all nine variables. We display the r values only when statistically significant (i.e., p values < 0.05). Figure 1b displays Pearson's partial correlation after removal of the effect of baseline ICP, measuring the strength of a linear relationship between two variables X and Y, whereas the influence of baseline ICP has been ruled out. Figures 1c–e and 2a–e represent partial correlation after removal of the influence of ICP plateau, AMP baseline, AMP plateau, PSS, static, and dynamic RCSF, CSF production rate, and elastance respectively.

Removing the influence of baseline ICP (Fig. 1b) does not modify the correlation between ICP plateau and AMP plateau. It suggests that the link between ICP plateau and AMP plateau is mainly causal, or more precisely not indirectly due to the influence of baseline ICP. In addition removing the influence of baseline ICP reinforces the correlation between ICP plateau and AMP plateau with the resistance to CSF outflow. Hence, the ICP plateau and AMP plateau seem to be linked to resistance to CSF outflow mainly by a causal process rather than by a simple correlation.

Conclusions

We question, by the use of partial correlations, the relation of causation between variables that are classically used to study ICP. This has been made possible by homogenizing the distributions of different variables. This approach may be an interesting tool for removing the influence of different variables when studying the relation between two specific variables and clarify their link. A deeper insight into the correlation/causation relationship between variables should help physicians or scientists to improve their understanding of biological or physiological processes and ameliorate patients' care. *Post hoc sed non semper propter hoc* (after this, but not always because of this).

Conflicts of interest statement We declare that we have no conflicts of interest.

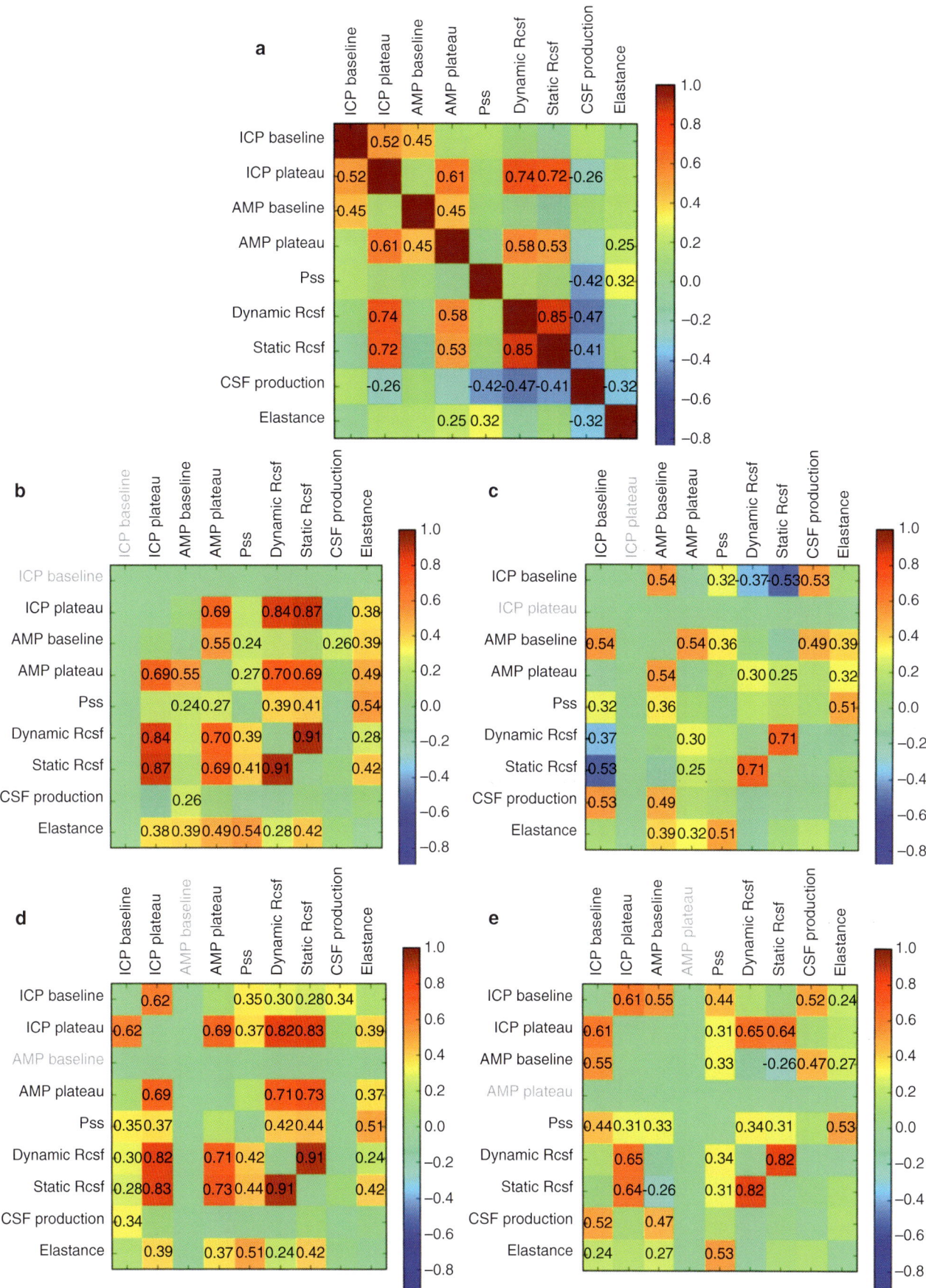

Fig. 1 Pearson correlation and partial correlations among the variables. The r values are displayed for p-values < 0.05. (**a**) Classic correlation. (**b–e**) Partial correlations after removing the effect of the ICP baseline, the ICP plateau, the AMP baseline, and the AMP plateau, respectively

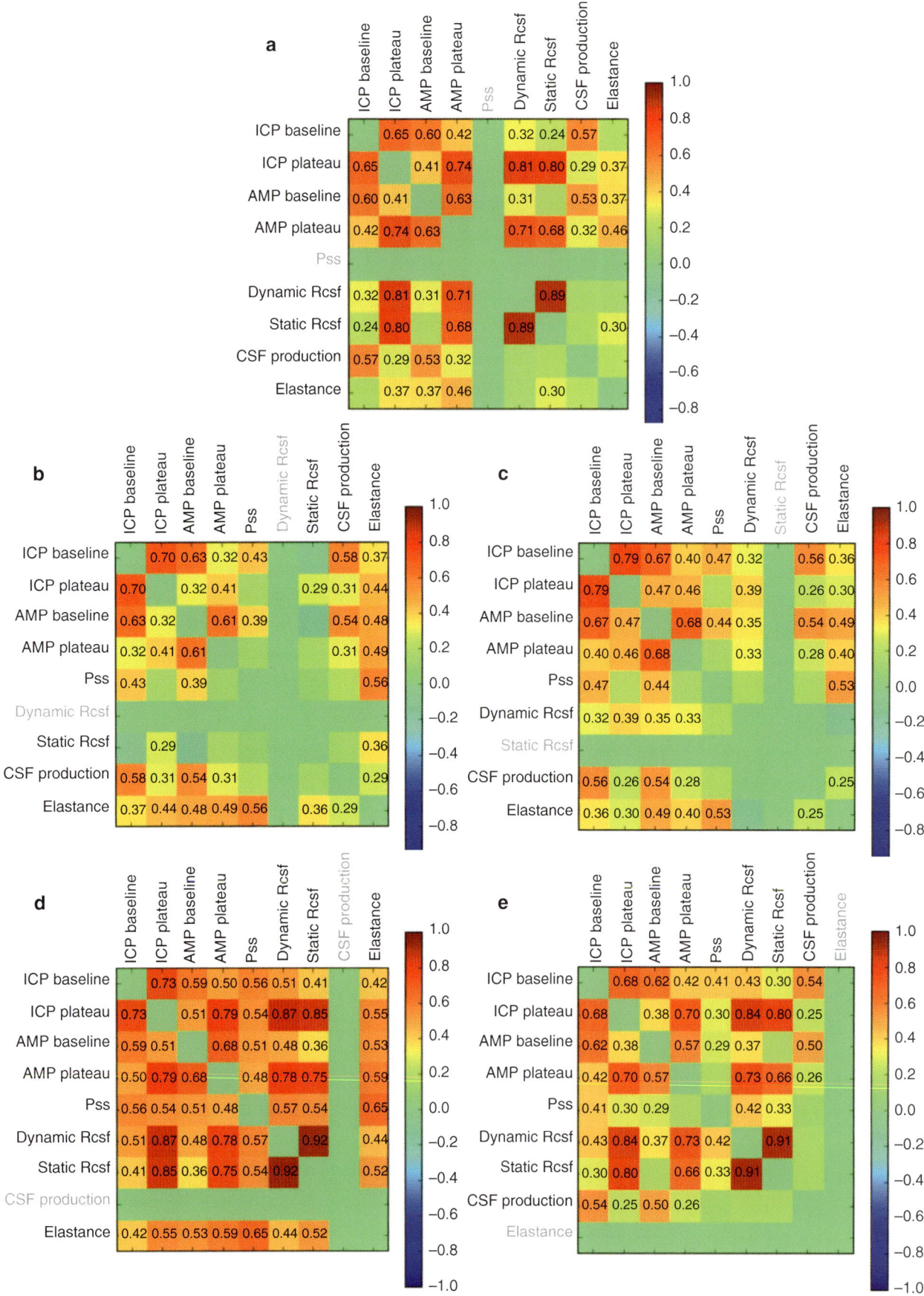

Fig. 2 Partial correlation among the variables. The *r* values are displayed for *p*-values < 0.05. (**a–e**) Partial correlations after removing the effect of the PSS, static and dynamic RCSF, CSF production rate, and elastance, respectively

References

1. Guilford JP, Fruchter B. Fundamental statistics in psychology and education. New York: McGraw-Hill; 1973.
2. Baba K, Shibata R, Masaaki Sibuya M. Partial correlation and conditional correlation as measures of conditional independence. Aust N Z J Stat. 2004;46(4):657–64.
3. Kendall MG, Stuart A. The advanced theory of statistics, volume 2. 3rd ed. Section 27.22. London: C. Griffin; 1973.

A Waveform Archiving System for the GE Solar 8000i Bedside Monitor

Andrea Fanelli, Rohan Jaishankar, Aristotelis Filippidis, James Holsapple, and Thomas Heldt

Abstract *Objectives*: Our objective was to develop, deploy, and test a data-acquisition system for the reliable and robust archiving of high-resolution physiological waveform data from a variety of bedside monitoring devices, including the GE Solar 8000i patient monitor, and for the logging of ancillary clinical and demographic information.

Materials and methods: The data-acquisition system consists of a computer-based archiving unit and a GE Tram Rac 4A that connects to the GE Solar 8000i monitor. Standard physiological front-end sensors connect directly to the Tram Rac, which serves as a port replicator for the GE monitor and provides access to these waveform signals through an analog data interface. Together with the GE monitoring data streams, we simultaneously collect the cerebral blood flow velocity envelope from a transcranial Doppler ultrasound system and a non-invasive arterial blood pressure waveform along a common time axis. All waveform signals are digitized and archived through a LabView-controlled interface that also allows for the logging of relevant meta-data such as clinical and patient demographic information.

Results: The acquisition system was certified for hospital use by the clinical engineering team at Boston Medical Center, Boston, MA, USA. Over a 12-month period, we collected 57 datasets from 11 neuro-ICU patients. The system provided reliable and failure-free waveform archiving. We measured an average temporal drift between waveforms from different monitoring devices of 1 ms every 66 min of recorded data.

Conclusions: The waveform acquisition system allows for robust real-time data acquisition, processing, and archiving of waveforms. The temporal drift between waveforms archived from different devices is entirely negligible, even for long-term recording.

Keywords Data acquisition · Intensive care · Data collection Waveform signals · Multi-modality monitoring

Introduction

Patients in neurocritical care tend to be heavily instrumented and their physiological state tracked very closely through a variety of bedside monitoring devices [1]. Such multimodality monitoring includes common signals such as the electrocardiogram (ECG), arterial blood pressure (ABP), central venous pressure (CVP), intracranial pressure (ICP), and arterial oxygen saturation (SpO_2). Additional instrumentation may include transcranial Doppler (TCD) ultrasound, near-infrared spectroscopy, or a variety of invasive sensors placed directly into the brain tissue to track local cerebral perfusion or metabolic markers.

Bedside monitors can typically acquire and display in real time such high-resolution data streams. However, most monitoring devices have limited capabilities for connecting to other bedside monitors. Additionally, they tend not to permanently archive the high-resolution waveform signals, although they may have a digital data interface that allows transmission of waveform and trend data in time-stamped data packets, often in proprietary data formats. In our experience, the time-stamping can be inaccurate and may lead to significant drift among waveforms archived from different devices, making accurate waveform archiving along a common time axis from digital data streams a challenging task. Such time-locked data archiving might best be achieved through the digitization of analog data streams.

In our work, we faced the need to archive high-resolution physiological waveforms from a variety of beside devices, including the GE Solar 8000i bedside patient monitor.

A. Fanelli, Ph.D. · R. Jaishankar, S.M. · T. Heldt, Ph.D. (✉)
Institute for Medical Engineering and Sciences, Massachusetts Institute of Technology, Cambridge, MA, USA
e-mail: thomas@mit.edu

A. Filippidis, M.D. · J. Holsapple, M.D.
Department of Neurosurgery, Boston University School of Medicine and Boston Medical Center, Boston, MA, USA

This bedside monitor does not have an analog interface for waveform archiving. Similarly, commercially available third-party solutions for real-time integrated monitoring and data archiving, such as the Moberg Component Neuromonitoring System [2] or the ICM+ software package [3], do not provide interfaces for archiving high-resolution waveforms from the GE Solar 8000i monitor. The lack of a readily available and robust archiving solution motivated the design, implementation, and deployment of our own data-acquisition system. Along with the physiological waveform data streams, the system also allows for the logging of important meta-data, such as clinical and patient demographic information.

Methods

The system (Fig. 1) consists of a GE Tram Rac 4A unit [4], connected to a standard GE Solar 8000i monitor, and a Windows-based computer (Intel® Core™2 Duo E7600, 3.06 GHz, 4 GB DDR3 SDRAM) for data archiving and control of the acquisition process. The Tram Rac serves as a port replicator for the GE monitor's patient data module (PDM). It can accommodate up to 13 front-end sensors and provides access to the associated signals through an analog data interface. In addition to the GE monitoring data streams, we needed to collect the cerebral blood flow velocity (CBFV) envelope from transcranial Doppler ultrasound (DWL Doppler-BoxX) and the ABP waveform from the BMEYE Nexfin monitor. Both devices provide analog output streams of the desired waveform signals. All analog waveforms are fed to an analog-to-digital converter (DAQ 6218, National Instruments) and are sampled at 250 samples/s at 16-bit amplitude resolution.

Data acquisition, visualization, and analysis are controlled by a custom-designed LabView interface that also allows for time-stamped logging of important patient, clinical, and study information. To interpret the waveform signals in the proper clinical context, we register:

1. Patient demographic information (age, gender, race, ethnicity).
2. Clinical information (diagnosis, type and site of injury, Glasgow Coma Scale score, hematocrit, medication information).
3. Study information (date and time of recordings, medical record number, study ID).
4. Important study meta-data (vertical height of pressure transducers to account for hydrostatic pressure differences; type and placement of ICP probes and other sensors; volume of CSF drained over study duration; state of ventricular drain (open or closed); and free text notes for time-stamped archiving of observations during the study period).

The entire acquisition system has been assembled on a small-footprint Ergotron medical cart [5] for space-saving and agile movement inside a potentially crowded ICU. The computer, TCD system, and Nexfin monitor are powered through a cart-based Tripp-Lite IS500HG isolation transformer [6] that guarantees patient isolation and protection from macroshock hazards [7].

For each recording session, the design outlined above requires the sensor cables to be disconnected from the GE PDM and then connected to the Tram-Rac 4A. A consequence of this step is that pressure signals need to be zeroed after disconnection/reconnection. This is an advantage for our purposes, as it ensures that all pressure sensors are properly zeroed at the beginning of each recording session. At the end of each session, the sensor cables are reconnected to the PDM and the pressure signals need to be zeroed again. Each reconnection takes approximately 30 s, during which the patient is disconnected from the bedside monitor.

All patient data are archived on an encrypted hard drive. The LabView software is configured to automatically duplicate data by creating both an identifiable and de-identified version of the recorded data, and the two copies are automatically organized in separate directory trees that reduce the risk for accidental access to and copying of protected health information. This approach also eliminates the need for *post hoc* de-identification of the archived data records. All waveform data are saved in ASCII and in the open-source waveform database format [8].

Results

The acquisition system was certified for hospital use by the Clinical Engineering team at Boston Medical Center, Boston, MA, USA. Over the course of one year, we successfully collected data from eleven patients, for a total of 57 distinct studies. The population so far includes five TBI patients, two patients affected by brain tumors, three by hydrocephalus, and one by subarachnoid hemorrhage. The average acquisition time is approximately 30 min per recording session.

Data acquisition has proceeded smoothly and without any complications. The system design proved to be sufficiently compact and agile for the cart to be maneuvered even in the most crowded and smallest of ICU bays. Even though our system requires sensor disconnection/reconnection and temporary interruption of patient monitoring, our study staff were able to execute these steps quickly and efficiently after minimal training. As our acquisition strategy relies on digitizing analog signal streams, the system performs well in aligning the input data along a common time axis (Fig. 2), with waveforms archived from different monitoring devices drifting by less than 1 ms, on average, over a period of 66 min.

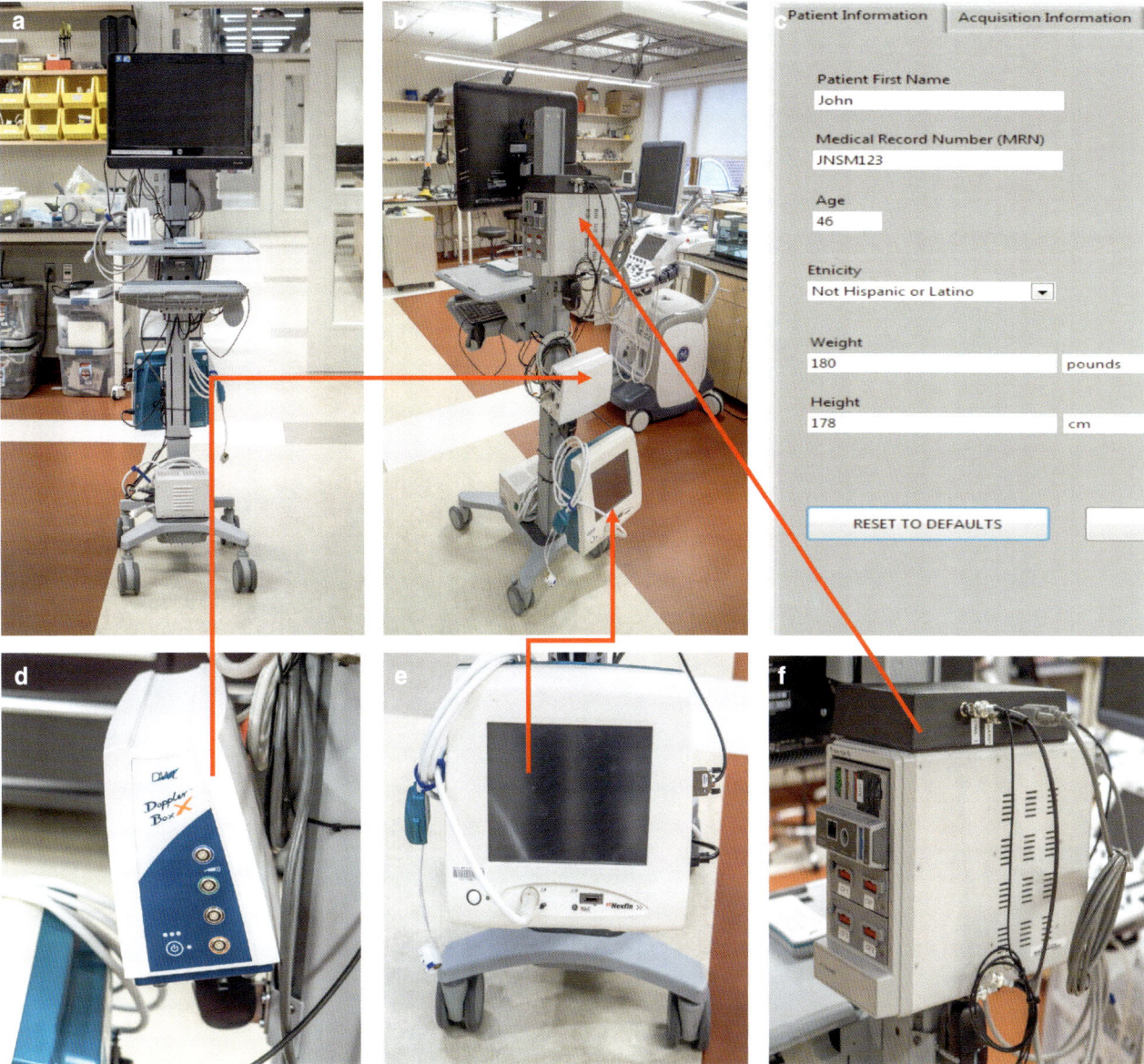

Fig. 1 System for collecting and archiving waveform data from GE Solar 8000i monitors. The figure shows (**a**) the front and (**b**) the back view of the acquisition system. (**c**) A LabView-based graphical user interface is used to archive patient information and for data analysis and visualization. (**d**) The DWL Doppler-BoxX is used to record the cerebral blood flow velocity from the patient. (**e**) The BMEYE Nexfin device is used for non-invasive arterial blood pressure (ABP) measurement. (**f**) A Tram Rac 4A replicates the GE monitor's patient data module and is connected to the electrocardiogram, ABP, central venous pressure, intracranial pressure, and arterial oxygen saturation sensors. (**f**) The *black box* contains the NI DAQ 6218, which collects and digitizes all waveforms, including the analog outputs of the DWL and Nexfin devices

Discussion

The data-acquisition and archiving system we developed allows for robust archiving of multimodality waveform data from the GE Solar 8000i bedside monitors. It has been used successfully to collect ABP, ECG, ICP, SpO_2, and CVP waveform signals from the GE 8000i series of bedside monitors, together with non-invasive ABP and the CBFV envelope waveform. Data collection has been successfully completed for eleven patients and 57 studies over the course of one year.

In the design of the system, we took into consideration a list of important prerequisites. Chiefly, we sought to ensure that the waveform data are archived with minimal temporal drift between signals from different bedside devices. This requirement led us to connect to the analog interfaces of our monitoring devices. The measured drift over time between archived waveform signals is entirely negligible, even for long-duration recordings, and therefore overcomes an

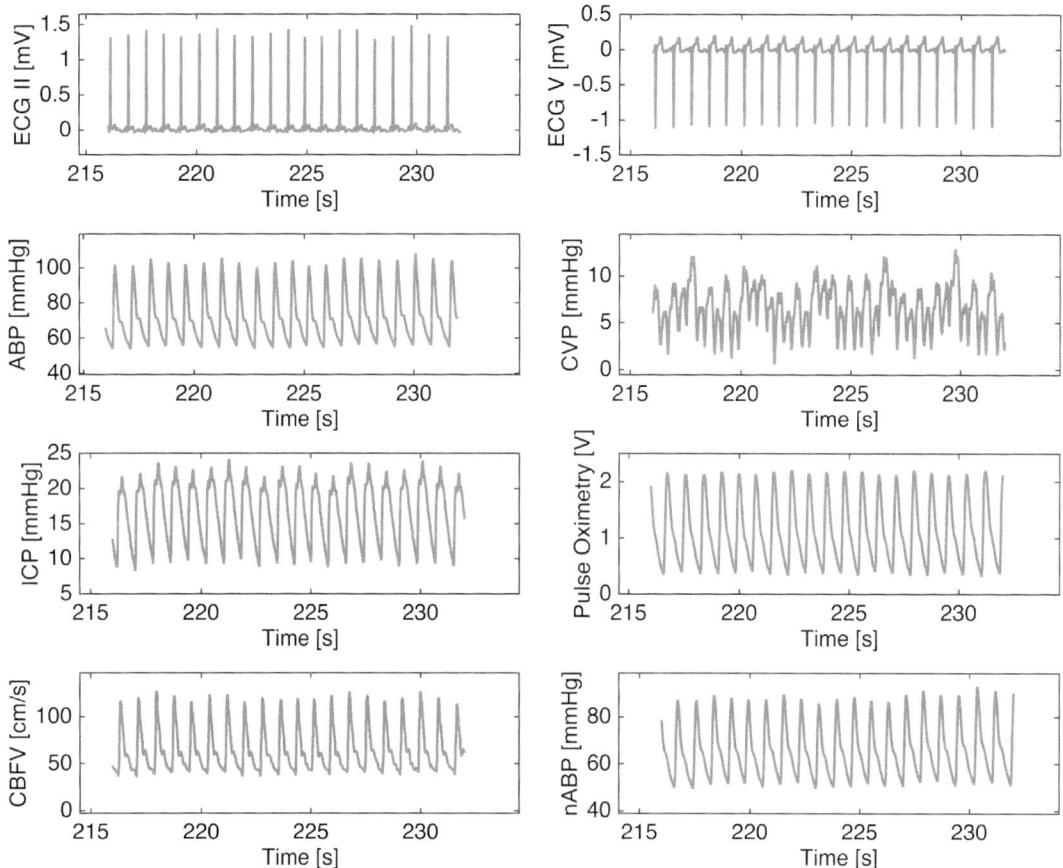

Fig. 2 Time-aligned ICU data collected with the data-acquisition system. Waveforms are noise-free and time-aligned. There is neglibible time drift between waveforms over the acquisition time

important limitation of digital data archiving from different bedside monitoring systems.

The system often needs to be used in space-limited ICUs. For this reason, it was designed to have a small footprint so that it can be easily transported into the narrow spaces of ICU rooms and to guarantee care providers access to both sides of the bed at all times in case of emergencies. Additionally, as the window for data acquisition sessions is often short and has to be coordinated around the clinical care of the patient, the set-up time has to be short and the user interface intuitive. Our clinical team has been trained so that the overall time spent at the bedside for each study is about 45 min, which allows us to collect approximately 30 min of stable waveform data.

Our system design has several limitations. The first is that it requires the sensors to be disconnected from the GE PDM and connected to the Tram Rac 4A before data collection can commence, and the sensor cables to be reconnected to the GE PDM at the end of each recording session. Each disconnection/reconnection takes approximately 30 s during which the patient is not monitored. The need for the re-routing of the sensor cables may limit the system to the collection of data from patients who are sufficiently stable. The second consequence of re-routing the sensor cables is the need to calibrate the pressure signals after each disconnect cycle. In our study, a care provider—either a member of the study staff or clinical team—is present at the bedside to perform the zeroing steps.

Conclusions

The waveform acquisition system we developed allows real-time data acquisition, processing, and archiving of waveforms from neurocritical care patients in ICUs employing the GE Solar 8000i series bedside monitors. The system was successfully deployed and has allowed us to collect data from eleven patients over twelve months, providing reliable and robust data collection from a variety of bedside monitoring devices.

Acknowledgements We would like to thank National Instruments for a donation of equipment under their campus donation program.

Conflicts of interest statement We declare that we have no conflicts of interest.

References

1. Mulvey JM, Dorsch NWC, Mudaliar Y, Lang EW. Multimodality monitoring in severe traumatic brain injury. Neurocritical Care. 2004;1(3):391–402.
2. CNS Monitor. Moberg ICU solutions. https://www.moberg.com/products/cns-monitor. Accessed on 7 March 2017.
3. ICM+. Brain monitoring software. Division of Neurosurgery, Department of Clinical Neurosciences, University of Cambridge. http://www.neurosurg.cam.ac.uk/pages/ICM/index.php. Accessed on 7 March 2017.
4. Tram-rac® 4A. Housing service manual. GE Medical Systems Information Technologies; 2007.
5. Ergotron. http://www.ergotron.com/en-us/. Accessed on 7 March 2017.
6. Goldberger AL, Amaral LAN, Glass L, Hausdorff JM, Ivanov PC, Mark RG, Mietus JE, Moody GB, Peng C-K, Stanley HE. PhysioBank, PhysioToolkit, and PhysioNet: components of a new research resource for complex physiologic signals. Circulation. 2000;101(23):e215–20.
7. Tripp-Lite. https://www.tripplite.com/. Accessed on 7 March 2017.
8. Webster JG. Medical instrumentation-application and design. Journal of Clinical Engineering. 1978;3(3):306.

Deriving the PRx and CPPopt from 0.2-Hz Data: Establishing Generalizability to Bedmaster Users

Murad Megjhani, Kalijah Terilli, Andrew Martin, Angela Velazquez, Jan Claassen, David Roh, Sachin Agarwal, Peter Smielewski, Amelia K. Boehme, J. Michael Schmidt, and Soojin Park

Abstract *Objective*: The objective was to explore the validity of industry-parameterized vital signs in the generation of pressure reactivity index (PRx) and optimal cerebral perfusion pressure (CPPopt) values.

Materials and methods: Ten patients with intracranial pressure (ICP) monitors from 2008 to 2013 in a tertiary care hospital were included. Arterial blood pressure (ABP) and ICP were sampled at 240 Hz (of waveform data) and 0.2 Hz (of parameterized data produced by heuristic industry proprietary algorithms). 240-Hz ABP were filtered for pulse pressure and diastolic ABP within the limits of 20–150 mmHg. The PRx was calculated as Pearson's correlation coefficient using 10-s averages of ICP and ABP over a 5-min moving window with 80% overlap. For ease of comparison, we used the naming convention of BMx for PRx values derived from 0.2-Hz data. A 5-min median cerebral perfusion pressure (CPP) trend was calculated, PRx or BMx values divided and averaged into CPP bins spanning 5 mmHg. The minimum Y value (PRx or BMx) of the parabolic function fit to the resulting XY plot of 4 h of data was obtained, and updated every 1 min. Pearson's R correlations were calculated for each patient. Linear mixed-effects models were used with a random intercept to assess the overall correlation between the PRx (outcome) and the BMx (fixed effect) or the CPPopt-PRx (outcome) and the CPPopt-BMx (fixed effect).

Results: The overall correlation between the PRx and BMx was 0.78 based on the linear mixed effects models ($p < 0.0001$), and the overall correlation for the CPPopt–PRx and CPPopt–BMx based on the linear mixed effects models

M. Megjhani • K. Terilli • A. Martin • A. Velazquez
J. Claassen • D. Roh • S. Agarwal • A.K. Boehme
J. Michael Schmidt • S. Park (✉)
Department of Neurology, Columbia University,
New York, NY, USA
e-mail: spark@columbia.edu

P. Smielewski
Department of Clinical Neurosciences, University of Cambridge,
Cambridge, UK

was 0.76 ($p < 0.0001$). One patient had low correlation of CPPopts derived from the PRx vs the BMx; this patient had the least number of hours of CPPopt data to compare.

Conclusions: The BMx shows promise in CPPopt derivation against the validated PRx measure. If further developed, it could expand the capability of centers to derive CPPopt goals for use in clinical trials.

Keywords Vasoreactivity index · Optimal CPP · Informatics Subarachnoid hemorrhage · Artifact filter

Introduction

Individualized targets for cerebral perfusion pressure (CPP) based on the pressure reactivity index (PRx) have been proposed since 2002 [1]. The PRx is a moving correlation coefficient between slow waves of intracranial pressure (ICP) and arterial blood pressure (ABP) to the order of 20–300 s [2]. In its original description and subsequent feasibility and validation studies, the PRx has been calculated as the moving correlation coefficient between consecutive 5- to 10-s averages of ICP and ABP (windows spanning 4–5.3 min) based on signal capture at a frequency of at least 30 Hz [1–6]. Plotting the PRx against CPP produces a U-shaped curve in 60% of patients, enabling CPPopt [1].

The PRx reflects illness severity in acute brain injury [2], and potentially provides targets for goal-directed therapy [1, 7]. Studies exploring their role in prospective management are warranted. A limiting step to widespread patient enrollment and eventual usability is high-frequency waveform data acquisition, storage, and manipulation. Meanwhile, intensive care unit-wide data solutions such as Bedmaster (BedmasterEX; Excel Medical Electronics, Jupiter, FL, USA) are propagating, along with the ability to more easily store and access parameterized low frequency 0.2-Hz (5 s) data. Although Bedmaster does collect high-frequency waveform data, they are stored in a binary format, which is unwieldy for transforming and processing at the bedside.

The impact of industry (e.g., General Electric) artifact filters and lower frequency sampling on the PRx and CPPopt is unknown. This study compares PRx and CPPopt derived from waveform and parameter data.

Materials and Methods

Study Population and Data Collection

Twenty-three patients admitted from June 2008 to January 2013 to a tertiary care hospital's neurointensive care unit with ICP and arterial blood pressure (ABP) monitors were prospectively enrolled in an observational cohort study of subarachnoid hemorrhage. The study was approved by the Columbia University Medical Center Institutional Review Board. ICP was monitored with a probe (Camino System, Integra Neurosciences) inserted into the frontal cortex. ABP was monitored through the radial artery using a pressure monitoring kit (Transpac IV Monitoring Kit; ICU Medical, San Clemente, CA USA), zeroed at the level of the phlebostatic axis. Digitized data were acquired utilizing Solar 8000i patient monitors on a General Electric (GE) Medical Systems Information Technologies' Unity Network (Port Washington, NY, USA). A high-resolution data acquisition and storage system (BedmasterEX; Excel Medical Electronics, Jupiter, FL, USA) using an open architecture of the Unity Network automatically acquired vital sign parameters and waveform data from GE monitors. Waveform data were stored at a resolution of 240 Hz in binary files. Parameter data were acquired every 5 s and recorded in an SQL database.

Notably, the 0.2-Hz (5 s) data are sampled from the nonwaveform values that are generated by and displayed on the GE patient monitors. These parameters are the result of a software package called EK-PRO project (http://clinicalview.gehealthcare.com/; Voith, PR, inventor; GE Medical Systems Information Technologies, assignee. US patent 6,731,973, 5/4/2004) that evolved over more than a decade to produce user-friendly monitors that eliminate clinically nonsignificant data that can result from simpler algorithms. The heuristic algorithm provides a representative clinical number, defending against outliers and influence from arrhythmias. There is hysteresis on the number to reduce flicker, and thus would be expected to have some time delay. The 0.2-Hz data acquired and stored in BedmasterEX is not synchronized when the number changes on the patient monitor, but is rather a view of what is displayed on the patient monitor at the moment of sampling.

Data Preprocessing

Data preprocessing was performed using ICM Plus software (University of Cambridge, Cambridge Enterprise, Cambridge, UK, http://www.neurosurg.cam.ac.uk/icmplus) [8]. 240 or 125 Hz sampled ABP were filtered for pulse pressure and diastolic ABP within the limits of 20–150 mmHg. No additional artifact filtering was performed beyond the industry black box heuristic algorithms on the 0.2-Hz sampled data. The PRx was calculated as Pearson's correlation coefficient using 10-s averages of ICP and ABP over a 5 min moving window with 80% overlap. For ease of comparison, we used the naming convention of BMx for the PRx values derived from 0.2-Hz data. A 5-min median cerebral perfusion pressure (CPP) trend was calculated, and the PRx or BMx values divided and averaged into CPP bins spanning 5 mm Hg. The minimum Y value (PRx or BMx) of the parabolic function fit to the resulting XY plot of 4 h of data was obtained, and updated every 1 min. (See Fig. 1 for an example of a calculation of BMx and CPPopt–BMx).

Statistical Analysis

Statistical analysis was performed using MATLAB (MATLAB and Statistics Toolbox Release 2015a; The Mathworks, Natick, MA, USA) and RStudio (RStudio Team 2015. RStudio: Integrated Development for R. RStudio, Boston, MA, USA; URL http://www.rstudio.com/). Pearson's R correlations for PRx to BMx, and the corresponding CPPopts were calculated for each patient. Linear mixed effects models with a random intercept were used to assess the overall correlation between the PRx (outcome) and the BMx (fixed effect) or the CPPopt–PRx (outcome) and the CPPopt–BMx (fixed effect), accounting for multiple measurements within each individual. p values <0.05 were considered statistically significant.

Results

Of the 23 patients, 13 were excluded because the duration of their recordings resulted in BMx or PRx calculations shorter than 4 consecutive hours, making CPPopt calculation unrealistic. Data were used from 10 patients, including 6 women, ranging in age from 47 to 73 years (median age, 59.5 years). The overall correlation between the PRx and BMx was 0.78 based on the linear mixed effects models ($p < 0.0001$), and the overall correlation for CPPOpt–PRx and CPPOpt–BMx based on the linear mixed effects models was 0.76 ($p < 0.0001$; Fig. 2). Patient 9 had low Pearson's R correlation of CPPopts derived from the PRx vs

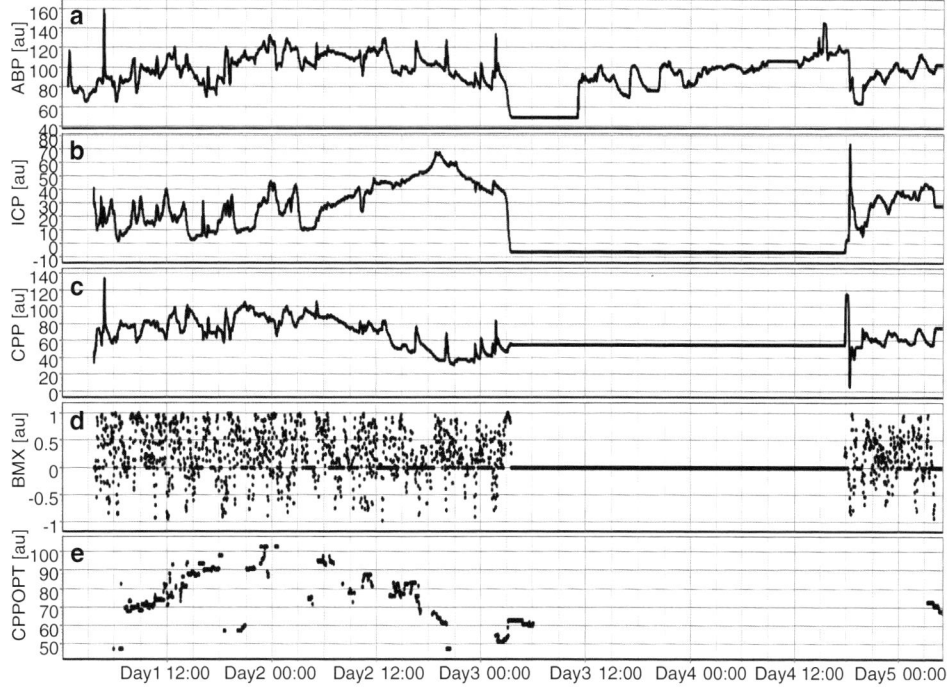

Fig. 1 Example of a calculation of the BMx and CPPopt (BMx-based). (**a**) Arterial blood pressure (ABP), (**b**) intracranial pressure (ICP), (**c**) cerebral perfusion pressure (CPP), (**d**) pressure reactivity Index derived using 0.2-Hz data (BMx), (**e**) optimal cerebral perfusion pressure (CPPopt)

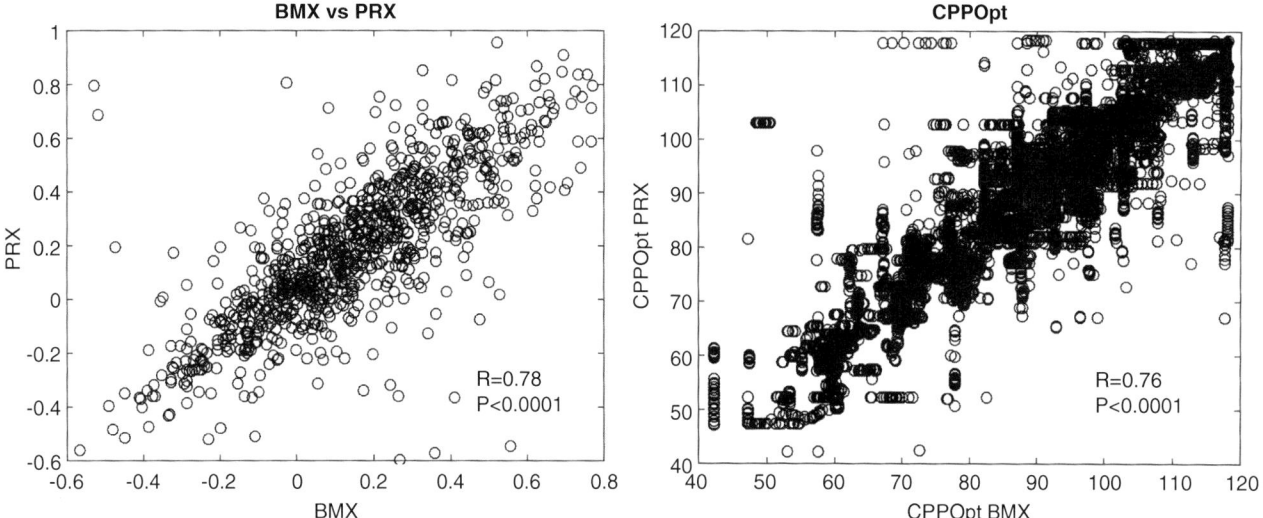

Fig. 2 Scatterplot of BMx vs PRx and CPPopt–BMx vs CPPopt–PRx

BMx; this patient had the least number of hours of CPPopt data (4 h) to compare (see Table 1 for detailed results).

Discussion

There is a growing interest in exploring the role of the PRx and CPPopt in the prospective management of acute brain injury. This effort is likely be meaningful only with the collaboration of multiple centers. A limiting step to such a project is the ability to acquire, store, and manipulate high-frequency waveform data. As centralized data acquisition systems enlarge their market share, it is useful to consider whether the PRx and CPPopt can be derived from opaquely derived parameters of industry patient monitors.

The BMx is derived from lower frequency parameters that have already been filtered for physiologically artifactual data (primarily arrhythmia-driven). The PRx is derived from

Table 1 Patient characteristics and Pearson's R correlation values

Patient	Hours of data	Age	Gender	MFS	HH	12-month mRS	PRx–BMx correlation, R (h)	CPPopt correlation, R (h)
1	52	60	Male	3	5	6	0.66 (47)	0.77 (17)
2	408	48	Female	3	2	3	0.54 (145)	0.66 (58)
3	456	73	Female	3	5	5	0.89 (16)	0.9 (9)
4	192	59	Male	4	5	6	0.69 (56)	0.67 (6)
5	72	57	Male	4	5	6	0.44 (55)	0.73 (23)
6	144	83	Female	3	4	5	0.88 (27)	0.76 (16)
7	192	72	Female	4	5	6	0.56 (152)	0.81 (57)
8	744	47	Male	3	5	5	0.81 (201)	0.78 (47)
9	312	71	Female	3	2	5	0.81 (7)	**0.18 (4)**
10	504	52	Female	4	5	5	0.53 (161)	0.8 (36)

MFS modified Fisher Scale, *HH* Hunt Hess Grade, *mRS* modified Rankin Scale, *PRx* pressure reactivity index derived from 240-Hz data, *BMx* pressure reactivity index derived from 0.2-Hz data, *CPPopt* optimal CPP

higher frequency waveforms that are post-processed for mechanical artifactual data. In our study of GE Solar 8000i-derived data, the PRx and BMx showed good correlation. CPPopt was calculated from 4 h of data, and these values also showed good correlation.

Determining the percentage of time that BMx and PRx and their respective CPPoptvs were able to be calculated was outside the scope of this project, given the complexities of data handling. This may warrant further analysis, as hypothetically, the BMx (and therefore the CPPopt–BMx) would be more frequently calculable.

One patient showed poor Pearson's R correlation for CPPopt derived from the PRx and BMx (patient 9). Incidentally, this patient only had 4 h of CPPopts to compare, the lowest of the batch. Additional examination with more patients would be needed to determine the factors that account for this mismatch.

Conclusions

The BMx shows promise against the validated PRx measure in the derivation of the CPPopt. If further developed, it could expand the capability of centers to measure pressure reactivity in the derivation of optimal CPP goals for use in clinical trials.

Acknowledgements SP is supported by grant funding NIH K01 ES026833.

Disclosures: None.

Conflicts of interest statement We declare that we have no conflicts of interest.

References

1. Steiner LA, Czosnyka M, Piechnik SK, Smielewski P, Chatfield D, Menon DK, et al. Continuous monitoring of cerebrovascular pressure reactivity allows determination of optimal cerebral perfusion pressure in patients with traumatic brain injury. Crit Care Med. 2002;30(4):733–8.
2. Czosnyka M, Smielewski P, Kirkpatrick P, Laing RJ, Menon D, Pickard JD. Continuous assessment of the cerebral vasomotor reactivity in head injury. Neurosurgery. 1997;41(1):11–7. discussion 7–9
3. Steiner LA, Coles JP, Johnston AJ, Chatfield DA, Smielewski P, Fryer TD, et al. Assessment of cerebrovascular autoregulation in head-injured patients: a validation study. Stroke. 2003;34(10):2404–9.
4. Zweifel C, Lavinio A, Steiner LA, Radolovich D, Smielewski P, Timofeev I, et al. Continuous monitoring of cerebrovascular pressure reactivity in patients with head injury. Neurosurg Focus. 2008;25(4):E2.
5. Consonni F, Abate MG, Galli D, Citerio G. Feasibility of a continuous computerized monitoring of cerebral autoregulation in neurointensive care. Neurocrit Care. 2009;10(2):232–40.
6. Brady KM, Shaffner DH, Lee JK, Easley RB, Smielewski P, Czosnyka M, et al. Continuous monitoring of cerebrovascular pressure reactivity after traumatic brain injury in children. Pediatrics. 2009;124(6):e1205–12.
7. Aries MJ, Czosnyka M, Budohoski KP, Steiner LA, Lavinio A, Kolias AG, et al. Continuous determination of optimal cerebral perfusion pressure in traumatic brain injury. Crit Care Med. 2012;40(8):2456–63.
8. Smielewski P, Czosnyka M, Zabolotny W, Kirkpatrick P, Richards H, Pickard JD. A computing system for the clinical and experimental investigation of cerebrovascular reactivity. Int J Clin Monit Comput. 1997;14(3):185–98.

Medical Waveform Format Encoding Rules Representation of Neurointensive Care Waveform Data

Ian Piper, Martin Shaw, Christopher Hawthorne, John Kinsella, and Laura Moss

Abstract *Objective*: Technology in neurointensive care units can collect and store vast amounts of complex patient data. The CHART-ADAPT project is aimed at developing technology that will allow for the collection, analysis and use of these big data at the patient's bedside in neurointensive care units. A requirement of this project is to automatically extract and transfer high-frequency waveform data (e.g. ICP) from monitoring equipment to high performance computing infrastructure for analysis. Currently, no agreed data standard exists in neurointensive care for the description of this type of data. In this pilot study, we investigated the use of Medical Waveform Format Encoding Rules (MFER—www.mfer.org-ISO 11073-92001) as a possible data standard for neurointensive care waveform data.

Materials and methods: Several waveform formats were explored (e.g. XML, DICOM waveform) and evaluated for suitability given existing computing infrastructure constraints, e.g. NHS network capacity and the processing capabilities of existing integration software.

Key requirements of the format included a compact data size and the use of a recognised standard. The MFER waveform format (ISO/TS 11073-92001) met both requirements. To evaluate the practicality of the MFER waveform format, seven waveform signals (ICP, ECG, ART, CVP, EtCO2, Pleth, Resp) collected over a period of 8 h from a patient at the Institute of Neurological Sciences in Glasgow were converted into MFER waveform format.

Results: The MFER waveform format has two main components: sampling information and frame information. Sampling information describes the frequency of the data sampling and the resolution of the data. Frame information describes the data itself; it consists of three elements: data block (the actual data), channel (each type of waveform data occupies a channel) and sequence (the repetition of the data). All seven waveform signals were automatically and successfully converted into the MFER waveform format. One MFER file was created for each minute of data (total of 479 files, 181 KB each).

Conclusions: The MFER waveform format has potential as a lightweight standard for representing high-frequency neurointensive care waveform data. Further work will include a comparison with other waveform data formats and a live trial of using the MFER waveform format to stream patient data over a longer period.

Keywords Medical waveforms · Standards · Neurointensive care

I. Piper (✉) · M. Shaw
Department of Clinical Physics and Bioengineering, Institute of Neurological Sciences, NHS Greater Glasgow and Clyde, Queen Elizabeth University Hospital, Glasgow, UK
e-mail: ian.piper@brainit.org

C. Hawthorne
Department of Neuroanaesthesia, Institute of Neurological Sciences, NHS Greater Glasgow and Clyde, Queen Elizabeth University Hospital, Glasgow, UK

J. Kinsella
Department of Anaesthesia, Pain and Critical Care, University of Glasgow, Glasgow, UK

L. Moss
Department of Clinical Physics and Bioengineering, Institute of Neurological Sciences, NHS Greater Glasgow and Clyde, Queen Elizabeth University Hospital, Glasgow, UK

Department of Anaesthesia, Pain and Critical Care, University of Glasgow, Glasgow, UK

Background

Technology in neurointensive care units can collect and store vast amounts of complex patient data. The CHART-ADAPT project [1, 2] is aimed at developing technology that will allow for the collection, analysis and use of these big data at the patient's bedside in neurointensive care units. CHART-ADAPT provides the technology to support the precision management of neurointensive care patients. It enables the simultaneous extraction of high-frequency data from devices monitoring the physiology of multiple patients, automatic integration of these data, provides data anonymisation services and allows the implementation of clinically useful physiological models and algorithms in real time at the patient's bedside. Further, the platform enables the analysis of patient data (both high and low frequency) to create new and novel closed loop diagnostic or therapeutic models/algorithms relevant to patient treatment. Additionally, the platform enables the assessment of these newly developed models/algorithms or existing models in the clinical environment.

A requirement of this project is to automatically extract and transfer high-frequency waveform data (e.g. ICP) from monitoring equipment to a high-performance computing infrastructure for analysis. Currently, no agreed data standard exists in neurointensive care for the description of this type of data. In this study we investigated the use of the Medical Waveform Encoding Rules (MFER) (www.mfer.org) as a possible data standard for neurointensive care waveform data. The MFER is an ISO-approved standard (ISO/TC 11073-92001). It is both an efficient yet affordable standard for storing waveform data. However, it is specific to medical waveform storage. There are no additional metadata fields for demographics or other patient-related information. Hence, the MFER, although efficient and standardised for medical waveforms, should be used in conjunction with other medical data standards such as HL7 and the Digital Imaging and Communications in Medicine (DICOM) standard.

Aims

The aims were to implement and assess the MFER standard for the storage of neurointensive care waveforms such as ECG, BP, ICP, etCO2 and pulse plethysmography signals.

Materials and Methods

Several waveform formats were explored (e.g. XML, DICOM Waveform) and evaluated for suitability given existing computing infrastructure constraints, e.g. NHS network capacity and the processing capabilities of existing integration software. Key requirements of the format included a compact data size and the use of a recognised standard. The MFER waveform format (ISO/TS 11073-92001) met both requirements.

The MFER waveform format contains a header and a body. The header contains a fixed width "preamble" field describing the source of the data (e.g. neuro ICU), a "manufacturer" field, where details about the equipment/monitor generating the waveform data are held, a flag indicating the byte order of data storage "Endian" and further fields indicating the number of channels collected and the number of data blocks in a sequence (see below).

The body has two main components: sampling information and frame information. Sampling information describes the frequency of the data sampling and the resolution of the

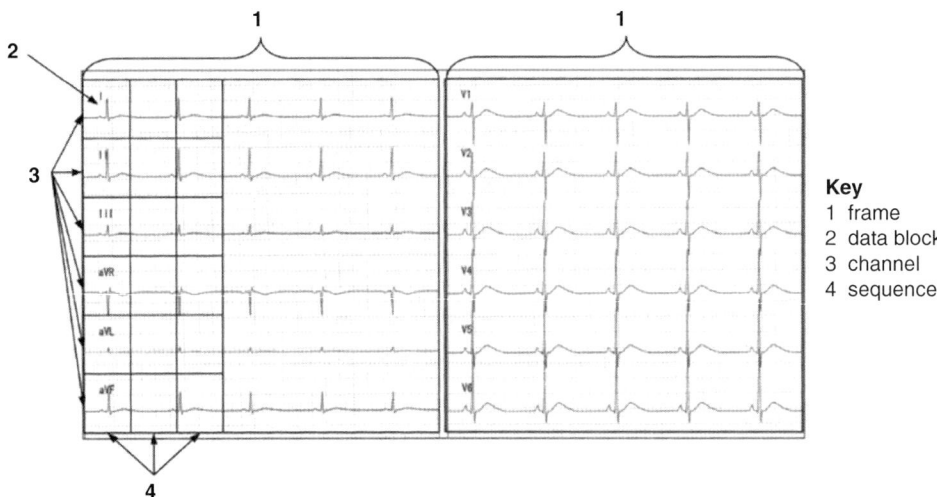

Fig. 1 Frame format. It consists of three elements: *data block* (the actual data), *channel* (each type of waveform data occupies a channel) and *sequence* (the repetition of the data). A sequence can contain one or more data blocks

data bit-size. Frame information describes the data itself and consists of three elements: *data block* (the actual data), *channel* (each type of waveform data occupies a channel) and *sequence* (the repetition of the data). A sequence can contain one or more data blocks. Figure 1 outlines the frame structure. All information in an MFER frame is encoded by a repeating sequence of one or more "*TLV*" sets where "*T*" is a two-byte code uniquely identifying the type of information (e.g. 0Bh = sampling frequency), followed by a two-byte "*L*" or length field describing the number of bytes contained within the data value, or "*V*" section. Each *channel* section contains information on the channel label, the source of the channel data (e.g. electrocardiography [ECG] monitor), sampling frequency, sampling resolution and finally how many bytes of data are stored per data block.

To evaluate the practicality of the MFER waveform format, up to seven waveform signals (ICP, ECG, ART, CVP, EtCO2, Pleth, Resp), collected from 12 patients at the Institute of Neurological Sciences in Glasgow, were converted into MFER. Waveform sampling frequency ranged from 500 Hz (for ECG) down to 60 Hz (Respiration, EtCO2). Most pressure channels (ART, CVP, ICP) were sampled at 125 Hz.

Results

Twelve patients (2 women, 10 men) admitted to the neuro-ICU at the Queen Elizabeth University Hospital between May and October 2016 had their data converted to the MFER format. Patient age ranged from 17 to 80 years (mean ± SD 42 ± 26 years). Admission diagnoses included: traumatic brain injury (4), maxillo-facial surgery (3), central nervous system tumour (2), seizures (2) and respiratory failure (1).

Over 62,000 MFER frames of data were generated from the ICU monitoring period of the 12 patients, which comprised up to seven waveform signals per MFER frame. One MFER file frame was created for approximately each minute of data, with a storage size of 181 KB each. Total database (Microsoft SQL server) file size for storage of this 12-patient dataset was 118 MB.

In this particular neuro-ICU, waveform data are captured from Philips Medical Intellivue MX800 bedside monitors. The iXellence (www.ixellence.com) "IxTrend Netserver" system is used to capture the waveform data. The Netserver system runs as a Windows service on an embedded PC within the MX800 monitor. One to two minutes of data are captured, compressed and sent via the local network to a proprietary IXtrend database (MS SQL). Java software designed in-house converts the IXtrend data file format into the open

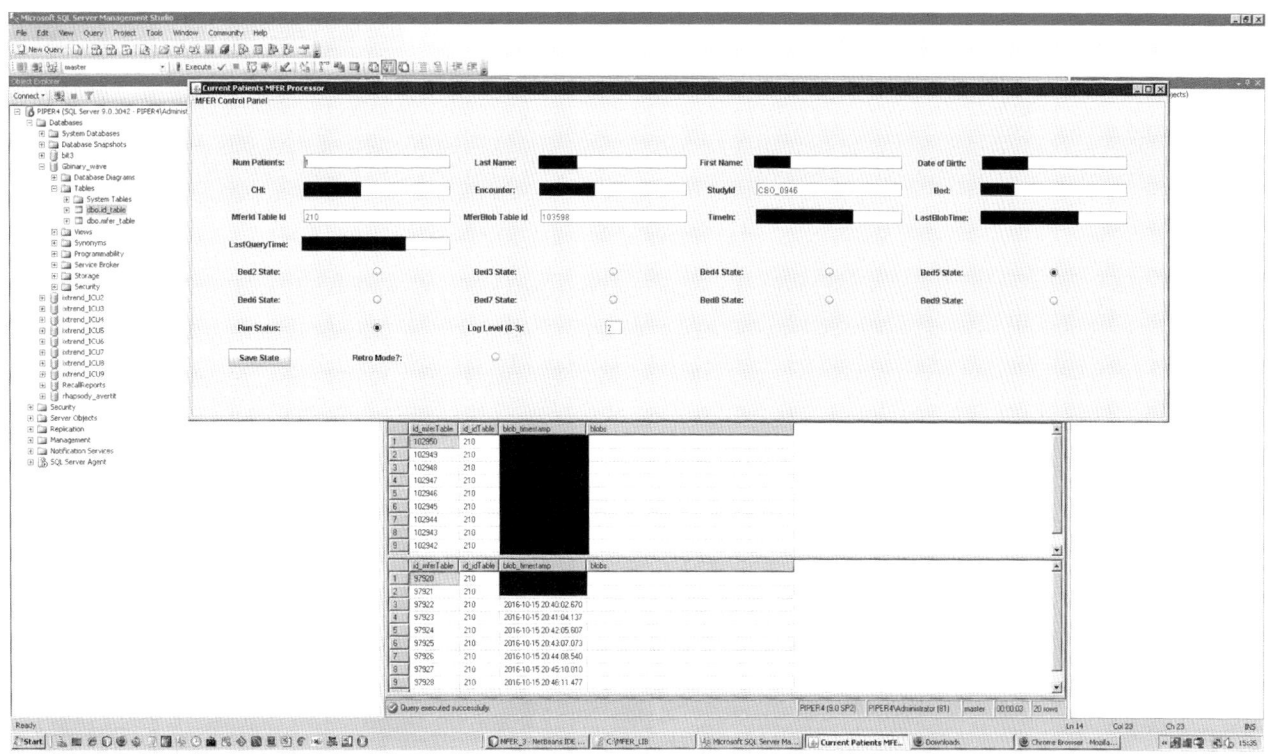

Fig. 2 Screen grab of in-house Java software that converts the IXtrend data file format into the open ISO standard Medical Waveform Format Encoding Rules (MFER) format on a minute-by-minute basis in real time

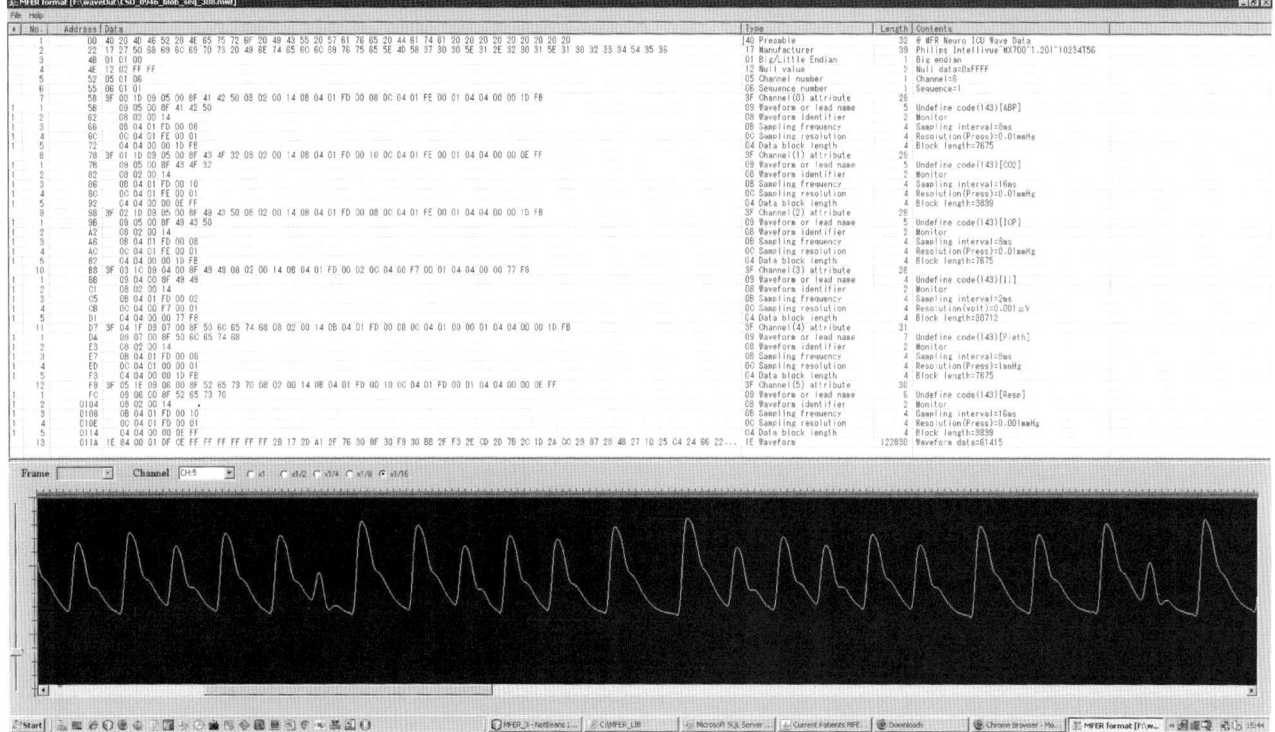

Fig. 3 A screen grab from the MFER data viewer showing one frame of MFER data. Viewable in the top section is the hex format byte information (with ASCII description fields to the right). This contains the header, channel description fields and finally the actual data block. At the bottom of the screen is a visualisation of one of the channels (arterial blood pressure [ABP])

ISO standard MFER format on a minute-by-minute basis in real time (Fig. 2).

Figure 3 is a screen grab from the MFRanz data viewer tool, which is free to download from the MFER site. The MFER viewer shows one frame of MFER data. Viewable in the top section is the hex format byte information (with ASCII description fields to the right). This contains the header, channel description fields and finally the actual data block. At the bottom of the screen is a visualisation of one of the channels (arterial blood pressure [ABP]). Note that no "data-padding" is required with this format. Figure 4 has been captured from the Philips Medical ICCA bedside e-Record system, which has been configured to have a "flow-sheet" with the usual hourly summary of patient data. In this example, using the CHART-ADAPT infrastructure, raw waveform data in MFER format is created, stored and then sampled and processed by the local server analytics cluster. Here, we see the results of six computer models (three running different variants of optimal CPP models, two running ABP hypotension models and one the highest modal frequency autoregulation model. Each model is calculated using the raw MFER waveform data and results sent once every 10 min to the patient's bed-space.

This example shows that the MFER format is an efficient waveform data format that can support "stream processing" of raw clinical waveform resolution data.

Discussion

Until recently, there has been a lack of cross-vendor (medical monitoring manufacturer) standard for the storage of high-resolution medical waveform data. This results in centres that wish to process waveform data purchasing or developing their own "format translator" from the equipment's native format to whichever analysis/archive system is in use. This approach adds cost, requires extra effort and is another potential point of failure.

It could be argued that before the MFER ISO format, there were other medical data standards that could encode medical waveform data. These include HL7, the Medical

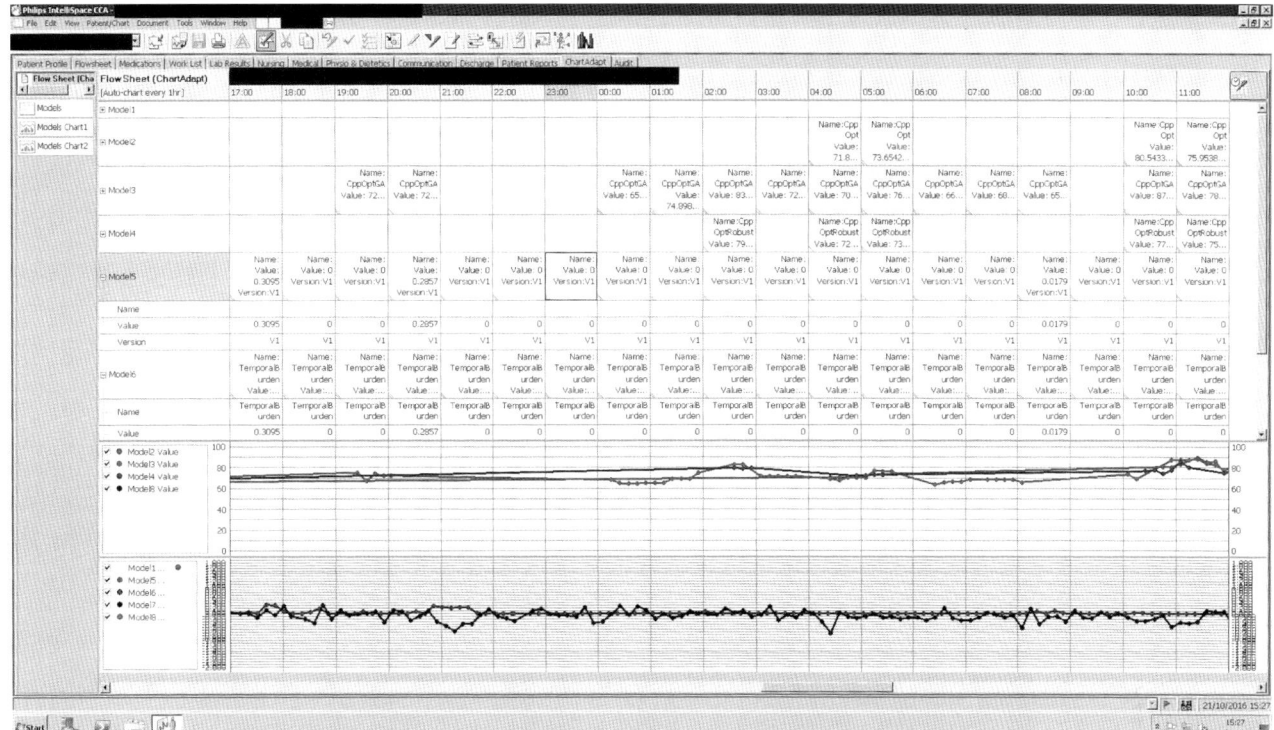

Fig. 4 Image from the Philips Medical ICCA bedside e-Record system. Using the CHART-ADAPT infrastructure, raw waveform data in MFER format are created, stored and then sampled and processed by the analytics cluster. Here, we see the results of six computer models (three running different variants of optimal cerebral perfusion pressure [CPP] models, two running ABP hypotension models and one the highest modal frequency autoregulation model). Each model is calculated using the raw MFER waveform data and results are sent once every 10 min to the patient's bed-space. This example shows that the MFER format is an efficient waveform data format that can support "stream processing" of clinical data

Information Bus (MIB) – ISO 11073, DICOM Waveform standard and the European Data Format (EDF). HL7 is a text-based format and any binary blob data inserted into V2 messages, for example, need to be base64-encoded and can lead to quite large messages. This is in fact how the CHART-ADAPT system transfers the MFER data between systems and demonstrates that standards can be mixed, using each for its own specialist purposes: MFER for waveform and HL7 for the other clinical data.

Although equipment manufacturers have come together to define a standard for device connectivity in the MIB (IEEE/ISO 11073), this standard does not define how waveform data are stored, only how it is represented and transferred. It is not ubiquitously adopted by device manufacturers. Furthermore, the standard is one that has been designed to be a general purpose medical data format and in some instances, does not adapt well to specific intensive care domain data fields (such as neuro-intensive care).

The DICOM standard is increasingly used by hospitals for radiological image management. It can store waveform data of any type, although it has focused on embedding ECG waveform data with some limitations to its functionality, such as a maximum of 13 waveform channels. However, similar to HL7 messaging, DICOM could also be adapted to embed the MFER data format within its structure, but this would need DICOM committee approval.

The European Data Format (EDF) has been designed for the exchange of multichannel biological and physical signals. Designed initially for supporting storage and annotation of multi-channel EEG, a version called EDF+ released in 2002 can represent most forms of electrophysiological recordings (electromyography, evoked potentials, ECG and sleep studies). Designed chiefly for electrophysiological testing, there is no reason why it could not be used to represent continuous intensive care bedside monitoring as well. It is a format most similar in concept to that of the MFER, its main limitations being that it is not widely adopted outside of the neurophysiological/electrophysiological community, nor has it achieved ISO standardisation.

Recently, specific to neuro-intensive care, is an initiative to create a "Smart Neuro ICU" – see www.SmartNeuroICU.org. This initiative is currently assessing new ways of representing and archiving neuro-ICU data that are frequently not well represented by other domain standards. One such format being considered by this initiative is the HDF5 format (see: www.hdfgroup.org/HDF5/). Again, this is a flexible format, which, similar to HL7 and DICOM could embed MFER data frames within its structure, again benefiting from the re-use of existing standards.

Conclusions

The MFER waveform format has potential as a lightweight standard for representing high-frequency neuro-intensive care waveform data. It should be used in conjunction with other existing and developing (e.g. HDF5) medical data standards that can encode the other key clinical data needed for clinical management, audit and research (e.g. HL7, DICOM).

Acknowledgements CHART-ADAPT (http://www.chartadapt.org) is an Innovate UK co-funded project and the project partners are: Aridhia, Philips Healthcare, University of Glasgow and NHS Greater Glasgow and Clyde.

Conflicts of interest statement We declare that we have no conflicts of interest.

References

1. Moss, L., Shaw, M., Piper, I., Hawthorne, C., Kinsella, J., Aridhia, Philips healthcare. Apache spark for the analysis of high frequency neurointensive care unit data: preliminary comparison of scala vs. R. Proceedings of American Medical Informatics Association 2016 Annual Symposium (AMIA 2016).
2. Moss, L., Shaw, M., Piper, I., Hawthorne, C., Kinsella, J., Aridhia, Philips healthcare. Enabling big data analysis in the neurointensive care unit. British Neurosurgical Research Group Meeting 2016, Cambridge, UK, March 2016.

Multi-Scale Peak and Trough Detection Optimised for Periodic and Quasi-Periodic Neuroscience Data

Steven M. Bishop and Ari Ercole

Abstract *Objectives*: The reliable detection of peaks and troughs in physiological signals is essential to many investigative techniques in medicine and computational biology. Analysis of the intracranial pressure (ICP) waveform is a particular challenge due to multi-scale features, a changing morphology over time and signal-to-noise limitations. Here we present an efficient peak and trough detection algorithm that extends the scalogram approach of Scholkmann et al., and results in greatly improved algorithm runtime performance.

Materials and methods: Our improved algorithm (modified Scholkmann) was developed and analysed in MATLAB R2015b. Synthesised waveforms (periodic, quasi-periodic and chirp sinusoids) were degraded with white Gaussian noise to achieve signal-to-noise ratios down to 5 dB and were used to compare the performance of the original Scholkmann and modified Scholkmann algorithms.

Results: The modified Scholkmann algorithm has false-positive (0%) and false-negative (0%) detection rates identical to the original Scholkmann when applied to our test suite. Actual compute time for a 200-run Monte Carlo simulation over a multicomponent noisy test signal was 40.96 ± 0.020 s (mean ± 95%CI) for the original Scholkmann and 1.81 ± 0.003 s (mean ± 95%CI) for the modified Scholkmann, demonstrating the expected improvement in runtime complexity from $\mathbb{O}(n^2)$ to $\mathbb{O}(n)$.

Conclusions: The accurate interpretation of waveform data to identify peaks and troughs is crucial in signal parameterisation, feature extraction and waveform identification tasks. Modification of a standard scalogram technique has produced a robust algorithm with linear computational complexity that is particularly suited to the challenges presented by large, noisy physiological datasets. The algorithm is optimised through a single parameter and can identify sub-waveform features with minimal additional overhead, and is easily adapted to run in real time on commodity hardware.

Keywords Peak detection · Trough detection · Algorithm design · Optimisation · Neuroinformatics · Intracranial pressure waveform analysis

Introduction

The reliable detection of peaks and troughs in physiological signals is essential to investigative techniques in medicine and computational biology and a prerequisite for many signal processing tasks. The challenge of accurate peak detection [1–3] is not unique to physiological signals and many solutions have been proposed in the literature, ranging from simple window-thresholding [4] and wavelet transform techniques [5] to Hidden Markov Models [6], k-means clustering [7] and entropy-based techniques [8].

In neuroscience data, the analysis of the intracranial pressure (ICP) waveform is a particular challenge and a number of algorithms [9, 10] have been proposed. In particular, algorithms suitable for ICP peak detection must be suited to multi-scale features, changing waveform morphology with time and poor signal-to-noise ratio.

There is a recognised trade-off between the generalisability of peak detection algorithms (degrees of freedom), accurate peak detection (false-positive and false-negative peak detection rates) and computational runtime performance [11]. For the most general algorithms to achieve a good domain-specific peak detection rate, they usually require significant parameter optimisation and long computational runtimes. The converse is also generally true, with algorithms designed exclusively for a domain-specific problem producing a better peak detection performance.

Scholkmann et al. [11] introduced an efficient and elegant algorithm for the automatic detection of peaks in noisy

S.M. Bishop (✉) • A. Ercole
Division of Anaesthesia, University of Cambridge, Cambridge University Hospitals NHS Foundation Trust, Cambridge, UK
e-mail: sbishop@doctors.org.uk

periodic and quasi-periodic signals, driven by their requirement to find peaks in near-infrared spectroscopy data. The Scholkmann algorithm (original Scholkmann) does not require any parameters, is fairly robust against high- and low-frequency noise and accurately detects peaks in quasi-periodic signals (provided that the highest frequency of oscillation is less than or equal to four times the frequency of the lowest in the signal). The algorithm is well-suited to ICP waveform peak detection tasks; however, it is hampered by an inefficient computational runtime and sizeable memory requirement.

In this work, we adapt the algorithm of Scholkmann et al. (modified Scholkmann) to dramatically improve runtime performance and memory storage requirements. We compare the peak detection rate and runtime performance of modified Scholkmann with original Scholkmann and provide further practical suggestions to improve performance when analysing ICP waveform data.

Materials and Methods

The Scholkmann Algorithm (Original Scholkmann)

The original Scholkmann algorithm begins by calculating a local maxima scalogram (LMS) over a linearly detrended signal X of length N, where $X = \{x_t \mid 1 \leq t \leq N\}$. The LMS is a matrix of $S_{max} = \left[\frac{N}{2}\right] - 1$ scales (rows) against N columns. If the value at time $t \in \{1 \ldots N\}$ and scale $s \in \{1 \ldots S_{max}\}$ is locally maximal, the matrix contains 0; otherwise, it contains $r + \alpha$ (where $r \in \Re$ is a uniformly distributed random variable and $\alpha \in \Re$ is a constant).

The LMS can be visualised more readily as an $S_{max} \times N$ matrix that marks the location of maxima at each scale (level of zoom). At scale $s = 1$ the matrix encodes a local maximum at time t if the signal value x_t is greater than the signal values at adjacent positions, i.e. $x_t > x_{t-1}$ and $x_t > x_{t+1}$. Likewise, at scale $s = 2$ the matrix encodes a local maximum at time t if the magnitude of the signal at position x_t is greater than the signals at times $t - 2$ and $t + 2$. This pattern continues up to scale S_{max}.

The LMS extends from the first scale ($s = 1$, highest or "finest" resolution) to scale $s = \left[\frac{N}{2}\right] - 1$ (a "low resolution" of approximately half the signal length). However, it is subsequently cropped to include only scales from 1 to $S_{cropped}$, where $S_{cropped}$ is the scale containing the greatest number of maxima. In the final step of the algorithm the column-wise standard deviation is calculated across scales, and time points with a standard deviation of zero identify the locations of maxima (peaks).

Optimisations Necessary to Produce Modified Scholkmann

A number of observations are necessary to optimise the original Scholkmann. First, the problem of peak and trough finding are equivalent: troughs are found by inverting the original signal and applying the peak-finding algorithm. Hence, trough-finding can occur simultaneously at minimal additional computational cost. Second, calculation of the LMS is costly; computational runtime and memory requirements have an $\mathbb{O}(n^2)$ upper complexity bound. Third, under most circumstances, calculation of the LMS using scales up to $S_{max} = \left[\frac{N}{2}\right] - 1$ is unnecessary. An appropriate upper scale bound can be parameterised in the algorithm and chosen using domain-specific knowledge. For ICP waveform data, the empirical maximum scale is equivalent to around one quarter signal wavelength, dramatically reducing the LMS search space. Fourth, calculation of uniform random numbers to populate the LMS is computationally expensive—the random numbers are only used during the final stage of the algorithm in the calculation of column-wise standard deviations. At the location of peaks, the corresponding column of the LMS is a zero vector and can be found through linear search, rendering the calculation of column-wise standard deviations and pseudo-random numbers unnecessary. Finally, the LMS should only be calculated once per signal and cached to allow subsequent runs of the algorithm to complete in $\mathbb{O}(n)$ time. This is extremely useful when working with ICP waveforms because recursive application of the algorithm can be employed to identify the ICP waveform sub-peaks P_1 to P_3 in linear time.

Comparing Original Scholkmann with Modified Scholkmann

The modified Scholkmann algorithm was developed and analysed in MATLAB R2015b (MathWorks, Natick, MA, USA) on a 16-core, 3.3-GHz Intel Xeon PC with 32GB RAM running Ubuntu Linux v12.04LTS. The algorithm code is found in Appendix.

Using a technique similar to that of Scholkmann et al. [11], synthesised waveforms (periodic, quasi-periodic and chirp sinusoids) were degraded with white Gaussian noise to achieve a range of test waveforms with signal-to-noise ratios as low as 5 dB. The synthesised waveforms were used to determine algorithmic performance and false-positive and false-negative peak detection rates were compared. The multicomponent simulated noisy signal defined by Scholkmann et al. [11] was used in a 200-run Monte

Carlo simulation to quantify the mean compute time with 95% confidence intervals for both algorithms. Further verification was performed using high-resolution electrocardiography, arterial blood pressure and intracranial pressure waveforms from a local neurointensive care waveform database.

Results

The modified Scholkmann algorithm applied to the test suite has false-positive (0%) and false-negative (0%) detection rates that are comparable with the original Scholkmann (Figs. 1 and 2), provided that a suitable maximum scale parameter is chosen (see section "Discussion" for details).

Actual compute time for a 200-run Monte Carlo simulation using the multicomponent noisy test signal was 40.96 ± 0.020 s (mean ± 95% CI) for original Scholkmann and 1.81 ± 0.003 s (mean ± 95% CI) for modified Scholkmann, showing the expected improvement in runtime complexity.

Discussion

In the test suites, a substantial improvement in compute time is seen from 40.96 s for original Scholkmann to 1.81 s for modified Scholkmann. The modified Scholkmann algorithm introduces a single parameter S_{max}, the maximum scale at which the LMS is computed, rather than deriving S_{max} from the signal data length. The LMS calculation in the original Scholkmann is the single most expensive computation and efficiency gains in the LMS calculation can lead to substantial gains in runtime performance. The improved performance in the modified Scholkmann relies on the periodic or quasi-periodic nature of physiological waveform signals—because of the periodicity of the signal, it is unnecessary to search the scalogram for peaks at a scale greater than one cycle length, allowing the limitation of S_{max} to a range much smaller than the signal length N. In this work an empirical range for S_{max} for ICP waveform data was found to be equivalent to one quarter of the waveform period. This reduces the algorithm's maxima search space, reducing space and time complexity

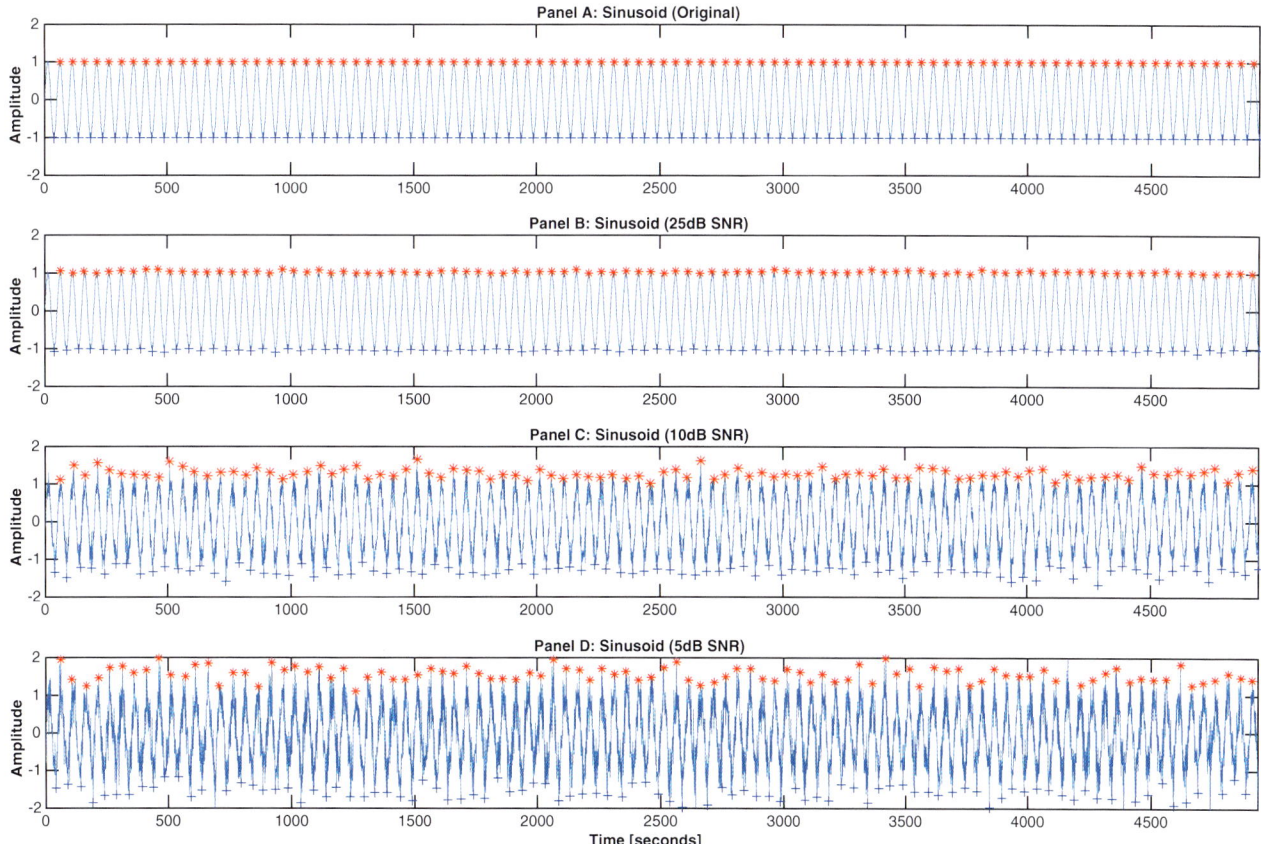

Fig. 1 (**a–d**) Modified Scholkmann algorithm. Detection of peaks (*red stars*) and troughs (*blue crosses*) in sinusoids degraded with white Gaussian noise to achieve signal-to-noise ratios (SNRs) down to 5 dB. Note that the algorithm can miss the first and/or last features in a signal owing to edge effects in the computed scalogram

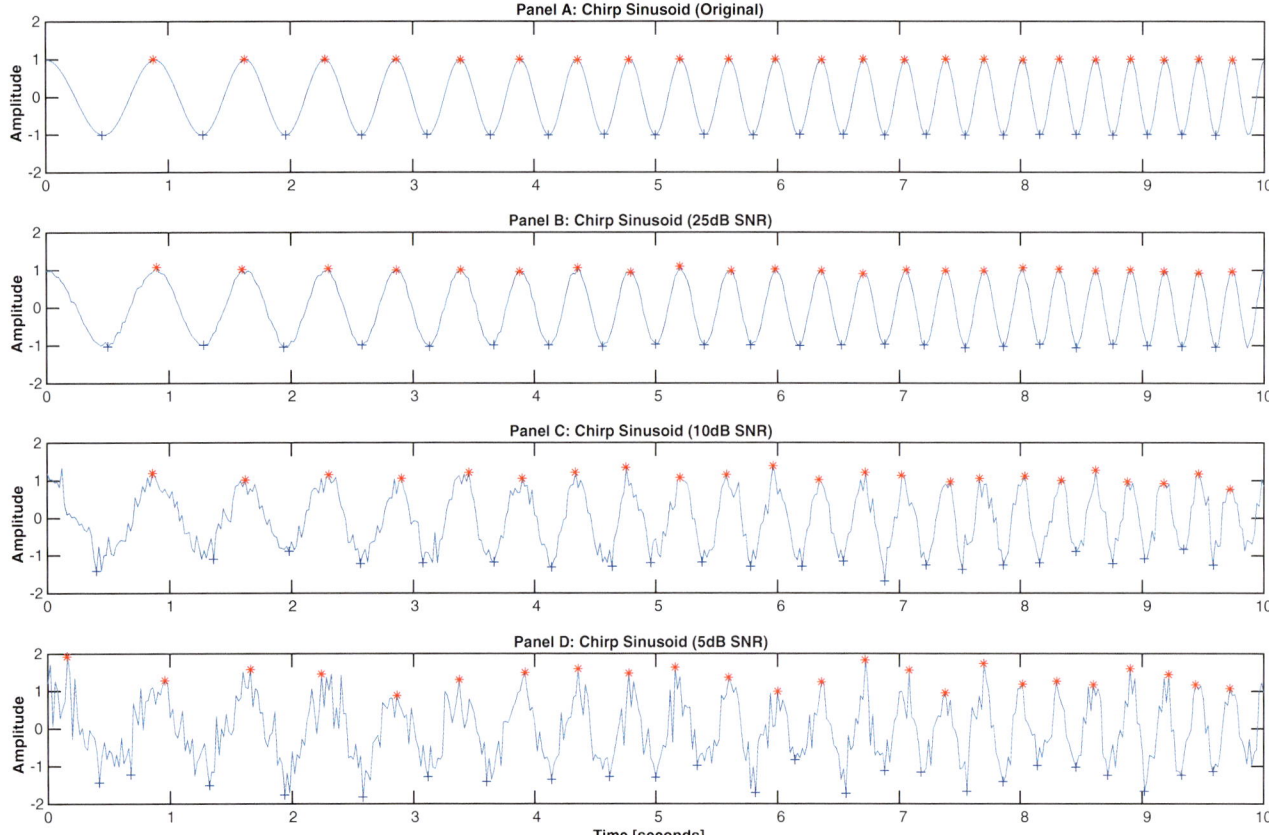

Fig. 2 (a–d) Modified Scholkmann algorithm. Detection of peaks (*red stars*) and troughs (*blue crosses*) in chirp sinusoids (frequency range 1–3.8 Hz) degraded with white Gaussian noise to achieve signal-to-noise ratios (SNRs) down to 5 dB. Note that the algorithm can miss the first and/or last features in a signal owing to edge effects in the computed scalogram

from $\mathbb{O}(n^2)$ in the original Scholkmann to $\mathbb{O}(kn) \equiv \mathbb{O}(n)$ in the modified Scholkmann. An improvement in efficiency of this magnitude is necessary to support real-time or near real-time analysis of neurological waveform data.

A widening edge artefact is seen in the LMS at increasing scales, because there is insufficient data to identify the location of "local" maxima. This is a limitation of both algorithms (original and modified Scholkmann); they both usually fail to identify the first and last peak or trough in the signal. The use of larger signal lengths and overlapping multiple windows can substantially mitigate this effect.

The original and modified algorithms are resistant to noise and operate at SNRs as low as 5 dB. At low SNRs both algorithms identify the expected peaks, but with reduced location accuracy. This results from the tendency of both algorithms to identify the most prominent local maxima in the expected sub-region of interest (which is a necessary constraint for quasi-periodic signals), allowing the algorithm to be misled by occasional high-magnitude noise.

The calculation of LMS is deterministic and results in a unique matrix for each signal that is amenable to memory or disk caching for later reuse. This acts as a simple method of improving runtime performance. Peak finding over a previously analysed signal can occur in linear time using the cached LMS.

An important benefit of the modified Scholkmann algorithm is the ability to identify sub-features within a signal. An example is the recursive application of the algorithm to identify ICP sub-peaks (Fig. 3), where the modified Scholkmann is used first to identify all troughs allowing individual waveforms to be spliced, and the modified Scholkmann is reapplied to each spliced waveform (which is efficient because of LMS caching) to identify the three largest sub-peaks P_1 to P_3. Here, the deliberate choice of a small

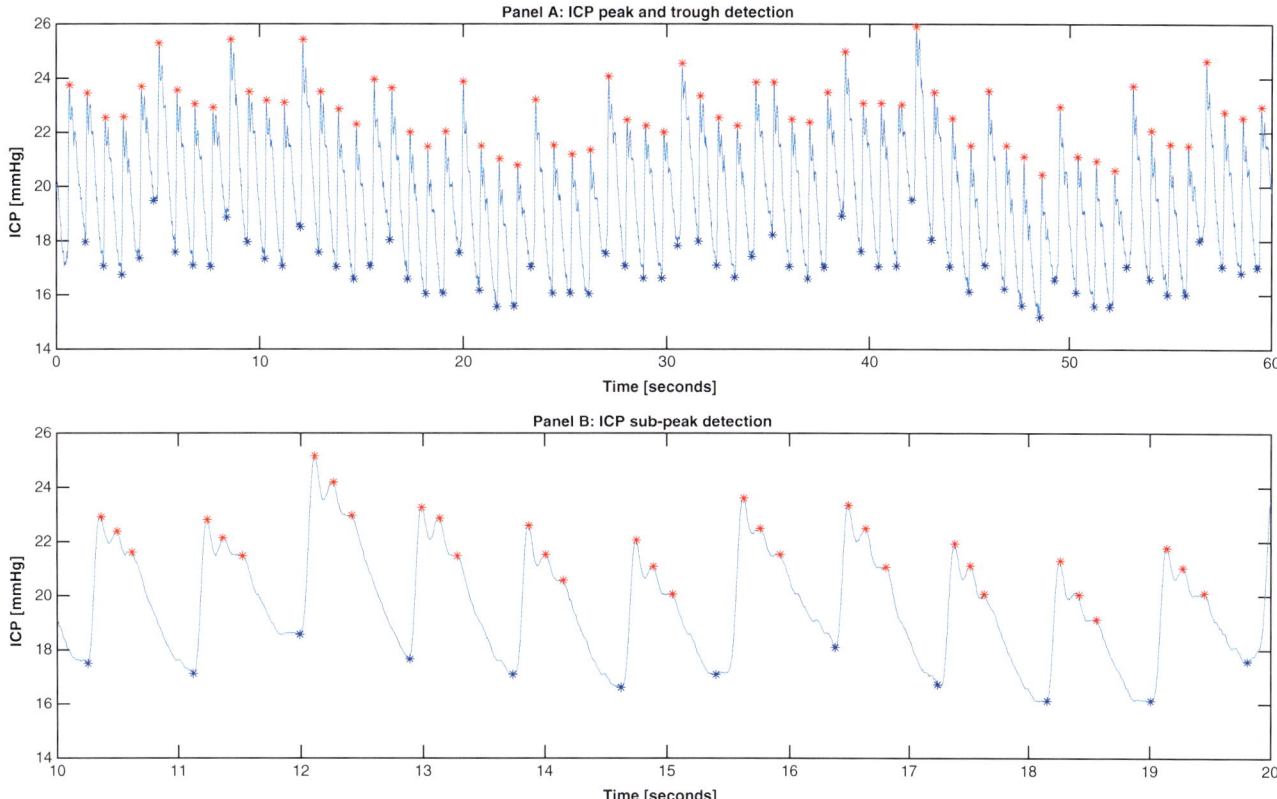

Fig. 3 (**a**) Modified Scholkmann algorithm. Detection of systole (*red stars*) and diastole (*blue stars*) in a continuous recording of intracranial pressure (ICP), sampled at 240 Hz via a Codman ICP Express Monitoring System (DePuy Syntheses, Raynham, Massachusetts, USA) and pre-processed with an unweighted 25 ms moving-average filter. A sliding window technique is used to mitigate scalogram edge effects and ensure that all peaks and troughs are accurately detected. (**b**) Modified Scholkmann algorithm. Recursive application of the algorithm to individual ICP waveforms delineated by trough–trough interval (*blue stars*) demonstrates the correct identification of individual ICP sub-peaks P1 to P3 (*red stars*)

maximum scale increases the false-negative detection rate, increasing the algorithm's sub-peak detection sensitivity.

Conflicts of interest statement We declare that we have no conflicts of interest.

Conclusions

The accurate interpretation of neuroscience waveform data to identify peaks and troughs is crucial in signal parameterisation, feature extraction and waveform identification tasks. Modification of a standard scalogram technique has produced a robust algorithm with linear computational complexity that is particularly suited to the challenges presented by large, noisy physiological datasets. The algorithm can be tuned for specific applications by optimising the optional parameter, can identify sub-waveform features with minimal additional overhead, and is easily adapted to run in real-time on commodity hardware.

Appendix

The MATLAB implementation of the modified Scholkmann algorithm (new_peak_trough.m):

```
% ----------
% Physiology Feature Extraction Toolkit
% Dr Steven Bishop, 2015-16
% Division of Anaesthesia, University of Cambridge, UK
% Email: sbishop {AT} doctors.org.uk
% ----------
% PEAK_TROUGH_FINDER
%
```

```
% Based upon the algorithm by (with up-
  dates and optimisations):
% Scholkmann F, Boss J, Wolk M. An
  Efficient Algorithm for Automatic Peak
% Detection in Noisy Periodic and Quasi-
  Periodic Signals. Algorithms 2012
% (5), p588-603; doi:10.3390/a5040588
% ----------
% [peaks,troughs,maximagram,minimagr
  am] = PEAK_TROUGH_FINDER(data, {max-
  interval})
% data: input data as vector
% sampling_frequency (optional): sam-
  pling frequency of input
% Returns: vectors [peaks, troughs, max-
  imagram, minimagram] containing
% indices of the peaks and troughs and
  the maxima/minima scalograms
function [peaks,troughs,maximagram,minim
agram] = new_peak_trough(data, varargin)
    N = length(data);
    if nargin == 2
        L = ceil(varargin{1}/2) - 1;
    else
        L = ceil(N/2) - 1;
    end
    %Detrend the data
    meanval = nanmean(data);
    data(isnan(data)) = meanval;
    data = detrend(data, 'linear');
    Mx = zeros(N, L);
    Mn = zeros(N, L);
    %Produce the local maxima scalogram
    for j=1:L
        k = j;
        for i=k+2:N-k+1
            if data(i-1) > data(i-k-1)
&& data(i-1) > data(i+k-1)
                Mx(i-1,j) = true;
            end
            if data(i-1) < data(i-k-1)
&& data(i-1) < data(i+k-1)
                Mn(i-1,j) = true;
            end
        end
    end
    maximagram = Mx;
    minimagram = Mn;
    %Form Y the column-wise count of
where Mx is 0, a scale-dependent distri-
bution of
    %local maxima. Find d, the scale
with the most maxima (== most number
    %of zeros in row). Redimension Mx to
contain only the first d scales
    Y = sum(Mx==true, 1);
    [~, d] = max(Y);
    Mx = Mx(:,1:d);
    %Form Y the column-wise count of
where Mn is 0, a scale-dependent distri-
bution of
    %local minima. Find d, the scale
with the most minima (== most number
    %of zeros in row). Redimension Mn to
contain only the first d scales
    Y = sum(Mn==true, 1);
    [~, d] = max(Y);
    Mn = Mn(:,1:d);
    %Form Zx and Zn the row-rise counts
of Mx and Mn's non-zero elements.
    %Any row with a zero count contains
entirely zeros, thus indicating
    %the presence of a peak or trough
    Zx = sum(Mx==false, 2);
    Zn = sum(Mn==false, 2);
    %Find all the zeros in Zx and Zn.
The indices of the zero counts
    %correspond to the position of peaks
and troughs respectively
    peaks = find(~Zx);
    troughs = find(~Zn);
end
```

References

1. Sezan MI. A peak detection algorithm and its application to histogram-based image data reduction. Comput Vision Graph Image Process. 1990;49(1):36–51. Available from: http://www.sciencedirect.com/science/article/pii/0734189X9090161N
2. Wilbanks EG, Facciotti MT. Evaluation of algorithm performance in ChIP-seq peak detection. PLoS One. 2010;5(7):e11471. Available from: http://dx.plos.org/10.1371/journal.pone.0011471
3. Du P, Kibbe WA, Lin SM. Improved peak detection in mass spectrum by incorporating continuous wavelet transform-based pattern matching. Bioinformatics. 2006;22(17):2059–65. Available from: http://www.ncbi.nlm.nih.gov/pubmed/16820428
4. Pan J, Tompkins WJ. A real-time QRS detection algorithm. IEEE Trans Biomed Eng. 1985;32(3):230–6. Available from: http://www.ncbi.nlm.nih.gov/pubmed/3997178
5. Wee A, Grayden DB, Zhu Y, Petkovic-Duran K, Smith D. A continuous wavelet transform algorithm for peak detection. Electrophoresis. 2008;29(20):4215–25. Available from: http://www.ncbi.nlm.nih.gov/pubmed/18924102

6. Coast DA, Stern RM, Cano GG, Briller SA. An approach to cardiac arrhythmia analysis using hidden Markov models. IEEE Trans Biomed Eng. 1990;37(9):826–36. Available from: http://www.ncbi.nlm.nih.gov/pubmed/2227969
7. Mehta SS, Shete DA, Lingayat NS, Chouhan VS. K-means algorithm for the detection and delineation of QRS-complexes in electrocardiogram. IRBM. 2010;31(1):48–54.
8. Palshikar GK. Simple algorithms for peak detection in time-series. In: First Int Conf advanced data analysis, business analytics and intelligence (ICADABAI2009), Ahmedabad, India, 6–7 June 2009. 2009.
9. Scalzo F, Asgari S, Kim S, Bergsneider M, Hu X. Robust peak recognition in intracranial pressure signals. Biomed Eng Online. 2010;9(1):61.
10. Scalzo F, Hamilton R, Hu X. Real-time analysis of intracranial pressure waveform morphology. CdnIntechopenCom. Available from: http://cdn.intechopen.com/pdfs/32480/InTech-Real_time_analysis_of_intracranial_pressure_waveform_morphology.pdf
11. Scholkmann F, Boss J, Wolf M. An efficient algorithm for automatic peak detection in noisy periodic and quasi-periodic signals. Algorithms. 2012;5(4):588–603.

Room Air Readings of Brain Tissue Oxygenation Probes

Stefan Wolf, Ludwig Schürer, and Doortje C. Engel

Abstract *Objective*: Brain tissue oxygenation ($p_{bt}O_2$) monitoring with microprobes is increasingly used as an important parameter in addition to intracranial pressure in acutely brain-injured patients. Data on accuracy and long-term drift after use are scarce. We investigated room air readings of used $p_{bt}O_2$ probes for their relationship with the duration of monitoring, geographic location of the center, and manufacturer type.

Methods: After finishing clinically indicated monitoring in patients, $p_{bt}O_2$ probes used in two centers in Berlin and Munich were explanted and cleaned to avoid blood contamination. Immediately afterward, room air readings of partial oxygen pressure ($p_{air}O_2$) from 44 Licox® and 10 Raumedic® $p_{bt}O_2$ probes were recorded. Assumed height above sea level was 42 m for Berlin and 485 m for Munich; this resulted in assumed theoretical $p_{air}O_2$ readings of 157.8 mmHg in Berlin and 149.9 mmHg in Munich.

Results: Licox® probes in Berlin showed a mean $p_{air}O_2$ of 160.5 (SD 14.4) mmHg and of 147.8 (11.9) mmHg in Munich. Raumedic® probes in Berlin showed a mean $p_{air}O_2$ of 170.5 (12.2) mmHg and the single Raumedic® probe used in Munich 155 mmHg. No significant drift was found over time for probes with up to 14 days of monitoring. Prolonged use of up to 20 days showed a clinically negligible drift of 1.2 mmHg per day of use for Licox® probes.

S. Wolf (✉)
Department of Neurosurgery, Charité Campus Virchow, Berlin, Berlin, Germany
e-mail: stefan.wolf@charite.de

L. Schürer
Department of Neurosurgery, Klinikum Bogenhausen, Technical University Munich, Munich, Germany

D.C. Engel
Department of Neurosurgery, Eberhard-Karls-University, Tübingen, Germany

Mean absolute deviation for $p_{air}O_2$ from expected values was 6.4% for Licox® and 9.7% for Raumedic® probes.

Conclusion: Room air partial oxygen pressure $p_{air}O_2$ may be utilized to assess the proper function of a $p_{bt}O_2$ probe. It provides a tool for quality control which is easy to implement. Probe readings are stable in the clinically relevant range, even after prolonged use.

Keywords Brain tissue oxygenation · Atmospheric pressure · Monitoring · Room air reading · Long-term assessment

Introduction

Monitoring brain tissue oxygenation ($p_{bt}O_2$) with intraparenchymal microprobes is an emerging tool and recommended in guidelines after traumatic brain injury and aneurysmal subarachnoid hemorrhage [1, 2]. A commonly proposed threshold is 20 mmHg: values below this margin are associated with a worse outcome [3]. As monitoring of critically injured patients may be required for days or even 1 or 2 weeks, it is crucial to know how accurate the readings of $p_{bt}O_2$ probes are over time and whether long-term drift is present. Currently, bench testing is available only for probes in mint condition and an assessment of $p_{bt}O_2$ devices after in vivo use is lacking [4, 5].

On earth, ambient dry air provides a stable environment with an oxygen fraction of 20.95% and a partial pressure of 159.21 mmHg at sea level. Therefore, a simple and ubiquitously available method of assessing the accuracy of a $p_{bt}O_2$ probe may be to use plain room air as a reference. Therefore, we investigated room air readings of used $p_{bt}O_2$ probes for their relationship with duration of monitoring, geographic location of the center, and manufacturer type.

Methods

Indications for $p_{bt}O_2$ monitoring were based on clinical considerations and were not part of the study. We investigated equipment from both vendors currently on the market; in particular, Licox CC1.SB probes (Integra Neuroscience, Saint Priest, France) and Neurovent PTO probes (Raumedic AG, Münchberg, Germany). We gathered data from probes used in two centers, located in Berlin and Munich, Germany. After finishing clinically indicated monitoring, $p_{bt}O_2$ probes were removed, superficially cleaned with a pad to prevent blood contamination and inspected for obvious mechanical damage. Immediately afterward, room air readings of partial oxygen pressure ($p_{air}O_2$) were recorded until a stable reading was achieved. As no patient data were used in this setup, the need for informed consent was waived.

Physical Laws and Considerations

Average standard atmospheric pressure at sea level is 1,013.25 kPa, equivalent to 760 mmHg (29.92 in), with a typical range between 670 mmHg (26.5 in) and 800 mmHg (31.5 in) on a mercury column barometer. Introduced by daily temperature fluctuations, atmospheric pressure shows a semicircadian rhythm. The amplitude of these fluctuations is dependent on latitude, with about 5 kPa (3.75 mmHg) at the equator, and 0.5–1 kPa (0.38–0.75 mmHg) at continental climate zones.

Simplified, atmospheric pressure decreases with altitude by:
$p_{height} \sim p_0 * \exp(-height/h_0)$,
with h_0 = 8435m. For low altitudes, this equals approximately about 1.2 kPa (0.9 mmHg) for every 100 m.

Assumed elevation above sea level was 42 m for Berlin, Germany, and 485 m for Munich, Germany. Using the stable oxygen fraction of 20.95%, this resulted in assumed theoretical $p_{air}O_2$ readings of 157.8 mmHg in Berlin and 149.9 mmHg in Munich [6].

Statistical Analysis

Data analysis was performed using R 3.3.1, R foundation for Statistical Computing, Vienna, Austria. The duration of previous use was plotted against the room air reading. Multivariate analysis was performed with linear regression using room air reading as a dependent variable, duration of use as an independent linear predictor, and probe type and center location as cofactors.

Results

Room air readings of $p_{air}O_2$ from 44 Licox® and 10 Raumedic® $p_{bt}O_2$ probes were available for analysis. One probe from the Munich center showed a $p_{air}O_2$ reading of 334 mmHg, more than 10 standard deviations off from the mean of all other probes. Although no mechanical damage was noted, this single probe was considered defective and excluded from analysis.

Licox® probes in Berlin showed a mean $p_{air}O_2$ of 160.5 (SD 14.4) mmHg and of 147.8 (11.9) mmHg in Munich. Raumedic® probes in Berlin showed a mean $p_{air}O_2$ of 170.5 (12.2) mmHg and a single Raumedic® probe used in Munich displayed 155 mmHg.

Licox® probes showed an increase of 1.28 mmHg ($p < 0.001$) per day of use when all data with up to 20 days of forgone monitoring time were considered. No significant trend was found if readings from probes with up to 14 days of previous use were examined. We found no significant increase per day of previous use for Raumedic® probes. Mean absolute deviation for $p_{air}O_2$ from expected values was 6.4% for Licox® and 9.7% for Raumedic® probes. Figure 1 shows the relationship among time, location of use, and type of probe with the acquired room air readings.

Discussion

Our findings show that room air may be utilized as a verification tool of proper function of a $p_{bt}O_2$ probe. Differences in geographic location and altitude are reflected accurately by room air readings of $p_{bt}O_2$ probes. For use of up to 14 days, readings of used probes remained stable. Even with prolonged utilization beyond that time period, the average drift of 1.2% per day of use translates to lower values than differences in measurement to be expected in vital brain tissue [7, 8]. Therefore, we consider probe drift per day of use to be clinically negligible.

The knowledge derived may help a clinician to decide whether previous readings obtained during clinical monitoring had been accurate. In the case of challenged low (or high) readings during previous clinical use, a finding compliant with proper probe function may trigger implantation of a new probe. Unfortunately, our findings do not represent an online function test for probes under consideration. The fragile nature of Licox® probes prohibits reinsertion after room air testing. In theory, this may be possible for the more rigid Raumedic® probes, but is strongly disadvised owing to potential breaches of sterility.

The main limitation of our study is that we did not the measure actual $p_{air}O_2$ with a dedicated and calibrated device. Rather, we relied on the theoretical calculated $p_{air}O_2$ value for

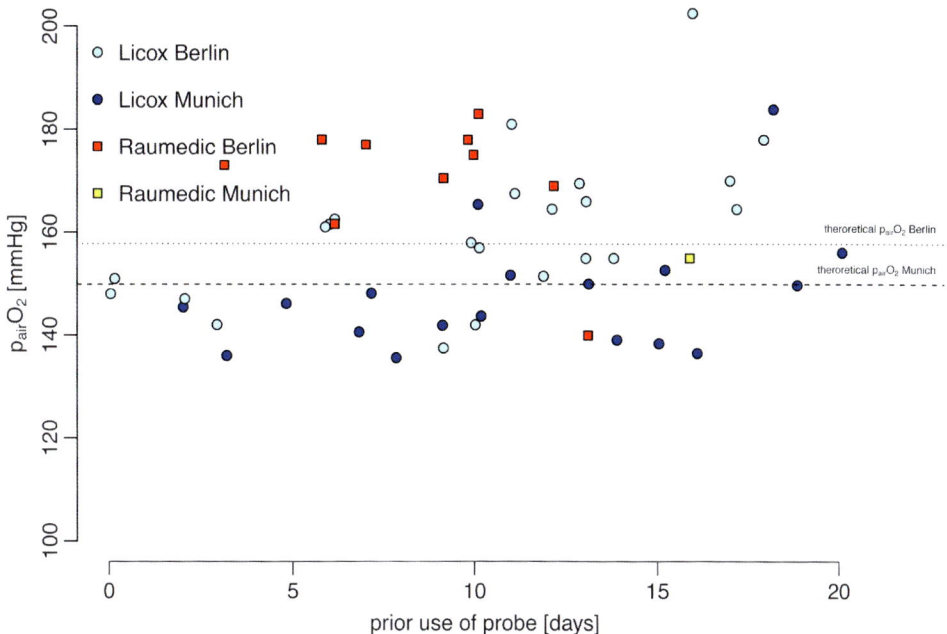

Fig. 1 Room air readings ($p_{air}O_2$) of brain tissue oxygenation probes from two manufacturers plotted versus days of previous use. Licox® probes are indicated by *circles*, Raumedic® probes by *squares*. *Dotted* and *dashed lines* indicate the theoretical readings in two centers, located in Berlin and Munich, Germany, respectively

the environment of the respective location. Daily fluctuations, in addition to high or low barometric pressures may subtly alter theoretical values of $p_{air}O_2$. Furthermore, it was assumed that it remained stable when measured indoors in the ICU with active air conditioning. Although both manufacturers perform adjustment of displayed pO_2 readings according to surrounding tissue temperature, the use of probes at room temperature is not at a level occurring in the living human body and outside of the manufacturers' specifications. Additionally, the cleansing process of the probes was not standardized and remnants of blood and tissue after clinical use may have contributed to unaccounted confounding. However, despite these limitations, the robustness of findings serve as important proof-of-principle of the validity of our analysis.

Conclusion

Room air partial oxygen pressure $p_{air}O_2$ may be utilized to assess the proper function of a $p_{bt}O_2$ probe. When the local altitude above sea level is considered, it provides a tool for quality control which is easy to implement. Probe readings are stable within the clinically relevant range, even after prolonged use.

Conflicts of interest statement We declare that we have no conflicts of interest.

References

1. Bratton SL, Chestnut RM, Ghajar J, et al. Guidelines for the management of severe traumatic brain injury. X. Brain oxygen monitoring and thresholds. J Neurotrauma. 2007;24(Suppl 1): S65–70.
2. Diringer MN, Bleck TP, Claude Hemphill J 3rd, et al. Critical care management of patients following aneurysmal subarachnoid hemorrhage: recommendations from the Neurocritical care society's multidisciplinary consensus conference. Neurocrit Care. 2011;15:211–40.
3. Ngwenya LB, Burke JF, Manley GT. Brain tissue oxygen monitoring and the intersection of brain and lung: a comprehensive review. Respir Care. 2016;61:1232–44.
4. Purins K, Enblad P, Sandhagen B, Lewén A. Brain tissue oxygen monitoring: a study of in vitro accuracy and stability of Neurovent-PTO and Licox sensors. Acta Neurochir. 2010;152:681–8.
5. Stewart C, Haitsma I, Zador Z, Hemphill JC, Morabito D, Manley G, Rosenthal G. The new Licox combined brain tissue oxygen and brain temperature monitor: assessment of in vitro accuracy and clinical experience in severe traumatic brain injury. Neurosurgery. 2008;63:1159–1164; discussion 1164–1165.
6. Atmospheric pressure. Wikipedia. https://en.wikipedia.org/wiki/Atmospheric_pressure. Accessed 15 November 2016.
7. Ponce LL, Pillai S, Cruz J, Li X, Julia H, Gopinath S, Robertson CS. Position of probe determines prognostic information of brain tissue PO2 in severe traumatic brain injury. Neurosurgery. 2012;70:1492–1502; discussion 1502–1503.
8. Hawryluk GWJ, Phan N, Ferguson AR, Morabito D, Derugin N, Stewart CL, Knudson MM, Manley G, Rosenthal G. Brain tissue oxygen tension and its response to physiological manipulations: influence of distance from injury site in a swine model of traumatic brain injury. J Neurosurg. 2016;125:1217–28.

What Do We Mean by Cerebral Perfusion Pressure?

Bart Depreitere, Geert Meyfroidt, and Fabian Güiza

Abstract *Introduction*: No consensus exists on the exact method for measuring mean arterial blood pressure (MAP) in the definition of cerebral perfusion pressure (CPP). The aim of the current study is to investigate how different MAP measurement methods have influenced the CPP recommendations in the Brain Trauma Foundation (BTF) guidelines.

Methods: All papers on which the chapter on CPP thresholds in the 2007 version of the BTF guidelines is based, were reviewed. If accurate descriptions of head of bed elevation and arterial pressure transducer height were lacking, the authors were emailed for clarification. Additionally, the effect of choosing the radial artery for MAP measurement and the potential effect of gravity were studied in the literature.

Results: Thresholds of CPP in the BTF guidelines are based on 11 studies. Head of bed elevation at 30° was part of the protocol in 5 studies, patients were nursed flat in 1 study, and this variable remained unknown for 5 studies. The arterial pressure transducer was at heart level in 5 studies, at ear level in 3 studies, and height was unknown in 3 studies. Measuring MAP in the radial artery underestimates carotid artery MAP by approximately 10 mmHg in the flat position, and in a nonflat position gravity influences MAP of the internal carotid artery.

Conclusion: There is no uniform definition for CPP, which may affect conclusions on proposed CPP targets in severe traumatic brain injury by ±10 mmHg.

B. Depreitere, M.D., Ph.D. (✉)
Department of Neurosurgery,
University Hospitals Leuven, Leuven, Belgium
e-mail: bart.depreitere@uzleuven.be

G. Meyfroidt, M.D., Ph.D. • F. Güiza, Ph.D.
Department of Intensive Care Medicine,
University Hospitals Leuven, Leuven, Belgium

Keywords Traumatic brain injury · Cerebral perfusion pressure · Mean arterial blood pressure · BTF guidelines · Radial artery

Introduction

Cerebral perfusion pressure (CPP) is the driving force for cerebral blood flow. CPP is defined as the difference between the mean arterial blood pressure (MAP) and the intracranial pressure (ICP). The venous pressure can be omitted from this formula, as it is generally lower than ICP. Although the recommendation for ICP thresholds has been quite consistent in initiating treatment for ICP above 20 mmHg in the first three editions of the Brain Trauma Foundation (BTF) guidelines on the management of severe traumatic brain injury (TBI) [1–3], different recommendations have been formulated regarding CPP after severe traumatic brain injury in the subsequent editions. In the first and second editions [1, 2], CPP was recommended to be kept at a minimum 70 mmHg, predominantly based on the Rosner studies [4], and the strength of this recommendation was "C" (option). In the third edition, this recommendation was changed to the recommendation, again with strength "C" (option), to target CPP within the range 50–70 mmHg [3].

No consensus exists on the exact measurement method of MAP in the CPP definition. Some centers install the arterial blood pressure transducer at the height of the atrium, whereas some correct for the effect of gravity on CPP when patients are nursed with the head at 30° by installing the arterial blood pressure transducer at ear level. The use of different measurement methods, and error ranges associated with these methods, may have affected the CPP thresholds in the guidelines. The aim of the current study is to investigate how different MAP measurement methods may have influenced the CPP recommendations in the BTF guidelines.

Methods

All 11 papers on which the chapter on CPP thresholds in the third edition (2007) of the BTF guidelines is based, were reviewed. If accurate descriptions of head of bed elevation and arterial pressure transducer height were lacking, the authors were emailed for clarification. Additionally, the literature was reviewed for comparison of MAP in the radial artery, internal carotid artery (ICA), and circle of Willis arteries, and for the effect of gravity on MAP measurements. Finally, an attempt was undertaken to adjust the CPP thresholds recommended in the 11 papers by correcting for gravity, for MAP estimation in the ICA, and for both.

Results

Eleven papers reporting on beneficial or nonbeneficial effects of CPP that is too low or too high are referenced in the third edition of the BTF guidelines [4–14]. Head of bed elevation at 30° was part of the protocol in 5 studies, patients were nursed flat in 1 study, and this variable remained unknown in 5 studies. The arterial pressure transducer was at heart level in 5 studies, at ear level in 3 studies, and height remained unknown in 3 studies (Table 1).

The baroreceptor reflex notwithstanding, in a nonflat position, MAP in the ICA is influenced by gravity [15]. If the patient is nursed with the head of bed raised 30°, the resulting hydrostatic pressure gradient is defined by the formula $x = $ [distance ear to atrium] $\times \sin(30°)$. For an adult of normal size, the distance from the ear to the atrium is approximately 30 cm. Hence, the hydrostatic pressure gradient is around 15 cmH$_2$O or approximately 10 mmHg (rounded), meaning that CPP will be approximately 10 mmHg less than based on MAP measured at atrium level. In addition, if MAP is measured by cannulation of the radial artery, it should be realized that actual MAP in the CA1 segment of the ICA in a flat position is approximately 10 mmHg higher than MAP in the radial artery [16, 17].

Table 1 shows the CPP recommendations resulting from each of the 11 papers and corrected figures when accounting for gravity, for MAP estimation in the ICA, and for both. When correcting for gravity, the range of advisable CPPs from these papers increases.

Table 1 Overview of publications in the cerebral perfusion pressure (CPP) threshold chapter of the Brain Trauma Foundation guidelines [3], their method of measuring CPP and corrections

Reference	Head of bed elevation	Arterial pressure transducer height	CPP recommendation	Correction for gravity	Correction for ICA MAP estimation	Correction for gravity and ICA MAP estimation
[5]	Unknown	Atrium	>80 mmHg ~ good outcome			
[6]	Unknown	Unknown	CPP-based strategy alone not sufficient			
[7]	Unknown	Atrium	>80 mmHg ~ good outcome			
[8]	30°	Ear	>70 mmHg no benefit	>70 mmHg no benefit	>80 mmHg no benefit	>80 mmHg no benefit
[4]	0°	Ear	>70 mmHg ~ better outcomes	>70 mmHg ~ better outcomes	>80 mmHg ~ better outcomes	>80 mmHg ~ better outcomes
[9]	30°	Atrium	<40 mmHg ~ poor outcome	<30 mmHg ~ poor outcome	<50 mmHg ~ poor outcome	<40 mmHg ~ poor outcome
[10]	30°	Atrium	<60 mmHg ~ poor outcome; >70 mmHg no benefit	<50 mmHg ~ poor outcome; >60 mmHg no benefit	<70 mmHg ~ poor outcome; >80 mmHg no benefit	<60 mmHg ~ poor outcome; >70 mmHg no benefit
[11]	30°	Ear	>70 mmHg ~ ARDS	>70 mmHg ~ ARDS	>80 mmHg ~ ARDS	>80 mmHg ~ ARDS
[12]	30°	Atrium	50–60 mmHg ~ better outcomes when deficient autoregulation	40–50 mmHg ~ better outcomes when deficient autoregulation	60–70 mmHg ~ better outcomes when deficient autoregulation	50–60 mmHg ~ better outcomes when deficient autoregulation
[13]	Unknown	Unknown	>60 mmHg no benefit			
[14]	Unknown	Unknown	CPP target is dynamic ~ autoregulation status			

ICA internal carotid artery, *MAP* mean arterial blood pressure, *ARDS* acute respiratory distress syndrome

Discussion

In the present study, it was shown that the measurement method for MAP was not uniform in the 11 studies on which the CPP thresholds in the third edition of the BTF guidelines are based. For some of the papers, correction for gravity affected the conclusion on CPP targets by approximately 10 mmHg.

A comment often made is that gravity reduces not only MAP, but also ICP, rendering a rather neutral effect on CPP. Although this is correct per se, ICP is monitored separately in patients with severe TBI, including the influence of gravity. Hence, correcting or not-correcting the MAP signal for gravity still influences the final calculated CPP. The current analysis not only illustrates that the lack of a uniform method with regard to correction of MAP for gravity may confuse the guidelines. It also emphasizes that MAP differs depending on the artery in which it is measured. Given this relativity, the question is not so much what is the true definition of CPP (radial artery cannulation should not be abandoned), but rather to aim at a uniform and accurate method that can be adopted in all ICUs. This is not necessarily easy. Even with the arterial blood pressure transducer aimed at ear level, it was found in an audit in Glasgow that incorrect height led to hydrostatic pressure gradients of more than 8 mmHg in over 35% (Ian Piper, personal communication). Replacing fixed CPP thresholds with dynamic targets based on autoregulation monitoring does provide a solution to this matter. However, in comparative trials testing optimal CPP methodology, a consensus on CPP in the control arm is needed. Also, even in dynamic targeting, the recommendation of safety limits may be useful.

The current analysis was presented at the ICP 2016 meeting in Boston. At that time, the fourth edition of the BTF guidelines [18] had not yet been released. The CPP threshold recommendation of the fourth edition includes 9 new studies and 4 studies were eliminated. Although the current study is based on the previous edition, this does not alter its message. This message is that it would be beneficial for comparing results of studies on severe TBI and benchmarking clinical outcomes if consensus were reached on an MAP measurement technique in the definition of CPP.

Conflicts of interest statement We declare that we have no conflicts of interest.

References

1. The Brain Trauma Foundation. The American Association of Neurological Surgeons. The Joint Section on Neurotrauma and Critical Care, et al. Guidelines for cerebral perfusion pressure. Brain Trauma Foundation. J Neurotrauma. 1996;13:693–7.
2. The Brain Trauma Foundation. The American Association of Neurological Surgeons. The Joint Section on Neurotrauma and Critical Care, et al. Guidelines for cerebral perfusion pressure. Brain Trauma Foundation. J Neurotrauma. 2000;17:507–11.
3. Brain Trauma Foundation; American Association of Neurological Surgeons; Congress of Neurological Surgeons; Joint Section on Neurotrauma and Critical Care, AANS/CNS, et al. Guidelines for the management of severe traumatic brain injury. IX. Cerebral perfusion thresholds. J Neurotrauma. 2007;24(Suppl 1):S59–64.
4. Rosner MJ, Daughton S. Cerebral perfusion pressure management in head injury. J Trauma. 1990;30:933–40.
5. Changaris DG, McGraw CP, Richardson JD, Garretson HD, Arpin EJ, Shields CB. Correlation of cerebral perfusion pressure and Glasgow Coma Scale to outcome. J Trauma. 1987;27:1007–13.
6. Cruz J. The first decade of continuous monitoring of jugular bulb oxyhemoglobin saturation: management strategies and clinical outcome. Crit Care Med. 1998;26:344–51.
7. McGraw CP. A cerebral perfusion pressure greater than 80 mm Hg is more beneficial. In: Hoff JT, Betz AL, editors. ICP VII. Berlin: Springer; 1989. p. 839–41.
8. Robertson CS, Valadka AB, Hannay HJ, Contant CF, Gopinath SP, Cormio M, et al. Prevention of secondary ischemic insults after severe head injury. Crit Care Med. 1999;27:2086–95.
9. Andrews PJ, Sleeman DH, Statham PF, McQuatt A, Corruble V, Jones PA, et al. Predicting recovery in patients suffering from traumatic brain injury by using admission variables and physiological data: a comparison between decision tree analysis and logistic regression. J Neurosurg. 2002;97:326–36.
10. Clifton GL, Miller ER, Choi SC, Levin HS. Fluid thresholds and outcome from severe brain injury. Crit Care Med. 2002;30:739–45.
11. Contant CF, Valadka AB, Gopinath SP, Hannay HJ, Robertson CS. Adult respiratory distress syndrome: a complication of induced hypertension after severe head injury. J Neurosurg. 2001;95:560–8.
12. Howells T, Elf K, Jones PA, Ronne-Engström E, Piper I, Nilsson P, et al. Pressure reactivity as a guide in the treatment of cerebral perfusion pressure in patients with brain trauma. J Neurosurg. 2005;102:311–7.
13. Juul N, Morris GF, Marshall SB, Marshall LF. Intracranial hypertension and cerebral perfusion pressure: influence on neurological deterioration and outcome in severe head injury. The Executive Committee of the International Selfotel Trial. J Neurosurg. 2000;92:1–6.
14. Steiner LA, Czosnyka M, Piechnik SK, Smielewski P, Chatfield D, Menon DK, et al. Continuous monitoring of cerebrovascular pressure reactivity allows determination of optimal cerebral perfusion pressure in patients with traumatic brain injury. Crit Care Med. 2002;30:733–8.
15. Gisolf J Postural changes in humans: effects of gravity on the circulation. Doctoral thesis February 25 2005, AMC, Amsterdam, The Netherlands.
16. Netlyukh AM, Shevaga VM, Yakovenko LM, Payenok AV, Salo VM, Kobyletskiy OJ. Invasive intracranial arterial pressure monitoring during endovascular cerebral aneurysms embolization for cerebral perfusion evaluation. Acta Neurochir Suppl. 2015;120:177–81.
17. Alastruey J, Parker KH, Sherwin SJ. Arterial pulse wave haemodynamics. Proc. BHR Group's 11th International Conference on Pressure Surges, Lisbon, Portugal, Oct. 2012.
18. Carney N, Totten AM, O'Reilly C, Ullman JS, Hawryluk GW, Bell MJ, et al. Guidelines for the management of severe traumatic brain injury, Fourth Edition. Neurosurgery. 2017;80(1):6–15.

Investigation of the Relationship Between the Burden of Raised ICP and the Length of Stay in a Neuro-Intensive Care Unit

Martin Shaw, Laura Moss, Chris Hawthorne, John Kinsella, and Ian Piper

Abstract *Objectives*: Raised intracranial pressure (ICP) is well known to be indicative of a poor outcome in traumatic brain injury (TBI). This phenomenon was quantified using a pressure time index (PTI) model of raised ICP burden in a paediatric population. Using the PTI methodology, this pilot study is aimed at investigating the relationship between raised ICP and length of stay (LOS) in adults admitted to a neurological intensive care unit (neuro-ICU).

Materials and methods: In 10 patients admitted to the neuro-ICU following TBI, ICP was measured and data from the first 24 h were analysed. The PTI is a bounded area under the curve, where the bound is the threshold limit of interest for the signal. The upper bound of 20 mmHg for ICP is commonly used in clinical practice. To fully investigate the relationship between ICP and LOS, further bounds from 1 to 40 mmHg were used during the PTI calculations. A backwards step Poisson regression model with a log link function was used to find the important thresholds for the prediction of full LOS, measured in hours, in the neuro-ICU.

Results: The fit was assessed using a Chi-squared deviance goodness of fit method, which showed a non-significant *p* value of 0.97, indicating a correctly specified model. The backwards step strategy, minimising the model's Akaike information criteria (AIC) at each change, found that levels 13–16, 18 and 20–21 combined were the most predictive. From this model it can be shown that for every 1 mmHg/h increase in burden, as measured by the PTI, the LOS has a base exponential increase of approximately 2 h, with the largest increases in the LOS given at the 20-mmHg threshold level.

Conclusions: This model demonstrates that increased duration of raised ICP in the early monitoring period is associated with a prolonged LOS in the neuro-ICU. Further validation of the PTI model in a larger cohort is currently underway as part of the CHART-ADAPT project. Second, further adjustment with known predictors of outcome, such as severity of injury, would help to improve the fit and validate the current combination of predictors.

Keywords ICP · Length of stay · Pressure time index · Neuro-intensive care

M. Shaw (✉) · L. Moss
Department of Clinical Physics and Bioengineering,
NHS Greater Glasgow and Clyde, Glasgow, UK

Academic Unit of Anaesthesia, Pain and Critical Care Medicine,
University of Glasgow, Glasgow, UK
e-mail: martin.shaw@nhs.net

C. Hawthorne
Department of Neuroanaesthesia, Institute of Neurological Sciences, Queen Elizabeth University Hospital, Glasgow, UK

J. Kinsella
Academic Unit of Anaesthesia, Pain and Critical Care Medicine,
University of Glasgow, Glasgow, UK

I. Piper
Department of Clinical Physics and Bioengineering,
NHS Greater Glasgow and Clyde, Glasgow, UK

Introduction

Patient length of stay (LOS) is a key factor in both clinical prognostic modelling and in guiding the overall management of a clinical environment. This has been shown in the intensive care unit (ICU) to be linked to initially poor, then subsequently improved, outcomes [1, 2]. The variability in outcome highlights the complex combination of factors that go into determining a patient's LOS.

A number of these factors, such as age, gender and cardiac complications, have all been investigated previously and shown to affect LOS [3, 4]. Age in particular is known to have a non-linear response with regard to LOS in the ICU [5]. This response translates in an elderly population into a 1-year decrease in survival, irrespective of ventilation status [6].

More specifically in a neurological intensive care unit (neuro-ICU), it is well documented that a raised intracranial pressure (ICP) is indicative of a poor outcome in traumatic brain injury (TBI) [7]. This phenomenon can be quantified using a dose- or burden-based analysis of the patient ICP [8, 9]. In Chambers et al. [8], they use an area under the ICP curve analysis, known as the pressure time index (PTI) model, to investigate the critical pressure values that are indicative of poor outcome based on a dichotomised Glasgow Outcome Scale (GOS).

The PTI methodology was initially validated in a paediatric population [8], subsequent work has shown its utility in an adult population [9]. An ICP value of 20 mmHg is commonly used in clinical practice as a critical ICP threshold in an adult population [7].

The aim of this pilot study is to investigate how the burden of raised ICP affects the neuro-ICU LOS by using a PTI modelling-based approach.

Materials and Methods

The PTI is a bounded area under the curve, where the bound is the threshold limit of interest for the signal [8]. This is normally implemented using Eq. (1) and is illustrated in Fig. 1.

$$\text{PTI} = \sum_{\forall t: \text{ICP}_t > \text{ICP}_{\text{thresh}}} \left(\text{ICP}_t - \text{ICP}_{\text{thresh}} \right) \Delta_{\text{time}} \quad (1)$$

where Δ_{time} is the time difference between the individual ICP values, measured in hours. The $\text{ICP}_{\text{thresh}}$ is the currently chosen ICP threshold. Finally, t is used to index all ICP values that are above the currently chosen threshold.

To evaluate any contribution, the new PTI value can add to an overall LOS prediction, ICP was measured in 10 patients admitted to the Glasgow Institute of Neurological Science's ICU following TBI and data from only the first 24 h were analysed. The main patient demographics can be seen in Table 1.

For the first 24 h of each patient's ICP recording, the PTI was calculated at threshold values ranging between 1 and 40 mmHg. This enables the threshold value influence on the model to be studied concurrently with the overall PTI value investigation. To this end, a backwards step Poisson regression modelling technique using a log link function was chosen.

Poisson regression is useful because each patient's LOS is bounded at the lower end by zero. If simple linear modelling was used, this fact could easily be violated by any subsequent predictions from the final model, which will not be the case when using a Poisson technique. The utility of each covariate estimate in the overall model is assessed by the standard z-test in Poisson regression.

Table 1 Summary of patient demographics used in the pilot study

Type	Value
Number of patients	10
Male, %	90
Age, median (IQR)	52 (45.75–57.75)
Length of stay, median hours (IQR)	43.37 (38.44–63.02)
Survival rate (%)	100

IQR interquartile range

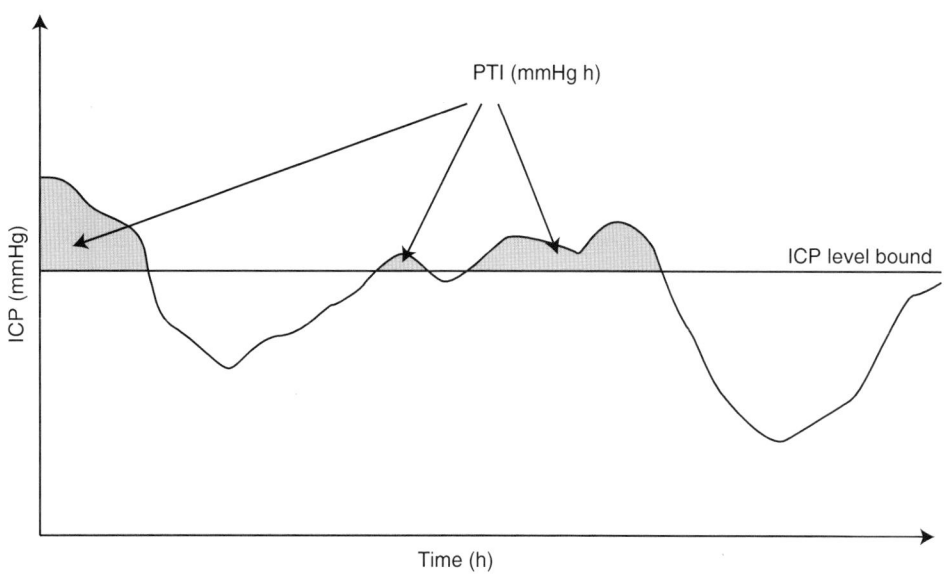

Fig. 1 Illustration of the main areas that would be included in the overall pressure time index calculation

The automated backwards step modelling strategy attempts to minimise Akaike information criteria (AIC) by systematically removing covariates. The AIC uses the likelihood of the model being correctly specified and penalises it by the number of covariates in the model. By searching for the smallest AIC, it chooses the best fitting model with the fewest covariates. In this specific case, the backwards step strategy finds the most predictive ICP thresholds when combined together into a single model.

To assess whether the final model output from the backward step modelling strategy is well specified, a Chi-squared deviance test was performed on the model. This test assumes a null hypothesis that the model is correctly specified; therefore, a non-significant p value for this test would imply that the model variables have been chosen correctly.

Table 2 Poisson regression model for length of stay with variable estimates for the pressure time index calculated at thresholds ranging between 13 and 21 mmHg

Variable	Estimate	Standard error	Adjusted p value
Intercept	0.135	0.53	0.8
Level = 13 mmHg	0.237	0.04	<0.001
Level = 14 mmHg	−0.585	0.15	<0.001
Level = 15 mmHg	1.060	0.37	0.004
Level = 16 mmHg	−0.621	0.29	0.031
Level = 18 mmHg	−1.184	0.16	<0.001
Level = 20 mmHg	3.091	0.33	<0.001
Level = 21 mmHg	−2.016	0.24	<0.001

Results

The modelling variable estimates and corresponding standard errors and p values are shown in Table 2. The Chi-squared deviance test gave a non-significant p value, in this case $p = 0.97$, which would imply that the final model variables have been chosen correctly.

The backwards step Poisson regression modelling strategy found that levels 13–16 mmHg, 18 mmHg and 20–21 mmHg combined were the most predictive, as shown in Eq. (2).

$$\text{LOS} = e^{(0.237 L_{13} - 0.585 L_{14} + 1.06 L_{15} - 0.621 L_{16} - 1.184 L_{18} + 3.091 L_{20} - 2.016 L_{21} + 0.135)} \quad (2)$$

where LN is the value of the PTI at a given threshold level of N.

Discussion

Interpreting the estimates in this model is a complex task, as it is multi-factorial with regard to the calculation of the PTI burden at a chosen threshold level. To simplify this significantly, analysis of the change in LOS, given a constant change in the PTI indices, could be performed.

It can then be shown that that for every 1 mmHg h increase in burden as measured by PTI the LOS has a base exponential increase of 1.12 h. However, this is likely to be an underestimation because of the nature of the simplification introduced. This probably implies that the approximate increase is closer to 2 h, with the largest increases in the LOS given by the 20-mmHg threshold level (as shown in Table 2).

This *critical* threshold value represents the turning point where the patient LOS begins to diverge from its optimal value because of the insult burden from the raised ICP. This value of 20 mmHg shown from the model is also in line with current clinical practice on the management of ICP.

This multi-factorial model shows promise for use in conjunction with the other known predictors from the current literature. However, owing to the pilot nature of this study, the model is close to being fully saturated. This results in a predilection towards overfitting during the modelling process. There is a definite need in this case to retune the model in a larger cohort of patients, enabling more accurate calculations of the model covariate estimates. This retuning would also address the issue that the model has been built on a cohort of patients who all survived and had a higher than average gender bias towards male subjects.

Conclusions

This model demonstrates that increased duration of raised ICP in the early monitoring period is associated with a prolonged LOS in the neuro-ICU. Further validation of the PTI model in a larger cohort is currently underway as part of the Connecting Healthcare and Research Through a Data Analysis Provisioning Technology (CHART-ADAPT) project [10]. Second, further adjustment with known predictors of outcome, such as severity of injury, would help to improve the fit and validate the current combination of predictors.

Conflicts of interest statement There are no conflicts of interest for any of the authors associated with this work.

References

1. Kisat MT, Latif A, Zogg CK, Haut ER, Zafar SN, Hashmi ZG, Oyetunji TA, Cornwell EE, Zafar H, Haider AH. Survival outcomes after prolonged intensive care unit length of stay among trauma patients: the evidence for never giving up. Surgery. 2016;160(3):771–80.

2. Stricker KH, Cavegn R, Takala J, Rothen HU. Does ICU length of stay influence quality of life? Acta Anaesthesiol Scand. 2005;49(7):975–83.
3. Almashra A, Elmontsri M, Aylin P. Systematic review of factors influencing length of stay in ICU after adult cardiac surgery. BMC Health Serv Res. 2016;16:318.
4. Moore L, Stelfox HT, Evans D, Hameed SM, Yanchar NL, Simons R, Kortbeek J, Bourgeois G, Clment J, Lauzier F, Turgeon AF. Hospital and intensive care unit length of stay for injury admissions: a pan-Canadian cohort study. Ann Surg. 2016. https://doi.org/10.1097/SLA.0000000000002036.
5. Zimmerman JE, Kramer AA, McNair DS, Malila FM, Shaffer VL. Intensive care unit length of stay: benchmarking based on acute physiology and chronic health evaluation (APACHE) IV. Crit Care Med. 2006;34(10):2517–29.
6. Moitra VK, Guerra C, Linde-Zwirble WT, Wunsch H. Relationship between ICU length of stay and long-term mortality for elderly ICU survivors. Crit Care Med. 2016;44(4):655–62.
7. Giza F, Depreitere B, Piper I, Citerio G, Chambers I, Jones PA, Lo T-YM, Enblad P, Nillson P, Feyen B, Jorens P, Maas A, Schuhmann MU, Donald R, Moss L, den Berghe GV, Meyfroidt G. Visualizing the pressure and time burden of intracranial hypertension in adult and paediatric traumatic brain injury. Intensive Care Med. 2015;41(6):1067–76.
8. Chambers IR, Jones PA, Lo TYM, Forsyth RJ, Fulton B, Andrews PJD, Mendelow AD, Minns RA. Critical thresholds of intracranial pressure and cerebral perfusion pressure related to age in paediatric head injury. J Neurol Neurosurg Psychiatry. 2006;77(2):234–40.
9. Sheth KN, Stein DM, Aarabi B, Hu P, Kufera JA, Scalea TM, Hanley DF. Intracranial pressure dose and outcome in traumatic brain injury. Neurocrit Care. 2013;18(1):26–32.
10. Connecting healthcare and research through a data analysis provisioning technology (CHART-ADAPT). 2015. http://www.chart-adapt.org/.

Pressure Reactivity-Based Optimal Cerebral Perfusion Pressure in a Traumatic Brain Injury Cohort

J. Donnelly, M. Czosnyka, H. Adams, C. Robba, L.A. Steiner, D. Cardim, B. Cabella, X. Liu, A. Ercole, P.J. Hutchinson, D.K. Menon, M.J.H. Aries, and P. Smielewski

Abstract *Objectives*: Retrospective data from patients with severe traumatic brain injury (TBI) indicate that deviation from the continuously calculated pressure reactivity-based "optimal" cerebral perfusion pressure (CPPopt) is associated with worse patient outcome. The objective of this study was to assess the relationship between prospectively collected CPPopt data and patient outcome after TBI.

Methods: We prospectively collected intracranial pressure (ICP) monitoring data from 231 patients with severe TBI at Addenbrooke's Hospital, UK. Uncleaned arterial blood pressure and ICP signals were recording using ICM+® software on dedicated bedside computers. CPPopt was determined using an automatic curve fitting procedure of the relationship between pressure reactivity index (PRx) and CPP using a 4-h window, as previously described. The difference between an instantaneous CPP value and its corresponding CPPopt value was denoted every minute as ΔCPPopt. A negative ΔCPPopt that was associated with impaired PRx (>+0.15) was denoted as being below the lower limit of reactivity (LLR). Glasgow Outcome Scale (GOS) score was assessed at 6 months post-ictus.

Results: When ΔCPPopt was plotted against PRx and stratified by GOS groupings, data belonging to patients with a more unfavourable outcome had a U-shaped curve that shifted upwards. More time spent with a ΔCPPopt value below the LLR was positively associated with mortality (area under the receiver operating characteristic curve = 0.76 [0.68–0.84]).

Conclusions: In a recent cohort of patients with severe TBI, the time spent with a CPP below the CPPopt-derived LLR is related to mortality. Despite aggressive CPP- and ICP-oriented therapies, TBI patients with a fatal outcome spend a significant amount of time with a CPP below their individualised CPPopt, indicating a possible therapeutic target.

Keywords Traumatic brain injury · Intracranial pressure · Cerebral hemodynamics · Autoregulation · Cerebral perfusion pressure

Introduction

Maintaining adequate cerebral perfusion pressure (CPP) is imperative for preventing cerebral hypoperfusion and ischaemia after severe traumatic brain injury (TBI). However, defining what might be an optimal CPP is uncertain: a CPP that is too low risks hypoperfusion, whereas a CPP that is too high risks cerebral hyperaemia. As such, the Brain Trauma Foundation recommends maintaining CPP somewhere between 60 and 70 mmHg [1]. However, applying rigid thresholds may not be appropriate for all patients [2].

Various physiological markers have been proposed as guides as to what may constitute an optimal CPP, including cerebral microdialysis, brain tissue oxygenation, or cerebral autoregulation. Estimating at which CPP cerebral autoregulation is most efficient is an attractive avenue as cerebral autoregulation per se is related to patient outcome and it can be estimated continuously using the pressure reactivity index (PRx) [3]. Previous investigations using retrospective datasets have ascertained that continuously estimating the optimal CPP (CPPopt) is feasible and is related to outcome [4–8].

The aim of this study was to ascertain whether prospectively collected optimal CPP data collected at the bedside, without any post-processing manual artefact removal, is at all related to patient outcome after severe TBI. This is a short version based on an oral presentation during the Intracranial Pressure 2016 Symposium in Boston, USA. The full paper, containing an extended analyses is available in *Critical Care Medicine* [9].

Materials and Methods

Patients

Two hundred and thirty-one patients with severe TBI who were at Addenbrooke's Hospital Neurocritical Care Unit between 2010 and 2015 and who underwent computerised intracranial pressure (ICP) monitoring were selected for this analysis. National ethical approval was obtained (30 REC 97/291) and patients were treated according to published protocolised guidelines [10], with attempts to maintain ICP < 20 and CPP between 60 and 70 mmHg [1]. The Glasgow Outcome Scale (GOS) was assessed at 6 months by outpatient assessment [11]. The primary outcome of this study was survival at 6 months.

Data Acquisition and Analyses

Intracranial pressure was monitored using an intraparenchymal sensor (Codman ICP Micro-Sensor; Codman & Shurtleff, Raynham, MA, USA) inserted into the frontal cortex via a burr hole and arterial blood pressure (ABP) was monitored in the radial or femoral artery zeroed at the level of the right atrium (Baxter Health-care CA, USA; Sidcup, UK). In patients with head elevation, no corrections were made for hydrostatic pressure differences. Data were sampled at 100 Hz using proprietary data acquisition software, which was also used to calculate the PRx and CPPopt on-line (ICM+©, http://www.neurosurg.cam.ac.uk/icmplus; Cambridge Enterprise, Cambridge, UK).

The PRx was calculated over a 5-min moving window as the Pearson correlation of 30 consecutive 10-s average values of ABP and ICP, as previously described [12] and CPPopt was also calculated as previously described (see appendix in Aries et al. [5]). ΔCPPopt was calculated as the mean CPP over a 5-min buffer, minus the current CPPopt value estimate.

Analysis of CPPopt Data

A method of incorporating information about the PRx into CPPopt assessment was developed based on initial exploratory analysis of the minute-by-minute ΔCPPopt and PRx data (Fig. 1). First, each PRx value was dichotomised into intact and impaired vascular reactivity using a threshold

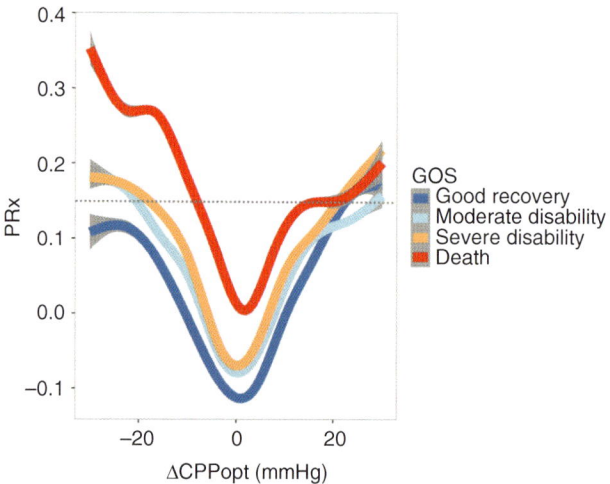

Fig. 1 Relationship between the difference between cerebral perfusion pressure (CPP) and optimal CPP (CPPopt; ΔCPPopt) and the pressure reactivity index (PRx), stratified by 6-month Glasgow Outcome Scale score. From *top* to *bottom* the fitted (generalised additive model) curves represent data from patients who subsequently died, had severe disability, had moderate disability, or had a good recovery. With increasing burden of disability, the U-shaped relationship between ΔCPPopt and PRx is shifted superiorly, indicating a narrower range of ΔCPPopt values associated with a good PRx. For subsequent calculations, an individualised dichotomisation of whether a patient's CPPopt value was below the individualised lower limit of reactivity (LLR) was devised. Using a cut-off for impaired PRx of 0.15 a.u. (*dotted line*), a CPP below the LLR was defined as CPP that was lower than CPPopt and was associated with a PRx greater than 0.15 a.u.

of +0.15 a.u. Then, each continuously derived ΔCPPopt value was coupled with its time-aligned dichotomised PRx value to give an estimate of whether the current CPP was above or below the limits of working cerebrovascular pressure reactivity. The percentage of time each patient spent with their CPP below the lower limit of reactivity (LLR) was calculated using the total time CPPopt was available as the denominator. These percentage times were compared across GOS groups.

Statistical Analysis

The relationship between time spent with CPP below the LLR and mortality was assessed using a ROC analysis with area under the curve descriptives. The ability of time spent below LLR to differentiate between survivors and non-survivors was compared with time spent with CPP below the fixed thresholds of 50, 60 and 70 mmHg by comparing area under the curve (AUC) values. The Delong test was used to detect statistically significant differences. All data manipulation and statistical analyses were conducted in the R language and software environment for statistical computation (version 2.12.1) [13]. The following packages were used: dplyr [14], ggplot2 [15], MASS [16] and pROC. The significance level was set at $p < 0.05$.

Results

Mean age of the cohort was 42 years and 19% were women. Of the 231 patients 21% died, 33 were severely disabled, 28% had moderate disability, and 17% had a good recovery.

The CPPopt calculated at the bedside was available on average 60% of total monitoring time (IQR 50.2–68.4).

When the difference between CPP and CPPopt was plotted against the PRx, a U-shaped curve was obtained, and the patients' eventual outcome seemed to determine the vertical position of these curves (Fig. 1). Those patients who died had a ΔCPPopt–PRx curve that was shifted upwards and had steeper edges, indicating in these patients a narrower range of CPP with adequate pressure reactivity.

Using a cut-off for an intact PRx of +0.15, those with a better outcome spent a shorter amount of time with a ΔCPPopt below the LLR (good recovery 13.7%, moderate disability 16.5%, severe disability 18.6%, dead 33.3%. The amount of time with CPP below the LLR was superior to using the fixed threshold of 50 or 70 mmHg in differentiating survivors from non-survivors and showed a tendency towards being superior to a fixed threshold of 60 mmHg (%time CPP < LLR AUC = 0.76 (0.68–0.84), %time CPP < 50 mmHg AUC = 0.64 (0.54–0.74), %time CPP < 60 AUC = 0.67

Table 1 Area under the receiver operating characteristic curve for differentiating survivors from non-survivors comparing the time spent with individualised CPP below LLR with time spent below fixed thresholds of CPP

% Time	AUC survivors vs non-survivors	p value fixed threshold vs individualised LLR
CPP < LLR	0.76 (0.68–0.84)	
CPP <50	0.64 (0.54–0.74)	0.046
CPP <60	0.67 (0.57–0.77)	0.11
CPP <70	0.58 (0.48–0.69)	<0.001

CPP cerebral perfusion pressure, *AUC* area under the curve, *LLR* lower limit of reactivity

(0.57–0.77), %time CPP < 70 mmHg AUC = 0.58 (0.48–0.69); Table 1).

Discussion

In this study, we demonstrate that CPPopt calculated at the bedside has prognostic importance after severe TBI. In addition, post-hoc analysis revealed that time spent with CPPopt below the individualised LLR may be a practical and prognostic metric for the adequacy of a patient's CPP.

Retrospective studies assessing a PRx-based CPPopt and outcome are limited to one large analysis (330 patients) [5] and several smaller pilot studies [6, 17, 18]. In addition, Depretiere et al. have shown the prognostic importance of an alternative method for determining CPPopt [7, 8]. For the current PRx-based method to be of practical use after TBI, the algorithm must be validated in a large cohort that is independent from the dataset used to derive the current CPPopt algorithm.

In this cohort, the time spent with a CPP below the LLR was associated with patient outcome. Importantly, the time spent with a CPP below the LLR was superior to fixed thresholds 50 or 70 mmHg and showed a tendency towards being superior to a threshold of 60 mmHg (Table 1). This provides evidence that individualised autoregulation-guided CPP management may be beneficial after severe TBI.

The precise threshold of PRx that indicates impaired cerebrovascular reactivity is largely unclear; a PRx < 0 is thought to indicate working pressure reactivity [19] and has been associated with a favourable outcome [20], whereas a PRx > 0.3 was strongly associated with mortality in TBI patients [20]. In light of these considerations, we used a value between these cut-off points (PRx = +0.15) as our threshold for dividing between working and impaired pressure reactivity.

In the current study, CPPopt was only available on average for 60% of the monitoring time. This low yield limits the practical utility of the current CPPopt methodology. However, one method has been proposed that produces a yield almost 100% of the time [7], and similar approaches are currently under development.

Furthermore, although the current study used prospectively collected CPPopt data from the bedside and showed an effect on outcome, whether targeting CPPopt improves outcome remains to be elucidated. Furthermore, the safety of a CPPopt based therapy is as yet unknown. Thus, studies investigating feasibility and clinical safety should be performed before conducting an outcome based randomised controlled trial of CPPopt-targeted therapy.

Conclusion

In this large severe TBI study, the time that CPP was below the lower limits of cerebral vascular reactivity was associated with increased mortality 6 months after ictus and seemed to be superior to time spent below the fixed thresholds of CPP. Further studies should focus on the clinical safety and feasibility of autoregulation-based CPP management.

Financial Support for This Project No specific funding for this study.

Conflicts of interest statement Authors MC and PS declare receiving a fraction of the licensing fees of the software, ICM+ (licensed by Cambridge Enterprise, United Kingdom), used for data collection and analysis in this study.

References

1. Carney N, Totten AM, O'reilly C, et al. Guidelines for the management of severe traumatic brain injury. Neurosurgery. 2017;80(1):6–15.
2. Le Roux P, Menon DK, Citerio G, et al. Consensus summary statement of the International Multidisciplinary Consensus Conference on Multimodality Monitoring in Neurocritical Care. Neurocrit Care. 2014;21:1189–209.
3. Donnelly J, Budohoski KP, Smielewski P, Czosnyka M. Regulation of the cerebral circulation: bedside assessment and clinical implications. Crit Care. 2016;20:129.
4. Steiner LA, Czosnyka M, Piechnik SK, Smielewski P, Chatfield D, Menon DK, Pickard JD. Continuous monitoring of cerebrovascular pressure reactivity allows determination of optimal cerebral perfusion pressure in patients with traumatic brain injury. Crit Care Med. 2002;30:733–8.
5. Aries MJH, Czosnyka M, Budohoski KP, et al. Continuous determination of optimal cerebral perfusion pressure in traumatic brain injury. Crit Care Med. 2012;40:2456–63.
6. Young AMH, Donnelly J, Czosnyka M, et al. Continuous multimodality monitoring in children after traumatic brain injury—preliminary experience. PLoS One. 2016;11:e0148817.
7. Depreitere B, Güiza F, Van den Berghe G, Schuhmann MU, Maier G, Piper I, Meyfroidt G (2014) Pressure autoregulation monitoring and cerebral perfusion pressure target recommendation in patients with severe traumatic brain injury based on minute-by-minute monitoring data. J Neurosurg 120:1451–1451457.
8. Guiza F, Depreitere B, Schuhmann M, Van Den Berghe G, Meyfroidt G. Development of a low-frequency autoregulation index for calculation of optimal CPP in severe traumatic brain injury. J Crit Care. 2013;28:e8.
9. Donnelly J, Czosnyka M, Adams H, et al. Individualizing thresholds of cerebral perfusion pressure using estimated limits of autoregulation. Crit Care Med. 2017;45(9):1464–71.
10. Menon DK. Cerebral protection in severe brain injury: physiological determinants of outcome and their optimisation. Br Med Bull. 1999;55:226–58.
11. Jennett B, Bond M. Assessment of outcome after severe brain damage: a practical scale. Lancet. 1975;1:480–1484.
12. Donnelly J, Aries MJH, Czosnyka M. Further understanding of cerebral autoregulation at the bedside: possible implications for future therapy. Expert Rev Neurother. 2015;15:169–85.
13. R Core Team. R: a language and environment for statistical computing. Vienna, Austria: R Foundation for Statistical Computing; 2015. http://www.r-project.org/
14. Wickham H, Francois R (2016) dplyr: a grammar of data manipulation. In: R Packag. version 0.5.0. http://cran.r-project.org/package=dplyr.
15. Wickham H. Elegant graphics for data analysis. New York: Springer; 2009. https://doi.org/10.1007/978-0-387-98141-3.
16. Venables WN, Ripley BD. Modern applied statistics with S. Technometrics. 2002. https://doi.org/10.1198/tech.2003.s33.
17. Lewis PM, Czosnyka M, Carter BG, Rosenfeld JV, Paul E, Singhal N, Butt W. Cerebrovascular pressure reactivity in children with traumatic brain injury. Pediatr Crit Care Med. 2015;16:739–49.
18. Dias C, Silva MJ, Pereira E, et al. Optimal cerebral perfusion pressure management at bedside: a single-center pilot study. Neurocrit Care. 2015. https://doi.org/10.1007/s12028-014-0103-8.
19. Brady KM, Lee JK, Kibler KK, Easley RB, Koehler RC, Shaffner DH (2008) Continuous measurement of autoregulation by spontaneous fluctuations in cerebral perfusion pressure: comparison of 3 methods. Stroke 39:2531–2532537.
20. Sorrentino E, Diedler J, Kasprowicz M, et al. Critical thresholds for cerebrovascular reactivity after traumatic brain injury. Neurocrit Care. 2012;16:258–66.

Hydrocephalus and CSF Biophysics

Spaceflight-Induced Visual Impairment and Globe Deformations in Astronauts Are Linked to Orbital Cerebrospinal Fluid Volume Increase

Noam Alperin and Ahmet M. Bagci

Abstract *Objective*: Most of the astronauts onboard the International Space Station (ISS) develop visual impairment and ocular structural changes that are not fully reversible upon return to earth. Current understanding assumes that the so-called visual impairments/intracranial pressure (VIIP) syndrome is caused by cephalad vascular fluid shift. This study assesses the roles of cerebrospinal fluid (CSF) and intracranial pressure (ICP) in VIIP.

Materials and methods: Seventeen astronauts, 9 who flew a short-duration mission on the space shuttle (14.1 days [SD 1.6]) and 7 who flew a long-duration mission on the ISS (188 days [SD 22]) underwent MRI of the brain and orbits to assess the pre-to-post spaceflight changes in four categories: VIIP severity measures: globe flattening and nerve protrusion; orbital and ventricular CSF volumes; cortical gray and white matter volumes; and MR-derived ICP (MRICP).

Results: Significant pre-to-post-flight increase in globe flattening and optic nerve protrusion occurred only in the long-duration cohort (0.031 [SD 0.019] vs −0.001 [SD 0.006], and 0.025 [SD 0.013] vs 0.001 [SD 0.006]; $p < 0.00002$ respectively). The increased globe deformations were associated with significant increases in orbital and ventricular CSF volumes, but not with increased tissue vascular fluid content. Additionally, a moderate increase in MRICP of 6 mmHg was observed in only two ISS astronauts with large ocular structure changes.

Conclusions: These findings are evidence for the primary role of CSF and a lesser role for intracranial cephalad fluid-shift in the formation of VIIP. VIIP is caused by a prolonged increase in orbital CSF spaces that compress the globes' posterior pole, even without a large increase in ICP.

Keywords Visual impairment/intracranial pressure syndrome · Globe flattening · Optic nerve protrusion · Quantitative MRI · Cephalad fluid shift

Introduction

In 2005, NASA recognized an ophthalmological health risk that evolves during long-duration spaceflight, and has affected some two thirds of US crew members who flew on the International Space Station (ISS) [1]. Crew members who have been classified as having the visual impairment/intracranial pressure (VIIP) syndrome experience visual performance decrements accompanied by ocular structural changes [2–4]. The most common features of VIIP are hyperopic shift, varying degrees of optic nerve protrusion (NP), optic disc edema, flattening of the posterior sclera, retrobulbar expansion of the optic nerve sheath, and choroidal folds. Following their return to Earth, these changes have partially reversed in some astronauts, but persist in others [2].

Attempts to explain VIIP focused on cephalad vascular fluid shift, in which the absence of gravitational force disrupts the balance between hydrostatic and local tissue pressures [5–7]. Mader et al. postulated that the cephalad fluid shift affects the eyes directly by causing swelling of the choroid and indirectly through increased ICP, through impaired cerebrospinal fluid (CSF) absorption, and/or through a hydrostatically driven increase in the interstitial fluid content of cerebral tissue [2].

One factor that hinders the elucidation of the mechanism leading to VIIP is a lack of quantitative, continuous, and reproducible measures of VIIP severity. The NASA-proposed VIIP clinical practice guideline (CPG) classifies the severity of VIIP using a four-class ordinal scale based on a refractive change greater than >0.5 diopter and subjective assessment

N. Alperin (✉)
Department of Radiology, Miller School of Medicine, University of Miami, Miami, FL, USA

Alperin noninvasive diagnostics, Miami, FL, USA
e-mail: Nalperin@med.miami.edu

A.M. Bagci
Department of Radiology, Miller School of Medicine, University of Miami, Miami, FL, USA

of the presence of orbital and ocular changes, such as nerve sheath distention and/or globe flattening (GF). VIIP CPG classes 1 and 2 are used when there is no evidence for optic disc edema, and CPG classes 3 and 4 are used when there is low-grade (Frisén scale 0–2), and high grade (Frisén scale 3 and above) optic disc edema.

The most consistent imaging signs of VIIP in affected astronauts are flattening of the posterior sclera and protrusion of the optic disc into the globe [2]. However, determining the magnitude of globe deformations by subjective visual inspection lacks consistency and sensitivity. This work incorporates novel enabling technology to quantify the 3D globe morphology [10] and derive continuous, objective, and reproducible measures of VIIP severity. Pre-to-post-flight-accumulated globe deformations in astronauts who flew short- and long-duration spaceflight missions were quantified and then tested for associations with changes in CSF and cerebral vascular volumes, in addition to MR-derived ICP to elucidate the mechanism of VIIP.

Materials and Methods

Participants and Imaging

All participating astronauts provided written informed consent. MRI scans of the brain and the orbits, performed using a 3-T scanner (Verio, Siemens Healthcare) in 16 astronauts before and shortly after their return from space, were analyzed to quantify pre-to-post flight cerebral and ocular changes. Findings in 7 astronauts (mean age 46.1 years [SD5.5]) who flew a long-duration mission on the ISS (mean duration of 188 days [SD 22]) were compared with those in 9 astronauts (mean age of 46.9 years [SD 2.6]) who flew a short-duration mission on the Space Shuttle (14.1 days [SD 1.6]). Five astronauts primarily from the short duration group had previously flown a long-duration mission on the ISS. Imaging of the brain included a T1-weighted 3D MPRAGE scan with 0.9-mm slice thickness and 1.0-mm in-plane resolution, and imaging of the orbits included three T2-weighted 3D TSE-FS scans, a bilateral scan with 0.8-mm isometric resolution, and a separate acquisition for each eye with 0.6-mm isotropic resolution.

Image Data Analysis

The deformations of the eye globes in astronauts with signs of VIIP are well illustrated by MRI [2, 3], although determining the magnitude of the deformations by subjective visual inspection has insufficient sensitivity for quantitation of the spaceflight-induced changes. A computerized approach to the quantitation of GF and NP, previously used in idiopathic intracranial hypertension (IIH) [8] was used as an objective measure of VIIP severity. Briefly, the computerized approach automatically segments the eye globe and converts the complex 3D curvature of the posterior wall into a 2D color map of the distances from the center of the globe to every point on the posterior hemisphere of the globe. A perfectly round hemisphere has a uniform color distance map, with all distances equal to the radius of that hemisphere. Measures of GF and NP are then derived from ratios of distances to the optic disc region, its surrounding region, and the peripheral regions. The respective roles of the CSF and vascular fluid in VIIP were then tested by determining associations between globe deformations, increases in ventricular and orbital CSF volumes, and/or with the vascular fluid content of brain tissue.

Determination of the Intra-Orbital CSF Volume

The CSF space around the extra-cranial segment of the optic nerve is adjacent to the posterior pole of the eye globe and therefore, expansion of this space can cause globe deformations. Reliable measurements of changes in this small CSF space shape and size are challenging and therefore a computerized approach developed for spinal CSF [9] was tailored for this purpose. Briefly, the algorithm first identifies the optic nerve path within the orbit. The surrounding CSF region is then segmented on perpendicular consecutive planes using 2D matched filters optimized to detect annular shapes.

Determination of Changes in Ventricular CSF, Cerebral Vascular Fluid Volumes, and MRICP

Volumes of the ventricles, cortical gray matter (GM) and white matter (WM) brain tissues were obtained using FreeSurfer software [10]. The segmented brain region includes the cellular, vascular and interstitial fluid compartments. Therefore, pre-to-post-flight changes in GM and WM volumes mainly represent the change in the cerebral vascular fluid content.

The previously described MRICP method was used to derive the intracranial compliance based on the ratios of the volume and pressure changes during the cardiac cycle. The ICP is then estimated using the inverse relationship between compliance and ICP [11].

Statistical Methods

Significance of differences in baseline measures and pre-to-post-flight changes between the short- and long-duration cohorts were assessed using an unpaired t test. The associations among individual measures were tested using Spearman's correlation coefficients (SCCs). SCCs were preferred over Pearson's correlation coefficient when a linear association between the variables was not necessarily expected and when a scatter plot of the variables indicated outlier data points. Statistical analyses were performed using MATLAB (The MathWorks, Natick, MA, USA).

Results

Baseline and Pre-to-Post-Flight-Accumulated VIIP-Related Changes

Preflight and pre-to-post-flight changes in VIIP measures (GF and NP indices), CSF volumes (orbital and ventricular), and brain tissue volumes (GM and WM) are listed in Table 1. Preflight baseline measures were similar in the short- and long-duration cohorts, except for GF. Baseline mean GF index was significantly larger in the short-duration cohort. The astronauts who had previously flown a long-duration mission had significantly increased GF and NP indices at baseline relative to the other astronauts with no previous long-duration spaceflight experience (1.12 [SD 0.03] vs 1.09 [SD 0.03]; $p = 0.03$, and 1.08 [SD 0.02] vs 1.05 [SD 0.01]; $p = 0.002$) respectively.

Post-flight, 6 of the 9 short-duration astronauts and 6 of the 7 long-duration astronauts were classified by NASA flight surgeons as having VIIP based on CPG classification. The 6 short-duration astronauts all had class 2 and of the 6 long-duration astronauts, 4 had class 2 and 2 had class 3 (with optic disc edema).

Pre-to-post-flight ocular changes measured using quantitative imaging demonstrated significant increases in GF and NP only in the long-duration cohort. The changes in the short-duration cohort were within the range of measurement variability.

Baseline and Pre-to-Post-Flight-Accumulated Change in CSF Volumes

There were no statistically significant differences in baseline orbital and ventricular CSF volumes between the short- and long-duration astronauts. Pre-to-post-flight change in the orbital and ventricular CSF volume was insignificant in the short-duration group, but significant in the long-duration cohort, with an average increase of 51 µl. Intracranial ventricular CSF volume demonstrated a similar behavior. Post-flight, ventricular CSF volume did not change in the short-duration cohort. However, a significant increase of 2.9 ml was measured in the long-duration cohort. In contrast to CSF volume, the post-flight GM and WM brain tissue volumes did not increase. The post-flight median GM and WM volumes were actually smaller in the long-duration cohort compared with the short-duration group, but the differences were not significant.

Associations Between Ocular Changes and Changes in CSF, Vascular Fluid Volumes, and MRICP

Testing for associations between the ocular changes and CSF volumes revealed significant positive associations with the orbital and ventricular CSF volumes. The changes in GF and NP were positively associated with the increase in the orbital CSF volume, with SCC of 0.58 ($p = 0.0005$) and 0.68 ($p < 0.00001$) respectively. The associations of the GF and NP with changes in the ventricular volume were also significant with SCC of 0.63 ($p = 0.0001$) and 0.71 ($p < 0.00001$) respectively. In contrast, the associations with cortical GM (SCC of -0.31, $p = 0.08$ and -0.33, $p = 0.07$) and WM volumes (SCC of -0.06, $p = 0.76$ and -0.18, $p = 0.33$) were not significant. Globe deformations were not associated with an increase in brain tissue volume.

Table 1 Mean and SD of preflight baseline measures and accumulated pre-to-post-flight changes for the short- and long-duration cohorts

	Preflight baseline						Pre-to-post-flight changes					
	GF	NP	Orbital CSF Vol. (µl)	Vent. CSF Vol. (ml)	GM Vol. (ml)	WM Vol. (ml)	Change in GF	Change in NP	Change in orbital CSF Vol. (µl)	Change in Vent. CSF Vol. (ml)	Change in GM Vol. (ml)	Change in WM Vol. (ml)
Short-duration ($n = 9$)	1.10 (0.03)	1.06 (0.02)	227 (156)	18.4 (13.5)	484 (38.7)	502 (37.7)	−0.001 (0.006)	−0.002 (0.007)	1.8 (29)	0.0 (0.4)	−1.8 (7.1)	3.9 (7.7)
Long-duration ($n = 7$)	1.08 (0.02)	1.05 (0.01)	239 (114)	19.8 (9.6)	492 (11.3)	516 (39.9)	0.031 (0.019)	0.026 (0.013)	51 (37)	2.9 (3.0)	−5.4 (6.3)	1.5 (8.7)
p value	0.03	0.16	0.79	0.82	0.59	0.47	0.00002	<0.00001	0.0005	0.048	0.31	0.58

GF globe flattening, *NP* nerve protrusion, *CSF* cerebrospinal fluid, *GM* gray matter, *WM* white matter

Finally, pre-to-post-flight MRICP was not statistically different in both cohort except for a moderate increase in of about 6 mmHg, that was observed in two ISS astronauts with large ocular structural changes.

Discussion

Using automated quantitation of the ocular structural changes observed in VIIP, namely GF and optic NP, and automated segmentation of the orbital CSF space around the optic nerve, this study documented that VIIP-associated ocular changes occur only during long-duration spaceflight and that the magnitude of the ocular changes correlate significantly with increases in the orbital CSF volume. The computerized quantitation of the globe deformations yields continuous and reproducible measures of GF and NP that have stronger statistical power compared with the ordinal measures available with subjective assessments. Therefore, the automated quantitation enabled the discovery of the correlations between the ocular changes and increased orbital CSF volume, even with a relatively small n, thereby establishing the primary role of CSF in the formation of VIIP.

Findings in this study also explain several VIIP-related symptoms. GF causes shortening of the optical axis leading to the hyperopic shift commonly experienced by astronauts on the ISS.

Another intriguing finding was the more flattened globes at baseline in the short-duration cohort compared with the long-duration group. We attribute this to the fact that 4 of the 9 short-duration astronauts had undertaken a previous long-duration mission on the ISS compared with only 1 from the long-duration cohort. Comparing the 4 short-duration astronauts who had undertaken a previous mission with the 5 short-duration astronauts who did not reveal that both the GF and the NP were significantly increased in the astronauts who had undertaken a previous long-duration mission several years back. This implies that the space-induced globe deformations do not fully reverse upon return to earth, at least not for several years. This also explains why short-duration astronauts were classified as having VIIP based on the CPG and the misconception that VIIP also occurs during short-duration spaceflight [2, 3].

Findings in this study lessen support for the role of intracranial cephalad vascular fluid shift in VIIP, as globe deformations were not positively associated with increases in brain tissue volumes. A pictorial summary of the proposed mechanism for VIIP formation contracted based on our findings is shown in Fig. 1.

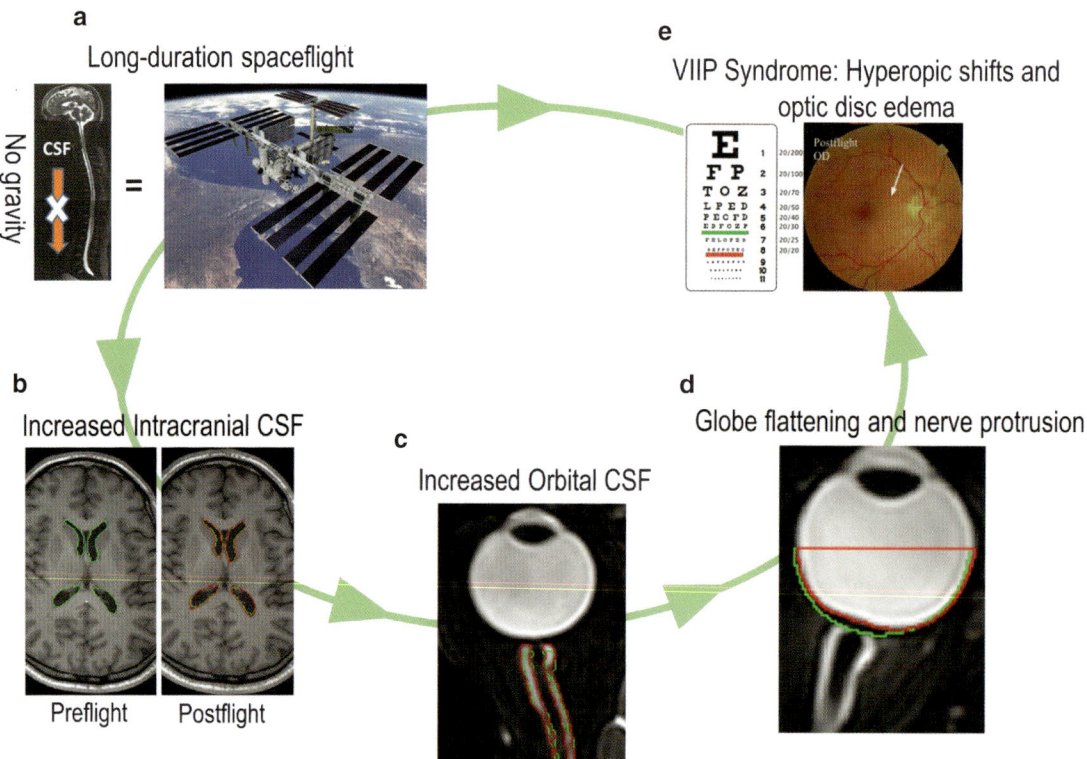

Fig. 1 A pictorial summary of the proposed mechanism for VIIP formation. (**a**) The lack of gravity in space eliminates movement of CSF from the cranium to the spinal canal. Significant pre-to-post-flight increase in ventricular (**b**) and orbital (**c**) CSF volumes occurred only in the long-duration astronauts (*green*- preflight, *red*- pre-to-post-flight CSF boundaries). (**d**) Expansion of the orbital CSF space likely compresses the posterior pole of the eye globe resulting with the observed ocular deformations. (**e**) VIIP symptoms linked with the observed ocular deformations

Conclusions

Using continuous, quantitative measures of VIIP-related ophthalmic deformations, this study provides evidence for the primary role of CSF in the formation of VIIP and a lesser role for intracranial cephalad vascular fluid-shift. The ocular changes occurring during long-duration exposure to microgravity are significantly associated with a large increase in orbital and ventricular CSF volumes, but not with brain tissue volumes.

Funding Information This work has been funded by NASA grants NNX14AB51G through a Cooperative Agreement to Alperin Noninvasive Diagnostics, Inc.

Conflicts of interest statement Noam Alperin is a shareholder in Alperin Noninvasive Diagnostics Inc.

References

1. NASA. Human Exploration Research Opportunities (HERO) NNJ14ZSA001N-MIXEDTOPICS Appendix E: Behavioral health & performance and human health countermeasures topics. 2015.
2. Mader TH, Gibson CR, Pass AF, Kramer LA, Lee AG, Fogarty J, et al. Optic disc edema, globe flattening, choroidal folds, and hyperopic shifts observed in astronauts after long-duration space flight. Ophthalmology. 2011;118(10):2058–69. doi: 10.1016/j.ophtha.2011.06.021
3. Kramer LA, Sargsyan AE, Hasan KM, Polk JD, Hamilton DR. Orbital and intracranial effects of microgravity: findings at 3-T MR imaging. Radiology. 2012;263(3):819–27. doi: 10.1148/radiol.12111986
4. Mader TH, Gibson CR, Pass AF, Lee AG, Killer HE, Hansen HC, et al. Optic disc edema in an astronaut after repeat long-duration space flight. J Neuroophthalmol. 2013;33(3):249–55.
5. Parazynski SE, Hargens AR, Tucker B, Aratow M, Styf J, Crenshaw A. Transcapillary fluid shifts in tissues of the head and neck during and after simulated microgravity. J Appl Physiol. 1991;71(6):2469–75.
6. Herault S, Fomina G, Alferova I, Kotovskaya A, Poliakov V, Arbeille P. Cardiac, arterial and venous adaptation to weightlessness during 6-month MIR spaceflights with and without thigh cuffs (bracelets). Eur J Appl Physiol. 2000;81(5):384–90.
7. Hargens AR, Richardson S. Cardiovascular adaptations, fluid shifts, and countermeasures related to space flight. Respir Physiol Neurobiol. 2009;169(Suppl 1):S30–3.
8. Alperin N, Bagci AM, Lam BL, Sklar E. Automated quantitation of the posterior scleral flattening and optic nerve protrusion by MRI in idiopathic intracranial hypertension. AJNR Am J Neuroradiol. 2013;34(12):2354–9. doi: 10.3174/ajnr.A3600
9. Alperin N, Bagci AM, Lee SH, Lam BL. Automated quantitation of spinal CSF volume and measurement of craniospinal CSF redistribution following lumbar withdrawal in idiopathic intracranial hypertension. AJNR Am J Neuroradiol. 2016.; doi: 10.3174/ajnr.A4837
10. Fischl B, Salat DH, Busa E, Albert M, Dieterich M, Haselgrove C, et al. Whole brain segmentation: automated labeling of neuroanatomical structures in the human brain. Neuron. 2002;33(3):341–55.
11. Alperin NJ, Lee SH, Loth F, Raksin PB, Lichtor T. MR-Intracranial pressure (ICP): a method to measure intracranial elastance and pressure noninvasively by means of MR imaging: baboon and human study. Radiology. 2000;217(3):877–85. doi: 10.1148/radiology.217.3.r00dc42877

Ventriculomegaly in the Elderly: Who Needs a Shunt? A MRI Study on 90 Patients

Marc Baroncini, Olivier Balédent, Celine Ebrahimi Ardi, Valerie Deken Delannoy, Gregory Kuchcinski, Alain Duhamel, Gustavo Soto Ares, Jean-Paul Lejeune, and Jérôme Hodel

Abstract *Objective*: In the case of ventriculomegaly in the elderly, it is often difficult to differentiate between communicating chronic hydrocephalus (CCH) and brain atrophy. The aim of this study is to describe the MRI criteria of CCH, defined by a symptomatic patient with ventriculomegaly and that improved after shunt placement.

Materials and methods: Magnetic resonance imaging was prospectively evaluated in 90 patients with ventriculomegaly. Patients were classified into three groups: patients without clinical signs of CCH (control, $n = 47$), patients with CCH treated by shunt placement with clinical improvement (responders, $n = 36$), and patients with CCH treated using a shunt without clinical improvement (nonresponders, $n = 7$). MRI parameters of the two groups of interest (responders vs. controls) were compared.

Results: Compared with controls, Evans' index ($p = 0.029$), ventricular area ($p < 0.01$), and volume ($p = 0.0001$) were higher in the responders. In this group, the callosal angle was smaller ($p \leq 0.0001$) and the aqueductal stroke volume (SVa) of CSF was higher ($p \leq 0.0001$) than in controls. On the ROC curves, the optimal cut-off values for differentiating between responders and controls were a ventricular area >33.5 cm^2, a callosal angle <90.8° and a SVa > 136.5 µL/R-R. In multivariate analysis, responders remained associated with SVa and callosal angle, with a c-statistic of 0.90 (95%CI, 0.83–0.98).

Conclusion: On suspicion of CCH, a large ventricular area, a small callosal angle, and an increased aqueductal stroke volume are important MRI arguments that can be associated with the clinical evaluation and dynamic testing of CSF to confirm the indication for a shunt.

Keywords Normal pressure hydrocephalus • Cerebrospinal fluid • MRI • Ventriculoperitoneal shunt • Ventriculomegaly

Introduction

Chronic communicating hydrocephalus (CCH) is a neurological disorder that is partially reversible if treated using shunt surgery. It is characterized by a triad of symptoms, i.e., gait disturbance, cognitive impairment, and urinary incontinence. Radiological diagnosis of CCH is often difficult to differentiate from normal aging and vascular dementia, in which brain atrophy with ventricular dilatation is present. Several quantitative parameters had been suggested as predictive of the shunt response. High-convexity tightness is a neuroimaging feature predictive of shunt response [1]. The callosal angle was first described by Benson et al. for the diagnostic finding of NPH on pneumoencephalography [2] and was then used by other teams [3]. More recently, Ishii et al. [4] found a smaller callosal angle in a group of hydrocephalus patients, in comparison with a group of patients with Alzheimer's disease. A sharp callosal angle, <90°, is produced by elevation of dilated lateral ventricles and compression by dilated lateral commissure. Virhammar et al. also reported that the callosal angle is smaller in shunt-responsive hydrocephalus patients than in non-responsive patients [5], with a very reproducible measurement.

Recently, our understanding of CSF dynamics has also been considerably improved by the use of phase-contrast magnetic resonance imaging (PCMRI). MRI may demonstrate CSF "flow void" in the aqueduct [6]. During the car-

M. Baroncini (✉) • J.-P. Lejeune
Neurosurgery, Lille University Hospital, Lille, France
e-mail: marc.baroncini@me.com

O. Balédent
Medical Imaging Unit, Amiens University Hospital, Amiens, France

C. Ebrahimi Ardi • G. Kuchcinski • G. Soto Ares • J. Hodel
Neuroradiology, Lille University Hospital, Lille, France

V. Deken Delannoy • A. Duhamel
Lille University Hospital, EA 2694 – Santé publique: épidémiologie et qualité des soins, Lille, France

diac cycle, the CSF oscillates between the intracranial compartment and spinal canal. In chronic hydrocephalus, the movement of CSF among the ventricular, intracranial subarachnoidal, and lumbar compartments may become disorganized. By using PCMRI it is possible and easy to measure the volume of CSF flowing through the aqueduct in either direction over a cardiac cycle (stroke volume). For some authors, a large aqueductal CSF stroke volume is a good indicator of a shunt placement, which should lead to the clinical improvement of dilated patients [6, 7]. However, the interest of these morphological and velocimetric criteria for the diagnosis of CCH have not been studied together. Our objective in this study was therefore to define multimodal MRI criteria of a shunt in symptomatic patients with ventriculomegaly and suspected CCH.

Methods

Patients and MRI

All subjects were over 18 and had ventriculomegaly, defined by Evans' index >0.3. We secondarily excluded patients with aqueductal stenosis. Clinical evaluation was performed with mini mental state examination and a score based on Larsson's work [8], which evaluate gait (normal gait: 0 points to wheelchair: 5 points), autonomy (independence: 0 points to hospitalized patient: 4 points), and urinary incontinence (1 point if present).

Brain MRI was performed at 3T (Achieva, Philips, Best, The Netherlands) and included the following sequences for each patient: 3D T1w, 3D heavily T2w TSE Brainview, phase contrast imaging (in and through planes at the level of the aqueduct and C2/C3). Sequence parameters are summarized in Table 1.

Image Analysis

The Evans' index and the ventricular area were calculated on an axial section situated 1 cm above the bi-commissural line (Fig. 1). The ventricular area was semi-automated, segmented and calculated using Osirix Lite software on the 3D T1w sequence. The callosal angle was measured on a coronal section perpendicular to the midline of the bi-commissural line.

A well-defined, disproportionately enlarged subarachnoid space corresponds to an enlargement of the lateral commissure and rarefaction of the subarachnoid spaces of the vertex. The CSF volumes within total, ventricular, and subarachnoid spaces were calculated using the available workstation (adw, General Electric) in addition to the ratio between ventricular and subarachnoid CSF volumes.

Finally, stroke volume of the cerebrospinal fluid (CSF) was evaluated through the aqueductal (SVa) and at C2C3 (SVc). Post-treatment was realized using Flow Software, which can be downloaded free at www.tidam.fr [9].

Complete post-treatment took <10 min by MRI and was realized after the classification of patients into one of the three groups. The data were therefore blinded from the clinicians until surgery and clinical follow-up had been performed.

Patients with clinical symptoms of chronic hydrocephalus (at least two elements of the Adams and Hakim triad [10] ± CSF tap test) were operated on by the same neurosurgeon (MB). A ventriculo-peritoneal shunt was performed with a regulated flow valve. Each patient was controlled before leaving the hospital with abdominal X-ray and head CT to control the position of the shunt. Clinical evaluation was performed at 3 months. Post-operative improvement was defined by at least 3 points more on the Mini-Mental State Examination or 2 points fewer on Larsson's modified score [8].

Statistical Analysis

Quantitative variables are expressed as mean (standard deviation) in the case of normal distribution or median (interquartile range: IQR) otherwise. Qualitative variables are expressed as numbers (percentage). Normality of distributions was assessed using histograms and Shapiro–Wilk test. Bivariate comparisons in MRI quantitative parameters between controls and responders were performed using Student's t test or Mann–Whitney U test for non-Gaussian distribution; comparison in a well-defined, disproportionally enlarged subarachnoid space was made using a Fisher's

Table 1 Sequence parameters

Sequence	TR (ms)	TE (ms)	Voxel size (mm)	FOV	Slices	Flip angle (°)
3D T1	9.8	4.6	$0.88 \times 1.19 \times 1$	$200 \times 239 \times 176$	176	8
T2 Brainview	2,500	700	$1.1 \times 1.1 \times 2.2$	$200 \times 239 \times 176$	164	90
Phase contrast MRI	15	10	$1.5 \times 1.5 \times 5$	$150 \times 102 \times 5$	1	10

TR repetition time, *TE* echo time, *FOV* field of view

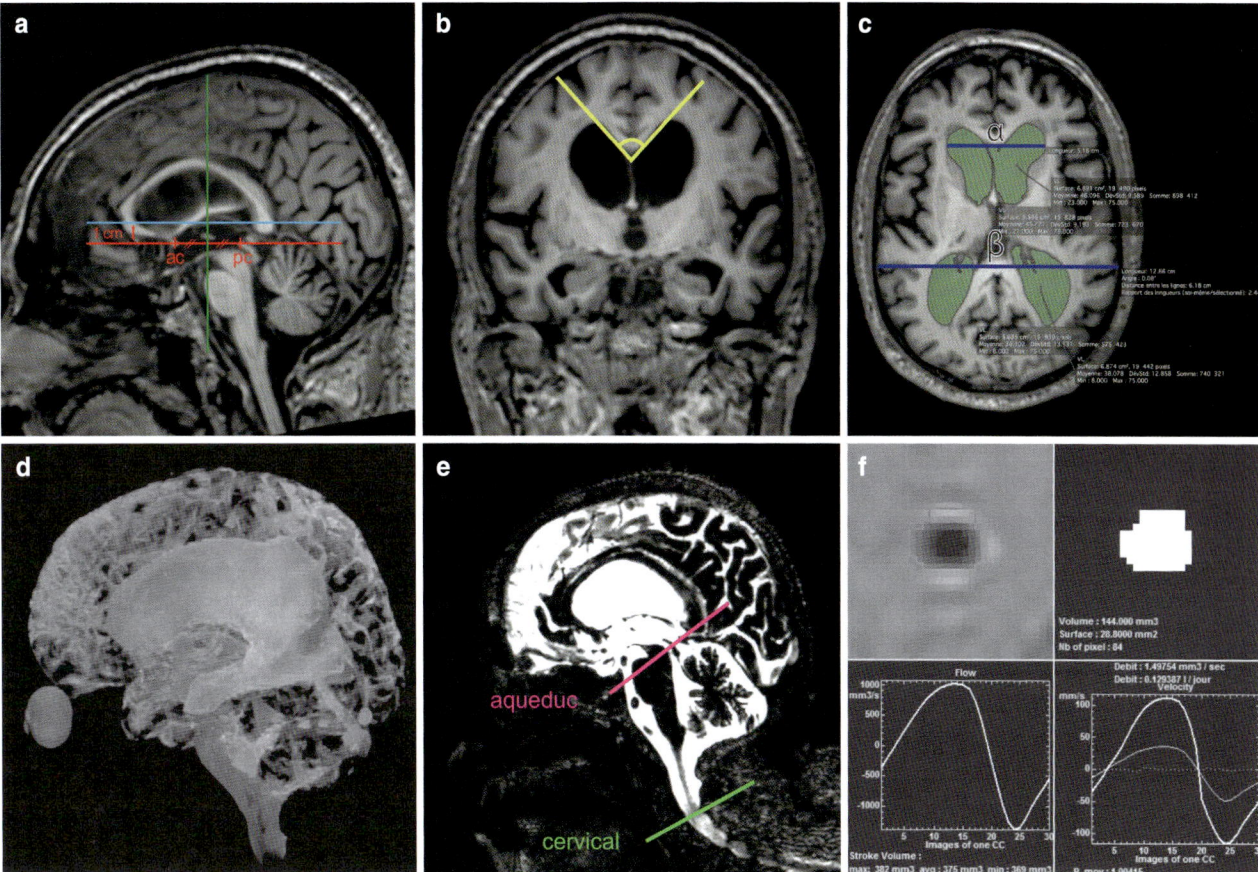

Fig. 1 Morphometric analysis. (**a**) Identification of the anterior (*ac*) and the posterior commissure (*pc*). *Green line*: coronal section perpendicular to the midline of the bi-commissural line (*red line*); *blue line*: axial section situated 1 cm above the bi-commissural line. (**b**) Callosal angle. (**c**) Evans' index (α/β) and ventricular surface. (**d**) 3D reconstruction of CSF volumes. (**e**) Sagittal section with planes at the level of the aqueduct and C2/C3 for phase contrast imaging. (**f**) Aqueductal stroke volume

exact test. Associations between MRI quantitative parameters were assessed by calculating Pearson's correlation coefficient. Receiver operating characteristics (ROC) curve analysis was carried out to assess the ability of relevant MRI quantitative parameters to discriminate between the two groups. The area under the ROC curve (AUC or c-statistic) values were calculated and the optimal cut-off values were determined using the Youden index. Sensitivity (Se) and specificity (Sp) for the optimal thresholds were calculated with their 95% exact confidence intervals (CIs).

Quantitative parameters of MRI, which differed significantly between the two groups (Evans' index, ventricular area, callosal angle, and SVa) were included in a backward-stepwise logistic regression analysis; ventricular volume was not included in the multivariate analysis owing to the collinearity with the ventricular area. The log-linearity assumption was checked for each MRI parameter using restricted cubic spline functions. We examined the performance of the final model by determining its calibration (using the Hosmer–Lemeshow test) and discrimination (using the c-statistic). This multivariate analysis was repeated after the exclusion of SVa.

Statistical testing was done at the two-tailed α level of 0.05. Data were analyzed using SAS software package, release 9.3 (SAS Institute, Cary, NC, USA). and GraphPad Prism version 6.00 for Mac OsX (GraphPad Software, La Jolla, CA, USA; www.graphpad.com).

Results

Based on clinical evaluation, the patients were classified into three groups (Fig. 2): 47 patients had no clinical signs of chronic hydrocephalus (control group), whereas 43 patients with symptoms were drained using a ventriculo-peritoneal shunt; 36 of them were clinically improved (responders), the 7 other patients were not significantly clinically improved after surgery (nonresponders). The distribution of each MRI parameter was described according to each study group in Fig. 3.

Compared with controls, Evans' index was slightly higher in responders and nonresponders, with a significant difference

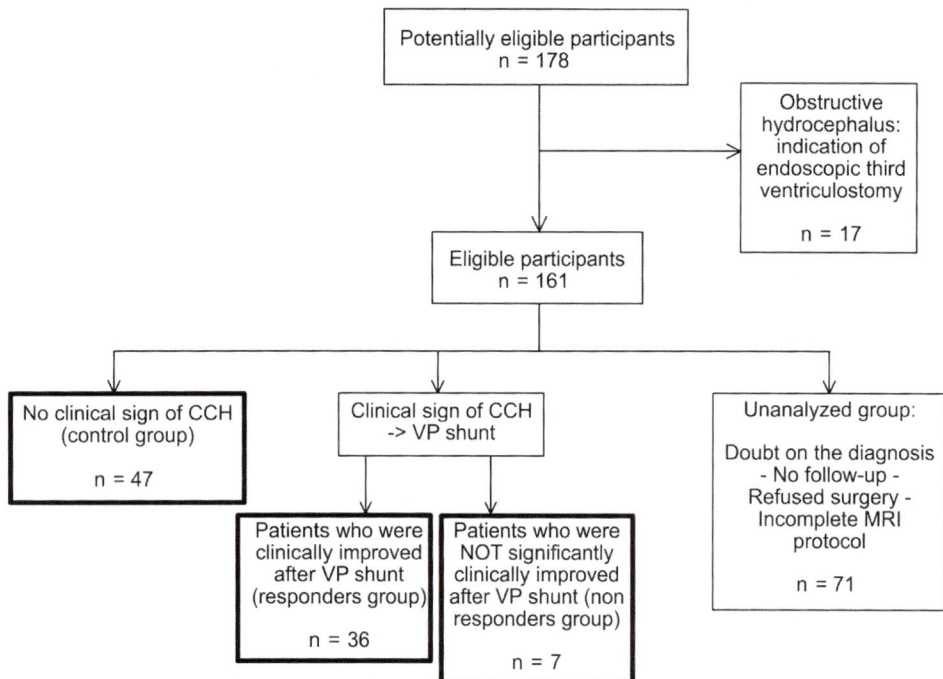

Fig. 2 Diagram of report flow of participants throughout the study

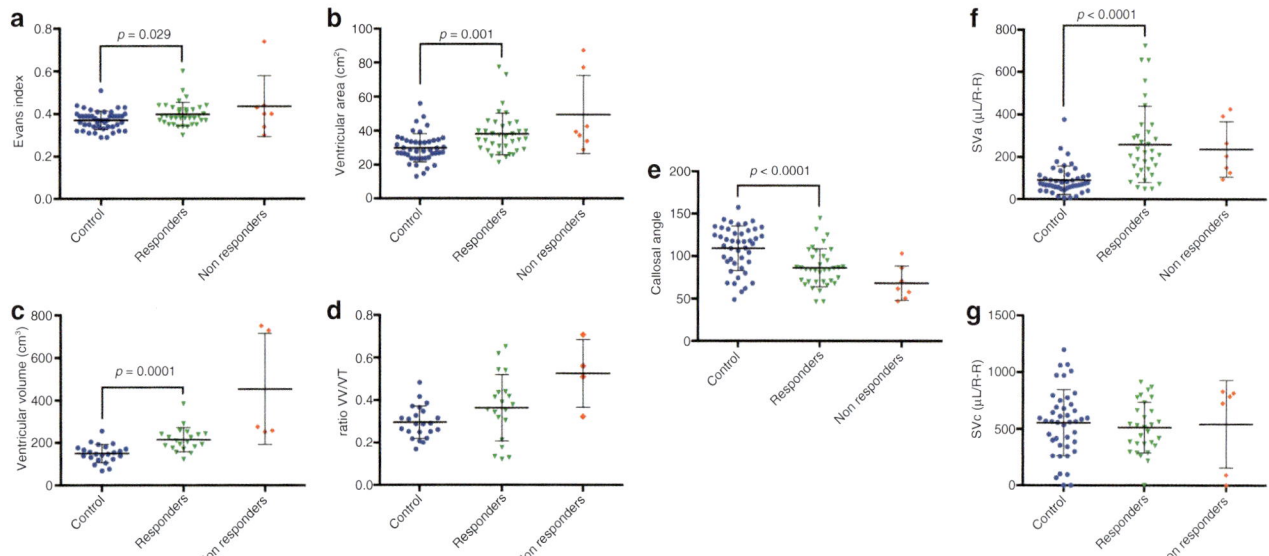

Fig. 3 Scatter plot graph of (**a**) Evans index, (**b**) ventricular areas, (**c**) ventricular volume, (**d**) ratio ventricular volume/total volume of CSF, (**e**) callosal angle, (**f**) aqueductal stroke volume, and (**g**) cervical stroke volume with comparisons between the two groups of interest (controls and responders)

between controls and responders (median [IQR]: 0.37 [0.34–0.39] vs 0.39 [0.37–0.43], $p = 0.029$). A greater difference between controls and surgical groups was found for ventricular area and volume values (Fig. 3b, c). The mean (±SD) ventricular area was 38 ± 12.2 cm^2 in responders and 29.8 ± 8.3 cm^2 in controls ($p = 0.001$). The corresponding values for ventricular volume were 215.2 ± 57.8 cm^3 vs 149.7 ± 42.8 cm^3 ($p = 0.0001$). There were no significant differences in the total volume of CSF and the ratio of ventricular volume/total volume of CSF between the two groups of interests (Fig. 3d). The ventricular area and the ventricular volume correlated strongly in controls ($r = 0.89$, $p < 0.0001$) and in responders ($r = 0.87$, $p < 0.0001$, Fig. 4a). In ROC analysis, the AUC of the ventricular area to differentiate controls and responders was 0.72

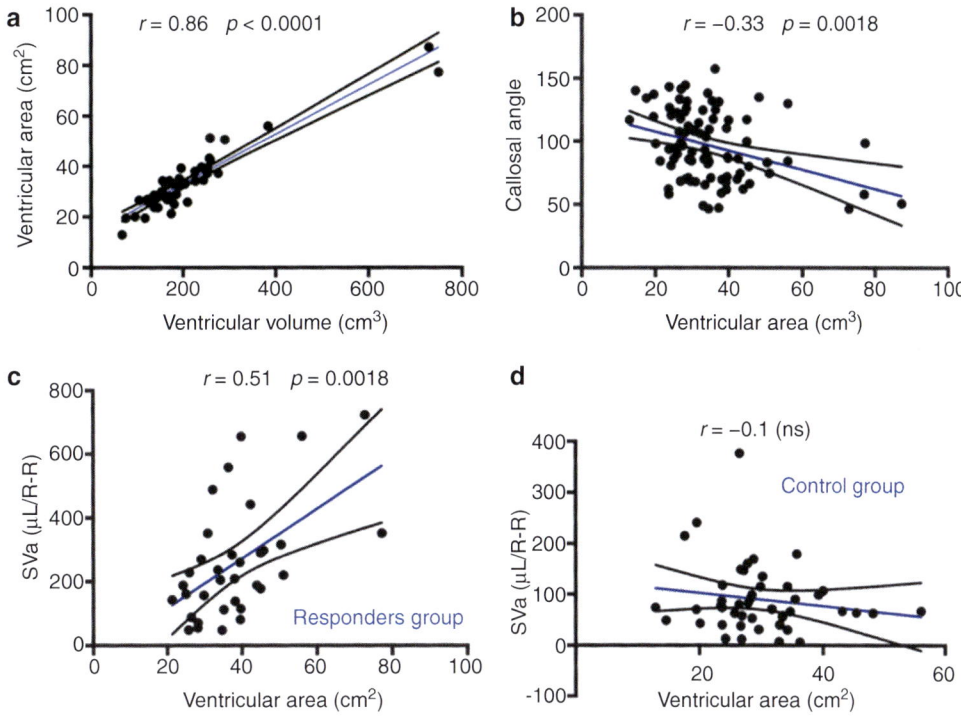

Fig. 4 Correlation graphics between ventricular area and (**a**) volume, (**b**) callosal angle and ventricular area, (**c**) SVa and ventricular area for the responders group, and (**d**) the control group

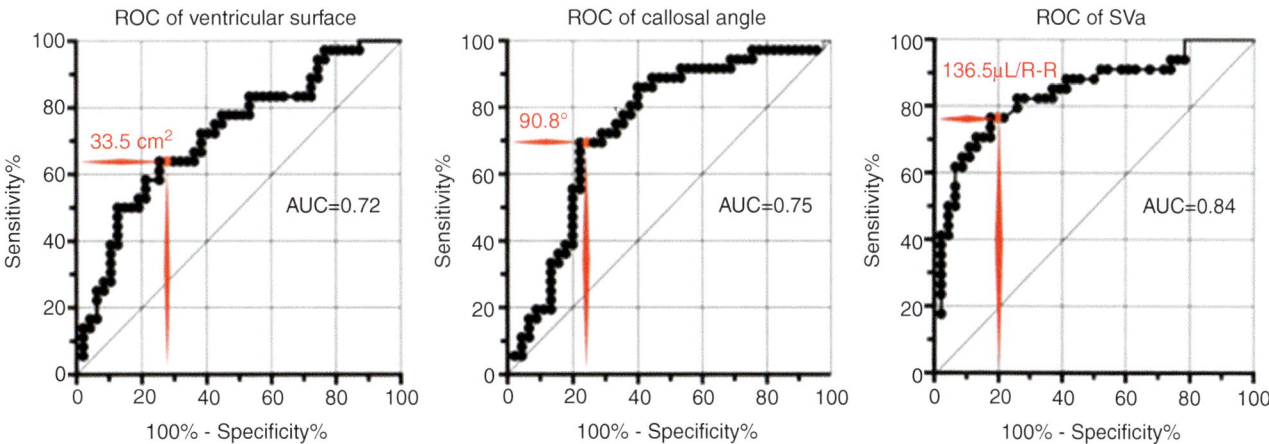

Fig. 5 Plot of the receiver operating characteristic analysis of the callosal angle, ventricular area, and SVa values for discrimination between control and responder patients. The optimal cut-off value according to the Youden index is in red on each figure

(95%CI, 0.609–0.831, Fig. 5). The optimal cut-off value according to the Youden index was found at >33.5 cm² (Fig. 5), with a specificity of 74.5% (95%CI, 59.6–86.1%) and a sensitivity of 63.9% (95%CI, 46.2–79.2%).

The callosal angle was smaller in surgical groups compared with controls (Fig. 3e). The mean callosal angle was 109.2° ± 26.2° in controls compared with 86.4° ± 22.2° in responders ($p < 0.0001$) and 68.4° ± 20.2° in nonresponders. The AUC of the callosal angle to differentiate controls and responders was 0.75 (95%CI, 0.635–0.855), with an optimal cut-off value of <90.8° (Fig. 3b, Sp: 77.8% (95%CI, 62.9–88.8%); Se: 69.4% (95%CI, 51.9–83.6%). The ventricular area and the callosal angle showed correlation ($r = -0.33$, $p = 0.0018$, Fig. 4b).

A well-defined disproportionately enlarged subarachnoid space was found in only 4 out of 46 patients of the control group, but in 13 out of 36 patients of the responders ($p = 0.007$) and 5 out of 7 patients of nonresponders (Fig. 6).

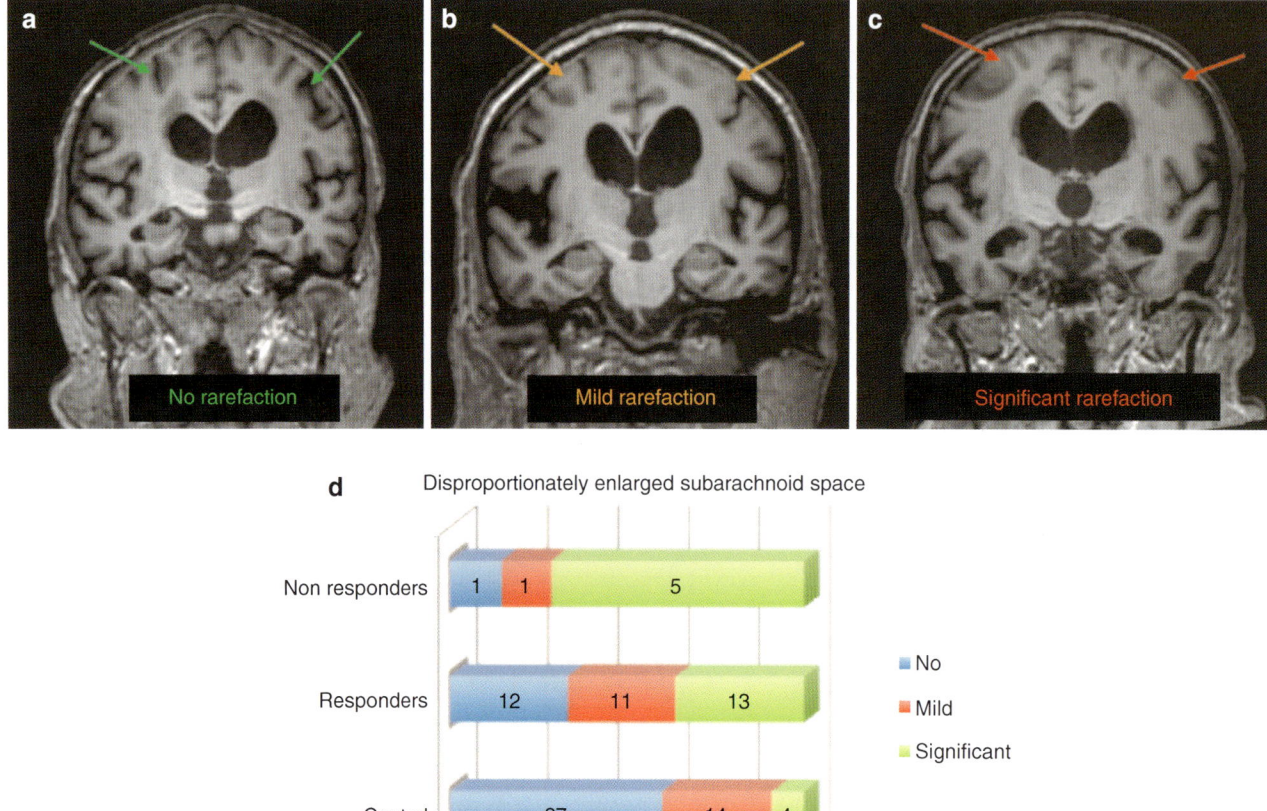

Fig. 6 Coronal slice (**a**) without rarefaction of subarachnoid spaces of the vertex, (**b**) with mild rarefaction or (**c**) with a significant rarefaction. (**d**) Histogram representation of patients

Concerning the velocimetry analysis, the SVa was lowest in the control group (median, 72.5 [IQR, 53–115] μL/cardiac cycle [R-R]) compared with responders (median, 214.5 [IQR, 138–317] μL/R-R, $p < 0.0001$) and nonresponders (median, 205 [IQR, 127–393]). There was no difference between the two groups of interest regarding SVc (Fig. 3g). We found a correlation between SVa and ventricular area in the responder group ($r = 0.54$, $p < 0.001$), but not in the controls ($r = -0.16$, $p = 0.29$). The AUC of the callosal angle to differentiate controls and responders of the SVa was 0.84 (95%CI, 0.75–0.93) with an optimal cut-off value of >136.5 μL/R-R (Sp: 82.6% [95%CI, 68.6–92.2%]; Se: 76.5% [95%CI, 58.8–89.3%]).

In backward-selection logistic regression analysis including Evans' index, ventricular area, callosal angle, and SVa, responders (compared with controls) remained significantly associated with SVa and callosal angle. Based on this model, we derived a first predictive score for CCH diagnosis using the regression coefficients ($1.8512 + 0.0169 \times$ SVa $- 0.0469 \times$ callosal angle). The optimal cut-off values for CCH diagnosis was ≥0.32 (Se = 85.3%; Sp = 86.4%). The AUC of this predictive score indicates an excellent discrimination (AUC: 0.90, 95%CI, 0.82–0.98) with a good calibration (Hosmer–Lemeshow test, $p = 0.26$). A second predictive score was derived from a backward-selection logistic regression analysis including the same MRI parameters except for the SVa parameters. This second score was constructed using the surface area and the callosal angle, both selected as significant prognostic factors in the second multivariate model (score = $0.4951 + 0.0740 \times$ ventricular area $- 0.0327 \times$ callosal angle). The optimal cut-off value for CCH diagnosis was ≥0.75 (Se = 88.9%; Sp = 57.8%), with a good calibration and a moderate discrimination (AUC: 0.79, 95% CI 0.69–0.89).

Discussion

One of the major challenges of the chronic hydrocephalus syndrome is to establish relevant tools to confirm a clinical diagnosis. Several studies are based on invasive tests. MRI has the advantage of the absence of morbidity and can serve as initial assessment before other more invasive explorations. We present in this study a radiological score based on the aqueductal stroke volume and the callosal angle that allows a good discrimination of patients.

Ventriculomegaly is a necessary but insufficient condition for the diagnosis of hydrocephalus. The concept of ventricular area seems original and can precisely quantify this ventriculomegaly. It correlated strongly with the ventricular volume, but it was much easier and faster to calculate. We agree with Holodny et al. who consider that volumetric analysis is time-consuming, difficult to perform and requires special equipment, making it impractical to perform in routine clinical practice [11]. The calculation of ventricular area is a good compromise and is also a much more accurate piece of data than the simple Evans' index.

The concept of the callosal angle was first described many years ago [2]. It is mainly a marker of ventricular size; moreover, we have found a correlation between the callosal angle and ventricular area. Virhammar et al. [5] also found a correlation between the callosal angle and the temporal horns ($r = -0.27, p < 0.001$).

Among other neuroimaging features predictive of shunt response, Narita et al. confirm that high convexity tightness is relevant [1]. Kojoukhova et al. found that visually evaluated disproportions between suprasylvian and sylvian subarachnoid spaces were also significantly associated with hydrocephalus diagnosis [12]. Another feature observed in patients with chronic hydrocephalus is that a few sulci over the convexity or medial surface of the hemisphere were dilated [13]. Disproportion can be considered to be caused by a suprasylvian block in relation to a low-grade asymptomatic meningeal disease, possibly fibrosing meningitis of undetermined origin [14]. However, this is a rather subjective criterion, based on a visual scale with no reproducibility.

Stroke volume is defined as the average of the volume of CSF moving craniocaudally during the cardiac cycle, and could be regarded as expressions of the compliance of the system [15]. The MRI flow measurement technique is noninvasive. A hyperkinetic CSF flow in the cerebral aqueduct in CCH has been described by several authors. In the mid-1990s, Bradley et al. evaluated 19 patients with symptoms of NPH who subsequently underwent shunt placement [6]. All 13 patients with an SVa of >42 μL on that particular MRI system responded to shunt placement, whereas only 3 of the 6 patients with a SVa < 42 μL responded. Later, Scollato et al. pointed out that some of these patients may, in fact, have been very early in their disease course, because their SVa 6 months later was increased [16]. We found, in our study, a significantly higher threshold, as in the study by Luetmer et al. [17].

Conclusion

We present here important MRI guidelines for the selection of patients requiring a ventricular shunt in cases of communicating chronic hydrocephalus: a ventricular area >33.5 cm^2, a callosal angle <90.8°, and a SVa > 136.5 μL/R-R are notable parameters that must be associated with the clinical evaluation and dynamic testing of CSF [18] to confirm the indication for a shunt. There remains no consensus as to what the best supplementary prognostic test is for chronic hydrocephalus [19], but it is certain that a multidisciplinary assessment is necessary and that a shunt decision cannot be decided only on MRI criteria.

Acknowledgements This prospective study was conducted in accordance with the Declaration of Helsinki, and the protocol was approved by the ethics committee of Amiens University Hospital, where the full study protocol can be accessed (no ID RCB: 2011-A01633-38), with funds from the interregional clinical research hospital program (IR11).

Conflicts of interest statement We declare that we have no conflicts of interest.

References

1. Narita W, Nishio Y, Baba T, Iizuka O, Ishihara T, Matsuda M, et al. High-convexity tightness predicts the shunt response in idiopathic normal pressure hydrocephalus. AJNR Am J Neuroradiol. 2016. Available from: http://www.ajnr.org/cgi/doi/10.3174/ajnr.A4838.
2. Benson DF, LeMay M, Patten DH, Rubens AB. Diagnosis of normal-pressure hydrocephalus. N Engl J Med. 1970;283:609–15. Available from: http://www.nejm.org/doi/abs/10.1056/NEJM197009172831201.
3. Sjaastad O, Nordvik A. The corpus callosal angle in the diagnosis of cerebral ventricular enlargement. Acta Neurol Scand. 1973;49:396–406. Available from: http://eutils.ncbi.nlm.nih.gov/entrez/eutils/elink.fcgi?dbfrom=pubmed&id=4542888&retmode=ref&cmd=prlinks.
4. Ishii K, Kanda T, Harada A, Miyamoto N, Kawaguchi T, Shimada K, et al. Clinical impact of the callosal angle in the diagnosis of idiopathic normal pressure hydrocephalus. Eur Radiol. 2008;18:2678–83. Available from: http://link.springer.com/10.1007/s00330-008-1044-4.
5. Virhammar J, Laurell K, Cesarini KG, Larsson E-M. The callosal angle measured on MRI as a predictor of outcome in idiopathic normal-pressure hydrocephalus. J Neurosurg. 2014;120:178–84. Available from: http://thejns.org/doi/abs/10.3171/2013.8.JNS13575.
6. Bradley WG, Scalzo D, Queralt J, Nitz WN, Atkinson DJ, Wong P. Normal-pressure hydrocephalus: evaluation with cerebrospinal fluid flow measurements at MR imaging. Radiology. 1996;198:523–9. Available from: http://pubs.rsna.org/doi/abs/10.1148/radiology.198.2.8596861.
7. Balédent O, Gondry-Jouet C, Meyer M-E, De Marco G, Le Gars D, Henry-Feugeas M-C, et al. Relationship between cerebrospinal fluid and blood dynamics in healthy volunteers and

patients with communicating hydrocephalus. Invest Radiol. 2004; 39:45–55. Available from: http://content.wkhealth.com/linkback/openurl?sid=WKPTLP:landingpage&an=00004424-200401000-00007.
8. Larsson A, Wikkelsö C, Bilting M, Stephensen H. Clinical parameters in 74 consecutive patients shunt operated for normal pressure hydrocephalus. Acta Neurol Scand. 1991;84:475–82. Available from: http://eutils.ncbi.nlm.nih.gov/entrez/eutils/elink.fcgi?dbfrom=pubmed&id=1792852&retmode=ref&cmd=prlinks.
9. Balédent O, Henry-Feugeas MC, Idy-Peretti I. Cerebrospinal fluid dynamics and relation with blood flow: a magnetic resonance study with semiautomated cerebrospinal fluid segmentation. Invest Radiol. 2001;36:368–77. Available from: http://eutils.ncbi.nlm.nih.gov/entrez/eutils/elink.fcgi?dbfrom=pubmed&id=11496092&retmode=ref&cmd=prlinks.
10. Adams RD, Fisher CM, Hakim S, Ojemann RG, Sweet WH. Symptomatic occult hydrocephalus with 'normal' cerebrospinal fluid pressure. N Engl J Med. 1965;273:117–26. Available from: http://www.nejm.org/doi/abs/10.1056/NEJM196507152730301.
11. Holodny AI, Waxman R, George AE, Rusinek H, Kalnin AJ, de Leon M. MR differential diagnosis of normal-pressure hydrocephalus and Alzheimer disease: significance of perihippocampal fissures. AJNR. Am J Neuroradiol. 1998;19:813–9. Available from: http://eutils.ncbi.nlm.nih.gov/entrez/eutils/elink.fcgi?dbfrom=pubmed&id=9613493&retmode=ref&cmd=prlinks.
12. Kojoukhova M, Koivisto AM, Korhonen R, Remes AM, Vanninen R, Soininen H, et al. Feasibility of radiological markers in idiopathic normal pressure hydrocephalus. Acta Neurochir. 2015;157:1709–19. Available from: http://link.springer.com/10.1007/s00701-015-2503-8.
13. Kitagaki H, Mori E, Ishii K, Yamaji S, Hirono N, Imamura T. CSF spaces in idiopathic normal pressure hydrocephalus: morphology and volumetry. AJNR. Am J Neuroradiol. 1998;19: 1277–84. Available from: http://eutils.ncbi.nlm.nih.gov/entrez/eutils/elink.fcgi?dbfrom=pubmed&id=9726467&retmode=ref&cmd=prlinks.
14. Adams RD. Recent observations on normal pressure hydrocephalus. Schweiz Arch Neurol Neurochir Psychiatr. 1975;116:7–15. Available from: http://eutils.ncbi.nlm.nih.gov/entrez/eutils/elink.fcgi?dbfrom=pubmed&id=1153967&retmode=ref&cmd=prlinks.
15. Bateman GA, Levi CR, Schofield P, Wang Y, Lovett EC. The pathophysiology of the aqueduct stroke volume in normal pressure hydrocephalus: can co-morbidity with other forms of dementia be excluded? Neuroradiology. 2005;47:741–8. Available from: http://link.springer.com/10.1007/s00234-005-1418-0.
16. Scollato A, Tenenbaum R, Bahl G, Celerini M, Salani B, Di Lorenzo N. Changes in aqueductal CSF stroke volume and progression of symptoms in patients with unshunted idiopathic normal pressure hydrocephalus. AJNR Am J Neuroradiol. 2008;29: 192–7. Available from: http://www.ajnr.org/cgi/doi/10.3174/ajnr.A0785.
17. Luetmer PH, Huston J, Friedman JA, Dixon GR, Petersen RC, Jack CR, et al. Measurement of cerebrospinal fluid flow at the cerebral aqueduct by use of phase-contrast magnetic resonance imaging: technique validation and utility in diagnosing idiopathic normal pressure hydrocephalus. Neurosurgery. 2002;50:534. Available from: http://eutils.ncbi.nlm.nih.gov/entrez/eutils/elink.fcgi?dbfrom=pubmed&id=11841721&retmode=ref&cmd=prlinks.
18. Czosnyka M, Pickard JD. Monitoring and interpretation of intracranial pressure. J Neurol Neurosurg Psychiatry. 2004;75:813–21. Available from: http://jnnp.bmj.com/cgi/doi/10.1136/jnnp.2003.033126.
19. Bergsneider M, Miller C, Vespa PM, Hu X. Surgical management of adult hydrocephalus. Neurosurgery. 2008;62(Suppl 2):643. Available from: http://content.wkhealth.com/linkback/openurl?sid=WKPTLP:landingpage&an=00006123-200802001-00021.

Is There a Link Between ICP-Derived Infusion Test Parameters and Outcome After Shunting in Normal Pressure Hydrocephalus?

Eva Nabbanja, Marek Czosnyka, Nicole C. Keong, Matthew Garnett, John D. Pickard, Despina Afroditi Lalou, and Zofia Czosnyka

Abstract *Objective*: The term "hydrocephalus" encompasses a range of disorders characterised by clinical symptoms, abnormal brain imaging and derangement of cerebrospinal fluid (CSF) dynamics. The ability to elucidate which patients would benefit from CSF diversion (a shunt or third ventriculostomy) is often unclear. Similar difficulties are encountered in shunted patients to predict the scope for improvement by shunt re-adjustment or revision.

Materials and methods: We compared retrospective pre-shunting infusion test results performed in 310 adult patients diagnosed with normal pressure hydrocephalus (NPH) and their improvement after shunting.

Results: Resistance to CSF outflow correlated significantly with improvement ($p < 0.05$). Other markers known from the literature, such as amplitude in CSF pulse pressure, the slope of the amplitude–pressure regression line, or elasticity did not show any correlation with outcome.

Conclusion: Outcome following shunting in adult NPH is associated with resistance to CSF outflow; however, the latter cannot be taken as an absolute predictor of shunt response.

Keywords Hydrocephalus · Infusion test · CSF outflow · Resistance

Introduction

The strict relationship between shunt responsiveness and increased resistance to cerebrospinal fluid outflow (Rout) was reported in 1981 by Børgesen and Gjerris [1]. Rout was measured using a lumbo-ventricular perfusion study, a method that potentially ensured a high level of accuracy, but is no longer in use because of its invasiveness. Predictive powers of 100% was observed for a threshold of 12 mmHg/(ml/min). Nearly 15 years later, the relationship between Rout and the results of shunting was investigated in the so-called Dutch Normal Pressure Hydrocephalus (NPH) trial [2]. The threshold for successful shunting was found to be at a higher level (17 mmHg/(ml/min)). The positive predictive power was 92%, but the negative predictive power was only 34%. Rout was measured using Katzman's lumbar infusion study [3]. Finally, quite recently, the "European NPH study" [4] reported no correlation between Rout (again, assessed using a lumbar test) and outcome following shunt surgery.

Is the result of shunting really dependent on cerebrospinal pressure volume compensation and CSF circulation? What happened between the timing of the three studies listed above, that the results changed so dramatically?

Is this a way that Rout is measured? Original lumbo-ventricular perfusion was compared with the "computerised constant rate lumbar study" and agreement between the two methods was found to be very satisfactory [5]. The "computerised infusion test" was a computer-supported single-rate Katzman's lumbar study and it is rather unlikely that such computer support was so decisive in the calculation of a relatively simple parameter such as Rout.

Perhaps the initial selection of the patients has changed. In 1981 more "pure hydrocephalus" was selected for a relatively invasive technique, whereas later, less invasive lumbar infusion study permitted patients with overlapping brain problems, such as small vessels disease, parkinsonism, Alzheimer's, etc., to be accepted.

We started our comprehensive program of CSF dynamics study in patients diagnosed with NPH in 1992. Recently, we reviewed our ongoing database to study patients with an initial diagnosis of NPH to compare the parameters describing CSF circulation and pressure–volume compensation and clinical improvement after shunting.

Materials and Methods

A total of 310 adult patients (aged 40–86) were eligible for retrospective analysis. All patients had probable NPH following clinical assessment and brain imaging. Patients underwent infusion tests and were available for follow-up via the multidisciplinary CSF clinic. Outcomes were assessed using the in-house pragmatic categorisation of patient cohorts into three groupings – sustained improvement, short-term improvement and no improvement.

The infusion test requires fluid infusion to be made into any accessible CSF compartment and monitoring of CSF pressure at the same time. Lumbar infusion, even if it has understandable limitations, is less invasive and therefore, more frequently performed. The second most frequent approach is an intraventricular infusion into a subcutaneously positioned reservoir, connected to an intraventricular catheter or shunt antechamber. In such cases, two hypodermic needles (gauge 25) are used: one for the pressure measurement and the second for the infusion.

During the infusion, the computer calculates and presents the mean pressure and pulse amplitude (with time along the X axis, Fig. 1). The resistance to CSF outflow can be calculated using simple arithmetic as the difference between the value of the plateau pressure during infusion and the resting pressure divided by the infusion rate. However, in many cases strong vasogenic waves or excessive elevation of the pressure above the safe limit of 40 mmHg do not allow the precise measurement of the final pressure plateau. Computerised analysis produces results, even in difficult cases when the infusion is terminated prematurely (i.e., without reaching the end-plateau). The algorithm utilizes a time series analysis for volume–pressure curve retrieval, the least-mean-squares model fitting and an examination of the relationship between the pulse amplitude and the mean CSF pressure. Apart from resting CSF pressure and the resistance to CSF outflow, the elastance coefficient or pressure–volume index, cerebrospinal compliance, CSF formation rate and the pulse wave amplitude of CSF pressure are calculated. All data recordings and calculations are performed using software ICM+ (https://icmplus.neurosurg.cam.ac.uk/).

Pulse amplitude increases proportionally to mean CSF pressure during the infusion study. The slope of the amplitude–pressure line (AMP/p) has been implicated as having a strong association with outcome following shunting [6]. Similarly,

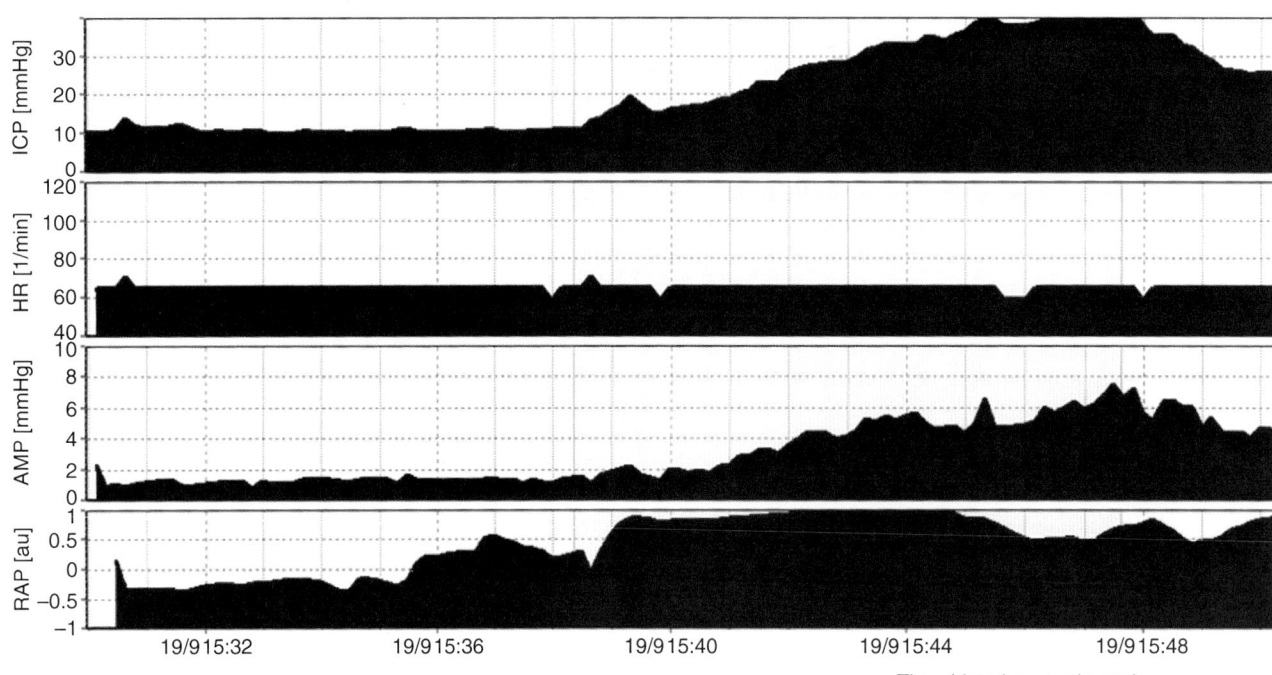

Fig. 1 Typical infusion study. Recording of mean cerebrospinal fluid (CSF) intracranial pressure (ICP). Heart rate, pulse amplitude of ICP (AMP) and index characterizing pressure volume compensatory reserve (RAP – correlation coefficient between slow changes in pulse amplitude and mean ICP). Infusion started at 15:37 with a rate of 1.5 ml/min and after 10 min, plateau pressure at 39 mmHg was reached. Elevated resistance to CSF outflow was demonstrated (21 mmHg/(ml/min)). The patient improved after shunting

pulse amplitude has been reported to be a strong predictor of outcome after surgery [7]. Consultants deciding on shunting were not blinded to the results of the infusion study.

Results

Baseline ICP was lower than 18 mmHg, median 9 mmHg. Median amplitude was 3 mmHg, median Rout 16 mmHg/(ml/min) and elasticity 0.3 (1/ml).

Seventy-nine percent of patients showed improvement after shunt insertion (60% sustainable, 19% temporary). Improvement rate increased from 1992 (60%) to 2013 (86%); $p = 0.0003$. Of all calculated CSF compensatory parameters, only Rout was associated with outcome ($p = 0.014$). Patients with Rout >13 mmHg/(ml/min) had an improvement rate of 79%, compared with 63% ($p = 0.011$) with Rout <13. Notably, none of the patients with low Rout (lower than 6 mmHg/(ml/min); $n = 7$) improved after shunting. Neither age nor sex correlated with outcome.

We investigated the best threshold value of Rout to differentiate between good and poor outcome.

On the X axis is a threshold value of Rout and on the y axis an F value of statistics for improvement.

This distribution presents two maxima (Fig. 2):
- at 13 mmHg/(ml/min)—close to the value as proposed by Børgesen and Gjerris [1]
- at 18 mmHg/(ml/min)—which was suggested in a Dutch study [3].

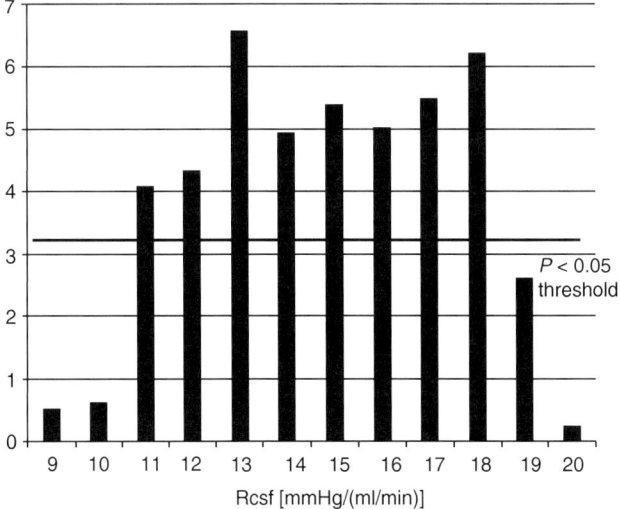

Fig. 2 Value of Kruskal–Wallis test statistics in testing the difference between improvement and no improvement after shunting as a function of estimated resistance to CSF outflow. Two maxima of distribution show the best thresholds for estimation of Rout

Discussion

Rout is related to outcome, but cannot be taken as a single discriminatory parameter in the making decision to shunt. If Rout was very low, lower than 6, we did not observe any improvement. However, between 6 and 13, the improvement rate was considerably higher. Other compensatory parameters are poorly related to outcome in our material. We need to search for better predictors for improvement after shunting in NPH. Rout was the only CSF compensatory parameter correlating with outcome following shunting. The relationship was weak but significant. Infusion studies appeared to be helpful in the assessment of the compensatory parameters both for diagnosing and yielding baseline values as a benchmark for further investigations in cases of suspected shunt malfunctions and complications.

Conclusion

- Rout is related to outcome, but cannot be taken as a yes/no parameter in decision-making about shunting.
- If Rout was very low, lower than 6, we did not observe any improvement.
- Other compensatory parameters are poorly related to outcome in our material.
- We need to continue searching for better predictors for improvement after shunting in NPH.

Conflicts of interest statement We declare that MC has a financial interest in a fraction of ICM+ software licensing fee (licensed by Cambridge Enterprise Ltd, UK).

References

1. Børgesen SE, Gjerris F. The predictive value of conductance to outflow of CSF in normal pressure hydrocephalus. Brain. 1982;105:65–86.
2. Katzman R, Hussey F. A simple constant infusion manometric test for measurement of CSF absorption. Neurology (Minneap). 1970;20:534–44.
3. Boon AJ, Tans JT, Delwel EJ, Egeler-Peerdeman SM, Hanlo PW, Wurzer HA, Avezaat CJ, de Jong DA, Gooskens RH, Hermans J. Dutch normal-pressure hydrocephalus study: prediction of outcome after shunting by resistance to outflow of cerebrospinal fluid. J Neurosurg. 1997;87(5):687–93.
4. Wikkelsø C, Hellström P, Klinge PM, Tans JT. European iNPH Multicentre Study Group. The European iNPH Multicentre Study on the predictive values of resistance to CSF outflow and the CSF Tap Test in patients with idiopathic normal pressure hydrocephalus. J Neurol Neurosurg Psychiatry. 2013;84(5):562–8.
5. Børgesen SE, Albeck MJ, Gjerris F, Czosnyka M, Laniewski P. Computerized infusion test compared to steady pressure constant

infusion test in measurement of resistance to CSF outflow. Acta Neurochir. 1992;119(1–4):12–6.
6. Anile C, De Bonis P, Albanese A, Di Chirico A, Mangiola A, Petrella G, Santini P. Selection of patients with idiopathic normal-pressure hydrocephalus for shunt placement: a single-institution experience. J Neurosurg. 2010;113(1):64–73.
7. Eide PK, Brean A. Intracranial pulse pressure amplitude levels determined during preoperative assessment of subjects with possible idiopathic normal pressure hydrocephalus. Acta Neurochir. 2006;148(11):1151–6.

Mathematical Modelling of CSF Pulsatile Flow in Aqueduct Cerebri

Zofia Czosnyka, Dong-Joo Kim, Olivier Balédent, Eric A. Schmidt, Peter Smielewski, and Marek Czosnyka

Abstract *Objective*: The phase-contrast MRI technique permits the non-invasive assessment of CSF movements in cerebrospinal fluid cavities of the central nervous system. Of particular interest is pulsatile cerebrospinal fluid (CSF) flow through the aqueduct cerebri. It is allegedly increased in hydrocephalus, having potential diagnostic value, although not all scientific reports contain unequivocally positive conclusions.

Methods: For the mathematical simulation of CSF flow, we used a computational model of cerebrospinal blood/fluid circulation designed by a former student as his PhD project. With this model, cerebral blood flow and CSF may be simulated in various vessels using a system of non-linear differential equations as time-varying signals.

Results: The amplitude of CSF flow seems to be positively related to the amplitude of pulse waveforms of intracranial pressure (ICP) in situations where mean ICP increases, such as during simulated infusion tests and following step increases of resistance to CSF outflow. An additional positive association between the pulse amplitude of ICP and CSF flow can be seen during simulated increases in the amplitude of arterial pulses (without changes in mean arterial pressure, MAP).

The opposite effect can be observed during step increases in the resistance of the aqueduct cerebri and with decreasing elasticity of the system, where the CSF flow amplitude and the ICP pulse amplitude are related inversely. Vasodilatation caused by both gradual decreases in MAP and by increases in PaCO2 provokes an elevation in the observed amplitude of pulsatile CSF flow.

Conclusions: Preliminary results indicate that the pulsations of CSF flow may carry information about both CSF-circulatory and cerebral vasogenic components. In most cases, the pulsations of CSF flow are positively related to the pulse amplitudes of both arterial pressure and ICP and to a degree of cerebrovascular dilatation.

Keywords Hydrocephalus · Mathematical modelling · Cerebrospinal fluid · Intracranial pressure · Pulsatile flow

Z. Czosnyka (✉)
Division of Neurosurgery, Addenbrookes Hospital, Cambridge, UK

Brain Physics Lab, Division of Neurosurgery,
Cambridge University Hospital, Cambridge, UK
e-mail: zc200@medachl.cam.ac.uk; zc200@medschl.cam.ac.uk

D.-J. Kim
Department Biomedical Engineering,
Korea University, Seoul, South Korea

O. Balédent
Department of Imaging and Biophysics,
Amiens University Hospital, Amiens, France

E.A. Schmidt
Department of Neurosurgery, Pourpan University Hospital,
Toulouse, France

P. Smielewski • M. Czosnyka
Brain Physics Lab, Division of Neurosurgery,
Cambridge University Hospital, Cambridge, UK

Introduction

In the last decade, pulsatile cerebrospinal fluid (CSF) flow has been studied non-invasively using the phase-contrast magnetic resonance imaging (MRI) technique [1, 2] and more recently with the time-spatial labeling inversion pulse methodology [3]. Pulsatile cerebrospinal fluid flow through the aqueduct cerebri has for quite a long time been advocated as a potential index of active hydrocephalus. Increased amplitude of flow, or increased stroke volume, was suggested to associate positively with a probability of improvement after shunting. However, there are some conflicting reports in the literature [3, 4]. The positive predictive power for improvement after shunting with a high amplitude of CSF void flow is rather agreed upon; however, low negative predictability is also emphasized [5]. The same can likely be said about both increased and low resistance to CSF outflow in lumbar infusion tests [6]—they carry good positive predictive power of increased resistance and poor negative predictive power for normal resistance to CSF outflow.

On the other hand, an increased amplitude of intracranial pressure (ICP) pulsation has been also advocated as a good indicator of improvement after shunt surgery [7]. One can possibly state that the increased pulsatility of ICP should be associated with an increased pulsatility of aqueductal CSF void flow. However, it is rather a pressure gradient between ventricles and cranial subarachnoid space which should drive aqueductal pulsatile CSF flow. Unfortunately, there is no evidence for the existence of such a gradient—neither in mean pressure nor in pressure pulsations [8].

Only the simultaneous assessment of both flow and pressure has the potential to mitigate speculation. Yet the high-intensity magnetic field of MRI creates difficulties in evaluating CSF pulse pressure and CSF flow at the same time. The indirect measurement of pressure pulsations derived from the Navier-Stokes equation [9] can produce results which are of doubtful value due to the repetitive use of the same input data (i.e. MRI-assessed flow) transformed mathematically.

Knowing that cerebrovascular conditions are strictly regulated by a rapid time response (9–12 s), we now need to determine how these conditions impact CSF void flow. Is a single time-point observation by the MRI magnet of CSF pulsatile flow sufficient for making an inference about responsiveness to shunting?

The mathematical modelling of cerebral blood flow (CBF) and CSF dynamics [10, 11] may be of assistance in shedding light on two fundamental questions: (1) Is there a direct link between the pulse amplitude of ICP and CSF void flow? (2) What is the relationship between cerebral haemodynamic parameters and CSF void flow?

Method

The mathematical model of cerebral blood and cerebrospinal fluid dynamics, described previously in detail [11], was used for this assessment. The blood pressure waveform is generated at the input and controls blood supply to the brain through two symmetrical neck arteries (ICA) with fragmentary blood mixing through the left-right communicating artery (ACoA). Main blood flow through major conductive vessels (MCAs) is directed to left and right resistive arterial pools (CVR), where autoregulation and PaCO2 regulation of CBF take place. Blood then flows through major veins to bridging veins, where an interaction between ICP and venous blood pressure takes place (venous blood follows ICP changes). Blood flows next through the dural sinuses and returns to the heart. CSF is formed at a constant rate from arterial blood, flowing through the resistance of both the aqueduct cerebri and the subarachnoid space to be passively absorbed by the sagittal sinuses. The compliance of CSF space (C_i) is associated mainly with the lumbar subarachnoid space.

Dedicated software allowing for controlled changes in various parameters in time was designed [11] on a personal computer; simulations were performed by the numerical integration of sets of differential equations describing the circuit.

Flow through the resistor symbolizing the aqueduct cerebri can be studied in the model. Its DC component is equal to the rate of CSF formation (approximately 0.3 mL/min), and its pulsations can be modulated according to the following studied conditions:

– Physiological manoeuvres: rise in ICP (infusion studies), arterial hypotension, and hypercapnia;
– Changes in parameters describing cerebrospinal dynamics: resistance to CSF outflow, resistance of aqueduct cerebri, and cerebrospinal elasticity;
– Change in overall 'brain pulsatility'.

This model is fully deterministic; therefore, results were presented as observations without any statistical evaluation.

Results

Response to Change in Cerebral Haemodynamics and ICP

The reduction of arterial blood pressure (ABP) from 120/80 mmHg in steps to 60/20 mmHg produced vasodilatation. Cerebrovascular resistance (CVR) decreased from 0.09 to 0.05 mmHg/(mL/min). The amplitude of CSF flow increased from 170 to 340 mm^3/s, and the amplitude of ICP pulsations also increased from 5 to 7 mmHg (Fig. 1—left panel).

Changing $PaCO_2$ from 35 to 60 mmHg while keeping blood pressure constant produced gradual vasodilatation (Fig. 1—right panel). Intracranial pressure increased slightly (from 10 to 17 mmHg), and its amplitude increased as well (from 7 to 15 mmHg). The amplitude of CSF flow increased (from 220 to 400 mm^3/s) proportionally with both changes in PaCO2 and decreased CVR.

Moderate intracranial hypertension has been modelled by intraventricular infusion tests (rate of 2 mL/min) in systems with normal resistance to CSF outflow (6 mmHg/(mL/min)). Mean ICP increased from 12 to 24 mmHg, and cerebral perfusion pressure decreased from 78 to 66 mmHg. The lower limit of autoregulation was set at 50 mmHg with a static rate of autoregulation at 60%. Unilateral blood flow decreased from 300 to 280 mL/min. The pulse amplitude of CSF flow increased from 152 to 178 mm^3/s. This increase was linearly correlated with both an increase in ICP pulse amplitude from 7 to 18 mmHg and a decrease in CVR.

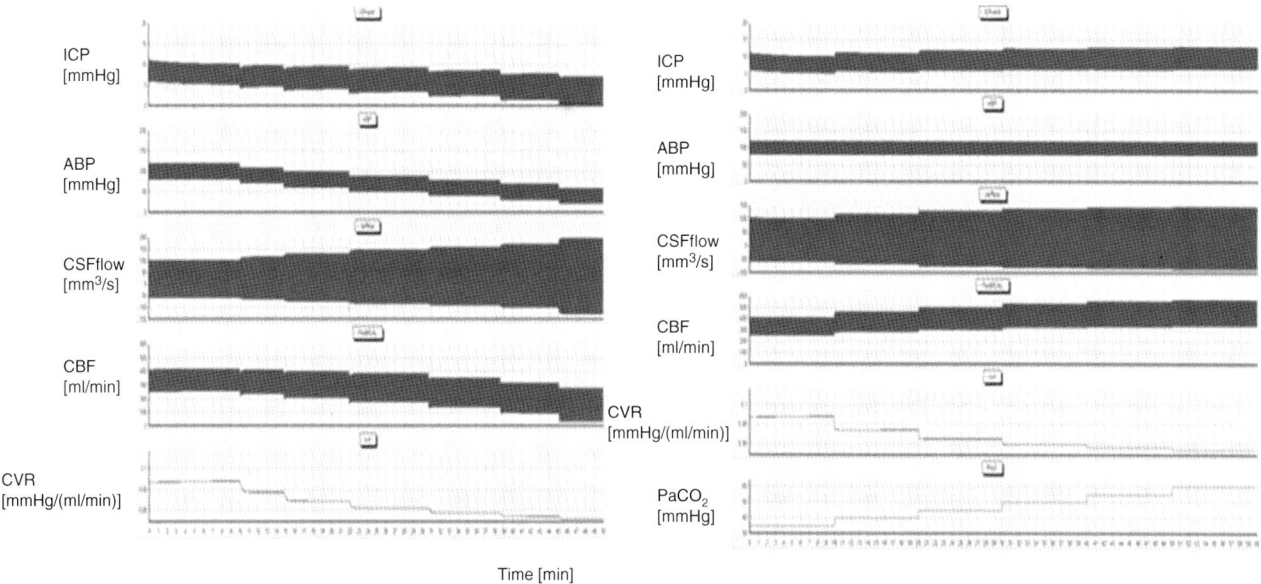

Fig. 1 *Left*: Simulation of a gradual decrease in arterial pressure (ABP). *Right*: Demonstration of gradual increase in PaCO2. Both manoeuvres caused a decrease in cerebrovascular resistance (CVR) and a gradual increase in the amplitude of cerebrospinal fluid (CSF) flow, seen here as an increase in distance between systolic and diastolic flow

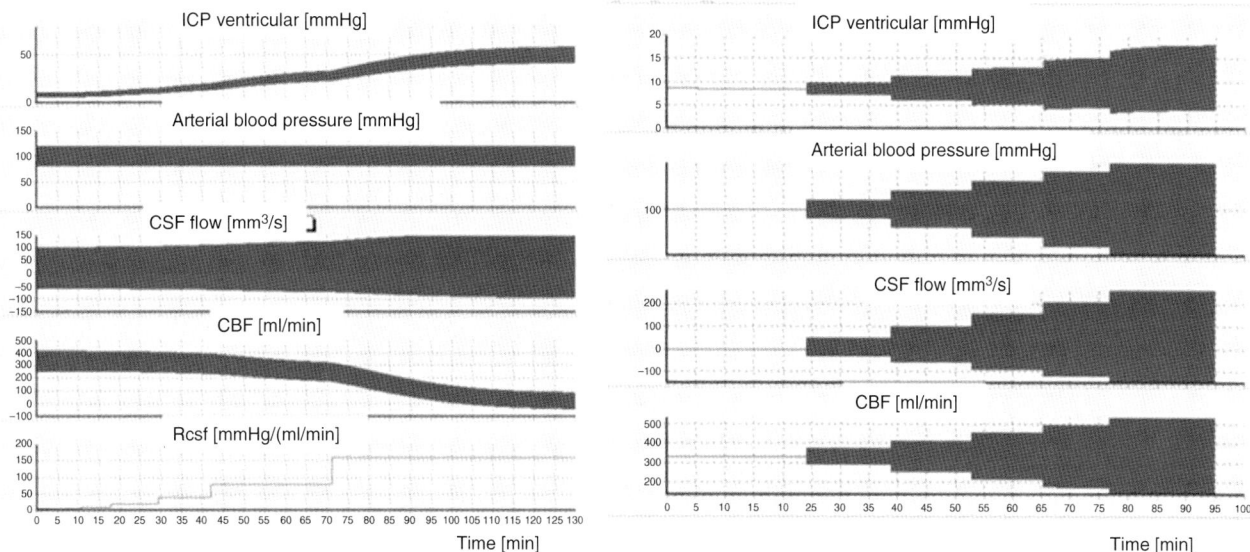

Fig. 2 *Left*: Simulation of elevating ICP by increasing resistance to CSF outflow (Rcsf). The ascending pulse amplitude of ICP caused a slight rise in the amplitude of pulsatile CSF flow. *Right*: Increasing the amplitude of ABP without eliciting changes in mean ABP produced synchronized changes in pulsatile CSF flow

Responses to Changes in CSF Dynamics

A gradual increase in the resistance to CSF outflow from 6 to 150 mmHg/(mL/min) mimics the development of acute hydrocephalus, for example, after subarachnoid haemorrhage. ICP increased to 50 mmHg. Both the pulse amplitude of ICP and the pulse amplitude of CSF flow changed proportionally with a rise in mean ICP (Fig. 2—left panel).

A gradual increase in the resistance of the aqueduct cerebri produced a minimal increase in ICP, but with a marked increase of its pulse amplitude from 7 to 22 mmHg. The pulse amplitude of CSF void flow decreased from 150 to 30 mm^3/s.

Decreasing the elasticity of brain produced a gradual increase in cerebrospinal compliance. Change in the pulsatility of ICP was minimal: it decreased from 5 to 4 mmHg. The CSF flow pulse amplitude increased slightly from 150 to 175 mm^3/s.

Response to Changes in Arterial Pressure Pulsatility

The pulse amplitude of ABP is certainly a major source of overall brain pulsatility for both blood and CSF flows. In the model, without changing mean ABP, a gradual increase in blood pressure pulsatility was simulated (Fig 2—right panel). All remaining signals (blood flow, CSF flow, and ICP) increased their pulsatile components proportionally with changes in the pulse amplitude of ABP. Mean values of CSF flow and CBF remained unchanged, and mean ICP increased slightly from 8 to 12 mmHg.

Discussion

This is a modelling study, and at present the experimental verification of findings is impossible. Even if the described changes in the pulsation of aqueductal CSF flow remain hypothetical, they have a common denominator.

First, changes in CSF pulsatile flow are in most situations proportional to changes in the pulse amplitude of ICP. It appears logical that any increase in the pulse amplitude of ventricular pressure should reflect a direct increase in the drive for increasing CSF void flow. The exception is an increase in the resistance of the aqueduct cerebri coupled with a decrease in the elasticity of CSF space. First case demonstrates that as CSF pulsatile flow decreases, ICP pulse amplitude increases. In a second case, we see exactly the inverse scenario, even though the changes in amplitudes are modest.

Conclusion

Results of mathematical simulation suggest that CSF pulsatile flow is both a function of cerebral haemodynamics and pressure-volume compensation.

Conflicts of interest statement We declare that we have no conflict of interest.

References

1. Balédent O, Gondry-Jouet C, Stoquart-Elsankari S, Bouzerar R, Le Gars D, Meyer ME. Value of phase contrast magnetic resonance imaging for investigation of cerebral hydrodynamics. J Neuroradiol. 2006;33(5):292–303.
2. Chiang WW, Takoudis CG, Lee SH, Weis-McNulty A, Glick R, Alperin N. Relationship between ventricular morphology and aqueductal cerebrospinal fluid flow in healthy and communicating hydrocephalus. Invest Radiol. 2009;44(4):192–9.
3. Yamada S, Miyazaki M, Kanazawa H, Higashi M, Morohoshi Y, Bluml S, McComb JG. Visualization of cerebrospinal fluid movement with spin labeling at MR imaging: preliminary results in normal and pathophysiologic conditions. Radiology. 2008;249(2):644–52.
4. Jaeger M, Khoo AK, Conforti DA, Cuganesan R. Relationship between intracranial pressure and phase contrast cine MRI derived measures of intracranial pulsations in idiopathic normal pressure hydrocephalus. J Clin Neurosci. 2016;33:169–72.
4. Yamada S, Tsuchiya K, Bradley WG, Law M, Winkler ML, Borzage MT, Miyazaki M, Kelly EJ, McComb JG. Current and emerging MR imaging techniques for the diagnosis and management of CSF flow disorders: a review of phase-contrast and time-spatial labeling inversion pulse. JNR. Am J Neuroradiol. 2015;36(4):623–30.
5. Poca MA, Sahuquillo J, Busto M, Rovira A, Capellades J, Mataró M, Rubio E. Agreement between CSF flow dynamics in MRI and ICP monitoring in the diagnosis of normal pressure hydrocephalus. Sensitivity and specificity of CSF dynamics to predict outcome. Acta Neurochir Suppl. 2002;81:7–10.
6. Boon AJ, Tans JT, Delwel EJ, Egeler-Peerdeman SM, Hanlo PW, Wurzer HA, Avezaat CJ, de Jong DA, Gooskens RH, Hermans J. Dutch normal-pressure hydrocephalus study: prediction of outcome after shunting by resistance to outflow of cerebrospinal fluid. J Neurosurg. 1997;87(5):687–93.
7. Eide PK, Brean A. Cerebrospinal fluid pulse pressure amplitude during lumbar infusion in idiopathic normal pressure hydrocephalus can predict response to shunting. Cerebrospinal Fluid Res. 2010;7:5.
8. Stephensen H, Tisell M, Wikkelsö C. There is no transmantle pressure gradient in communicating or noncommunicating hydrocephalus. Neurosurgery. 2002;50(4):763–71.
9. Alperin NJ, Lee SH, Loth F, Raksin PB, Lichtor T. MR-Intracranial pressure (ICP): a method to measure intracranial elastance and pressure noninvasively by means of MR imaging: baboon and human study. Radiology. 2000;217(3):877–85.
10. Ursino M. A mathematical model of overall cerebral blood flow regulation in the rat. IEEE Trans Biomed Eng. 1991;38(8):795–807.
11. Piechnik SK, Czosnyka M, Harris NG, Minhas PS, Pickard JD. A model of the cerebral and cerebrospinal fluid circulations to examine asymmetry in cerebrovascular reactivity. J Cereb Blood Flow Metab. 2001;21(2):182–92.

Cerebrospinal Fluid and Cerebral Blood Flows in Idiopathic Intracranial Hypertension

Cyrille Capel, Marc Baroncini, Catherine Gondry-Jouet, Roger Bouzerar, Marek Czosnyka, Zofia Czosnyka, and Olivier Balédent

Abstract *Objectives*: Cerebrospinal fluid (CSF) and blood flows have a strong relationship during a cardiac cycle. Idiopathic intracranial hypertension (IIH) is a pathology that seems to present hemodynamic and hydrodynamic disturbance. The aim of this study was to establish CSF and blood interaction in IIH.

Material and methods: We retrospectively studied cerebral hydrodynamic and hemodynamic flows by phase-contrast MRI (PCMRI) in 13 IIH subjects (according Dandy's criteria) and 16 controls. We analyzed arterial peak flow, pulsatility index, and resistive index in arterial and venous compartments (PFart, PIart, RIart, PFvein, PIvein, RIvein) and measured arteriovenous and CSF peak flow and stroke volume (PFav, SV_{VASC}, PF_{CSF}, SV_{CSF}).

Results: We found no significant difference between IIH and control groups in arterial and venous parameters. Arteriovenous flow analysis showed higher PFav and SV_{VASC} in the IIH group than in the control group (respectively 369 ± 27 mL/min and 286 ± 47 mL/min, $p = 0.02$; and 1085 ± 265 μL/cardiac cycle and 801 ± 226 μL/cardiac cycle, $p = 0.007$). PF_{CSF} and SV_{CSF} were higher in the IIH group than in the control group (respectively 206 ± 50 mL/min and 126.6 ± 24.8 mL/min, $p = 0.04$; and 570 ± 190 μL/cardiac cycle and 430 ± 100 μL/cardiac cycle, $p = 0.0007$).

Conclusion: Although no significant change was found in arterial and venous flows, we showed that a small phase shift of venous outflow might cause an increase in the arteriovenous pulsatility and an increasing brain expansion during the cardiac cycle. This arteriovenous flow increase would result in an increase of CSF flushing through the foramen magnum and an increased ICP.

Keywords Intracranial hypertension · Phase-contrast MRI · Cerebral hydrodynamic · Cerebral hemodynamic

C. Capel, M.D. (✉)
Neurosurgery Department, Hospital University Center of Amiens-Picardie, Amiens, France

BioFLOW Image Research Group, Hospital University Center of Amiens-Picardie, Amiens, France

Neurosurgery Department, CHU Amiens—Picardie, Salouel, Amiens, France
e-mail: capel.cyrille@chu-amiens.fr

M. Baroncini, M.D., Ph.D.
Neurosurgery Department, Hospital University Center of Lille, Lille, France

C. Gondry-Jouet, M.D.
Radiology Department, Hospital University Center of Amiens-Picardie, Amiens, France

R. Bouzerar, Ph.D. • O. Balédent, Ph.D.
BioFLOW Image Research Group, Hospital University Center of Amiens-Picardie, Amiens, France

M. Czosnyka, Ph.D. • Z. Czosnyka, Ph.D.
Neurosciences Department, University of Cambridge, Cambridge, UK

Introduction

Idiopathic intracranial hypertension (IIH) is a well-studied but still poorly understood pathology. Clinical presentation typically involves a young obese woman with headaches and bilateral papilledema [1]. Papilledema could generate visual disturbance, which could move toward a progressive blindness [2]. No anatomic explanation can be found in cerebral imaging, and ventricle size must be normal or slit [1]. During intracranial pressure (ICP) monitoring, mean cerebrospinal fluid (CSF) pressures are elevated. CSF component analysis is normal. IIH diagnosis is one of exclusion.

The physiopathology of IIH is unknown. The relationship between IIH and venous drainage is described in the literature [3, 4, 5]. In up to 26% of all chronic intracranial hypertension cases, dural sinus stenosis can be identified [6]. Nevertheless, cerebral venous thrombosis seems to be overlooked when intracranial hypertension is isolated [7].

Dural venous stenosis was found in 90% of IIH patients and in 6.8% of the control group [8]. Transverse sinus is the main site of stenosis [8], but all dural sinuses could be affected [9]. A recent mathematical model [10] proposes a collapsible sinus hypothesis.

Phase contrast magnetic resonance imaging MRI (PCMRI) is a unique tool that can be used to analyze arterial and venous flows and CSF flows. Many studies have analyzed arterial and venous cerebral blood flow by PCMRI in many pathologies (hydrocephalus, intracranial hypertension, obesity). In IIH, most of these studies focused on venous pulsatility and arteriovenous interactions [3, 4, 10]. No study considered blood and CSF interactions. The aim of this study was to establish CSF and blood interactions in intracranial hypertension patients.

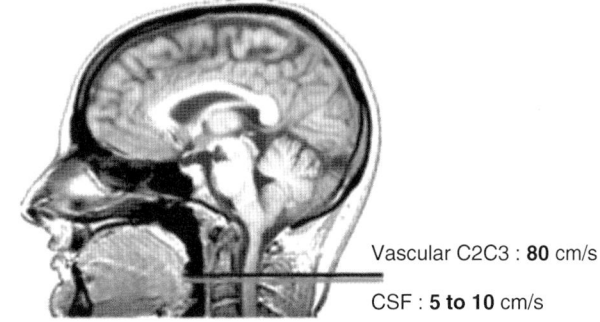

Fig. 1 Slice placement. Vascular and blood acquisition was placed at the cervical level with a parallel plane to C2–C3 intervertebral disc

Material and Methods

We retrospectively studied 13 patients with IIH and 16 healthy controls at University Hospital of Amiens.

IIH Group

The IIH group was composed of 13 patients (31 ± 11 years old). Inclusion criteria were headaches or visual impairment with bilateral papilledema and normal MR scan morphologically (no ventricular dilation, no venous thrombosis, no other pathologies); CSF composition was normal.

Control Group

This group was composed of 16 volunteers (37 ± 7 years old). They had no neurological or functional pathologies; morphological MR scans were normal.

MRI Acquisition

All patients underwent an MRI scan for a conventional clinical diagnosis assessment. The MRI was performed more than three months after the lumbar puncture. In addition to conventional clinical sequences, we add two PCMRI sequences (additional acquisition time: 3 min).

Cerebral MRIs were performed on a 3T scanner (GE Healthcare, Milwaukee, WI, USA) with the following parameters: repetition time (TR) and echo time (TE) = minimum depending on heart rate; field of view = 2 cm; matrix = 256 mm² or 128 × 256 mm²; slice thickness = 5 mm; flip angle = 30°; 2 excitations; 2 views per segment. Peripheral cardiac synchronization was achieved with retrospective gating (either foot or finger) to reconstruct 32 phases and reproduce a mean of all cardiac cycles. For CSF flow, we selected velocity encoding (VENC) of 5 cm/s at the cervical level (increased to 10 cm/s if aliasing occurred). For cervical blood flows, we selected VENC = 80 cm/s. CSF and blood flow acquisition slices were positioned perpendicular to the presumed direction of the flows (Fig. 1).

Data Analysis

Data were analyzed using in-house software (www.tidam.fr).

Stroke volumes were defined as the average of craniocaudal and caudo-cranial volumes displaced through the region of interest during the cardiac cycle. They were measured for CSF in the cervical level.

Cerebral arterial blood flow (CBF_a) was defined as the sum of the internal carotids and vertebral artery flows. It was measured at the level of the intervertebral disc C2–C3.

Cerebral venous blood flow (CBF_v) was also measured at the same level and was defined as the sum of jugular vein flow at the cervical level. Since blood volume that fills the brain during a cardiac cycle by the arteries completely flush out by the veins, CBF_v measures were adjusted to provide $_{corrected}CBF_v$; thus, $(_{corrected}CBF_v)$ = mean (CBF_a) [11].

Arteriovenous flow (Figs. 2 and 3) was calculated by the sum of arterial inflow CBF_a and corrected venous outflow $_{corrected}CBF_v$. Consequently, we were able to generate the vascular flow curve during a cardiac cycle. Arteriovenous stroke volumes were calculated by the time integral of both positive and negative parts of the arteriovenous flow to provide the intracranial blood volume change during the cardiac cycle. The flow curves were presented as a percentage of the cardiac cycle.

We calculated some derived parameters (peak flow, pulsatility index, and resistive index) for venous and arterial blood flow. Peak flow (PF) was defined by the highest value of flow measured in a compartment during a cardiac cycle.

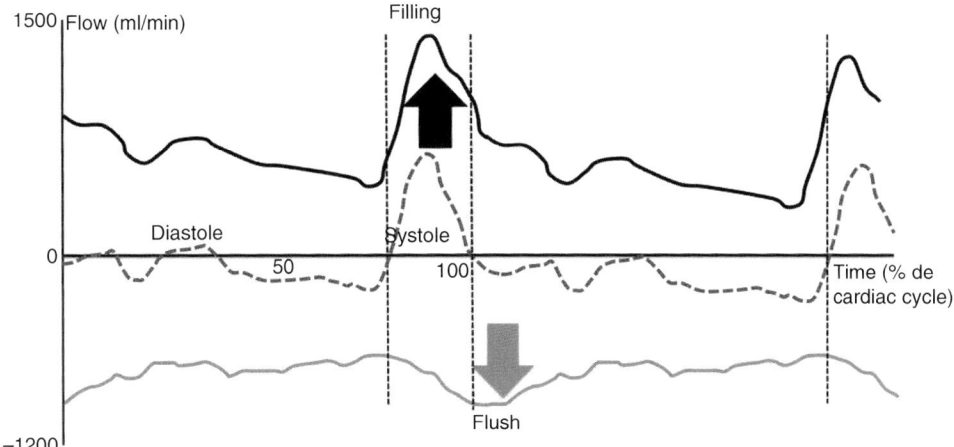

Fig. 2 Blood flow curves during two cardiac cycles. Arterial flow curve (*black solid curve*) analysis showed a sudden and high blood inflow during the systole. This inflow was compensated by a venous outflow (*solid gray line*). This outflow was not instantaneous. This was the arteriovenous delay. Consequently, arteriovenous curve (*broken gray line*) was not constant, and we observed an inflow during the systole (positives values), and blood was flushing (negative values) during the diastole. Intracranial vascular volume was not constant

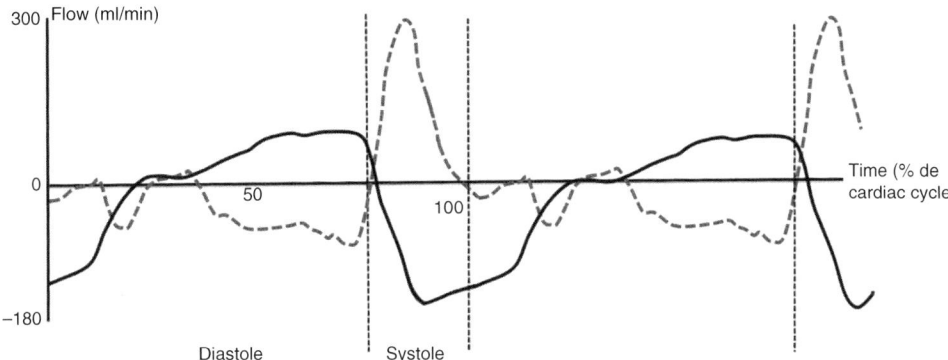

Fig. 3 Arteriovenous and CSF flow interactions. Arteriovenous flow (*broken gray curve*) and cervical CSF flow (*solid black line*) are interacting. During the systole, vascular volume increases. We observed a CSF flush to the spinal subarachnoid spaces that compensated for this increase in vascular volume. During the diastole, vascular volume increases and CSF is filled in the cranium

The pulsatility index (PI) was calculated by the quotient between the amplitude of the flow curve and the average value during one cardiac cycle in one compartment. The resistive index (RI) was calculated as the quotient between the amplitude of the velocity curve and the average value during one cardiac cycle.

In summary, we measured the stroke volume of CSF in cervical subarachnoid spaces (SV_{CSF}) and of the arteriovenous compartment (SV_{VASC}). We measured peak flows in an arterial compartment (PFart), in a venous compartment (PFvein), in an arteriovenous compartment (PFav), and in a cervical CSF compartment (PF_{CSF}). We calculated pulsatility index in venous and arterial compartments (PIart and PIvein) and RI in the same compartment (RIart and RIvein).

A Wilcoxon test ($p = 0.05$) was performed to compare all mean flows between these groups.

Results

The results of arteriovenous and cervical CSF flow measurements are shown in Table 1.

PFart was not significantly different between the IIH group and the control group (respectively 1166 ± 174 mL/min and 1258 ± 174 mL/min; $p = 0.09$). Similarly, PIart was not different between the IIH group and the control group (respectively 1.24 ± 0.36 and 0.98 ± 0.24; $p = 0.6$). RIart was higher in the IIH group than in the control group (0.57 ± 0.10 and 0.49 ± 0.10; $p = 0.03$).

PFvein was not different between the IIH and control groups (respectively 617 ± 201 mL/min and 554 ± 227 mL/min; $p = 0.25$). PIvein was not different between the IIH and control groups (respectively 0.50 ± 0.20 and 0.54 ± 0.12; $p = 0.5$). RIvein was not different between the IIH group and the control group (0.38 ± 0.14 and 0.38 ± 0.17; $p = 0.91$).

Table 1 Comparison of flow parameters between IIH and control groups (results in bold front are significant)

	Control group	IIH group	p
PFart (mm³/s)	1166 ± 174	1258 ± 174	0.09
PIart	0.98 ± 0.24	1.24 ± 0.36	0.60
RIart	**0.49 ± 0.10**	**0.57 ± 0.10**	**0.03**
PFvein (mm³/s)	554 ± 227	617 ± 201	0.25
PIvein	0.54 ± 0.12	0.50 ± 0.20	0.50
PIvein	0.38 ± 0.17	0.38 ± 0.14	0.91
PFav (mm³/s)	**286 ± 47**	**369 ± 27**	**0.02**
SVVASC (μl/cc)	**801 ± 226**	**1085 ± 265**	**0.007**
PFCSF (mL/min)	**126.6 ± 24.8**	**206.0 ± 50.0**	**0.004**
SVCSF (μl/cc)	**430 ± 100**	**570 ± 190**	**0.0007**

Arteriovenous flow analysis showed higher PFav and SV_{VASC} values in the IIH group than in the control group (respectively 369 ± 27 mL/min and 286 ± 47 mL/min; $p = 0.02$; 1085 ± 265 μL/cardiac cycle and 801 ± 226 μL/cardiac cycle; $p = 0.007$). PF_{CSF} and SV_{CSF} were higher in the IIH group than in the control group (respectively 206 ± 50 mL/min and 126.6 ± 24.8 mL/min; $p = 0.04$; 570 ± 190 μL/cardiac cycle and 430 ± 100 μL/cardiac cycle; $p = 0.0007$).

Discussion

In IIH, we observed significant alterations of arteriovenous and CSF flows. Our data confirmed that CSF flows and arteriovenous flows are closely related. CSF flow is the consequence of vascular volume changes in a cardiac cycle. Arterial and venous flow analysis is a necessary prerequisite to CSF and global intracranial fluid flow analysis.

Arterial and Venous Flows

In IIH, arterial flow is not frequently studied in isolation. We found no difference between the control and IIH groups in PFart and PIart. A difference in RIart was found. Nevertheless, this result tempermay be due to the low number of patients in our groups and the low level of significance ($p = 0.03$). The alteration of pulsatility and resistance in extracranial arteries was never identified in the literature. An increase in these parameters was measured in intracranial arteries by transcranial doppler [12].

In venous analysis, we found no study of cervical venous flow in the literature. Bateman studied venous blood flow in the superior sagittal sinus and the straight sinus. In this study, a reduction of pulsatility in the superior sagittal sinus was found. In our study, we found no change in PFvein, PIvein, or RIvein. The dural venous sinus has a strong wall, and pulsatility is mainly due to the pressure inside. Greitz [13] suggested that the compliance of sinuses wall was due to arachnoid granulation. Pulsatility depends on the pressure gradient at the walls of the sinuses. In IIH, pressur in the superior sagittal sinus is slightly lower than CSF pressure but both of them increase [5]. In IIH the pressure gradient at the sinus walls decreases and causes a decrease in the pulsatility. The extracranial venous wall is mainly compliant because of its histological composition. Pulsatility is probably dampened by the inherent compliance of the venous wall.

No difference was clearly identified in separate analyses of arterial and venous flows. Nevertheless, we found significant differences in arteriovenous parameters (SV_{VASC}, PF_{VASC}). During a cardiac cycle, arterial inflow is almost immediately compensated by CSF outflow. Venous outflow is shifted in time on average 90–100 ms later than arterial systolic peak flow [14]. This is called arteriovenous delay. The intracranial vascular volume changes during a cardiac cycle [11]. SV_{VASC} reflects this intracranial vascular volume variation. By a very simple mathematical model, we increased the arteriovenous delay. As a result of this manipulation, we observed a substantial increase in SV_{VASC} and PF_{VASC}. This shows an increase in intracranial vascular volume variation during a cardiac cycle.

CSF Flows

The Monroe-Kellie doctrine states that intracranial volume is stable during a cardiac cycle [8]. A volume change in an intracranial compartment causes an opposite change in another. During the systolic phase, we observed a blood inflow by arterial circulation. This increased flow is not immediately compensated by a venous outflow [11, 13]. This results in an increase of the volume of the vascular compartment. Consequently, CSF passively flushes through the foramen magnum from intracranial subarachnoid spaces to the spinal subarachnoid spaces. This phenomenon is secondary to vascular volume variations and partially preserves the intracranial volume.

In our study, we observed an increase in PF_{CSF} and SV_{CSF} in the IIH group. CSF flows are passive and secondary to vascular volume changes. An increase in the CSF pulsatility during a cardiac cycle is therefore a consequence of an increase in intracranial volume variations.

Conclusion

On a small population of IIH patients, arterial and venous flow analysis showed no significantly abnormal oscillations while the CSF flows in cervical subarachnoid spaces were increased. Although no significant changes in arterial and venous flows were found, we showed that a small phase shift of venous outflow might cause an increase in both the arteriovenous pulsatility and brain expansion during the cardiac cycle. This arteriovenous flow increase would result in an increase in CSF flushing through the foramen magnum and an increased ICP.

Conflicts of interest statement We declare that we have no conflict of interest.

References

1. Gross CE, Tranmer BI, Adey G, Kohut J. Increased cerebral blood flow in idiopathic pseudotumour cerebri. Neurol Res. 1990;12(4):226–30.
2. Wall M. Idiopathic intracranial hypertension. Semin Ophthalmol. 1995;10(3):251–9.
3. Alperin N, Ranganathan S, Bagci AM, Adams DJ, Ertl-Wagner B, Saraf-Lavi E, Sklar EM, Lam BL. MRI evidence of impaired CSF homeostasis in obesity-associated idiopathic intracranial hypertension. AJNR Am J Neuroradiol. 2013;34(1):29–34.
4. Bateman GA. Vascular hydraulics associated with idiopathic and secondary intracranial hypertension. AJNR Am J Neuroradiol. 2002;23(7):1180–6.
5. Pickard JD, Czosnyka Z, Czosnyka M, Owler B, Higgins JN. Coupling of sagittal sinus pressure and cerebrospinal fluid pressure in idiopathic intracranial hypertension – a preliminary report. Acta Neurochir Suppl. 2008;102:283–5.
6. Leker RR, Steiner I. Features of dural sinus thrombosis simulating pseudotumor cerebri. Eur J Neurol. 1999;6(5):601–4.
7. Biousse V, Ameri A, Bousser MG. Isolated intracranial hypertension as the only sign of cerebral venous thrombosis. Neurology. 1999;53(7):1537–42.
8. Farb RI, Vanek I, Scott JN, Mikulis DJ, Willinsky RA, Tomlinson G, terBrugge KG. Idiopathic intracranial hypertension: the prevalence and morphology of sinovenous stenosis. Neurology. 2003;60(9):1418–24.
9. Rohr A, Dörner L, Stingele R, Buhl R, Alfke K, Jansen O. Reversibility of venous sinus obstruction in idiopathic intracranial hypertension. AJNR Am J Neuroradiol. 2007;28(4):656–9.
10. Bateman GA, Stevens SA, Stimpson J. A mathematical model of idiopathic intracranial hypertension incorporating increased arterial inflow and variable venous outflow collapsibility. J Neurosurg. 2009;110(3):446–56.
11. Balédent O, Henry-Feugeas MC, Idy-Peretti I. Cerebrospinal fluid dynamics and relation with blood flow: a magnetic resonance study with semiautomated cerebrospinal fluid segmentation. Invest Radiol. 2001;36(7):368–77.
12. Wang Y, Duan Y-Y, Zhou H-Y, Yuan L-J, Zhang L, Wang W, Li L-H, Li L. Middle cerebral arterial flow changes on transcranial color and spectral Doppler sonography in patients with increased intracranial pressure. J Ultrasound Med. 2014;33(12):2131–60.
13. Greitz D, Wirestam R, Franck A, Nordell B, Thomsen C, Ståhlberg F. Pulsatile brain movement and associated hydrodynamics studied by magnetic resonance phase imaging. The Monro-Kellie doctrine revisited. Neuroradiology. 1992;34(5):370–80.
14. Bateman GA. Vascular compliance in normal pressure hydrocephalus. AJNR Am J Neuroradiol. 2000;21(9):1574–85.

Significant Association of Slow Vasogenic ICP Waves with Normal Pressure Hydrocephalus Diagnosis

Andreas Spiegelberg, Matthias Krause, Juergen Meixensberger, Burkhardt Seifert, and Vartan Kurtcuoglu

Abstract *Objective*: We aimed to test whether there is an association of slow vasogenic wave (SVW) occurrence with positive response to external lumbar drainage (ELD) and ventriculoperitoneal shunting and to design a method for the recognition and quantification of SVWs in the intracranial pressure (ICP) signal.

Materials and methods: We constructed SVW templates using normalized sine waves. We calculated the cross-correlation between the respective SVW template and the ICP signal. This was followed by shifting the templates forward and performing the cross-correlation analysis again until the end of the recording. Cross-correlation values above a threshold were considered to be indicative of SVWs. This threshold was previously determined and validated on a sample of ICP records of six patients. We calculated the root mean square of the recognized SVW periods as a measure of signal strength. Time-averaged signal strength was calculated over the full recording time (ICP_{Smean}) and over the wave periods (ICP_S).

Results: We determined ICP_S and ICP_{Smean} in recordings of 2 groups of patients presenting with Hakim's triad: 26 normal pressure hydrocephalus (NPH) patients and 20 non-NPH patients. We then tested whether there was an association between ICP_S or ICP_{Smean} and the respective diagnosis using a Mann–Whitney test. We found significant association between ICP_S ($p = 0.014$) and ICP_{Smean} ($p = 0.022$) and the diagnoses.

Conclusions: The described method based on pattern recognition in the time domain is suitable for the detection and quantification of SVWs in ICP signals. We found a significant association between the occurrence of SVWs and independent NPH diagnosis.

Keywords Intracranial pressure · B-waves · Slow waves · Vasogenic waves · Waveform analysis

Introduction

The B-wave is a feature of the intracranial pressure (ICP) waveform, reflecting vasogenic activity of cerebral autoregulation. B-waves were originally defined to occupy a frequency range of 0.5–2 cycles per minute [1]. Recently renamed and redefined as slow vasogenic waves (SVWs) with an extended range of 0.33–3 cycles per minute [2], specific changes in their pattern of occurrence are considered to be indicative of reduced intracranial compliance.

Beyond visual inspection, computerized methods for the detection and quantification of B-waves have been described [3–5]. However, there is no general agreement on the quantitative description of B-waves [6]. Nor is there agreement on a possible correlation between shunt responsiveness and B-wave occurrence: while Pickard et al. [7], Symon et al. [8], Lenfeldt et al. [9], and Poca [10] describe such a correlation, Woodworth [11], Stephenson et al. [12], and Williams [13] report that there is no or only poor correlation. The idiopathic normal pressure hydrocephalus (INPH) guidelines provide a review of those and of other publications on the topic [14].

Our aim was to test whether there is an association of SVW occurrence with the diagnosis of normal pressure hydrocephalus (NPH) as indicated by positive response to

A. Spiegelberg (✉)
The Interface Group, Institute of Physiology, University of Zurich, Zürich, Switzerland
e-mail: andreas.spiegelberg@uzh.ch

M. Krause • J. Meixensberger
Klinik und Poliklinik für Neurochirurgie,
Universitaetsklinikum Leipzig AoeR, Leipzig, Germany

B. Seifert
Department of Biostatistics, Epidemiology, Biostatistics and Prevention Institute (EBPI), University of Zurich, Zurich, Switzerland

V. Kurtcuoglu
The Interface Group, Institute of Physiology, University of Zurich, Zürich, Switzerland

Zurich Center for Integrative Human Physiology and Neuroscience Center Zurich, University of Zurich, Zurich, Switzerland

external lumbar drainage (ELD) and ventriculoperitoneal (VP) shunting. To this end, we designed a method for the recognition and quantification of SVWs in the ICP signal of patients with suspected NPH.

Materials and Methods

We used cross-correlation to compare the ICP signal with templates of SVWs. The cross-correlation is a measure of the similarity between two signals. We constructed SVW signal templates (TMP) covering the full frequency range of SVWs. Each template consisted of two full sine wave periods, as illustrated in Fig. 1. Starting at the beginning of an ICP record, we calculated one by one for all SVW templates the cross-correlation between the respective SVW template and the normalized ICP signal (ICPn). This was followed by shifting the templates forward in time and calculating the cross-correlation again until the end of the recording was reached. Fig. 1 illustrates the calculation of the cross-correlation between the normalized ICP (ICPn, mmHg) and a template TMP (no dimension) according to Eq. (1), n being the number of samples in the template TMP:

$$CC(t) = \frac{\sum_{i=0}^{n-1}\left(\text{ICP}n_{(t+i\cdot\Delta t)}\cdot\text{TMP}_{(i\cdot\Delta t)}\right)}{\sqrt{\sum_{i=o}^{n-1}\left(\text{ICP}n_{(t+i\cdot\Delta t)}\right)^2}\cdot\sqrt{\sum_{i=o}^{n-1}\left(\text{TMP}_{(i\cdot\Delta t)}\right)^2}}. \quad (1)$$

Cross-correlation values above a certain threshold were considered to be indicative of SVWs. This threshold was adjusted in a stepwise manner such that the recognition rate and the rate of false positives were optimized when

Table 1 Number, sex, age, and preoperative Kiefer score ± standard deviation (SD) of NPH (normal pressure hydrocephalus) and NNPH (non-NPH) patient groups

	NNPH	NPH
Number of patients	20	26
Males/females	9/11	18/8
Age ± SD (years)	70.7 ± 7.1	73.1 ± 6.0
Kiefer Score preop. ± SD	6.9 ± 3.4	7.2 ± 3.4

comparing the decision of the algorithm to the decision by visual inspection. The criterion used for the decision by visual inspection was a peak-to-peak amplitude >1 mmHg. The threshold was validated on a sample of ICP records of six patients by comparing the SVW periods recognized by the new algorithm to the SVW periods recognized by visual inspection. The person performing the visual inspection was blinded to the diagnoses of said six patients.

We calculated the root mean square (RMS) of the recognized SVW periods as a measure of signal strength. Time-averaged signal strength was calculated over the full recording time (denoted by ICP$_{Smean}$) and over the wave periods (denoted by ICP$_S$).

We determined ICP$_S$ and ICP$_{Smean}$ in recordings of two groups of patients presenting with Hakim's triad: 26 NPH patients (with positive response to ELD and sustained neurological improvement 12 months after VP shunting) and 20 non-NPH (NNPH) patients (without positive response to ELD or irresponsive to VP shunt therapy). Written informed consent was obtained from the patients before participation in the study. The recordings of the six patients used for the validation were not included in the samples. Table 1 indicates the sex, age, and preoperative Kiefer score [15] of the patient groups. We then tested whether there was an association between ICP$_S$ or ICP$_{Smean}$ and the corresponding diagnosis. A Mann–Whitney test was used for this purpose because the samples were not normally distributed.

Results

The SVW recognition rate determined in the aforementioned six patients was 97%. The rate of false positive recognitions was 1.4%.

Using the Mann–Whitney test we found significant association between ICP$_S$ and the diagnoses ($p = 0.014$) and between ICP$_{Smean}$ and the diagnoses ($p = 0.022$). Table 2 indicates the values of ICP$_S$ and ICP$_{Smean}$ as well as the time fraction with slow waves (TF$_S$) for the individual patients, the mean values, and standard deviations with the corresponding p-values.

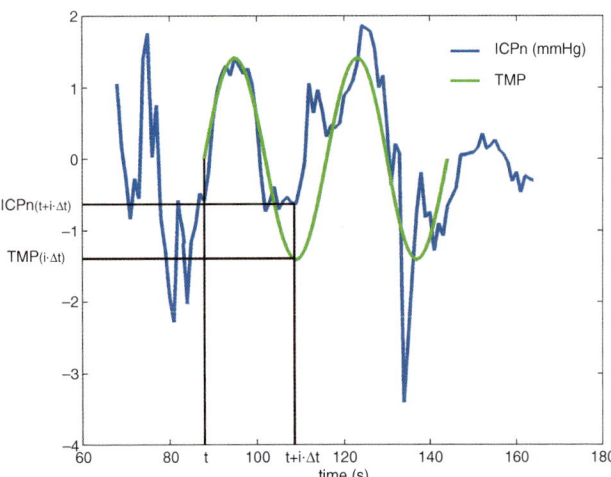

Fig. 1 Calculation of cross-correlation between normalized ICP (ICPn, mmHg) and a template TMP (no dimension) at time t, with Δt being the sampling interval and n the number of samples per template

Table 2 ICP_S, ICP_{Smean}, and TF_S of individual patients identified by patient number (Pat. no.) as well as the mean values, standard deviations (SD), and p-values

NNPH				NPH			
Pat. no.	ICP_{Smean} (mmHg)	TF_S	ICP_S (mmHg)	Pat. no.	ICP_{Smean} (mmHg)	TF_S	ICP_S (mmHg)
1	0.496	0.397	1.250	21	0.321	0.197	1.632
2	0.251	0.503	0.498	22	0.172	0.203	0.845
3	0.473	0.307	1.542	23	0.512	0.343	1.494
4	0.447	0.522	0.857	24	0.476	0.548	0.868
5	0.143	0.152	0.941	25	0.313	0.214	1.460
6	0.406	0.296	1.373	26	0.508	0.487	1.044
7	0.465	0.500	0.931	27	0.054	0.046	1.189
8	0.375	0.487	0.769	28	1.884	0.468	4.026
9	0.233	0.370	0.629	29	0.053	0.045	1.176
10	0.464	0.479	0.967	30	0.446	0.553	0.807
11	0.170	0.237	0.716	31	0.231	0.321	0.719
12	0.010	0.025	0.404	32	0.797	0.529	1.506
13	0.337	0.455	0.742	33	0.263	0.225	1.171
14	0.305	0.322	0.946	34	0.925	0.487	1.897
15	0.399	0.351	1.135	35	0.336	0.368	0.912
16	0.691	0.565	1.223	36	0.707	0.474	1.493
17	0.238	0.277	0.858	37	0.476	0.328	1.451
18	0.010	0.007	1.575	38	0.387	0.486	0.798
19	0.398	0.348	1.146	39	0.472	0.473	0.998
20	0.311	0.352	0.883	40	0.508	0.389	1.306
				41	0.287	0.224	1.278
				42	0.493	0.480	1.029
				43	1.224	0.571	2.144
				44	0.520	0.464	1.121
				45	0.623	0.426	1.464
				46	0.588	0.569	1.034
Mean	0.331		0.969		0.522		1.341
SD	0.164		0.309		0.370		0.636

p-Value Mann–Whitney Test ICP_{Smean} NPH vs. NNPH	0.022

p-Value Mann–Whitney Test ICP_S NPH vs. NNPH	0.014

Discussion

The described method based on a pattern recognition technique in the time domain is suitable for the detection and quantification of SVWs in ICP signals. We consider the SVW recognition rate of 97% and the false positive recognition rate of 1.4% to be promising. However, while both ICP_S and ICP_{Smean} show clear association with the diagnoses, the method in its current form could not be proven to be suitable for determination of a cutoff point with good specificity and sensitivity.

The recognition algorithm can be further improved by using a larger database for the definition of the threshold beyond which SVW is indicated and by having multiple operators perform the visual inspection of the waveforms in this database. This extended parameterization and validation is likely to be of particular relevance for noisy and artifact-laden ICP signals.

Conclusions

The method described herein is suitable for the detection and quantification of SVWs in ICP signals. Using this method, we found a significant association between the occurrence of SVWs and independent NPH diagnosis. We conclude that recognition and quantitative analysis of SVWs may be considered a component in the diagnosis of NPH.

Acknowledgement We gratefully acknowledge partial funding by the Swiss National Science Foundation through NCCR Kidney.CH.

Conflicts of interest statement We declare that we have no conflict of interest.

References

1. Lundberg N. Continuous recording and control of ventricular fluid pressure in neurosurgical practice. Acta Psychiatr Scand. 1959;36(Suppl):1–193.
2. Momjian S, Czosnyka Z, Czosnyka M, Pickard JD. Link between vasogenic waves of intracranial pressure and cerebrospinal fluid outflow resistance in normal pressure hydrocephalus. Br J Neurosurg. 2004;18:56–61.
3. Mueller JU, Schmidtke J, Woertgen C, Gaab MR. ICP analysis in normal pressure hydrocephalus – a prospective comparison between conventional and automatic online analysis. Zentralblatt Neurochir. 2000;61(Suppl):14.
4. Eklund A, Ågren-Wilsson A, Andersson N, Bergenheim AT, Koskinen LO, Malm J. Two computerized methods used to analyze intracranial pressure B waves: comparison with traditional visual interpretation. J Neurosurg. 2001;94:392–6.
5. Kasprowicz M, Asgari S, Bergsneider M, Czosnyka M, Hamilton R, Hu X. Pattern recognition of overnight intracranial pressure slow waves using morphological features of intracranial pressure pulse. J Neurosci Methods. 2010;190:310–8.
6. Spiegelberg A, Preuss M, Kurtcuoglu V. B-Waves revisited. Interdiscip Neurosurg Adv Tech Case Manag. 2016;6:13–7.
7. Pickard JD, Teasdale G, Matheson M, Lindsay K, Galbraith S, Wyper D, Macpherson P. Intraventricular pressure waves—the best predictive test for shunting in normal pressure hydrocephalus. Intracranial pressure IV. New York, NY: Springer; 1980. p. 498–500.
8. Symon L, Dorsch NWC, Stephens RJ. Pressure waves in so-called low-pressure hydrocephalus. Lancet. 1972;300:1291–2.
9. Lenfeldt N, Andersson N, Ågren-Wilsson A, Bergenheim AT, Koskinen LO, Eklund A, Malm J. Cerebrospinal fluid pulse pressure method: a possible substitute for the examination of B waves. J Neurosurg. 2004;101:944–50.
10. Poca MA, Gandara D, Mestres O, Canas V, Radoi A, Sahuquillo J. Resistance to outflow is an unreliable predictor of outcome in patients with idiopathic normal pressure hydrocephalus. Int ICP Symp. 2013;XV:Abstr: 42–3.
11. Woodworth GF, McGirt MJ, Williams MA, Rigamonti D. Cerebrospinal fluid drainage and dynamics in the diagnosis of normal pressure hydrocephalus. Neurosurgery. 2009;64:919–26.
12. Stephensen H, Andersson N, Eklund A, Malm J, Tisell M, Wikkelsoe C. Objective B wave analysis in 55 patients with non-communicating and communicating hydrocephalus. J Neurol Neurosurg Psychiatry. 2005;76:965–70.
13. Williams MA, Razumovsky AY, Hanley DF. Comparison of Pcsf monitoring and controlled CSF drainage diagnose normal pressure hydrocephalus. Intracranial pressure X. New York, NY: Springer; 1998. p. 328–30.
14. Marmarou A, Bergsneider M, Klinge P, Relkin N, Black PM. The value of supplemental prognostic tests for the preoperative assessment of idiopathic normal-pressure hydrocephalus. Neurosurgery. 2005;57:2–17.
15. Kiefer M, Eymann R, Komenda Y, Steudel WI. Ein Graduierungssystem für den chronischen Hydrozephalus. Zentralbl Neurochir. 2003;64:109–15.

ICP Monitoring and Phase-Contrast MRI to Investigate Intracranial Compliance

A. Lokossou, O. Balédent, S. Garnotel, G. Page, L. Balardy, Z. Czosnyka, P. Payoux, and E.A. Schmidt

Abstract *Objective*: The amplitude of intracranial pressure (ICP) can be measured by ICP monitoring. Phase-contrast magnetic resonance imaging (PCMRI) can quantify blood and cerebrospinal fluid (CSF) flows. The aim of this work was to investigate intracranial compliance at rest by combining baseline ICP monitoring and PCMRI in hydrocephalus patients.

Materials and methods: ICP monitoring was performed before infusion testing to quantify ΔICP_rest at the basal condition in 33 suspected hydrocephalus patients (74 years). The day before, patients had had a PCMRI to assess total cerebral blood flow (tCBF), intracranial blood volume change (stroke volume SVblood), and cervical CSF volume change (the stroke volume CSV). Global (blood and CSF) intracranial volume change (ΔIVC) during each cardiac cycle (CC) was calculated. Finally, Compliance: C_rest = ΔIVC/ΔICP_rest was calculated. The data set was postprocessed by two operators according to blind analysis.

Results: Bland–Altman plots showed that measurements presented no significant difference between the two operators. ΔICP_rest = 2.41 ± 1.21 mmHg, tCBF = 469.89 ± 127.54 mL/min, SVblood = 0.82 ± 0.32 mL/cc, CSV = 0.50 ± 0.22 mL/cc, ΔIVC = 0.44 ± 0.22 mL, and C_rest = 0.23 ± 0.15 mL/mmHg. There are significant relations between SVblood and CSV and also SVblood and tCBF.

Conclusions: During "basal" condition, the compliance amplitude of the intracranial compartment is heterogeneous in suspected hydrocephalus patients, and its value is lower than expected! This new parameter could represent new information, complementary to conventional infusion tests. We hope that this information can be applied to improve the selection of patients for shunt surgery.

Keywords ICP monitoring · PCMRI · Physiological · Intracranial compliance · Rest · Hydrocephalus

Introduction

Hydrocephalus is associated with cerebrospinal fluid (CSF) dynamic disturbances [1, 2]. It is characterized by gait disturbance, urinary incontinence, cognitive impairment, and ventricle enlargement [3]. The guidelines for the management of patients with hydrocephalus recommend intracranial pressure (ICP) monitoring and infusion studies [4] and the placement of a shunt as the treatment of reference.

From ICP monitoring and infusion tests, many parameters, like resistance to CSF absorption (Ro), mean ICP wave amplitude (MWA), mean ICP, elastance coefficient or

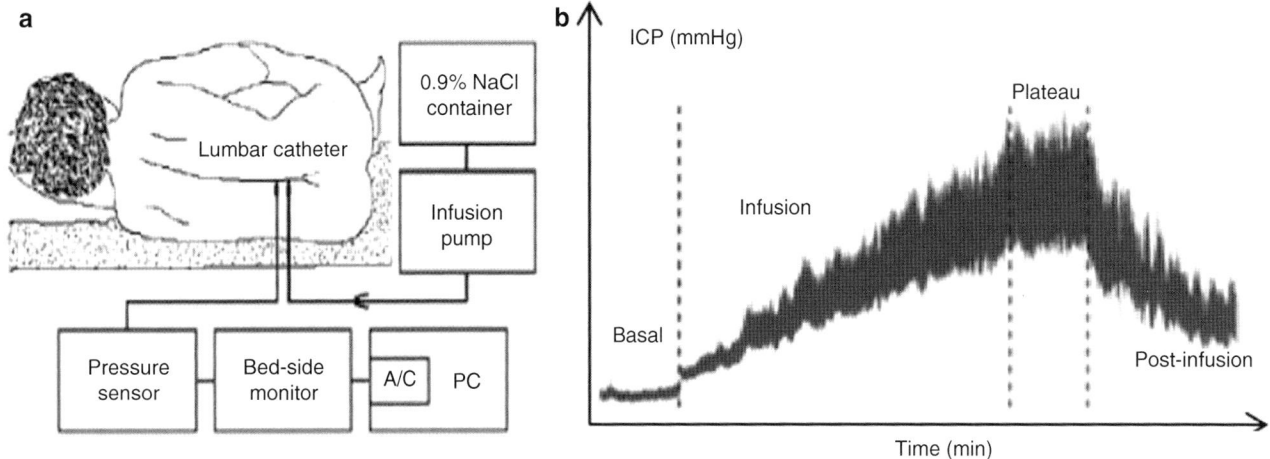

Fig. 1 (**a**) ICP monitoring system used during infusion test [15]. (**b**) Typical recording of mean ICP during constant-rate infusion test. Resting ICP was monitored at basal period. During infusion, ICP increases, reaches a plateau, and decreases after infusion

intracranial compliance, can be assessed. Some authors have suggested the usefulness of these parameters in identifying shunt responders [5], while others did not find this benefit [6]. Intracranial compliance determines the ability of the cranio-spinal system to accommodate an increase in volume without an increase in pressure [7, 8].

Intracranial compliance is obtained by dividing a known external volume infused in the subarachnoid spaces by the amplitude of ICP in response to this volume [9]. However, although this way of assessing intracranial compliance is recognized worldwide, it appears that infusion is a kind of disruption of intracranial volume [10] and does not reflect the physiological behavior of the intracranial compartment.

Phase-contrast magnetic resonance imaging (PCMRI) is the only imaging technique that is able to quantify the CSF and blood oscillations in physiological conditions during the cardiac cycle (CC) [11–13]. These volume changes are directly related to ICP oscillations during the CC [14].

We hypothesized that it was possible to calculate ICP changes during the CC before an infusion using ICP monitoring and to calculate intracranial volume change (blood and CSF) during the CC by PCMRI. The aim of this study was to quantify the intracranial compliance of hydrocephalus patients in physiological conditions without an infusion.

Materials and Methods

Study Population

Thirty-three patients suspected of probable hydrocephalus (15 women and 18 men) with a mean age of 74 ± 8 years (range 52–85) were prospectively included in the "Proliphyc" research program in Toulouse Hospital. They were included on the basis of chronic hydrocephalus symptoms: gait disturbance, cognitive impairment, urinary incontinence, and ventricular dilation. These patients underwent a lumbar constant-rate infusion test and PCMRI the day before.

ICP Study: Infusion Test Protocol

The lumbar constant-rate infusion test protocol described previously was used [15]. The test is performed with a constant-rate infusion (1.5 mL min^{-1}) using a lumbar catheter. The measuring system is presented in Fig. 1a. The lumbar catheter is connected to two needles: a pressure sensor and an infusion pump. A syringe infusion pump is connected to the second needle to infuse normal saline. After about 10 min of the basal pressure measurement, the infusion is started. The constant-rate infusion is continued until ICP reaches the plateau, and then the infusion is stopped. After infusion, the descending ICP is recorded for about 10 min (Fig. 1b). The signal is sampled, stored, analyzed, and displayed during the infusion test by using purpose-designed software ICM+ [16].

ICP Study: Postprocessing

We used homemade software to assess the resting ICP amplitude (ΔICP_rest) during the CC before the injection in the basal period (Fig. 1b). The software overcomes a patient's respiratory modulations and calculates the curve of evolution of ICP during the CC at rest. Then, ΔICP_rest was calculated during the rest period: ΔICP_rest = ICP$_{max}$-ICP$_{min}$ (Fig. 2).

Fig. 2 Determination of resting ICP amplitude during CC. Using MRiCP software, we focus on basal ICP measurement (**a**); the software overcomes the respiratory modulations and focuses on patient cardiac frequency (**b**). Then, mean ICP with standard deviation was calculated over the entire CC, and the ICP amplitude at rest during the CC (ΔICP_rest) was also determined (**c**)

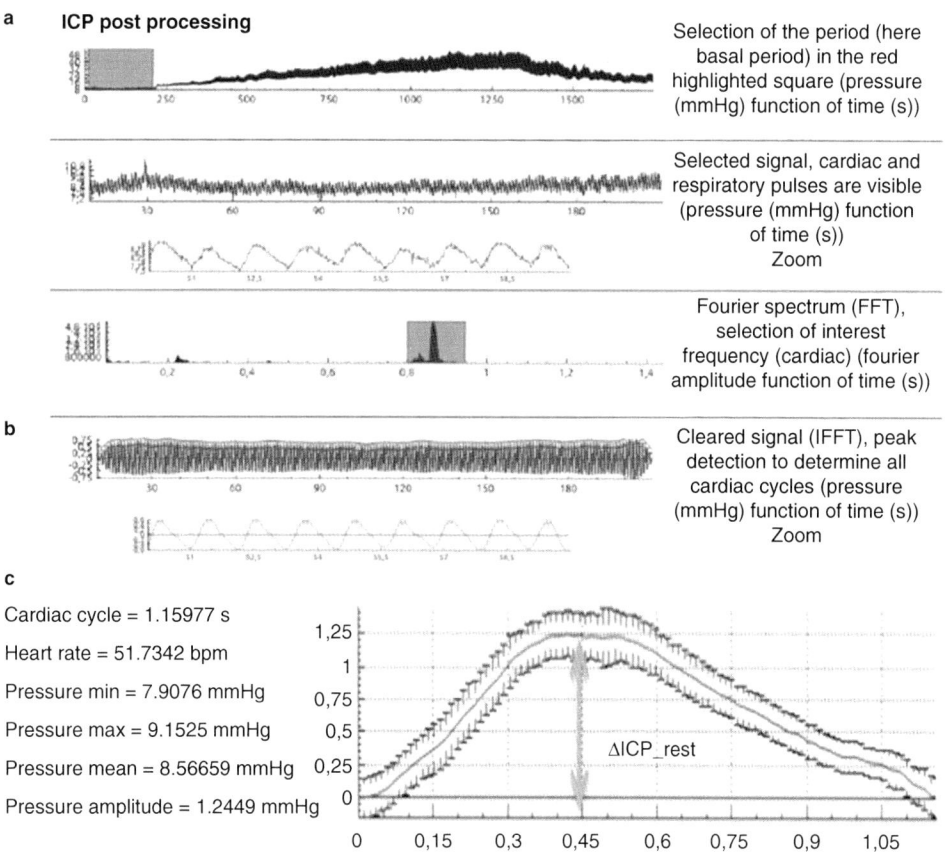

PCMRI Study: Flow Acquisitions

The same patients had PCMRI the day before the infusion test. It was performed on a 3T MRI machine. The PCMRI planes were perpendicular to the assumed direction of the CSF and blood flows to assess: (1) arterial blood flow in the internal carotid arteries (ICAs) and basilar artery (BA), and venous flow in the sinuses (sagittal and straight); (2) cervical CSF flow at the C2–C3 level. PCMRI parameters included a repetition time of 23 ms, echo time of 5 ms, a 150 × 150 mm field of view, a section thickness of 5 mm, and a flip angle of 15°. Velocity sensitization was set to 80 cm/s for the blood vessels and 5 cm/s for the CSF around the spine. Retrospective cardiac gating was used, and 32 images per CC were reconstructed. For each flow series, the acquisition time was approximatively 2 min, depending on the cardiac period (Fig. 3).

PCMRI Study: Flow Measurements

PCMRI acquisitions were postprocessed using flow analysis software [11]. This software automatically determines the flow curve over the CC for a given region of interest. The flow in the left and right internal carotid and basilar arteries were added in each individual to determine the total cerebral blood flow (tCBF). The flows in the sagittal and straight sinuses were summed to obtain the measured cerebral venous outflow. Given that the entire cerebral venous outflow must equal the tCBF, the measured venous flow was corrected taking account of tCBF. Arteriovenous flow was determined by subtracting the corrected venous flow from the tCBF. Cervical CSF flow during the CC was also determined. Cervical CSF stroke volume (CSV) and blood stroke volume (SVblood) were calculated by integrating respectively the cervical CSF flow and arteriovenous flow along the CC. These stroke volumes correspond to the volume of fluid moving inside and outside the cranium during the CC and represent the area under and over the curves of the cervical CSF and arteriovenous flows, respectively (Fig. 4a).

Arteriovenous flow and cervical CSF flow were summed, and the global intracranial flow change in the system during the CC was obtained. This global intracranial flow change was integrated along the CC, and the global (blood and CSF) intracranial volume change (ΔIVC) during the same CC was calculated (Fig. 4b).

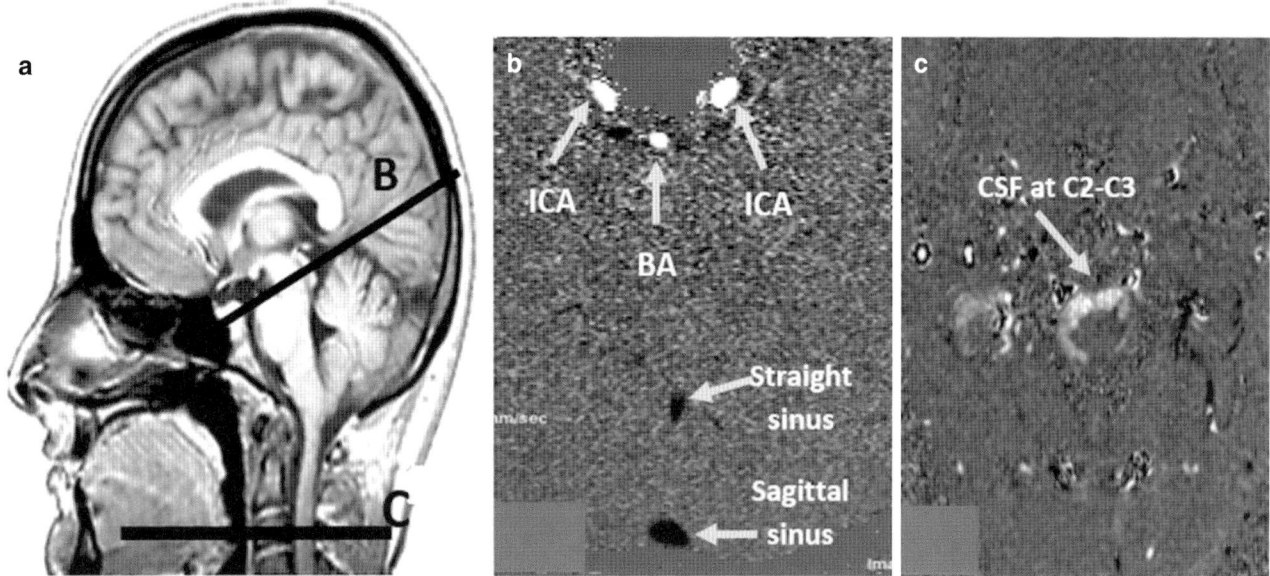

Fig. 3 (a) Data acquisition by PCMRI. The selected acquisition planes were perpendicular to the presumed flow direction. By convention, cranial–caudal flow was negative, whereas caudal–cranial flows were positive. Sections through the intracranial level (b) were used to quantify flows in right and left internal carotid arteries (ICAs), basilar artery (BA), and sinuses (sagittal and straight); a section through the cervical level (c) was used to quantify CSF at C2–C3 around the spine

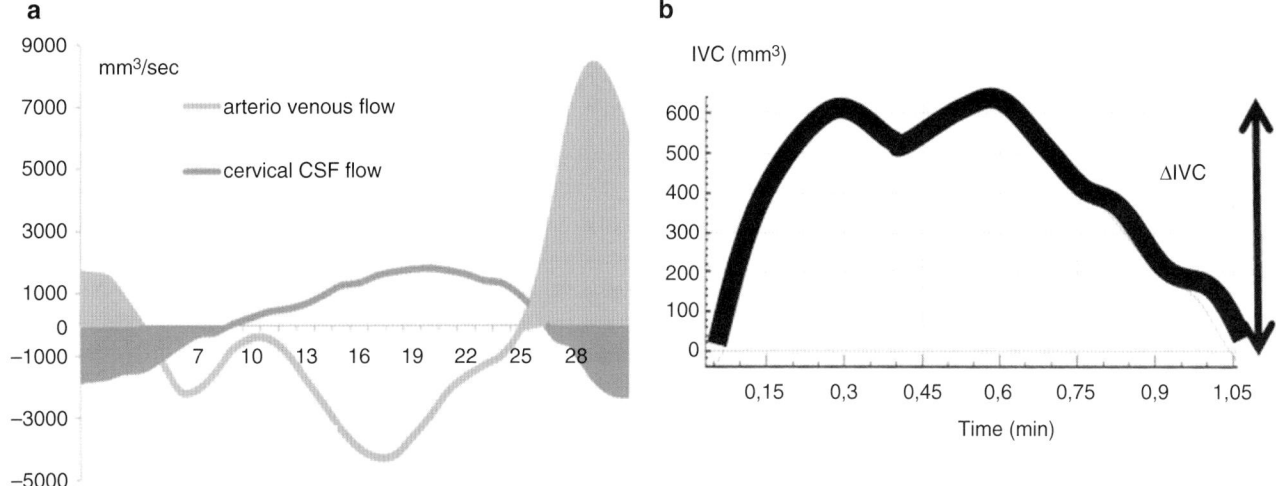

Fig. 4 (a) Arteriovenous and cervical CSF flow curves during CC. The areas under and over the curves represent the stroke volume. These two flows during the CC were summed and integrated, and global (blood + CSF) intracranial volume change (ΔIVC) was obtained (b)

Compliance of Intracranial Compartment

Finally, compliance at rest (C_rest) in mL/mmHg was calculated:

$$C\_rest = \frac{\Delta IVC}{\Delta ICP\_rest}.$$

Statistical Analysis

Statistical analysis was performed using *R* statistical and *Excel* software. Two independent operators postprocessed these data by blinding analysis. To evaluate the agreement between the measurements (tCBF, ΔIVC, ΔICP_rest) performed by both of them, we used Bland–Altman plots and

Pearson correlation coefficients. After this step, we used the mean value of the measurements of both operators. We also determined the correlation between (1) tCBF and SVblood and (2) SVblood and CSV. Statistical significance was set at $p < 0.05$.

Results

The Bland–Altman plots showed that the measurements presented no significant difference between the two operators (Fig. 5). The Pearson correlation coefficient presented a good correlation between the measurements of the two operators: $r = 0.87$, $p < 0.001$; $r = 0.69$, $p < 0.001$; and $r = 0.96$, $p < 0.001$ for tCBF, ΔIVC, and ΔICP_rest, respectively. The mean value of two measurements were synthetized in Table 1. As shown in Fig. 6, there is a strong correlation between CSV and SVblood ($r = 0.76$, $p < 0.0001$) and between tCBF and SVblood ($r = 0.53$, $p < 0.001$). We found a heterogeneous value of compliance in our cohort: C_rest = 0.23 ± 0.15 mL/mmHg (range 0.04–0.63 mL/mmHg).

Discussion

This study proposes a new approach to assessing physiological intracranial compliance at rest in hydrocephalus patients.

First, our results showed that the quantification of intracranial volume change (ΔIVC) and resting intracranial amplitude (ΔICP_rest) could be acquired and calculated with good reproducibility even if the values are small. The obtained intracranial volume change during the CC is a small volume resulting from multiple measurements, which can generate additional errors. Nevertheless, the values obtained

Table 1 Mean values and standard deviation of parameters calculated by two blind operators

Parameter	Mean value
tCBF (mL/min)	469.89 ± 127.54
CSV (mL/cc)	0.50 ± 0.22
SVblood (mL/cc)	0.82 ± 0.32
ΔIVC (mL)	0.44 ± 0.22
ΔICP_rest (mmHg)	2.41 ± 1.21

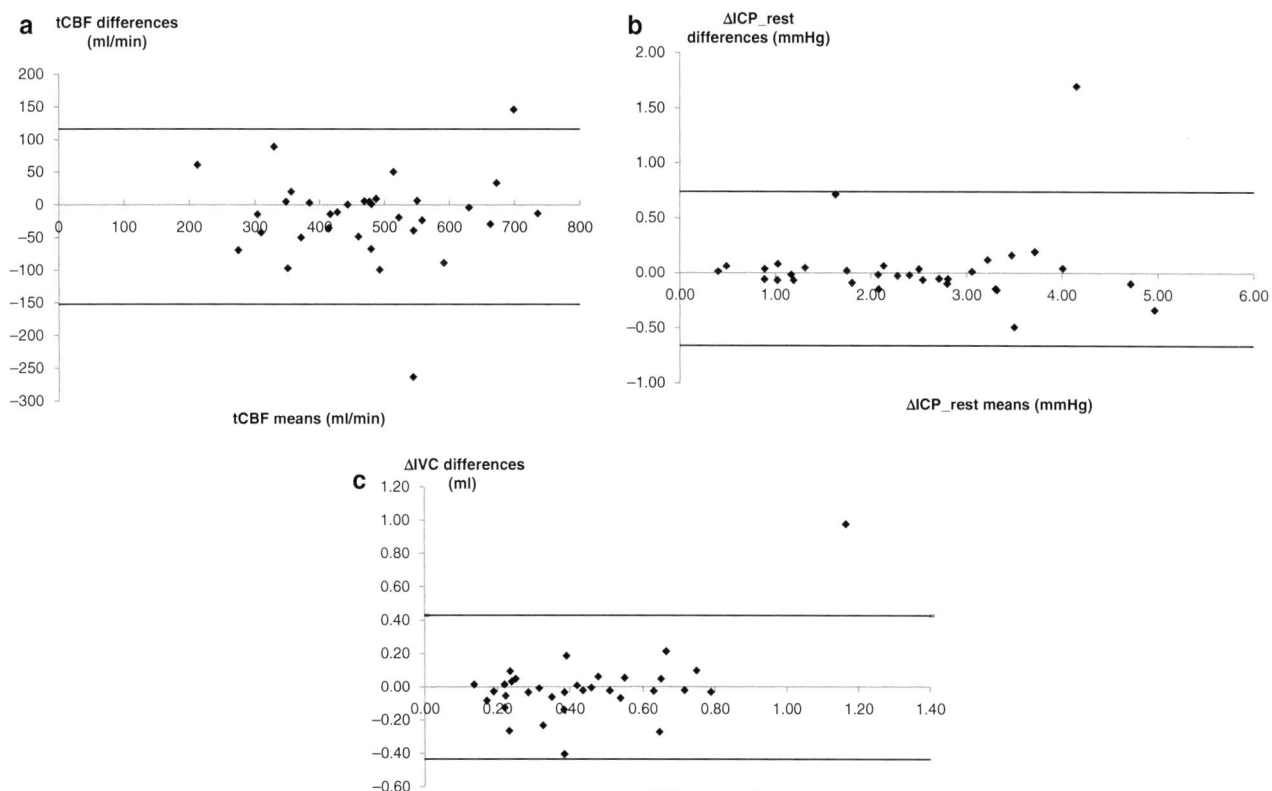

Fig. 5 Bland–Altman analysis plots of measurements performed by two independent operators for total cerebral blood flow (**a**), intracranial pressure amplitude at rest (**b**), and intracranial volume change (**c**). The difference between the two measurements lay with the limits of agreement, and the bias was close to zero for all estimations

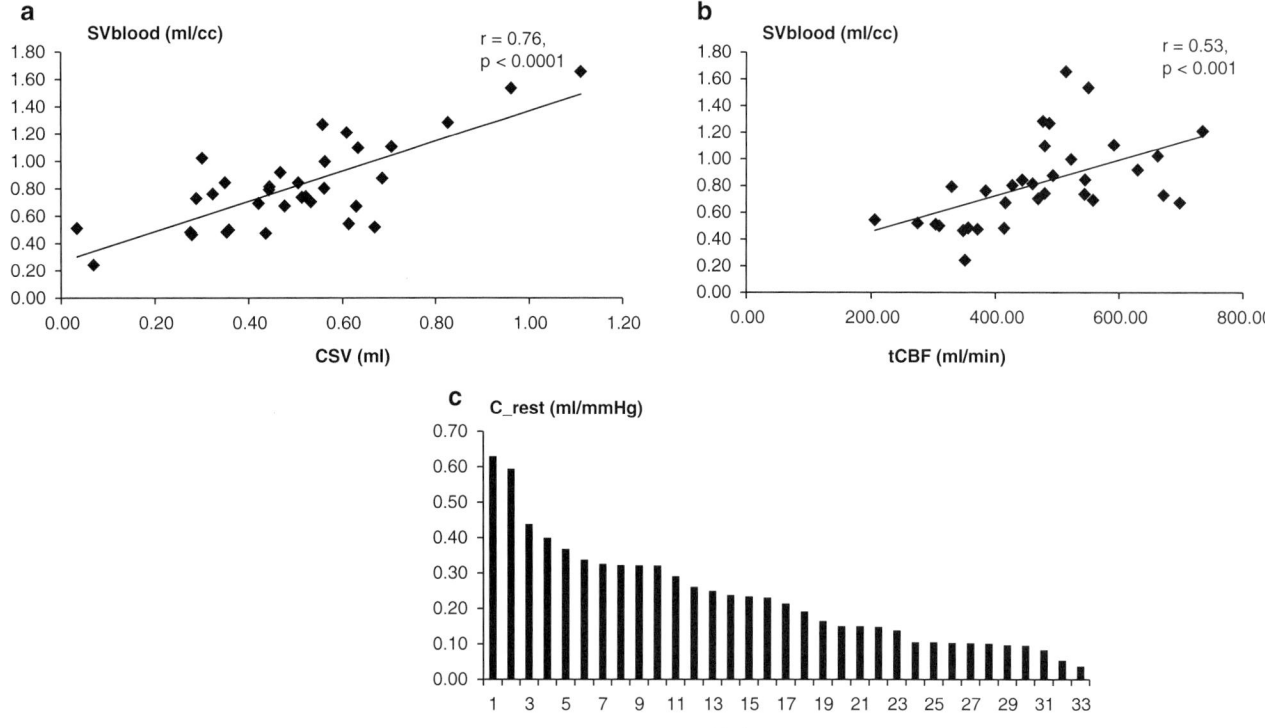

Fig. 6 (a) Correlation between arteriovenous stroke volume (SVblood) and cervical stroke volume (CSV) in patients. SVblood was positively correlated with CSV. (b) Correlation between SVblood and total cerebral blood flow (tCBF) in patients. SVblood was positively correlated with tCBF. (c) Compliance values at rest were heterogeneous in patients with suspected hydrocephalus

were in accordance with previous works [11, 17, 18]. Using a phantom, some authors have shown that PCMRI is an accurate technique for measuring small flow [18], while others have used this methodology to propose a noninvasive method to calculate ICP [17]. Another limit is that ICP monitoring and PCMRI were not performed at the same moment because ICP monitoring remains unavailable under MRI.

The mean value of compliance calculated at rest (C_rest = 0.23 ± 0.15 mL/mmHg) in our hydrocephalus patients was smaller than 0.5 mL/mmHg, a value that corresponds to altered intracranial compliance [19, 20]. C_rest was for the most part smaller than the values of intracranial compliance calculated using the infusion procedure in hydrocephalus patients (0.809 ± 0.085 mL/mmHg) [20] or in patients with severe head injury (0.68 ± 0.3 mL/mmHg) [8].

The differences in intracranial compliances observed may be related to the method used to measure intracranial compliance at rest. To measure C_rest, we used the intrinsic physiological intracranial volume change during the CC. Thus, this is a quick (1 s) and small volume change (less than 1 mL) in comparison with the infusion procedure. These results highlight the fact that intracranial compliance is a complex concept, and we hypothesize that intracranial compliance is time and volume dependent and use different mechanisms to maintain ICP mean value and amplitude.

The compliances calculated reflect the brain behavior at rest during one CC. In our population, we found heterogeneous values of C_rest. This indicates that the physiological intracranial compliance calculated could be a new biomarker to differentiate patients with hydrocephalus.

Taking into account that the patients included in this study underwent an infusion test, our future research will compare intracranial compliance at rest with other parameters like resistance to CSF absorption (Ro) and the following of patients. Future studies will seek for if physiological intracranial compliance may be helpful for selecting shunting patients.

Conclusion

This study shows that by combining the record of ICP monitoring at the basal period before injection and PCMRI, we are able to measure physiological intracranial compliance at rest. In hydrocephalus patients, this compliance is heterogeneous and lower than the impairment limit of compliance measured after infusion. This result indicates that the mechanism involved during a CC to respond to an increase in intracranial volume differs from that implicated during an infusion test.

Conflicts of interest statement We declare that we have no conflict of interest.

References

1. Balédent O, et al. Relationship between cerebrospinal fluid and blood dynamics in healthy volunteers and patients with communicating hydrocephalus. Investig Radiol. 2004;39:45–55.
2. Bradley WG, et al. Normal-pressure hydrocephalus: evaluation with cerebrospinal fluid flow measurements at MR imaging. Radiology. 1996;198:523–9.
3. Hakim S, Adams RD. The special clinical problem of symptomatic hydrocephalus with normal cerebrospinal fluid pressure. Observations on cerebrospinal fluid hydrodynamics. J Neurol Sci. 1965;2:307–27.
4. Marmarou A, Black P, Bergsneider M, Klinge P, Relkin N. Guidelines for management of idiopathic normal pressure hydrocephalus: progress to date. Acta Neurochir Suppl. 2005;95:237–40.
5. Kim D-J, et al. Thresholds of resistance to CSF outflow in predicting shunt responsiveness. Neurol Res. 2015;37:332–40.
6. Delwel EJ, de Jong DA, Avezaat CJJ. The prognostic value of clinical characteristics and parameters of cerebrospinal fluid hydrodynamics in shunting for idiopathic normal pressure hydrocephalus. Acta Neurochir. 2005;147:1037–1042-1043.
7. Tain R-W, Ertl-Wagner B, Alperin N. Influence of the compliance of the neck arteries and veins on the measurement of intracranial volume change by phase-contrast MRI. J. Magn. Reson. Imaging JMRI. 2009;30:878–83.
8. Portella G, et al. Continuous cerebral compliance monitoring in severe head injury: its relationship with intracranial pressure and cerebral perfusion pressure. Acta Neurochir (Wien). 2005;147:707–713.; discussion 713.
9. Marmarou A, Shulman K, LaMorgese J. Compartmental analysis of compliance and outflow resistance of the cerebrospinal fluid system. J Neurosurg. 1975;43:523–34.
10. Marmarou A, Shulman K, Rosende RM. A nonlinear analysis of the cerebrospinal fluid system and intracranial pressure dynamics. J Neurosurg. 1978;48:332–44.
11. Balédent O, Henry-Feugeas MC, Idy-Peretti I. Cerebrospinal fluid dynamics and relation with blood flow: a magnetic resonance study with semiautomated cerebrospinal fluid segmentation. Investig Radiol. 2001;36:368–77.
12. Enzmann DR, Ross MR, Marks MP, Pelc NJ. Blood flow in major cerebral arteries measured by phase-contrast cine MR. AJNR Am J Neuroradiol. 1994;15:123–9.
13. Marks MP, Pelc NJ, Ross MR, Enzmann DR. Determination of cerebral blood flow with a phase-contrast cine MR imaging technique: evaluation of normal subjects and patients with arteriovenous malformations. Radiology. 1992;182:467–76.
14. Miller K. Biomechanics of the brain. New York, NY: Springer; 2011.
15. Juniewicz H, et al. Analysis of intracranial pressure during and after the infusion test in patients with communicating hydrocephalus. Physiol Meas. 2005;26:1039.
16. Smielewski P, et al. ICM+: software for on-line analysis of bedside monitoring data after severe head trauma. Acta Neurochir Suppl. 2005;95:43–9.
17. Alperin NJ, Lee SH, Loth F, Raksin PB, Lichtor T. MR-intracranial pressure (ICP): a method to measure intracranial elastance and pressure noninvasively by means of MR imaging: baboon and human study. Radiology. 2000;217:877–85.
18. Wåhlin A, et al. Phase contrast MRI quantification of pulsatile volumes of brain arteries, veins, and cerebrospinal fluids compartments: repeatability and physiological interactions. J Magn Reson Imaging JMRI. 2012;35:1055–62.
19. Kiening KL, Schoening WN, Lanksch WR, Unterberg AW. Intracranial compliance as a bed-side monitoring technique in severely head-injured patients. Acta Neurochir Suppl. 2002;81:177–80.
20. Yau Y, et al. Multi-centre assessment of the Spiegelberg compliance monitor: interim results. Acta Neurochir. 2002;81(Suppl):167–70.

Numerical Cerebrospinal System Modeling in Fluid-Structure Interaction

Simon Garnotel, Stéphanie Salmon, and Olivier Balédent

Abstract *Objective*: Cerebrospinal fluid (CSF) stroke volume in the aqueduct is widely used to evaluate CSF dynamics disorders. In a healthy population, aqueduct stroke volume represents around 10% of the spinal stroke volume while intracranial subarachnoid space stroke volume represents 90%. The amplitude of the CSF oscillations through the different compartments of the cerebrospinal system is a function of the geometry and the compliances of each compartment, but we suspect that it could also be impacted be the cardiac cycle frequency. To study this CSF distribution, we have developed a numerical model of the cerebrospinal system taking into account cerebral ventricles, intracranial subarachnoid spaces, spinal canal and brain tissue in fluid-structure interactions.

Materials and methods: A numerical fluid-structure interaction model is implemented using a finite-element method library to model the cerebrospinal system and its interaction with the brain based on fluid mechanics equations and linear elasticity equations coupled in a monolithic formulation. The model geometry, simplified in a first approach, is designed in accordance with realistic volume ratios of the different compartments: a thin tube is used to mimic the high flow resistance of the aqueduct. CSF velocity and pressure and brain displacements are obtained as simulation results, and CSF flow and stroke volume are calculated from these results.

Results: Simulation results show a significant variability of aqueduct stroke volume and intracranial subarachnoid space stroke volume in the physiological range of cardiac frequencies.

Conclusions: Fluid-structure interactions are numerous in the cerebrospinal system and difficult to understand in the rigid skull. The presented model highlights significant variations of stroke volumes under cardiac frequency variations only.

Keywords Cerebrospinal fluid · Intracranial pressure · Stroke volume · Fluid-structure interaction · Finite-element method

Introduction

Cerebrospinal fluid (CSF) stroke volume in the aqueduct (SV_{aq}) is widely used to evaluate CSF dynamics disorders. In healthy population, SV_{aq} represents around 10% of the spinal stroke volume (SV_{spi}), while intracranial subarachnoid space (SAS) stroke volume (SV_{sas}) represents around 90% of SV_{spi} [1]. The amplitude of the CSF oscillations through the different compartments of the cerebrospinal system is a function of the geometry and the compliances of each compartment, but we suspect that it could also be impacted by cardiac frequency. To study the CSF distribution, a numerical model of the cerebrospinal system was developed taking into account cerebral ventricles, intracranial SASs, spinal canal, and brain tissue in fluid-structure interactions.

Numerical models of the cerebrospinal system have already been developed using fluid equations only [2] or fluid and porous media equations [3], but they are not relevant in this study, so a new numerical framework is introduced. Model geometry and parameters are detailed and numerical simulations are run. A first step of validation is done before the presentation of the results and discussion.

S. Garnotel · O. Balédent (✉)
Equipe de recherhce BioFlowImage, Université de Picardie Jules Verne, Amiens, France

Unité de traitement de l'image médicale,
Centre Hospitalo-Universitaire de Picardie, Amiens, France
e-mail: olivier.baledent@chu-amiens.fr

S. Salmon
Laboratoire de Mathematiques EA 4535 - FR CNRS ARC 3399, Université de Reims Champagne-Ardenne, Reims, France

Materials and Methods

Numerical Framework

A numerical fluid-structure interaction model is implemented using the finite-element-method library FreeFem++ [4] to model the cerebrospinal system and its interactions with the brain. This model is based on fluid mechanics equations, Navier-Stokes equations, solid mechanics equations, and linear elasticity equations coupled in a monolithic formulation [5].

The Navier-Stokes equations that describe the fluid behavior in a moving domain read as follows:

$$\rho^F \frac{\partial u}{\partial t} + \rho^F \left((u-U).\nabla \right) u - 2\mu^F \nabla.\epsilon(u) + \nabla p = f^F$$

$$\nabla.u = 0,$$

where u is velocity, p pressure, U domain velocity, f^F volumetric external force (taken here to be zero, meaning gravity is neglected), ρ^F density, and μ^F fluid dynamic viscosity, and where

$$\epsilon(u) = \frac{1}{2}\left(\nabla u + (\nabla u)^T \right).$$

The linear elasticity equations that describe solid deformations read as follows:

$$\rho^S \frac{\partial^2 d}{\partial t^2} - \nabla.\sigma^S(d) = f^S,$$

where d is the displacement, f^S the volumetric external force (taken here to be zero, meaning gravity is neglected), and ρ^S the density of the solid, and where

$$\sigma^S(d) = \lambda (\nabla.d) I + 2\mu^S \epsilon(d)$$

where λ and μ^S are Lamé's coefficients and I is the identity matrix.

Lamé's coefficients are defined using the Young's modulus and Poisson's ratio as follows:

$$\lambda = \frac{\nu E}{(1-2\nu)(1+\nu)}$$

$$\mu^S = \frac{E}{2(1+\nu)},$$

where E is the Young's modulus and ν Poisson's ratio.

To couple these two equations, the continuity of velocity and stress is imposed at the fluid-structure interface as follows:

$$u = \frac{\partial d}{\partial t}$$

$$\sigma^F(u,p) n = -\sigma^S(d) n,$$

where n is the normal vector and

$$\sigma^F(u,p) = -pI + 2\mu^F \epsilon(u).$$

The monolithic formulation of this problem leads to the following matrix form, where fluid and structure problems are strongly coupled and solved at the same time:

$$\begin{pmatrix} A & B^T & 0 \\ B & \epsilon & 0 \\ 0 & 0 & \epsilon \end{pmatrix} \begin{pmatrix} U \\ P^F \\ P^S \end{pmatrix} = \begin{pmatrix} L \\ 0 \\ 0 \end{pmatrix},$$

where ϵ is a stabilization term, A and B are the representatives matrix of the problem, U is the fluid velocity, P^F is the fluid pressure, P^S is the solid pressure (equal to zero), and L represents external and coupling conditions.

Geometry

The model geometry, simplified in a first approach, is deigned in accordance to realistic volume ratios of the different compartments of the cerebrospinal system. Brain, intracranial SASs, and ventricles are designed using two-dimensional disks, and a thin tube is used to mimic the high flow resistance of the aqueduct (Fig. 1).

The cranium has a radius of 10 cm, intracranial SASs have a thickness of 0.75 cm, ventricles have a radius of 3 cm, the aqueduct has a radius of 0.2 cm, and the spinal canal has a radius of 1 cm.

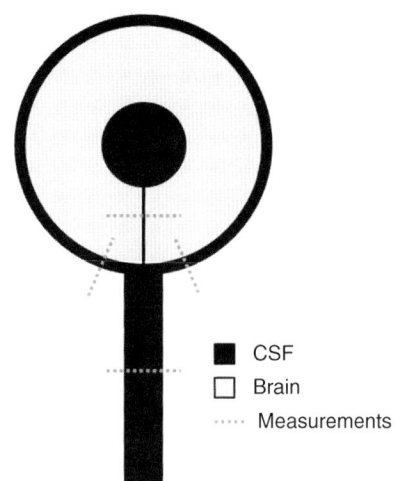

Fig. 1 Model geometry

Parameters

Fluid and structure parameters, provided from the literature [6], are taken in accordance with the CSF and brain mechanical physiological parameters (Table 1).

The model input is located on the spinal canal end where a velocity profile, close to the physiological one, is imposed:

$$v = A \sin\left(\frac{2\pi t}{p}\right),$$

where A is the velocity amplitude and p the period of the cardiac cycle.

Remark 1

In physiological conditions, CSF oscillations come from brain expansion at each cardiac cycle. In our model, this is the inverse phenomenon: CSF oscillations cause brain deformations. This behavior has been chosen, for future use of physiological measures, because CSF flow is easily measured by phase-contrast magnetic resonance imaging (PC-MRI); contrariwise, brain deformations are hard to obtain.

Simulations are performed with different values of the heart rate period (p), keeping the same SV_{spi} (Fig. 2). Twenty cardiac cycles are simulated and the results are extracted from the last cardiac cycle. CSF velocity and pressure and brain displacements are obtained as simulation results, and CSF flow and stroke volume are calculated on the basis of these results.

Remark 2

Many cardiac cycles are simulated to ensure the stabilization of the system.

Results

Validation

Model validity is successfully performed on numerical benchmarks (specific cases) to ensure the correct agreement of the algorithm. In addition, flow conservation is calculated in the used model geometry during a cardiac cycle; the net flow error is 1.4% ± 1.3 SD.

Study Case

As a second validation, geometry and flow are measured in a healthy subject by MRI to design the model and impose an input velocity. Simulation results (Figs. 3 and 4) show good agreement with the PC-MRI measured data and with the physiological intracranial pressure curve shape and amplitude.

Cardiac Cycle Impact

Simulation results (Figs. 5 and 6) show significant variability of SV_{aq} and SV_{sas} in the physiological range of cardiac frequencies; an inversion of the distribution is even observed for

Table 1 Mechanical parameters

Parameter	Symbol	Value	Unity
Fluid density	ρ^F	1	g cm^{-3}
Fluid viscosity	μ^F	0.001	g cmcm^{-1} s^{-1}
Solid density	ρ^S	1.1	g cm^{-3}
Solid Young's modulus	E	4.10^3	g cm^{-1} s^{-2}
Fluid Poisson's ratio	ν	0.35	–

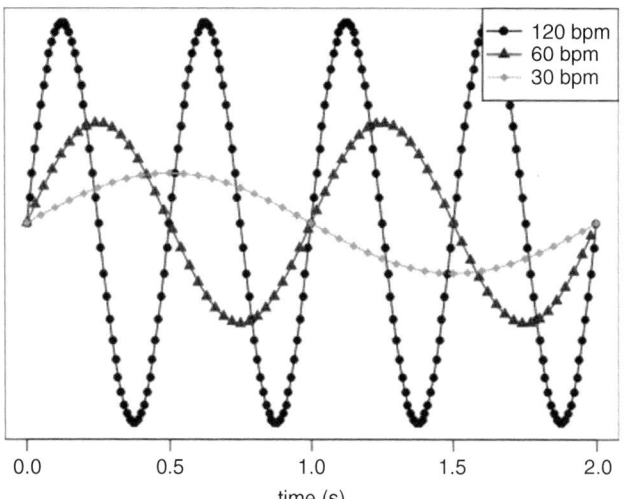

Fig. 2 Input of model

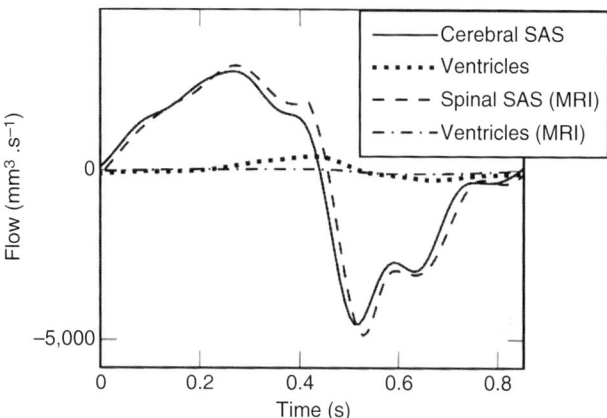

Fig. 3 Simulation results and PC-MRI measurements of flow

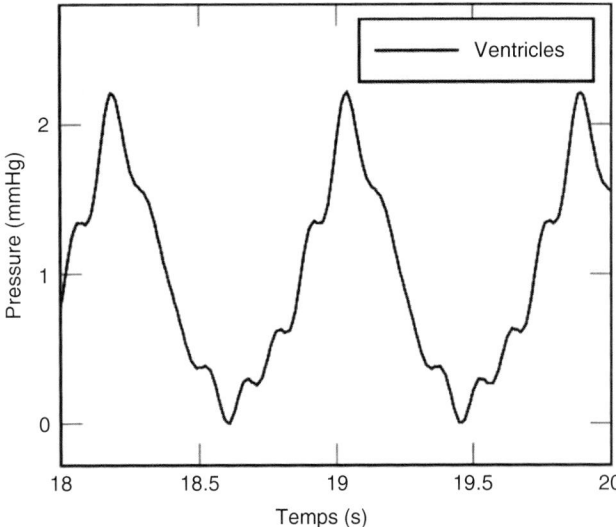

Fig. 4 Simulation results of pressure

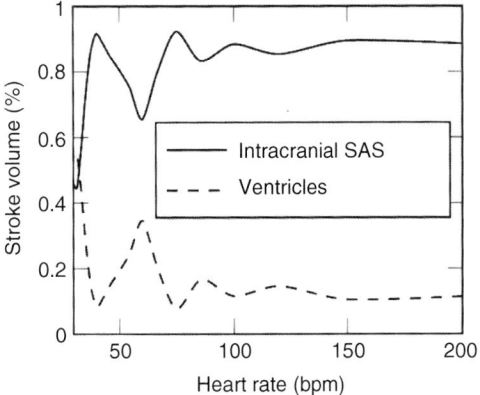

Fig. 5 Stroke volume function of cardiac frequency

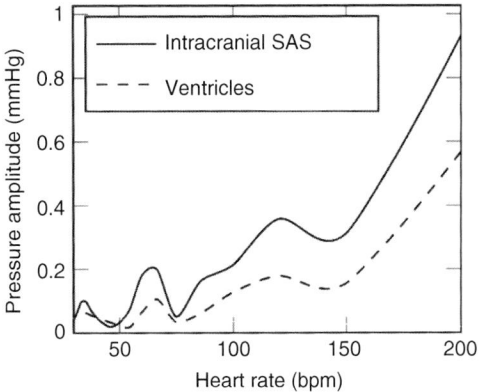

Fig. 6 Pressure gradient function of cardiac frequency

slow cardiac frequencies. The pressure gradient (maximum pressure minus minimum pressure during a cardiac cycle) is likewise modified by the cardiac frequency variations; it is exponentially increased with cardiac frequency growth.

Discussion

Linear elasticity is justified in this application since small deformations are obtained in the simulation results. The proposed model is validated from numerical (benchmark) and physiological (flow conservation) points of view.

Numerical results in the study case are in accordance with PC-MRI measured data. In addition, the pressure curve presents a physiological amplitude and shape (peaks and valleys).

Cardiac frequency affects the CSF distribution between the two main intracranial compartments: ventricles and intracranial SASs; stroke volume distribution is in a physiological range for normal (around 60–100 bpm) and high cardiac frequencies; contrariwise, the stroke volume distribution tends to be equal in the two main compartments as cardiac frequency decreases.

Likewise, cardiac frequency affects the pressure gradient in the two compartments; the pressure gradient grows as cardiac frequency increases. Because the SV_{spi} is conserved, a high cardiac frequency causes a rapid inflow of CSF into the intracranial compartment, which can explain this phenomenon.

Because the absolute pressure term does not appear in the Navier-Stokes formulation (only its gradient), it is impossible to obtain information about the absolute pressure of the CSF; only the gradient of the intracranial pressure is calculated.

Conclusions

A numerical model is presented taking into account the numerous fluid-structure interactions in the cerebrospinal system closed in the rigid skull. This model highlights significant variations in stroke volume distribution under cardiac frequency variations only.

In the future, spatial distribution of the intracranial pressure gradient in all the cranio spinal compartments will be studied over the time. Improvements will be introduced to the model, including with respect to arterial and venous flow.

Another improvement could be the determination of the absolute intracranial pressure in connection with Marmarou's studies and the pressure volume curve [7, 8].

Acknowledgement This research was partially funded by Agence Nationale de la Recherche (Grant Agreement ANR-12-MONU-0010).

Conflicts of interest statement We declare that we have no conflict of interest.

References

1. Balédent O, Gondry-Jouet C, Meyer ME, De Marco G, Le Gars D, Henry-Feugeas MC, Idy-Peretti I. Relationship between cerebrospinal fluid and blood dynamics in healthy volunteers and patients with communicating hydrocephalus. Invest Radiol. 2004;39:45–55.
2. Alperin NJ, Lee SH, Loth F, Raksin PB, Lichtor T. MR-intracranial pressure (ICP): a method to measure intracranial elastance and pressure noninvasively by means of MR imaging: baboon and human study. Radiology. 2000;217:877–85.
3. Linninger AA, Xenos M, Zhu DC, Somayaji MR, Kondapalli S, Penn RD. Cerebrospinal fluid flow in the normal and hydrocephalic human brain. IEEE Trans Biomed Eng. 2007;54:291–302.
4. Hecht F. New development in FreeFem++. J Numer Math. 2012;20:251–65.
5. Sy S, Murea, CM. Algorithme for solving fluid-structure interaction problem on a global moving mesh. In: Proceedings of IV European conference on computational mechanics. 2010
6. Dutta-Roy T, Wittek A, Miller K. Biomechanical modelling of normal pressure hydrocephalus. J Biomech. 2008;41(2269):2271.
7. Marmarou A, Sulman K, LaMorges J. Compartmental analysis of compliance end outflow resistance of the cerebrospinal fluid system. J Neurosurg. 1975;43:523–34.
8. Marmarou A, Shulman K, Rosende RM. A nonlinear analysis of the cerebrospinal fluid system and intracranial pressure dynamics. J Neurosurg. 1978;48:332–44.

Cerebrovascular Autoregulation

Differential Systolic and Diastolic Regulation of the Cerebral Pressure-Flow Relationship During Squat-Stand Manoeuvres

Jonathan D. Smirl, Alexander D. Wright, Philip N. Ainslie, Yu-Chieh Tzeng, and Paul van Donkelaar

Abstract *Objective*: Cerebral pressure-flow dynamics are typically reported between mean arterial pressure and mean cerebral blood velocity. However, by reporting only mean responses, potential differential regulatory properties associated with systole and diastole may have been overlooked.

Materials and methods: Twenty young adults (16 male, age: 26.7 ± 6.6 years, BMI: 24.9 ± 3.0 kg/m^2) were recruited for this study. Middle cerebral artery velocity was indexed via transcranial Doppler. Cerebral pressure-flow dynamics were assessed using transfer function analysis at both 0.05 and 0.10 Hz using squat-stand manoeuvres. This method provides robust and reliable measures for coherence (correlation index), phase (timing buffer) and gain (amplitude buffer) metrics.

Results: There were main effects for both cardiac cycle and frequency for phase and gain metrics ($p < 0.001$). The systolic phase (mean ± SD) was elevated at 0.05 (1.07 ± 0.51 radians) and 0.10 Hz (0.70 ± 0.46 radians) compared to the diastolic phase (0.05 Hz: 0.59 ± 0.14 radians; 0.10 Hz: 0.33 ± 0.11 radians). Conversely, the systolic normalized gain was reduced (0.05 Hz: 0.49 ± 0.12%/%; 0.10 Hz: 0.66 ± 0.20%/%) compared to the diastolic normalized gain (0.05 Hz: 1.46 ± 0.43%/%; 0.10 Hz: 1.97 ± 0.48%/%).

Conclusions: These findings indicate there are differential systolic and diastolic aspects of the cerebral pressure-flow relationship. The oscillations associated with systole are extensively buffered within the cerebrovasculature, whereas diastolic oscillations are relatively unaltered. This indicates that the brain is adapted to protect itself against large increases in systolic blood pressure, likely as a mechanism to prevent cerebral haemorrhages.

Keywords Cerebral blood flow · Middle cerebral artery · Cerebral autoregulation · Cardiac cycle · Transfer function analysis · Blood pressure

J.D. Smirl, Ph.D. (✉) · P. van Donkelaar
Sports Concussion Research Lab, School of Health and Exercise Sciences, University of British Columbia, Kelowna, BC, Canada
e-mail: jonathan.smirl@ubc.ca

A.D. Wright
Sports Concussion Research Lab, School of Health and Exercise Sciences, University of British Columbia, Kelowna, BC, Canada

MD/PhD Program, University of British Columbia, Vancouver, BC, Canada

Southern Medical Program, University of British Columbia, Kelowna, BC, Canada

Experimental Medicine Program, University of British Columbia, Vancouver, BC, Canada

P.N. Ainslie
Centre for Heart, Lung and Vascular Health, School of Health and Exercise Sciences, University of British Columbia, Kelowna, BC, Canada

Y.-C. Tzeng
Cardiovascular Systems Laboratory, Centre for Translational Physiology, University of Otago, Wellington, New Zealand

Introduction

Cerebral blood flow (CBF) is regulated independently of peripheral circulation through a process commonly known as cerebral autoregulation (CA) [1, 2]. The underlying relationship between blood pressure (BP) and CBF effectively functions as a high-pass filter [2–5]. Very-low-frequency (VLF: 0.02–0.07 Hz) and low-frequency (LF: 0.07–0.20 Hz) oscillations in BP are extensively buffered within the cerebrovasculature, while high-frequency (HF) oscillations (>0.20 Hz) are passed through comparatively unhindered [1–5]. The most common method to quantify this relationship is the application of linear transfer function analysis (TFA) between mean BP and mean cerebral blood velocity (CBV) [2, 3, 5–7]. TFA provides several key metrics (coherence–linear correlation coefficient, phase–timing buffer and gain–amplitude modulation) that are useful when interpreting the input (BP) and output (CBV) nature of this dynamic relationship [1–5, 7, 8].

Traditionally, mean BP and mean CBV are employed as the input and output parameters for quantifying the cerebral pressure-flow response [2, 4, 5, 9–11]. Although this approach provides useful information in terms of cerebral perfusion pressure (~*mean BP*) and an index of total CBF (~*mean CBV*), it provides no additional information about the limitations of the CA system, which can be observed when examining the systolic and diastolic aspects of the cardiac cycle [12]. Previous research has examined the CA relationship in both systole and diastole [12], but it was evaluated under spontaneous conditions, which have been shown to greatly limit the interpretability of results [5]. Therefore, the aim of this study was to re-examine the findings reported by Ogoh et al. [12], which demonstrated there were no changes associated with phase and gain metrics across the cardiac cycle in healthy humans at rest. In severe unilateral carotid stenosis patients, the diastolic correlation coefficient autoregulatory index was augmented in the ipsilateral cerebral artery (systolic was unchanged) [13], indicating there are differential CA regulatory properties across the cardiac cycle. Therefore, it was hypothesized there would be reductions in gain and increases in phase during systole, relative to diastole.

Methods and Materials

Ethical Approval

This study was approved by the University of British Columbia Clinical Research Ethics Board, and written informed consent was obtained prior to the initiation of data collection.

Subjects

Twenty healthy younger adult (16 male, 26.7 ± 6.6 years, body mass index: 24.9 ± 3.0 kg/m^2) subjects were recruited for this study. All subjects had a clear history of cardiorespiratory and cerebrovascular diseases and were not taking any form of medication, and had abstained from exercise, caffeine and alcoholic beverages for at least 12 h prior to data collection.

Experimental Protocols

Squat-stand manoeuvres were employed at 0.05 and 0.10 Hz for assessing the cerebral pressure-flow response, as previous research has demonstrated this to be the *gold-standard* method to enhance the interpretability of associated transfer function metrics [5]. The frequencies for the point estimates were selected as they are within the range where CA is thought to have its greatest influence on cerebral pressure-flow dynamics [2].

Instrumentation

Subjects were equipped with a three-lead electrocardiogram (ECG) for measurement of R-R intervals. Finger photoplethysmography was used to continuously track BP (Finometer; Finapres Medical Systems, Amsterdam, The Netherlands). Bilateral middle cerebral arteries were insonated by placing 2 MHz Doppler probes (Spencer Technologies, Seattle, WA, USA) over the temporal window to obtain CBV. The partial pressure of end-tidal carbon dioxide ($P_{ET}CO_2$) was sampled with a mouthpiece and monitored via an online gas analyser (ML206; AD Instruments, Colorado Springs, CO, USA). Figure 1 provides representative traces from squat-stand manoeuvres (A: BP, B: CBV, C: $P_{ET}CO_2$). Heart rate was calculated from the ECG. All data were recorded at 1000 Hz via an analog-to-digital converter and stored for subsequent analysis using commercially available software (Powerlab 16/30 ML880; LabChart version 7.1; AD Instruments, Colorado Springs, CO, USA).

Data Processing

Real-time, beat-to-beat systolic, mean and diastolic values of BP and CBV were determined from each R-R interval. All data were processed and analysed with custom-designed software in LabView 11 (National Instruments, Austin, TX, USA) as previously described [5, 9–11, 14]. Phase wrap-around was not present at any of the point estimates at 0.05 and 0.10 Hz. Impulse step responses were derived as the inverse Fourier transform of the transfer function at the point estimates (0.05 or 0.10 Hz) of the driven BP oscillations at the systolic, mean and diastolic phases of the cardiac cycle.

Statistical Analysis

Statistical analyses were performed using SPSS version 23.0. A 3 (cardiac cycle: systole, mean, diastole) × 2 (frequency: 0.05 Hz, 0.10 Hz) repeated measures ANOVA was conducted to examine the main effects on BP, CBV, cross-

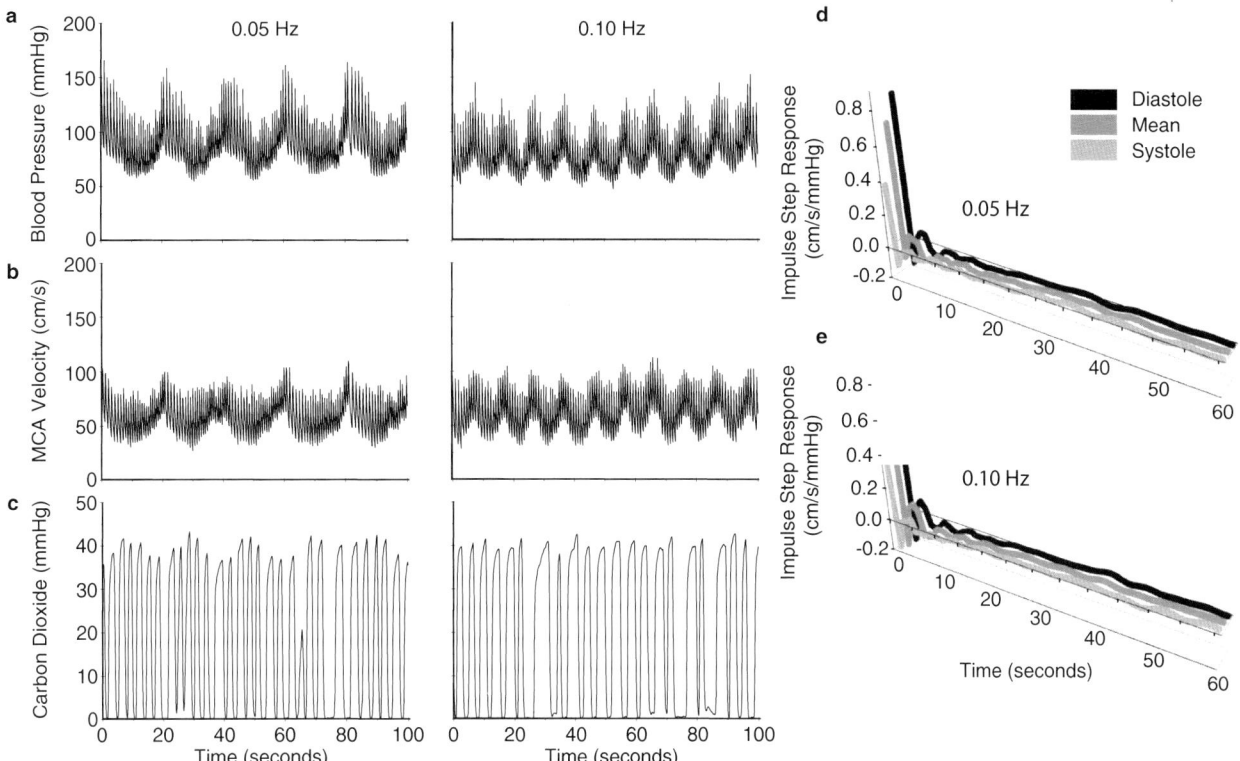

Fig. 1 Representative time series for blood pressure (BP) (**a**), middle cerebral artery blood velocity (MCAv) (**b**) and expired carbon dioxide (**c**) during 100 s of squat-stand manoeuvres performed at 0.05 and 0.10 Hz. Mean impulse step responses from the squat-stand manoeuvres at 0.05 (**d**) and 0.10 Hz (**e**)

spectral power and TFA metrics. Where appropriate, Bonferroni-corrected post hoc comparisons were performed to determine simple effects. Comparisons between frequencies for heart rate and $P_{ET}CO_2$ were performed with two-tailed paired T-tests. Data are presented as mean ± standard deviation (SD). Significance was set a priori to achieve an experiment-wide $p < 0.05$.

Results

Haemodynamic and Cerebrovascular Responses

There was a main effect of frequency on cardiac cycle for BP ($p = 0.020$) which was not present for CBV measurements ($p = 0.850$). Examining simple effects revealed a 5.9% elevation in systolic BP ($p = 0.006$) during the 0.10 Hz squat-stand manoeuvres. No significant differences were noted between frequencies in any other haemodynamic or cerebrovascular responses.

Fourier and Transfer Function Analysis (Table 1)

Impulse step response: The systolic impulse step response (Fig. 1d: 0.05 Hz, E: 0.10 Hz) slope was ~40% and ~50% less than the mean ($p < 0.001$) and diastolic ($p < 0.001$) components of the cardiac cycle, respectively.

Power spectrum: The absolute power spectrum of systolic BP was approximately double the diastolic BP power spectrum at both frequencies (Fig. 2a: $p < 0.001$), and nearly triple when normalized (Fig. 2b: $p < 0.001$). In contrast, the absolute systolic CBV power spectrum was only 42% of the diastolic point estimate at 0.05 Hz and just 29% at 0.10 Hz (Fig. 2c: $p < 0.001$). For normalized data, the systolic CBV power spectrum was reduced to just 7 and 5% of the normalized diastolic power spectrum at 0.05 Hz and 0.10 Hz respectively (Fig. 2d: $p < 0.001$).

Transfer function analysis: Systolic coherence was reduced at both 0.05 Hz (−5%) and 0.10 Hz (−3%) (Fig. 2e: $p < 0.001$). All TFA phase (Fig. 2f) and gain (Fig. 2g, h) metrics across the cardiac cycle were consistent with the high-pass-filter model. At 0.05 Hz the phase lead associ-

Table 1 TFA of driven data between blood pressure and MCAv during different aspects of cardiac cycle

	Systole	Mean	Diastole	p-Value
0.05 Hz BP power (mmHg^2)/Hz	58,121 ± 37,757	37,601 ± 17,167[a]	25,212 ± 14,670[a,b]	0.000
0.10 Hz BP power (mmHg^2)/Hz	32,050 ± 20,895	25,436 ± 10,688	17,899 ± 8142[a,b]	0.002
0.05 Hz BP power (%^{2})/Hz	28,456 ± 17,988	51,969 ± 29,410[a]	57,561 ± 42,390[a]	0.002
0.10 Hz BP power (%^{2})/Hz	14,958 ± 11,066	31,988 ± 22,629[a]	44,545 ± 41,781[a,b]	0.002
0.05 Hz MCAv power (cm/s)^2/Hz	7404 ± 5606	18,506 ± 9526[a]	17,391 ± 10,657[a]	0.000
0.10 Hz MCAv power (cm/s)^2/Hz	6711 ± 5419	21,448 ± 12,772[a]	22,862 ± 12,815[a]	0.000
0.05 Hz MCAv power (%^{2})/Hz	7735 ± 6575	53,635 ± 25,711[a]	112,491 ± 70,625[a,b]	0.000
0.10 Hz MCAv power (%^{2})/Hz	8374 ± 7867	56,512 ± 27,817[a]	147,558 ± 71,162[a,b]	0.000
0.05 Hz coherence	0.94 ± 0.06	0.99 ± 0.01[a]	0.99 ± 0.01[a]	0.001
0.10 Hz coherence	0.97 ± 0.03	0.99 ± 0.01[a]	1.00 ± 0.00[a]	0.001
0.05 Hz phase (rad)	1.07 ± 0.51	0.61 ± 0.12[a]	0.59 ± 0.14[a]	0.000
0.10 Hz phase (rad)	0.70 ± 0.46	0.34 ± 0.10[a]	0.33 ± 0.11[a]	0.001
0.05 Hz gain (cm/s/mmHg)	0.35 ± 0.07	0.71 ± 0.13[a]	0.86 ± 0.21[a,b]	0.000
0.10 Hz gain (cm/s/mmHg)	0.44 ± 0.13	0.91 ± 0.24[a]	1.14 ± 0.28[a,b]	0.000
0.05 Hz gain (%/%)	0.49 ± 0.12	1.04 ± 0.19[a]	1.46 ± 0.43[a,b]	0.000
0.10 Hz gain (%/%)	0.66 ± 0.20	1.35 ± 0.33[a]	1.97 ± 0.48[a,b]	0.000
0.05 Hz impulse step response slope (cm/s/mmHg)	−0.50 ± 0.16	−0.81 ± 0.23[a]	−1.01 ± 0.34[a,b]	0.000
0.10 Hz impulse step response slope (cm/s/mmHg)	−0.64 ± 0.20	−1.10 ± 0.28[a]	−1.19 ± 0.36[a,b]	0.000

Values are means ± SD. Blood pressure (BP); middle cerebral artery velocity (MCAv). Statistical significance was set at $p < 0.05$
[a]Significance from systole
[b]Significance from mean

ated with systole was ~3.4 s and ~1.9 s for both the mean and diastolic components of the cardiac cycle. These phase leads were further reduced at 0.10 Hz to 1.1 s for systole and 0.5 s for mean and diastole. TFA gain was blunted during systole at both 0.05 and 0.10 Hz compared with all other aspects of the cardiac cycle for both absolute ($p < 0.001$) and normalized ($p < 0.001$) values. The absolute gain associated with systole at both driven frequencies was ~40% ($p < 0.001$) of the diastolic cardiac cycle, a ratio that was reduced even further to 33% ($p < 0.001$) when the data were normalized.

Discussion

Employing the gold-standard squat-stand manoeuvres to augment the signal-to-noise ratio, thereby maximizing the reliability of the linear relationship between arterial BP and CBV [5], revealed differential regulatory properties between the systolic and diastolic components of the cerebral pressure-flow relationship. These data reveal that oscillations associated with systole are extensively buffered within the cerebrovasculature, whereas diastolic BP oscillations are passed along to the cerebrovasculature essentially unaltered (Table 1). These findings are in stark contrast to the work by Ogoh et al. [12], which revealed there to be no alterations to the BP–CBV relationship across the cardiac cycle under resting conditions. The discrepancy in the findings of these two studies is likely a result of the augmented signal-to-noise ratio associated with the squat-stand manoeuvres employed in the current study design. Squat-stand manoeuvres raise the coherence from 0.50–0.70 obtained with resting data [12] to >0.90 in the current study (Table 1).

The current findings indicate the brain is adapted to protect itself against large increases in systolic BP, which we speculate is a protective mechanism to prevent cerebral hyperperfusion and haemorrhages. During acute elevations in intracranial pressure, it has been demonstrated that increased central venous pressure can provide a protective mechanism to prevent increases in cerebrovascular transmural pressure, thereby avoiding cerebrovascular damage [15]. Although the exact protective mechanisms between the current study and the work of Haykowsky et al. [15] differ in time courses, their function is essentially the same—to protect the brain from surges in CBF. Therefore, previous studies which employed TFA to examine CA likely overlooked valuable insight into the mechanisms which underlie CBF control.

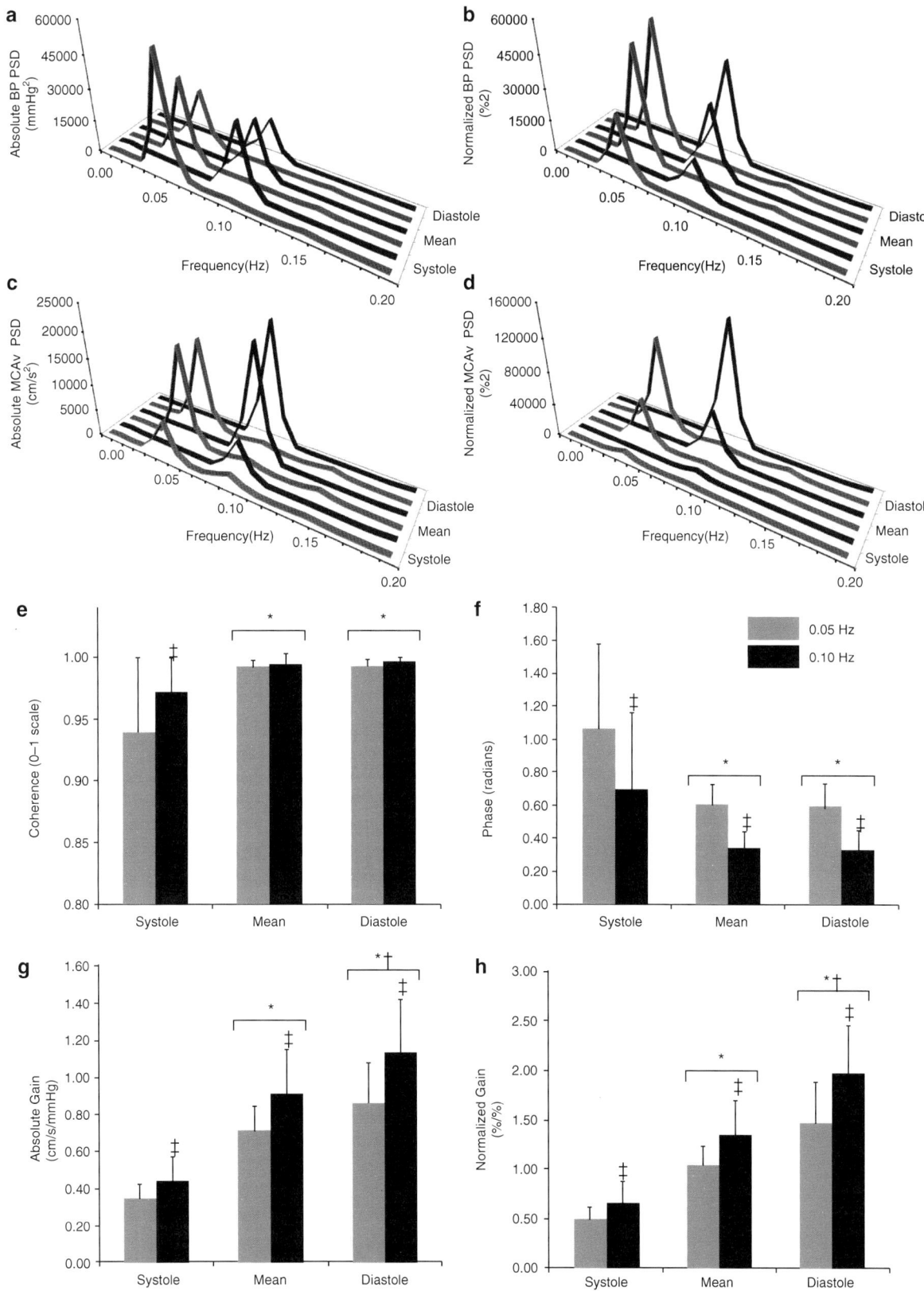

Fig. 2 Mean power spectrum densities (PSDs) for absolute blood pressure (BP) (**a**), normalized BP (**b**), absolute middle cerebral artery velocity (MCAv) (**c**) and normalized MCAv (**d**). TFA outcome metrics (mean ± SD) for coherence (**e**), phase (**f**), absolute gain (**g**) and normalized gain (**h**) for systole, mean and diastole during squat-stand manoeuvres performed at 0.05 and 0.10 Hz. *Asterisk* denotes significance from systole, *dagger* denotes significance from mean, *double dagger* denotes significance from 0.05 Hz

Conclusion

The differential systolic and diastolic aspects of the cerebral pressure-flow relationship can be accurately quantified through the application of squat-stand manoeuvres. Systolic BP oscillations are extensively buffered within the cerebrovasculature, whereas diastolic oscillations are relatively unaltered. This indicates the brain is adapted to protect itself against large increases in systolic BP, likely as a mechanism to prevent cerebral haemorrhages. In clinical situations in which individuals are able to perform a squat-stand manoeuvre (e.g. mild traumatic brain injury, concussion, chronic obstructive pulmonary disease, heart failure), we recommend that investigators employ this technique to examine the CA response across the cardiac cycle. This approach will provide additional insight into the regulatory mechanisms within the cerebrovasculature.

Conflicts of interest statement We declare that we have no conflict of interest.

References

1. Aaslid R, Lindegaard KF, Sorteberg W, Nornes H. Cerebral autoregulation dynamics in humans. Stroke. 1989;20(1):45–52.
2. Zhang R, Zuckerman JH, Giller CA, Levine BD. Transfer function analysis of dynamic cerebral autoregulation in humans. Am J Phys. 1998;274(1 Pt 2):H233–41.
3. Tzeng YC, Ainslie PN, Cooke WH, Peebles KC, Willie CK, MacRae BA, et al. Assessment of cerebral autoregulation: the quandary of quantification. Am J Physiol Heart Circ Physiol. 2012;303(6):H658–71.
4. Claassen JAHR, Levine BD, Zhang R. Dynamic cerebral autoregulation during repeated squat-stand maneuvers. J Appl Physiol. 2009;106(1):153–60.
5. Smirl JD, Hoffman K, Tzeng YC, Hansen A, Ainslie PN. Methodological comparison of active and passive driven oscillations in blood pressure; implications for the assessment of cerebral-pressure flow relationships. J Appl Physiol. 2015;119(5):487–501.
6. Giller CA. The frequency-dependent behavior of cerebral autoregulation. Neurosurgery. 1990;27(3):362–8.
7. Birch AA, Dirnhuber MJ, Hartley-Davies R, Iannotti F, Neil-Dwyer G. Assessment of autoregulation by means of periodic changes in blood pressure. Stroke. 1995;26(5):834–7.
8. Hughson RL, Edwards MR, O'Leary DD, Shoemaker JK. Critical analysis of cerebrovascular autoregulation during repeated head-up tilt. Stroke. 2001;32(10):2403–8.
9. Smirl JD, Tzeng YC, Monteleone BJ, Ainslie PN. Influence of cerebrovascular resistance on the dynamic relationship between blood pressure and cerebral blood flow in humans. J Appl Physiol. 2014;116(12):1614–22.
10. Smirl JD, Lucas SJE, Lewis NCS, Dumanior GR, Smith KJ, Bakker A, et al. Cerebral pressure-flow relationship in lowlanders and natives at high altitude. J Cereb Blood Flow Metab. 2013;34(2):248–57.
11. Smirl JD, Haykowsky MJ, Nelson MD, Tzeng YC, Marsden KR, Jones H, et al. Relationship Between Cerebral Blood Flow and Blood Pressure in Long-Term Heart Transplant Recipients. Hypertension. 2014;64(6):1314–20.
12. Ogoh S, Fadel PJ, Zhang R, Selmer C, Jans O, Secher NH, et al. Middle cerebral artery flow velocity and pulse pressure during dynamic exercise in humans. Am J Physiol Heart Circ Physiol. 2005;288(4):H1526–31.
13. Reinhard M, Roth M, Muller T, Czosnyka M, Timmer J, Hetzel A. Cerebral autoregulation in carotid artery occlusive disease assessed from spontaneous blood pressure fluctuations by the correlation coefficient index. Stroke. 2003;34(9):2138–44.
14. Smirl JD, Hoffman K, Tzeng YC, Hansen A, Ainslie PN. Relationship between blood pressure and cerebral blood flow during supine cycling: influence of aging. J Appl Physiol. 2016;120(5):552–63.
15. Haykowsky MJ, Eves ND, R Warburton DE, Findlay MJ. Resistance exercise, the Valsalva maneuver, and cerebrovascular transmural pressure. Med Sci Sports Exerc. 2003;35(1):65–8.

Normative Ranges of Transcranial Doppler Metrics

Solventa Krakauskaite, Corey Thibeault, James LaVangie, Mateo Scheidt, Leo Martinez, Danielle Seth-Hunter, Amanda Wu, Michael O'Brien, Fabien Scalzo, Seth J. Wilk, and Robert B. Hamilton

Abstract *Objective*: To determine normal ranges for traditional transcranial Doppler (TCD) measurements for two age groups (14–19 and 20–29 years) and compare to existing literature results. The development of a normal range for TCD measurements will be required for the development of diagnostic and prognostic tests in the future.

Materials and Methods: We performed TCD on the middle cerebral artery on 147 healthy subjects aged 18.9 years (SD = 2.1) and calculated mean cerebral blood flow velocity (mCBFV) and pulsatility index (PI). The study population was divided into two age populations (14–19 and 20–29 years).

Results: There was a significant decrease in PI ($p = 0.015$) for the older age group with no difference in mCBFV.

Conclusion: Age-related, normal data are a prerequisite for TCD to continue to gain clinical acceptance. Our correlation of age-related TCD findings with previously published results as the generally accepted "gold standard" underlines the validity and sensitivity of this ultrasound method.

Keywords Transcranial Doppler · Ultrasound · Traumatic brain injury · Pulsatility index

S. Krakauskaite
Kaunas University of Technology, Kaunas, Lithuania

C. Thibeault · J. LaVangie · M. Scheidt · L. Martinez
D. Seth-Hunter · A. Wu · M. O'Brien · S.J. Wilk · R.B. Hamilton (✉)
Neural Analytics, Los Angeles, CA, USA
e-mail: Robert@NeuralAnalytics.com

F. Scalzo
UCLA, Los Angeles, CA, USA

Introduction

Transcranial Doppler (TCD) ultrasound was developed in the early 1980s and is a safe and noninvasive alternative to costly imaging diagnostics for measuring cerebral hemodynamics [1]. TCD has been widely used for a number of neurological conditions, including assessing the status of the arteries after a subarachnoid hemorrhage (SAH) [2], aiding preventive maintenance in children with sickle cell anemia [3–5], facilitating risk assessment in embolic stroke patients [6, 7], and monitoring changes in cerebral blood flow velocity (CBFV) following a traumatic brain injury (TBI).

Compared with more advanced imaging modalities (e.g., MRI, CT, PET), TCD provides high temporal resolution information about cerebral hemodynamics while being low-cost and portable. However, to use TCD as a general diagnostic tool for TBI or other neurological conditions, normative ranges of CBFV for healthy populations must be established.

Two traditional TCD metrics calculated from CBFV are mean cerebral blood flow velocity (mCBFV) and pulsatility index (PI). mCBFV is derived through the spectral envelope of the Doppler signal as

$$mCBFV = (PSV + [EDV \times 2])/3,$$

where PSV is peak systolic velocity and EDV is end-diastolic blood flow velocity [8]. Gosling's PI is calculated as

$$PI = (PSV - EDV)/mCBFV.$$

The reference range of Gosling's PI is between 0.5 and 1.19 [9]. The main advantage of PI is that it is a ratio and not affected by the angle of insonation. Therefore, PI may be a very sensitive parameter for early detection of intracranial hemodynamic changes.

Previous studies evaluated CBFV within different subject groups using TCD [6, 8, 10–12]. Here, we provide an overview of the basic ranges of traditional features for different

Table 1 Summary of mCBFV and PI for TCD studies performed on healthy subjects published in current literature

Age	MCA Mean Velocity (SD)							Pulsatility Index (SD)			
	Hennerici	Khoja	Ringelstein	Demirkaya	Bode	Tegeler	This work	Demirkaya	Bode	Tegeler	This work
1									0.69 (0.19)		
2					85 (10)						
3					94 (10)				0.87 (0.22)		
4											
5				75.7 (8.7)				0.75 (0.21)			
6					97 (9)				0.73 (0.18)		
7											
8											
9											
10			70 (16.4)		81 (11)				0.85 (0.26)		
11				63.6 (12.1)				0.86 (0.36)			
12											
13											
14							70.71 (13.0)				0.79 (0.11)
15											
16											
17											
18		68 (13)				66.6 (14.4)				0.85 (0.13)	
19											
20							67.53 (11.1)				0.74 (0.11)
21	58.4 (8.4)			57.4 (8.7)				0.97 (0.44)			
25											
29											
30			57 (11.2)			64.6 (8.8)			0.80 (0.15)		
31				57.9 (11.2)				0.80 (0.40)			
34											
35											
39											
40	57.7 (11.5)	57 (12)				60.0 (11.2)			0.76 (0.10)		
41				65.9 (14.5)				0.75 (0.41)			
44											
45											
49											
50			51 (9.7)			56.6 (9.4)			0.80 (0.10)		
51				51.3 (12.7)				0.82 (0.37)			
54											
55											
59											
60						51.2 (10.0)			0.85 (0.10)		
61	44.7 (11.1)	54 (18)									
64											
65											
69											
70						49.6 (10.5)			0.95 (0.17)		
74											
75											
80											

Values reported as mean and SD

age ranges found in the current literature and include our recent results (Table 1). In general, all studies combined show that CBFV decreases with increasing age and that PI is not age dependent.

Tegeler et al. completed a comprehensive study of TCD velocities in a large, healthy population consisting of 364 healthy subjects aged 18–80 [6]. There was no difference in the mCBFV between left- and right-side segments of the circle of Willis, with the exception of the distal M1 ($p = 0.022$) and the C1 ($p < 0.0001$), both slightly higher on the left.

Bode et al. performed a cross-sectional study on 112 healthy children between 1 day and 18 years of age [8]. A rapid linear increase of flow velocities was found within the first 20 days, with higher velocities in neonates of higher birth weight and gestational age. Maximal CBFV values were recorded between the ages of 5 and 6 years. After years 5 and 6, velocities decreased linearly to 81 cm/s (standard deviation (SD) = 11) at the age of 18 years, 70% of their maximum.

Ringelstein and colleagues examined 106 normal volunteers and 59 patients with subclavian steal mechanisms [10] who showed a decrease in CBFV with increasing age.

A study investigating the age dependence of CBFV by Grolimund and Seiler [11] was completed that consisted of 535 subjects with a mean age of 54.9 years (SD = 16.0) years. They reported no significant difference between right and left sides with a mean velocity of 57.3 cm/s (SD = 14.8). None of these patients showed any neurological deficit at the time of the investigation.

Demirkaya et al. studied the influence of age and gender on normal values of flow velocities in 63 healthy volunteers (30 male and 33 females; age range 5–69 years old) [12]. Contrary to [6], they did not find a difference in gender. Results showed a decrease with advancing age that was significant above 40 years of age.

Hennerici et al. presented a study with 50 subjects ranging from 21 to 79 years of age and proposed a scanning system to help reduce interindividual variation for peak flow measurements [13]. This work noted that the variation in mean flow velocities was lower.

We have compiled a comparison table that includes our new measurements (Table 1). Additional data from a workshop presented by Khoja are also included [14].

Material and Methods

Study subjects (or parent/guardian) were asked to complete a brief medical questionnaire to ensure inclusion in the study, and informed consent was obtained for each subject. Study inclusion and exclusion criteria are described below. Subjects were then moved to a private area to reduce distraction during the study, where an acclimatization period of approximately 5–10 min prior to the beginning of the study protocol. Subjects sat upright (70–90°) in a high-back chair with arm and head rests to provide comfort. TCD ultrasonography was used to monitor CBFV in the middle cerebral artery (MCA) bilaterally using a U.S. Food and Drug Administration–cleared headset (Doppler BoxX, DWL USA, Inc.). Ultrasound probes (2 MHz) were positioned over the right and left temporal bones superior to the zygomatic arch. Ultrasound gel was applied to enhance signal quality.

All results are reported as mean and SD. The clinical study enrolled 147 healthy subjects 18.9 (2.09) years of age who had not suffered a TBI within the last 90 days. TCD measurements were taken for 5 min during normal breathing, and mCBFV and PI were then calculated. TCD metrics were compared with the Mann–Whitney test at a significance of 0.05. The study was approved by the local Western Institutional Review Board (20141111). Exclusion criteria included the following: individuals younger than 14 years of age, a person from a vulnerable group (cognitively impaired individuals, prisoners, and pregnant women), open head injury, skull fracture, soft tissue trauma to the temporal region, subjects with a history of moderate or severe TBI, stroke, seizure disorder (epilepsy), brain tumor, brain abscess or brain infection, meningitis, blood clotting disorder, sickle cell disease, systolic arterial blood pressure greater than 140 mmHg (hypertension), asthma, emphysema, bronchitis, pneumonia, chronic obstructive pulmonary disease, and other pulmonary diseases and disorders.

Results

Normal ranges for mCBFV and PI measured in this study are shown in Table 2 and Fig. 1. They suggest that there is a significant decrease in PI ($p = 0.015$) between the two age groups but no significant change in mean CBFV.

Table 2 Summary of normative TCD data measured at baseline, rest conditions

Age range	Male/female, n	Age, years	Mean CBFV, cm/s	Mean PI, unitless
14–19	86/10	16.5 (1.3)	71.0 (13.0)	0.79 (0.11)
20–29	36/15	23.5 (3.1)	68.5 (11.1)	0.74 (0.11)

Values reported as mean and SD

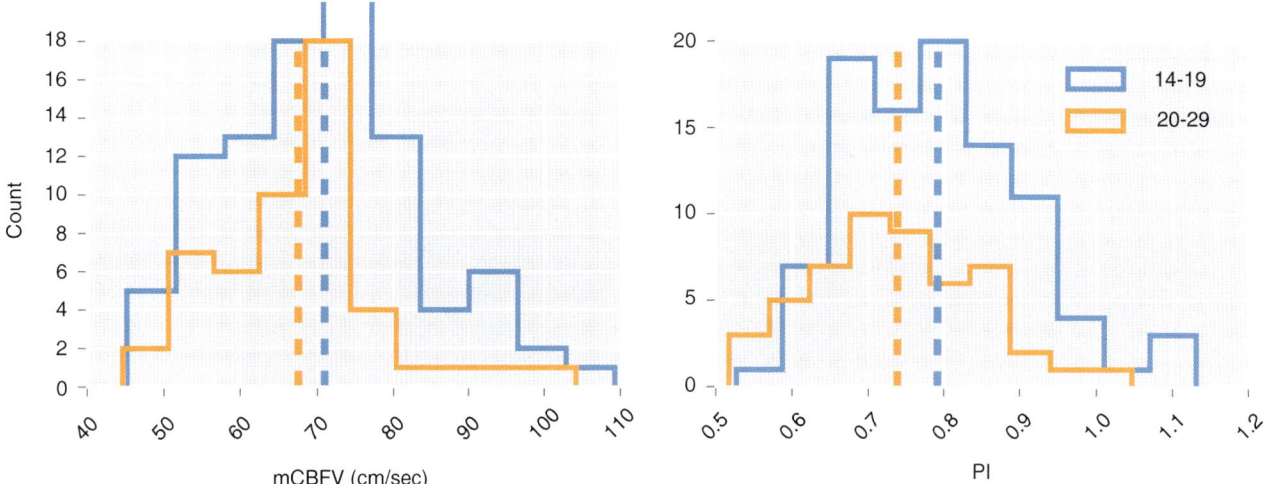

Fig. 1 Histogram summary of normative TCD data for subjects aged 14–19 and 20–29 measured in this study: (**a**) mean velocity and (**b**) PI, both measured at baseline rest conditions

Discussion

The present study was designed to establish normal reference values of different age groups for the mCBFV and PI in the MCA as determined with TCD. According to the existing literature, the range of mCBFV for children under the age of 18 is 66.6–97.0 cm/s and healthy adults 18 and older 57.4–81.0 cm/s. In general, mCBFV in the MCA is higher among women than men [6]. mCBFV decreased with advancing age in both men and women. Measured results reported here show similar findings to those in published work for normative ranges. In particular, our results correlate well with those reported by Tegeler and Ringelstein in their study of a large, healthy population. This work and cited references support the need for additional age-matched cerebral hemodynamic data, including the traditional TCD metrics mCBFV and PI for relevant comparisons.

Current literature describes the TCD monitoring process of pinpointing arteries as a difficult task that requires considerable expertise [15, 16]. The technical limitations of TCD include user variability both intra- and interoperator. The standard TCD method is performed by manual handheld monitoring. Manual monitoring is typically useful for recording flow data for 5–50 cardiac cycles. Longer periods may result in signal loss owing to operator fatigue, loss of interface from operator hand, or subject head movements, all leading to increased variability in measurements. To address this issue, a number of different TCD headsets, such as the one used for our study, have been designed that improve the stability of measurements. The ultrasound probe is no longer held manually by the operator. Instead, a headset with an attached probe is secured to the subject's head and then the probe is adjusted manually until a sufficient signal is found. However, current headset designs can become cumbersome and uncomfortable to wear and lack consistent stability for continuous monitoring owing to the numerous points of contact around the head. Widespread use in the clinical realm for continuous monitoring requires significant strides in the design of a device that simplifies continuous TCD signal acquisition through fast localization of vessels, stabilization, and real-time tracking.

In addition to the technical difficulties of TCD, many physiological factors affect CBFV, including age, hematocrit, gender, fever, metabolic factors, pregnancy, menstruation, ethnicity, exercise, and brain activity [9, 17–19]. Of these, age is the most important factor affecting measured TCD values in men and women. The lack of side-to-side differences in TCD parameters may offer another normative parameter to use for patients with severe unilateral conditions where contralateral TCD measurements may serve as control values. Moreover, the CBFV in a given artery is inversely related to the cross-sectional area of the same artery [16, 20]. Hence, TCD ultrasonography gives an indirect evaluation of the diameter of an intracranial vessel through the analysis of blood flow velocity, which can be used to determine constriction as well as obstructions that effectively reduce the diameter. Finally, it is estimated that approximately 10–20% of patients have inadequate transtemporal acoustic windows, which would impact the ability to acquire a true CBFV signal [21].

Conclusion

Age-related, normal data are a prerequisite for TCD to continue to gain clinical acceptance. The high sensitivity of TCD in identifying abnormally high or low CBFVs demonstrates that TCD represents an excellent first-line examination method to identify patients who may need urgent aggressive treatment. Results presented here and in recent publications for mCBFV show significant decreases with increasing age, which need to be considered when trying to understand hemodynamic changes with age and pathology.

TCD studies in large multiethnic populations are still required to determine differences in cerebral hemodynamics across various ethnic groups. The data arising from our retrospective study on adolescents and adults without cerebral and cerebrovascular disease may serve as preliminary, normal data until a prospective TCD study of this age group strengthens or elaborates our findings. Additionally, methods and techniques to simplify and automate measurements with TCD will improve both its utility and acceptance in clinical settings.

Acknowledgments This work was supported partially by the National Institutes of Health Small Business Innovation Research (NINDS 1R43NS092209-01) and private funds from Neural Analytics Inc.

Conflicts of interest statement Solventa Krakauskaite – No Conflict of interest, Corey Thibeault – Employee and shareholder of Neural Analytics, James LaVangie – Employee and shareholder of Neural Analytics, Mateo Scheidt – Employee and shareholder of Neural Analytics, Leo Martinez – Employee and shareholder of Neural Analytics, Danielle Seth-Hunter – Employee and shareholder of Neural Analytics, Amanda Wu – Employee and shareholder of Neural Analytics, Michael O'Brien – Employee and shareholder of Neural Analytics, Fabien Scalzo – Contractor and shareholder of Neural Analytics, Seth J. Wilk – Employee and shareholder of Neural Analytics, Robert B. Hamilton – Employee and shareholder of Neural Analytics.

References

1. Aaslid R, Markwalder TM, Nornes H. Noninvasive transcranial Doppler ultrasound recording of flow velocity in basal cerebral arteries. J Neurosurg. 1982;57(6):769–74.
2. Rasulo FA, De Peri E, Lavinio A. Transcranial Doppler ultrasonography in intensive care. Eur J Anaesthesiol Suppl. 2008;42:167–73.
3. Nichols FT, Jones AM, Adams RJ. Stroke prevention in sickle cell disease (STOP) study guidelines for transcranial Doppler testing. J Neuroimaging. 2001;11(4):354–62.
4. Pavlakis SG, Rees RC, Huang X, Brown RC, Casella JF, Iyer RV, Kalpatthi R, Luden J, Miller ST, Rogers ZR, Thornburg CD, Wang WC, Adams RJ, Investigators BH. Transcranial doppler ultrasonography (TCD) in infants with sickle cell anemia: baseline data from the BABY HUG trial. Pediatr Blood Cancer. 2010;54(2):256–9.
5. Krejza J, Chen R, Romanowicz G, Kwiatkowski JL, Ichord R, Arkuszewski M, Zimmerman R, Ohene-Frempong K, Desiderio L, Melhem ER. Sickle cell disease and transcranial Doppler imaging: inter-hemispheric differences in blood flow Doppler parameters. Stroke. 2011;42(1):81–6.
6. Tegeler CH, Crutchfield K, Katsnelson M, Kim J, Tang R, Griffin LP, Rundek T, Evans G. Transcranial Doppler velocities in a large, healthy population. J Neuroimaging. 2013;23(3):466–72.
7. North American Academy of Neurology. Assessment of transcranial Doppler ultrasonography. AAN guideline summary for clinicians assessment, 2007. Chicago, IL: North American Academy of Neurology; 2007. https://www.aan.com/Guidelines/home/GetGuidelineContent/147
8. Bode H, Wais U. Age dependence of flow velocities in basal cerebral arteries. Arch Dis Child. 1988;63(6):606–11.
9. Moppett IK, Mahajan RP. Transcranial Doppler ultrasonography in anaesthesia and intensive care. Br J Anaesth. 2004;93(5):710–24.
10. Ringelstein EB, Kahlscheuer B, Niggemeyer E, Otis SM. Transcranial doppler sonography: anatomical landmarks and normal velocity values. Ultrasound Med Biol. 1990;16(8):745–61.
11. Grolimund P, Seiler RW. Age dependence of the flow velocity in the basal cerebral arteries—a transcranial Doppler ultrasound study. Ultrasound Med Biol. 1988;14(3):191–8.
12. Demirkaya S, Uluc K, Bek S, Vural O. Normal blood flow velocities of basal cerebral arteries decrease with advancing age: a transcranial Doppler sonography study. Tohoku J Exp Med. Feb. 2008;214(2):145–9.
13. Hennerici M, Rautenberg W, Schwartz A. Transcranial Doppler ultrasound for the assessment of intracranial arterial flow velocity—part 2. Evaluation of intracranial arterial disease. Surg Neurol. 1987;27(6):523–32.
14. Khoja W, "Transcranial Doppler made easy," first Saudi transcranial Doppler workshop, 2012. [Online]. http://ssa.org.sa/TCD Pocket Guide/Front Cover.htm. Accessed 2 Sept 2017.
15. Baumgartner RW. Handbook on neurovascular ultrasound. Berlin: Karger; 2006.
16. Nicoletto HA, Burkman MH. Transcranial Doppler series part II: performing a transcranial Doppler. Am J Electroneurodiagnostic Technol. Mar. 2009;49(1):14–27.
17. Droste DW, Harders AG, Rastogi E. A transcranial Doppler study of blood flow velocity in the middle cerebral arteries performed at rest and during mental activities. Stroke. 1989;20(8):1005–11.
18. Patel PM, Drummond JC. Cerebral physiology and the effects of anesthetic drugs. In: Miller's Anesthesia. 7th ed. New York, NY: Churchill Livingstone; 2009. p. 305–40.
19. Shahlaie K, Keachie K, Hutchins IM, Rudisill N, Madden LK, Smith KA, Ko KA, Latchaw RE, Muizelaar JP. Risk factors for posttraumatic vasospasm. J Neurosurg. 2011;115(3):602–11.
20. Arnolds BJ, von Reutern GM. Transcranial Doppler sonography. Examination technique and normal reference values. Ultrasound Med Biol. 1986;12(2):115–23.
21. Naqvi J, Yap KH, Ahmad G, Ghosh J, Naqvi J, Yap KH, Ahmad G, Ghosh J. Transcranial Doppler ultrasound: a review of the physical principles and major applications in critical care. Int J Vasc Med. 2013;2013:629378.

Autoregulating Cerebral Tissue Selfishly Exploits Collateral Flow Routes Through the Circle of Willis

Flora A. Kennedy McConnell and Stephen J. Payne

Abstract *Objective*: Ischemic stroke is a leading cause of death and disability. Autoregulation and collateral blood flow through the circle of Willis both play a role in preventing tissue infarction. A steady-state model of the cerebral arterial network was used to investigate the interaction of these mechanisms when autoregulation is impaired ipsilateral to an occluded artery.

Materials and methods: Twelve structural variants of the circle of Willis were modelled with left internal carotid artery occlusion and coupled with (1) a passive model of the cerebral vascular bed, (2) a steady-state model of an autoregulating cerebral vascular bed, and (3) a model in which the contralateral hemisphere autoregulates and the ipsilateral hemisphere does not.

Results: Results showed that if the autoregulatory response is impaired ipsilaterally, then, in the autoregulating hemisphere, cerebral flows are preserved at the expense of those on the ipsilateral side.

Conclusions: Thus, although autoregulation is an essential facilitator of collateral flow through the circle of Willis, contralateral autoregulation can exacerbate flow reductions if not balanced by the same response in the vascular beds on the ipsilateral side. The status of the autoregulatory response in both hemispheres can strongly influence cerebral blood flows and tissue survival and should, therefore, be monitored in stroke.

Keywords Collateral flow · Impaired autoregulation · Ischemia · Arterial occlusion · Cerebral haemodynamics

F.A. Kennedy McConnell (✉) • S.J. Payne
Institute of Biomedical Engineering, Department of Engineering Science, University of Oxford, Oxford OX1 3PJ, UK
e-mail: flora.kennedy-mcconnell@eng.ox.ac.uk

Introduction

During stenosis or occlusion of an artery supplying the brain, the health of cerebral tissue is primarily dependent on the severity and duration of ischemia. Because brain tissue has only very small stores of glucose [1], reductions in cerebral blood flow rapidly lead to a depletion of energy stores, resulting in tissue damage. Blood is supplied to the brain via the circle of Willis, an arterial ring at the base of the cranium (Fig. 1a). Through the communicating arteries the circle of Willis provides the brain with primary collateral (i.e. alternative) flow pathways. These pathways potentially enable blood to bypass a vessel blockage and to continue to supply hypoperfused tissue [2], thereby reducing the severity of ischemia.

However, the structure of the circle of Willis varies from one individual to the next [3, 4], meaning that its potential to provide collateral flow routes is also variable. In a clinical context, vascular surgeries such as aortic arch repair [5] and carotid endarterectomy [6] rely on collateral flow through the circle of Willis to perfuse cerebral tissue adequately while one or both of the ipsilateral afferent arteries are intentionally occluded. Furthermore, the presence of good collateral routes on angiography has been shown to be associated with smaller infarct volumes [7] and improved outcomes of endovascular recanalisation therapies [8, 9].

Cerebral autoregulation is another system which protects cerebral blood flows after arterial occlusion. This physiological mechanism can maintain constant flows over wide ranges of arterial blood pressure [10]. Autoregulation is enacted through dilation of resistance vessels, primarily the small arteries and arterioles in response to blood pressure reduction, and constriction of these vessels in response to raised blood pressure.

Many modelling studies have been conducted on collateral flow through the circle of Willis and on cerebral autoregulation, discussions of which can be found in Refs. [10, 11]. However, it seems that only [12, 13] have investigated

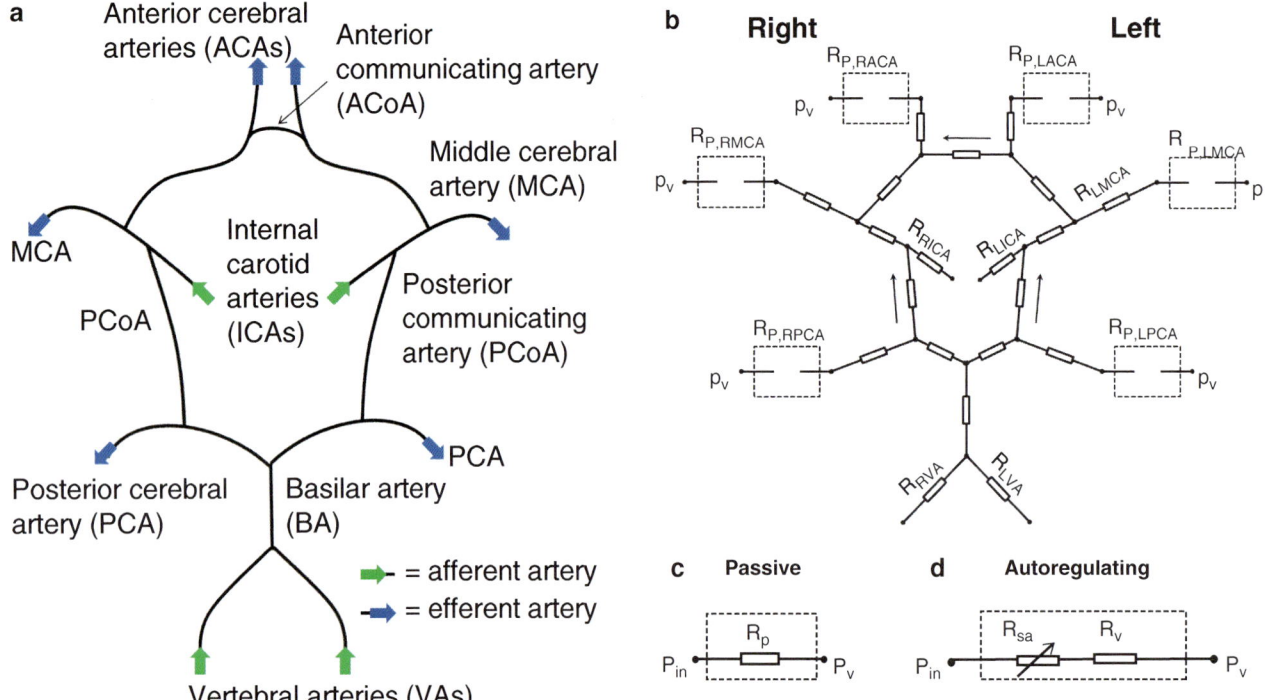

Fig. 1 The cerebral blood supply arises from (**a**) the circle of Willis. The network of resistances used to represent the *circle* is shown in (**b**), where the *dashed boxes* contain one of two models of the peripheral cerebral vasculature: (**c**) passive; (**d**) autoregulating

the interaction between the two mechanisms, and neither work considered the impact of impaired autoregulation ipsilateral to an occluded vessel.

Understanding the interaction between cerebral autoregulation and collateral flow is vital, especially because autoregulation can be impaired in the ipsilateral hemisphere in stroke patients [10]. Hence, this work will investigate the extent to which impaired cerebral autoregulation affects collateral flow and, thereby, affects flows to the cerebral arteries in the event of afferent vessel occlusion. An understanding of these factors may allow combined assessments of collateral flow and autoregulation to be used as better predictors of outcome in cerebrovascular diseases and interventions.

Materials and Methods

The arterial network model, including all the parameters used to define it, are outlined in [11]. The network was modelled as a steady-state electrical circuit using

$$\frac{\Delta P}{Q} = \frac{8\mu l}{\pi r^4} = R \tag{1}$$

to define the resistance R of each vessel to blood flow Q, based on its length l, radius r, the viscosity of blood μ, and ΔP the pressure drop across the vessel. Thus, the cerebral arterial network was modelled as a system of linear equations. The circle of Willis portion of the model is shown in Fig. 1b. Through the elimination of circulus arteries, by setting $r=0$, variants of the structure of the circle of Willis thought to convey high risk of ischemia during left internal carotid artery (LICA) occlusion (Fig. 3) [5, 11] were modelled.

Passive cerebral vascular territories were simulated using a fixed peripheral resistance, R_p, between the efferent cerebral artery and the venous system (Fig. 1c):

$$p = p_v + R_p Q, \tag{2}$$

where p_v is the pressure of the venous system, which was taken to be 5 mmHg.

Autoregulation, particularly unilaterally impaired autoregulation, was of interest in this work. Autoregulating cerebral vascular territories were modelled as described in [11], wherein the peripheral resistance was divided into a variable arteriolar resistance, R_{sa}, and a fixed capillary and venous resistance, R_v (Fig. 1d):

$$R_p = R_{sa} + R_v. \tag{3}$$

Negative feedback, based on deviations from reference blood flow rates, caused changes in arteriolar compliance, which in turn led to changes in arteriolar volume and, therefore, resistance. The reference blood flow rates were specific to each circle of Willis configuration: they were set at the flow to the same cerebral territory under non-autoregulating conditions when all of the afferent arteries were open, i.e. no occlusions.

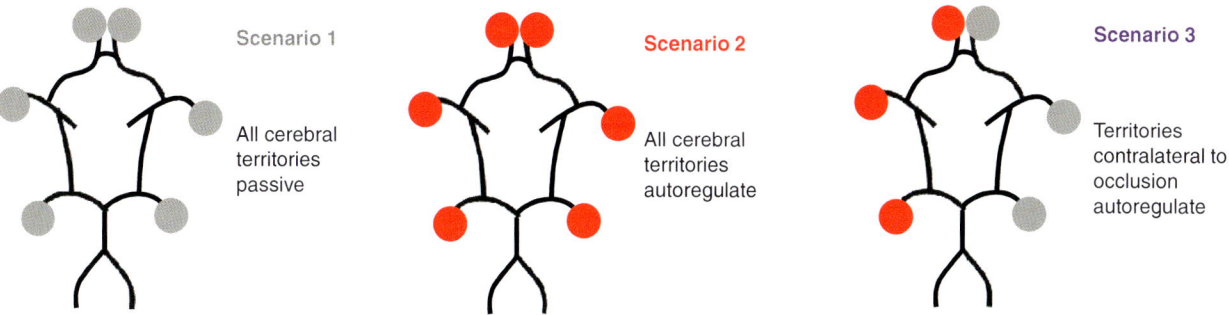

Fig. 2 Three autoregulation scenarios were simulated in 12 circle of Willis variants

The network model forms a system of linear equations, which was solved by matrix inversion using Gaussian elimination. The network and autoregulation equations were solved iteratively, as described in [11], until the model converged on a solution.

Simulations

For each circle of Willis configuration of interest three scenarios concerning the status of the cerebral autoregulatory response were considered (Fig. 2): Scenario 1—none of the cerebral territories autoregulates; Scenario 2—all of the cerebral territories autoregulate; and Scenario 3—only those cerebral territories contralateral to the occluded afferent artery autoregulate. The three scenarios were simulated under baseline conditions, i.e. when all of the afferent arteries were open, then simulated with the LICA occluded.

Results

Figure 3 shows the effects of LICA occlusion on flows through the efferent arteries of the 12 circle of Willis configurations of interest in this work. For example, in Fig. 3, Scenario 1 shows that in the complete circle of Willis occlusion of the LICA results in a 7.1% reduction in blood flow to the left middle cerebral artery if none of the cerebral territories autoregulates, a 1.0% reduction if all of the territories autoregulate, and a 7.2% reduction if only the territories on the right side autoregulate.

Figure 3 demonstrates that collateral flow alone (Scenario 1) is unable to ensure adequate (>90%) cerebral flows in all but three variants of the circle of Willis (1, 2 and 4). It is also evident that autoregulation locally enhances maintenance of blood flow to cerebral tissue. Complete autoregulation (Scenario 2) preserves flows in all but two circle variants (8 and 10), whereas incomplete autoregulation (Scenario 3) preserves flows contralateral to the occlusion at the expense of the cerebral territories most at risk.

Discussion

A simplified cerebral arterial network was modelled in steady state. The model had previously been shown to compare well with 1D flow models of the same network and with data of measured flow rates in the cerebral arteries [11]. The results of simulations of LICA occlusion show that autoregulating cerebral arteriolar networks exploit available collateral flow routes through the circle of Willis to preserve flow; however, this occurs at the expense of cerebral territories that cannot autoregulate. The Scenario 3 simulations in which autoregulation is active contralateral to and impaired ipsilateral to the ICA occlusion show that the autoregulating territories are protected, often more so than in Scenario 2, in which all of the cerebral territories autoregulate. Conversely, in Scenario 3, the passive cerebral territories of the left hemisphere receive even lower blood flow than in Scenario 1, in which none of the cerebral territories autoregulates.

In [11], the 12 circles of Willis were categorised as low, medium or high risk based on the magnitude of the flow reductions seen after LICA occlusion when the 6 cerebral territories were either all passive or all autoregulating. Circles 1, 2 and 4 were classed as low risk because flow reductions were limited to less than 10%, regardless of the status of autoregulation. Circles 3, 5, 6, 7, 9, 11 and 12 were classed as medium risk because all efferent flow reductions of greater than 10% in Scenario 1 were reduced to below 10% when autoregulation was active globally (Scenario 2). Only circles 8 and 10 were considered high risk because they saw flow reductions which remained greater than 10%, even when complete autoregulation was taken into account. However, the results presented in Fig. 3 demonstrate that all circle of Willis structures classified as medium risk in [11] are high risk when autoregulation is only active contralateral to the occluded ICA (Scenario 3).

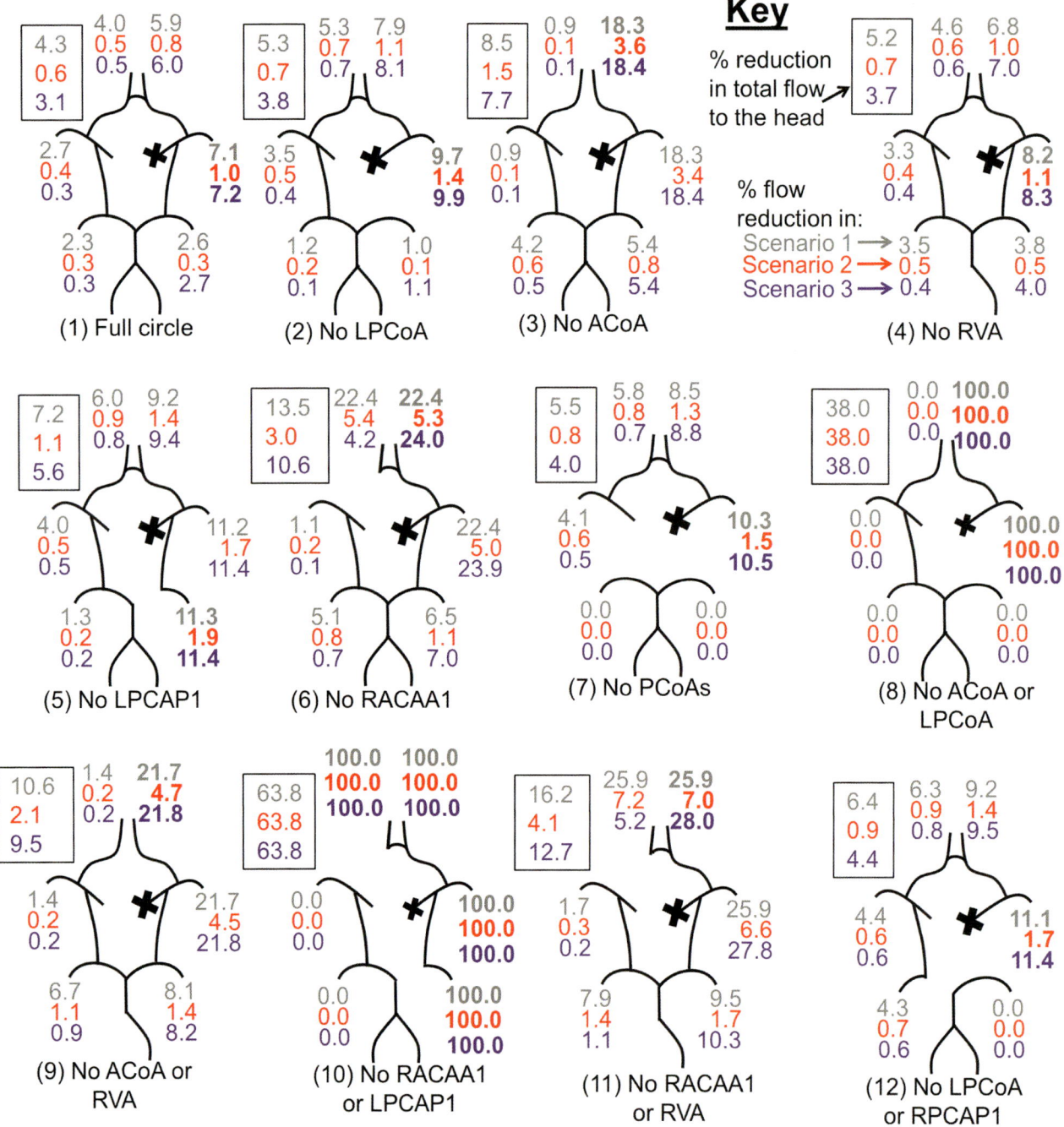

Fig. 3 Percentage reductions in flow rates through the cerebral arteries of 12 circle of Willis variants. *Black crosses* denote arterial occlusion. Flow reductions are listed with Scenario 1 on top, 2 in the middle and 3 on the bottom. *Boxed numbers* give the total percentage reduction in flow to the brain. Maximum reductions in each case are highlighted in *bold*

Conclusions

There is evidence that good collateral flow routes can reduce stroke risk [7] and improve outcomes of endovascular therapies [8, 9]. However, this work demonstrates that, in the case of ICA occlusion, the potential benefit of collateral flow is substantially undermined when autoregulation is impaired in the ipsilateral hemisphere. Thus, knowledge of autoregulatory status in both hemispheres is vitally important when assessing collateral flow, and that status may be a good predictor of outcome in cerebrovascular disease.

Acknowledgements FKM gratefully acknowledges support from Research Councils UK Digital Economy Programme: Grant EP/G036861/1 (Oxford Centre for Doctoral Training in Healthcare Innovation).

Conflicts of interest statement We declare that we have no conflict of interest.

References

1. Markus H. Cerebral perfusion and stroke. J Neurol Neurosurg Psychiatry. 2004;75(3):353–61.
2. Liebeskind DS. Collateral circulation. Stroke. 2003;34(9):2279–84.
3. Alpers BJ, Berry RG, Paddison RM. Anatomical studies of the circle of Willis in normal brain. AMA Arch Neurol Psychiatry. 1959;81(4):409–18.
4. Riggs HE, Rupp C. Variation in form of circle of Willis: the relation of the variations to collateral circulation: anatomic analysis. Arch Neurol. 1963;8:8–14.
5. Papantchev V, Stoinova V, Aleksandrov A, Todorova-Papantcheva D, Hristov S, Petkov D, Nachev G, Ovtscharoff W. The role of Willis circle variations during unilateral selective cerebral perfusion: a study of 500 circles. Eur J Cardiothorac Surg. 2013;44(4):743–53.
6. Romero JR, Pikula A, Nguyen TN, Nien YL, Norbash A, Babikian VL. Cerebral collateral circulation in carotid artery disease. Curr Cardiol Rev. 2009;5(4):279–88.
7. Angermaier A, Langner S, Kirsch M, Kessler C, Hosten N, Khaw AV. CT-angiographic collateralization predicts final infarct volume after intra-arterial thrombolysis for acute anterior circulation ischemic stroke. Cerebrovasc Dis. 2011;31(2):177–84.
8. Bang OY, Saver JL, Kim SJ, Kim GM, Chung CS, Ovbiagele B, Lee KH, Liebeskind DS. Collateral flow predicts response to endovascular therapy for acute ischemic stroke. Stroke. 2011;42(3):693–9.
9. Bang OY, Saver JL, Kim SJ, Kim GM, Chung CS, Ovbiagele B, Lee KH, Liebeskind DS. Collateral flow averts hemorrhagic transformation after endovascular therapy for acute ischemic stroke. Stroke. 2011;42(8):2235–9.
10. Payne SJ. Cerebral autoregulation. SpringerBriefs in bioengineering. New York, NY: Springer; 2016.
11. Kennedy McConnell F, Payne SJ. The dual role of cerebral autoregulation and collateral flow in the circle of Willis after major vessel occlusion. IEEE Trans Biomed Eng. 2016;64(8):1793–802.
12. Alastruey J, Moore S, Parker K, David T, Peiró J, Sherwin S. Reduced modelling of blood flow in the cerebral circulation: coupling 1-D, 0-D and cerebral auto-regulation models. Int J Numer Meth Fl. 2008;56(8):1061–7.
13. Liang F, Fukasaku K, Liu H, Takagi S. A computational model study of the influence of the anatomy of the circle of willis on cerebral hyperperfusion following carotid artery surgery. Biomed Eng Online. 2011;10:84.

ICP Monitoring by Open Extraventricular Drainage: Common Practice but Not Suitable for Advanced Neuromonitoring and Prone to False Negativity

Konstantin Hockel and Martin U. Schuhmann

Abstract *Objective*: A drawback in the use of an external ventricular drain (EVD) originates in the fact that draining cerebrospinal fluid (CSF) (open system) and intracranial pressure (ICP) monitoring can be done at the same time but is considered to be unreliable regarding the ICP trace. Furthermore, with the more widespread use of autoregulation monitoring using blood pressure and ICP signals, the question arises of whether an ICP signal from an open EVD can be used for this purpose. Using an EVD system with an integrated parenchymal ICP probe we compared the different traces of an ICP signal and their derived parameters under opened and closed CSF drainage.

Methods: Twenty patients with either subarachnoid or intraventricular hemorrhage and indication for ventriculostomy plus ICP monitoring received an EVD in combination with an air-pouch-based ICP probe. ICP was monitored via an open ventricular catheter (ICP_evd) and ICP probe (ICP_probe) simultaneously. Neuromonitoring data (ICP, arterial blood pressure, cerebral perfusion pressure, pressure reactivity index (PRx)) were recorded by ICM+ software for the time of ICU intensive care treatment. Routinely (at least every 4 h) ICP was recorded with a closed CSF drainage system for at least 15 min. ICP, ICP amplitude, and the autoregulation parameters (PRx_probe, PRx_evd) were evaluated for every episode with closed CSF drainage and during the 3 h prior with an open drainage system.

Results: One hundred and forty-four episodes with open/closed drainage were evaluated. During open drainage, overall mean ICP_evd levels were nonsignificantly different from those of ICP_probe, with 9.8 + 3.3 versus 8.2 + 3.2 mmHg, respectively. Limits of agreement ranged between 5.2 and −8.3 mmHg. However, 51 increases of ICP >20 mmHg with a duration of 3–30 min were missed by ICP_evd, and in 101 episodes the difference between ICPs was greater than 10 mmHg. After closure of the EVD, ICP increased moderately using both methods. Mean PRx_evd was significantly higher (falsely indicating impaired autoregulation) and more subjected to fluctuations than PRx_probe.

Conclusion: The general practice of draining CSF and monitoring ICP via a (usually open) EVD plus frequently performed catheter closure for ICP reading is feasible for assessment of overall ICP trends. However, it does have clinically relevant drawbacks, namely, a significant amount of undetected increases in ICP above thresholds, and continuous assessment of cerebrovascular autoregulation is less reliable. In conclusion, all patients who need CSF drainage plus ICP monitoring due to the severity of their brain insult need either an EVD with integrated ICP probe or an EVD line plus a separate ICP probe.

Keywords ICP monitoring · Intraparenchymal ICP probe · Probe · Extraventricular drainage · Cerebral autoregulation

Introduction

When patients are admitted with intraventricular or subarachnoid hemorrhage (SAH), they frequently receive a ventriculostomy for the treatment of acute hydrocephalus by an extraventricular drainage (EVD) line. At the same time, especially if the clinical condition is poor or other reasons for continued sedation are present, continuous monitoring of intracranial pressure (ICP) and, nowadays more frequently employed, assessment of cerebrovascular autoregulation, e.g., by pressure reactivity index (PRx), is warranted [1–3].

K. Hockel, M.D. (✉) · M.U. Schuhmann, M.D., Ph.D.
Department of Neurosurgery, University Hospital Tübingen, University of Tübingen, Tübingen, Germany
e-mail: konstantin.hockel@med.uni-tuebingen.de

The available ICP monitoring devices differ in the location (intraventricular, intraparenchymal, sub- and epidural) and the sensor technology for ICP detection (fluid-coupled pressure transducer, piezo-electric, stain-gauge, and fiber-optic sensors) [4–7]. By conventional means a continuous cerebrospinal fluid (CSF) drainage and simultaneous continuous ICP-based neuromonitoring can only be achieved by implantation of both an EVD and a separate, for example intraparenchymal ICP, probe, doubling the costs, the invasiveness, and the rate of potential complications thereafter, e.g., for infection [8].

To reduce these drawbacks, a compromise solution is often used as general practice in many neurocritical care units (NCCUs), i.e., to use the EVD for both CSF diversion and sole ICP monitoring device via connection by a fluid-filled line to a conventional pressure transducer. In this setting, there are two possible options, as outlined previously [9]:

1. Monitor first: The EVD is generally kept closed and connected to the ICP transducer, allowing for continuous ICP measurement until a certain threshold is reached, then opening would enable CSF drainage for a certain time period until the ICP returns to below the threshold.
2. Drainage first: The EVD is generally open, allowing for continuous CSF drainage, and closed at certain intervals to assess the "true" ICP because with an open EVD system the pressure gradient along the catheter may produce erroneous false low ICP results.

In general, both options are employed, although either the risk for underdrainage and unnecessary high ICPs or misjudgment of ICP (false low ICP) is conceivable [10–12].

Besides assessment and display of an accurate ICP, the calculated cerebral perfusion pressure (CPP), and its trends, modern neuromonitoring requires high-resolution recording of the ICP signal to facilitate, for example, wave form analysis, ICP amplitude analysis, and bedside monitoring of cerebrovascular autoregulation, for example by PRx, which has proven feasible via an EVD-mediated ICP signal [1, 13]. Nevertheless, it is unclear whether the aforementioned practice of alternating open/closed EVD guarantees reliable data collection. Therefore, we compared the neuromonitoring of ICP and associated parameters (ICP amplitude and PRx) by an EVD in open and closed settings with a direct intraparenchymal ICP probe measurement via a combined EVD with an air-pouch-based integrated probe.

Patients and Methods

The standard NCCU management of patients with intraventricular hemorrhage or aneurysmal SAH includes ventriculostomy in case of acute hydrocephalus and monitoring of ICP in patients who cannot be subjected to neurological assessment owing to their poor clinical condition, which mandates continuous analgosedation. Intensive care management was conducted according to our current NCCU standards. This means that mechanical ventilation is regulated to keep arterial pO_2 at 110 ± 5 mmHg and arterial pCO_2 between 35 and 40 mmHg, fluid balance aims at normovolemia, and catecholamines (noradrenalin) are titrated to ensure cerebral perfusion pressures of ≥ 70 mmHg.

Extraventricular Drainage, ICP Monitoring, and Assessment of Cerebral Autoregulation

When the decision to do a ventriculostomy and ICP monitoring was made, an extraventricular silver drain with a combined air-pouched-based ICP probe (Silverline Ventricular probe®, Spiegelberg GmbH & Co.KG, Hamburg, Germany) was implanted in the right frontal horn of the lateral ventricle via a one-lumen bolt. While the catheter tip is placed in the ventricle, the air pouch is located about 2 cm more proximal in the parenchyma of the frontal white matter. The drainage system was set at (5)–10–(15) cm above the foramen of Monro (depending on the clinically desired ICP levels that should be maintained) and permitted continuous CSF drainage ("drainage first" protocol).

ICP was continuously assessed by both the ICP probe via an air pressure–mediating line to a bedside ICP monitor (Spiegelberg GmbH & Co.KG, Hamburg, Germany) (ICP_probe) and the EVD via a fluid-coupled pressure transducer (xtrans, CODAN pvb Critical Care GmbH, Forstinning, Germany) referenced as closely as possible to the foramen of Monro (ICP_evd). Mean arterial pressure (MAP) was continuously monitored by a radial artery catheter with the transducer equally referenced to the foramen of Monro.

ICP_evd and MAP were continuously recorded on a bedside mounted device (Datalogger MPR, Raumedic AG, Helmbrechts, Germany) and transmitted to the bedside hospital monitoring system. The ICP_probe signal was not visualized on the hospital monitor but was visible only at the Spiegelberg monitor and thus indirectly accessible to the staff of the intensive care unit (ICU).

Blood pressure and ICP_evd taken from the Datalogger MPR and ICP_probe from the Spiegelberg monitor were additionally digitally sampled at a rate of 100 Hz by a notebook PC running ICM+ software (Cambridge Enterprise, Cambridge, UK). The ICM+ software was used for both online display of data and retrospective analysis of recorded neuromonitoring parameters. CPP_probe and CPP_evd were calculated as the difference between MAP and the respective ICP. ICP amplitude was calculated by the ICM+ software following Fourier transformation of the ICP signal as the ICP amplitude corresponding to the first harmonic, which is the heart rate (AMP).

The ICP/ABP-derived PRx as a parameter of cerebrovascular autoregulatory capacity was calculated as both PRx_probe and PRx_evd, as described elsewhere [14]. In short, PRx was computed as a moving Pearson correlation coefficient between averaged (60 s periods) ICP and MAP calculated over the moving window length of 5 min. PRx may vary between −1 and 1. Intact cerebral autoregulation can be assumed when index values are close to or below zero, meaning that no or a negative correlation between ICP and MAP exists.

CSF Drainage and Intermittent EVD Closure

The practice of intermittent EVD closure to assess the true ICP was investigated. For this the EVD was kept open for continuous drainage of CSF while monitoring ICP_evd, and on several occasions EVD was closed for at least 15 min. ICU nursing staff is generally required to close EVDs at least three times per 8 h shift and more frequently if that is deemed necessary. In parallel, EVD closure was marked as an event in the ICM+ record file.

Data Analysis and Statistics

The local ethics committee's approval was obtained for computerized neuromonitoring and data collection for retrospective data analysis. The local ethics committee granted a waiver for patient consent.

For retrospective analysis ICP and MAP data were subjected to manual artifact detection and removal. Events of EVD closure were identified in the ICM+ data files, and a baseline of 3 h monitoring prior to closure and time of EVD closure were evaluated for each event. Besides the overall mean values of MAP, ICP, ICP amplitude, CPP, PRx (evd and probe) for the 3 h baseline and 15 min period of closed EVD a 1 min mean value was calculated for ICP and ICP amplitude (evd and probe) for the 3 h baseline period as well as the period of EVD closure.

For a comparison of methods for ICP monitoring and assessment of PRx, Bland-Altman plots were used [15]. Data analysis was performed using Sigmaplot 12.5 software (Systat Software GmbH, Erkrath, Germany).

Results

Patient and General ICP Monitoring Characteristics

ICP monitoring data of 20 patients with either intraventricular hemorrhage ($n = 1$) or SAH ($n = 19$) in the year 2015 was retrospectively evaluated. Mean age was 55 years, with 60% of the patients being female. Monitoring was initiated within 48 h of ICU admission, and the duration ranged from several hours to more than 23 days.

Overall, 144 episodes of open/closed EVD were recorded and evaluated.

Neuromonitoring Parameters and Cerebral Autoregulation

Open Drainage

Mean ICP_evd levels were moderately higher than ICP_probe, with 9.8 ± 3.3 and 8.2 ± 3.2 mmHg, respectively, $p > 0.05$. Limits of agreement according to Bland-Altman analysis ranged between 5.2 and −8.3 mmHg. ICP amplitude (AMP) did not differ significantly between the two methods, with 1.5 ± 0.6 and 1.8 ± 0.9 mmHg for ICP_evd and ICP_probe, respectively, $p > 0.05$.

During open EVD, ICP_evd did not detect 51 episodes of ICP_probe values above 20 mmHg. These episodes ranged between 5 and 30 min, in one case 77 min. In one case, the reason for the missed detection was EVD obstruction due to ventricular collapse (e.g., Fig. 1). For the remaining episodes

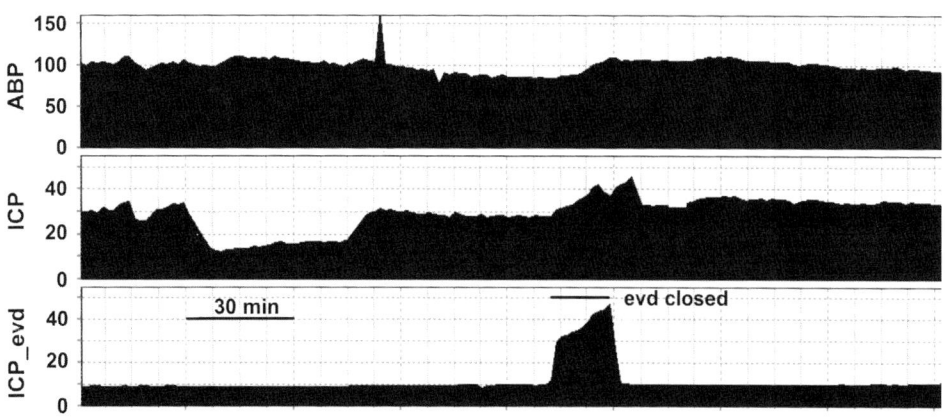

Fig. 1 Example of 4 h ICP monitoring with presumed EVD catheter blockage due to ventricular collapse. Discrepancy of ICP recordings, ICP (probe) vs. ICP_evd during "open" but blocked EVD and assessment of true ICP after closure of EVD

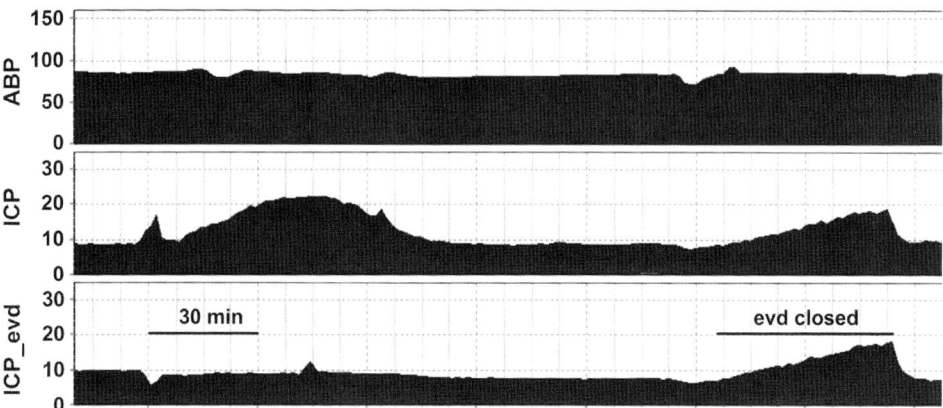

Fig. 2 Example of 4 h ICP monitoring with normally functioning EVD. During open EVD an approximately 25 min episode of ICP_probe >20 mmHg is missed by ICP_evd

ventricular drainage was considered undisturbed (e.g., Fig. 2). Furthermore, 101 episodes were identified in which the absolute difference between ICP_evd and ICP_probe was greater than 10 mmHg. In 85% of the cases, ICP_probe was higher than ICP_evd.

Assessment of pressure reactivity by PRx was feasible with both ICP_evd and ICP_probe. Cerebral autoregulation of all analyzed 3 h time segments as quantified by PRx taken from ICP_probe showed preserved vasoreactivity with mean values around zero (PRx_probe 0.01 ± 0.09). If calculated from the ICP_evd, PRx_evd was assessed with 0.12 ± 0.20, $p > 0.05$ vs. PRx_probe. The much greater variance for PRx_evd is also visualized by the increasing discrepancy for higher PRx values (around 0.2) in Bland-Altman analysis (Fig. 3).

Closed EVD

When EVD was closed, both ICP_evd and ICP_probe increased moderately, but insignificantly, to 11.3 ± 4.1 and 9.0 ± 3.1 mmHg, respectively, at 15 min after closure, compared to baseline and between each other, $p > 0.05$ vs. baseline and between methods (Fig. 4). Limits of agreement for 15 min mean values of ICP ranged between 4.6 and −9.0 mmHg (Fig. 5). Mean ICP amplitude did not change significantly, with 1.9 ± 0.9 and 2.0 ± 0.9 mmHg for ICP_evd and ICP_probe, respectively, $p > 0.05$ vs. baseline.

Autoregulation assessment was not significantly affected by EVD closure with a 15 min mean PRx_evd of 0.16 ± 0.23 and PRx_probe of 0.01 ± 0.18, $p > 0.05$ to baseline. Limits of agreement remain wide, with a remaining greater variance for PRx_evd.

Discussion

Our data once again demonstrate that ICP readings via a CSF pressure transducer in the setting of an opened EVD can be erroneous [10–12]. Even if the CSF drainage system is at a

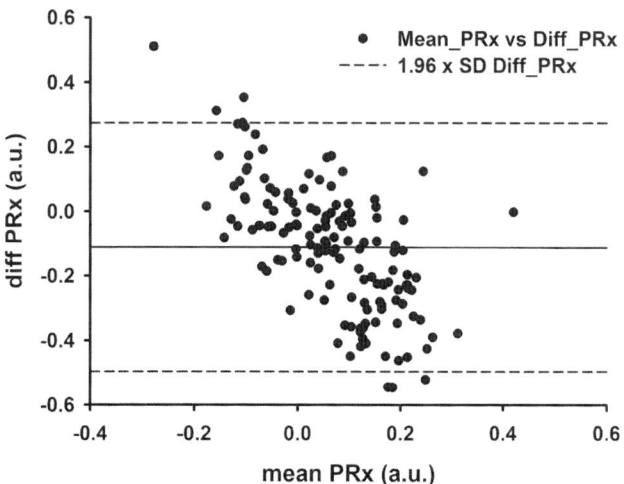

Fig. 3 Bland-Altman analysis of PRx_probe vs. PRx_evd under open EVD. Especially for higher PRx (>0.2), where autoregulation assessment is critical, the discrepancy of the two methods is increased

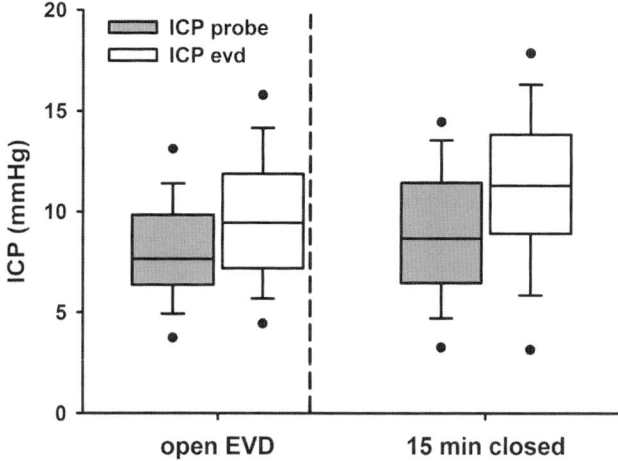

Fig. 4 Box plots of overall mean ICP values, both ICP_probe and ICP_evd, for open and closed EVD. In this cohort there exists fair agreement of ICP assessment between the methods. EVD closure leads to a minor increase of both ICP_probe and ICP_evd

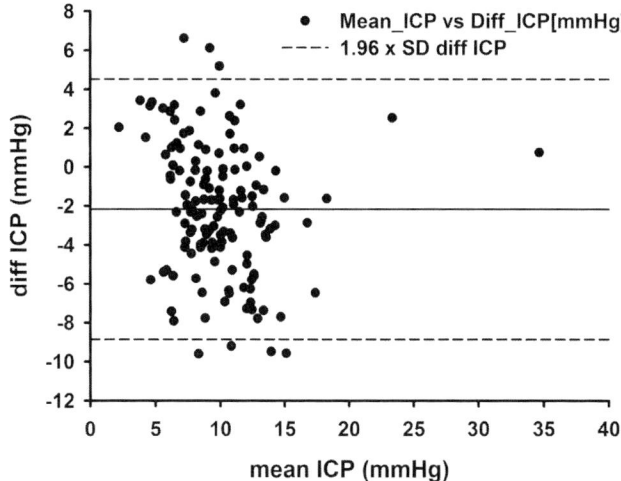

Fig. 5 Bland-Altman analysis of ICP_probe vs. ICP_evd under closed EVD. Limits of agreement for 15 min mean values of ICP ranged between 4.6 and −9.0 mmHg

medium level, i.e., in our ICU usually 10 cm above the foramen of Monro (corresponding to 7.3 mmHg), the intracranial compliance is well preserved, and ICP is mostly below the pathological range, there are periods of temporal ICP increase, e.g., during nursing maneuvers, decreased sedation levels, or during vasogenic waves, where the induced increased CSF outflow creates a pressure gradient via the catheter, and correct ICP assessment by EVD is impossible. In 19 of our 20 patients, ICP levels were not substantially elevated during the monitoring period, which explains the high agreement of ICP assessment (between ICP_probe and ICP_evd).

Nevertheless 51 episodes were detected with temporal ICP values above 20 mmHg, in which those temporal increases in ICP were missed by the ICP_evd reading. The episodes were usually short, less than 1 h, and not life threatening, however effectively decreasing the CPP. In one of the 20 patients, however, who was suffering from progressive brain swelling, a persistent high ICP level above 30 mmHg developed. The resulting CSF outflow led to a ventricular collapse and a loss of fluid coupling within the EVD system. Therefore, ICP_evd showed constantly low values, but with a suspiciously silent and nonfluctuating ICP trace, and the high ICP values were only noticed when the EVD was closed (Fig. 1). This is a typical example of false negative ICP readings via EVD, which seems to occur especially in the most critical situation of brain edema/brain swelling.

The identification of a total of 101 episodes with an ICP difference of >10 mmHg between the open (EVD) and closed (air pouch) system underscores the dangers of false low ICU determination and, thus, false high CPP calculation using an open EVD system for ICP monitoring.

With the drainage system of the EVD closed, ICP increased only mildly within 15 min, as can be expected in patients with preserved intracranial reserve capacity at ICP values below 20 mmHg. The bias and discrepancy of the two methods (ICP_evd and ICP_probe) can be considered acceptable (Fig. 5) and correlated to other comparative studies of different ICP monitors [11], where differences of 5 mmHg are found frequently and were considered to have no significant clinical impact. Thus, with a closed drainage system, EVD-based ICP monitoring seems to be sufficient, but our study only compared 15 min intervals as opposed to 3 h intervals with an open drainage system. Since all patients had acute posthemorrhagic occlusive hydrocephalus, a monitor-first approach with closed EVD was most of the time not possible because of rapid ICP increase.

The air-pouch-based parenchymal ICP monitor provided continuous, reliable, and high-frequency assessment of ICP [16]. The failure rate for this device was determined to be zero in these 20 patients. Fluid-coupled ICP monitoring, in contrast, is susceptible to artifacts and several possible human handling errors, like undetected partial or complete catheter blockage, air bubbles in the line, or incorrect height adjustment of the transducer with false zeroing [11]. Moreover, in patients with reduced compliance, frequent EVD closure might be critical.

As other authors have pointed out, continuous bedside determination of cerebrovascular autoregulatory state has become a well-recognized tool in ICU treatment. The PRx uses the extent of correlation between slow frequency waves in the ICP and ABP signals in a closed system, i.e., the cranium, to establish a statement about the state of cerebrovascular autoregulation [3, 14]. It has been disputed whether an open EVD already abolishes the requirement for a closed system since the ICP waveform is altered in this setting. Recently, Aries et al. not only showed that autoregulation assessment by PRx is feasible in the setting of an open EVD; they also demonstrated that the ICP signal from an open EVD, otherwise corrupted for estimation of ICP, carries sufficient information, i.e., low-frequency waves, to produce a reliable PRx [1].

From the present data we can confirm that PRx can be assessed by the ICP_evd signal, and, although it is difficult to draw a definitive conclusion from 15 min of recording, EVD closure did not change the PRx_evd value significantly. Nevertheless, when comparing PRx_evd with PRx_probe, we assume that PRx_probe is the more precise variable because its variance of the 3 h mean values is much less. In parallel, PRx_probe did not differ between EVD opening and closure.

The fact that our PRx_evd variable was not as reliable and comparable to ICP_probe as in the Aries et al. study [1] might be explained by the fact that we used a longer fluid-filled line connected to the ICP pressure transducer, which is a well-known source of signal artifact. From the presented data in this specific setup, PRx_probe seems to be the preferred method for reliable continuous assessment of cerebral autoregulation.

A concern expressed previously referred to a possible dampening of the ICP signal by the air-pouch-based technique of ICP measurement, which transfers changes in ICP to an air-filled balloon and line connected to the ICP monitor. From the signal assessment of the ICP_probe wave with preserved ICP amplitude (AMP) especially compared to the signal via a closed EVD, we conclude that this presumed dampening effect can be neglected.

Conclusion

In summary, if current NCCU treatment standards require an accurate, high-resolution ICP recording, which furthermore makes continuously collected data available for online evaluation, and if the ICP signal is used for the assessment of indices for autoregulation and cerebrospinal compliance, then a combined EVD with a drainage-independent, parenchymal ICP monitoring system is most suitable.

As stated earlier, this can be achieved as well by an EVD plus a separate ICP probe. The compromise of using one EVD only requires an elaborate technique and the highest surveillance and alertness of the nursing staff to minimize false recordings and artifacts. This still has the disadvantage that a truly continuous signal recording cannot be achieved when open and closed intervals alternate.

Lastly, continuous assessment of cerebrovascular autoregulation (via PRx) by EVD gives less reliable information with a high likelihood of having false positive results, meaning that autoregulatory capacities would be considered nonfunctional at a much earlier time point.

Conflicts of interest statement We declare that we have no conflict of interest.

References

1. Aries MJH, de Jong SF, van Dijk JMC, Regtien J, Depreitere B, Czosnyka M, Smielewski P, Elting JWJ. Observation of autoregulation indices during ventricular CSF drainage after aneurysmal subarachnoid hemorrhage: a pilot study. Neurocrit Care. 2015;23(3):347–54.
2. Jaeger M, Schuhmann MU, Soehle M, Nagel C, Meixensberger J. Continuous monitoring of cerebrovascular autoregulation after subarachnoid hemorrhage by brain tissue oxygen pressure reactivity and its relation to delayed cerebral infarction. Stroke. 2007;38(3):981–6.
3. Le Roux P, Menon DK, Citerio G, et al. Consensus summary statement of the international multidisciplinary consensus conference on multimodality monitoring in neurocritical care: a statement for healthcare professionals from the Neurocritical Care Society and the European Society of Intensive C. Neurocrit Care. 2014;21(Suppl 2):S1–26.
4. Citerio G, Piper I, Chambers IR, Galli D, Enblad P, Kiening K, Ragauskas A, Sahuquillo J, Gregson B, BrainIT Group. Multicenter clinical assessment of the raumedic neurovent-P intracranial pressure sensor: a report by the BrainIT group. Neurosurgery. 2008;63(6):1152–8. discussion 1158
5. Czosnyka M, Czosnyka Z, Pickard JD. Laboratory testing of three intracranial pressure microtransducers: technical report. Neurosurgery. 1996;38(1):219–24.
6. Piper I, Barnes A, Smith D, Dunn L. The Camino intracranial pressure sensor: is it optimal technology? An internal audit with a review of current intracranial pressure monitoring technologies. Neurosurgery. 2001;49(5):1158–64. discussion 1164–5
7. Raabe A, Stöckel R, Hohrein D, Schöche J. Reliability of intraventricular pressure measurement with fiberoptic or solid-state transducers: avoidance of a methodological error. Neurosurgery. 1998;42(1):74–9. discussion 79–80
8. Dimitriou J, Levivier M, Gugliotta M. Comparison of complications in patients receiving different types of intracranial pressure monitoring: a retrospective study in a single center in Switzerland. World Neurosurg. 2016;89:641–6.
9. Kim GS, Amato A, James ML, Britz GW, Zomorodi A, Graffagnino C, Zomorodi M, Olson DM. Continuous and intermittent CSF diversion after subarachnoid hemorrhage: a pilot study. Neurocrit Care. 2011;14(1):68–72.
10. Birch AA, Eynon CA, Schley D. Erroneous intracranial pressure measurements from simultaneous pressure monitoring and ventricular drainage catheters. Neurocrit Care. 2006;5(1):51–4.
11. Vender J, Waller J, Dhandapani K, McDonnell D. An evaluation and comparison of intraventricular, intraparenchymal, and fluid-coupled techniques for intracranial pressure monitoring in patients with severe traumatic brain injury. J Clin Monit Comput. 2011;25(4):231–6.
12. Wilkinson HA, Yarzebski J, Wilkinson EC, Anderson FA. Erroneous measurement of intracranial pressure caused by simultaneous ventricular drainage: a hydrodynamic model study. Neurosurgery. 1989;24(3):348–54.
13. Howells T, Johnson U, McKelvey T, Ronne-Engström E, Enblad P. The effects of ventricular drainage on the intracranial pressure signal and the pressure reactivity index. J Clin Monit Comput. 2016;31(2):469–78. https://doi.org/10.1007/s10877-016-9863-3.
14. Czosnyka M, Smielewski P, Kirkpatrick P, Laing RJ, Menon D, Pickard JD. Continuous assessment of the cerebral vasomotor reactivity in head injury. Neurosurgery. 1997;41(1):11–7. discussion 17–9
15. Bland JM, Altman DG. Statistical methods for assessing agreement between two methods of clinical measurement. Lancet (London). 1986;1(8476):307–10.
16. Chambers IR, Siddique MS, Banister K, Mendelow AD. Clinical comparison of the Spiegelberg parenchymal transducer and ventricular fluid pressure. J Neurol Neurosurg Psychiatry. 2001;71(3):383–5.

Comparison of Intracranial Pressure and Pressure Reactivity Index Obtained Through Pressure Measurements in the Ventricle and in the Parenchyma During and Outside Cerebrospinal Fluid Drainage Episodes in a Manipulation-Free Patient Setting

Samuel Patrick Klein, Dominike Bruyninckx, Ina Callebaut, and Bart Depreitere

Abstract

Objective: We investigated the effect of cerebrospinal fluid (CSF) drainage on the intracranial pressure (ICP) signal measured in the parenchyma and the ventricle as well as the effect on the pressure reactivity index (PRx) calculated from both signals.

Methods: Ten patients were included in this prospective study. All patients received a parenchymal ICP sensor and an external ventricular drain (EVD) for CSF drainage. ICP signals (ICP-p and ICP-evd) were captured. Part of the study was a period of 90 min during which the patient was free from any manipulation, consisting of 30 min of drainage (O1), 30 min EVD closed (C) and 30 min of drainage (O2).

Results: Mean ICP-evd and mean AMP-evd increased (3.03 and 0.46 mmHg) from O1 to C and decreased (2.12 and 0.43 mmHg) from C to O2. ICP-p and AMP-p changes were less pronounced (closing EVD: +0.81 mmHg/+0.22 mmHg; opening EVD: −0.22 mmHg/−0.05 mmHg). Mean difference between PRx-evd and PRx-p was 0.12 for O1, 0.02 for C and −0.02 for O2. The intraclass correlation coefficient for absolute agreement of single measures was 0.66 for O1, 0.77 for C and 0.69 for O2. Mean PRx differences demonstrated a significant difference between O1 versus C and O1 versus O2 but not between C versus O2.

Conclusion: Drainage of CSF reduces ICP magnitude and amplitude through the EVD. This effect was only marginal in parenchymal ICP measurements. In manipulation-free circumstances, agreement of PRx obtained through parenchymal and ventricular measurements was moderate to good, depending on the statistical method, and was not necessarily influenced by drainage.

Keywords Intracranial pressure · Autoregulation · External ventricular drain · Cerebrospinal fluid drainage

Introduction

Intracranial pressure (ICP) is an important parameter in neurointensive care medicine due to the ability to diagnose and treat raised ICP [1]. Raised ICP is associated with poor clinical outcomes [2]. Measurement of ICP allows for the determination and therapeutic adjustment of cerebral perfusion pressure (CPP) [3]. Furthermore, ICP can be used to assess cerebrovascular autoregulation by calculation of cerebral pressure reactivity. The pressure reactivity index (PRx) is considered to be a measure of continuous autoregulation by quantifying the relationship between slow fluctuations in mean arterial blood pressure (ABP) and ICP [4]. High PRx values have been shown to be a predictor of poor clinical outcome [4, 5]. Continuous determination of the state of autoregulation can potentially be used to direct CPP-oriented therapy by calculation of the optimal CPP at a given point in time [6]. The correct measurement of ICP is thus essential for the guidance of therapy. ICP can be measured using various methods. The gold standard for ICP measurement involves the placement of an external ventricular drain (EVD) and measurement of intraventricular pressure using a fluid-filled pressure transducer. Measurement of ICP using an EVD is potentially vulnerable to external artefacts confounding the signal such as patient positioning, tracheal suctioning and drainage of cerebrospinal fluid (CSF). Drainage of CSF may attenuate ICP signals by decreasing the pressure gradient in the EVD. Alternatively, ICP measured using a parenchymal probe is less sensitive to artefacts. In patients diagnosed with a subarachnoid haemorrhage, it was recently shown that an open EVD system could be used to calculate dynamic autoregulation indices owing to preserved slow fluctuations in ICP signals [7]. The aim of the present study is to investigate the effect of CSF drainage on ICP signals

S.P. Klein, M.D. (✉) • D. Bruyninckx • I. Callebaut, Ph.D.
B. Depreitere, M.D., Ph.D.
Department of Neurosurgery, University Hospitals Leuven, Leuven, Belgium
e-mail: sam.klein@kuleuven.be

measured in the parenchyma and the ventricle as well as the influence on PRx calculated from both signals.

Materials and Methods

Patients and Management

Ten patients with severe traumatic brain injury admitted to the Department of Neurosurgery between December 2014 and March 2015 were included. The study was approved by the local ethics committee. At University Hospitals Leuven, the protocol for the management of severe traumatic brain injury includes the placement of both a microstrain gauge transducer (Codman ICP MicroSensor; Codman & Shurtleff, Inc., Raynham, MA) for parenchymal ICP monitoring and an EVD for the drainage of CSF as a treatment for raised ICP. The parenchymal probe was inserted ipsilaterally in proximity to the EVD using the same burr hole.

Data Collection

All patients underwent monitoring of ABP and ICP signals from both parenchymal (ICP-p) and ventricular recordings (ICP-evd). Waveform data were captured continuously with ICM+ software (Cambridge Enterprise, University of Cambridge, Cambridge, UK) at a frequency of 60 Hz. ABP was monitored from the radial artery using a fluid-coupled pressure transducer placed at the level of the heart. The fluid-filled pressure transducer from the EVD was placed at the level of the external auditory meatus to record ICP. The most proximal part of the EVD was used for ICP recording.

Study Protocol

Data for analysis were recorded during critical care admission. Part of the study protocol was a period of 90 min during which the patient was free from any manipulation. The manipulation-free period intended to minimise confounding of data by external artefacts such as patient positioning or tracheal suctioning, for example. During that period of 90 min, a study collaborator was present to confirm no manipulations occurred. If urgent manipulation was necessary, the data were excluded for this part of the study. The correct position of ABP and EVD pressure transducers, as well as fluid-transducer patency, was verified before the start of the manipulation-free period (MFP). During the MFP, the EVD was opened for drainage of CSF during the first 30 min (O1), followed by 30 min of closure of the EVD for drainage (C), and finally opening of the EVD for drainage for 30 min (O2). The MFP was performed once per patient.

Calculation of PRx, AMP and RAP

The PRx was calculated as moving Pearson correlation coefficients, using 300 s time windows, between 10 s averages of ABP and ICP signals (separate calculations using ICP-p and ICP-evd). ICP pulse amplitude (AMP) was calculated using a fast Fourier transform to convert the signals into the frequency domain and to extract the fundamental first harmonic from consecutive 10 s time windows. The RAP index (correlation coefficient [R] between AMP [A] and mean ICP [P]), was calculated as a moving Pearson correlation coefficient between mean ICP and AMP from a 5 min window, updated every 60 s.

Statistical Analysis

Statistical analysis was performed using the statistical software SPSS 20 (IBM/SPSS, Inc., Armonk, NY, USA). Normality of data was assessed using a Shapiro-Wilk statistic, and, if necessary, logarithmic transformation was applied.

Results

Patients

All patients were sedated and ventilated during data gathering. The MFP was performed on days 1–14 after trauma with a median of 3.5 days. The mean age was 51.9 (standard deviation (SD) = 19.2). Two patients were female and eight were male.

ICP, AMP and RAP During EVD Drainage States

Mean ICP-evd and ICP-p increased with 3.03 mmHg (SD = 5.9, $p < 0.001$) and 0.81 mmHg (SD = 1.68, $p < 0.001$) respectively from O1 to C. Reopening of the EVD resulted in a mean ICP-evd and ICP-p decrease of 2.12 mmHg (SD = 6.23, $p < 0.001$) and 0.22 mmHg (SD = 1.71, $p = 0.023$) respectively.

Table 1 Mean ICP and ICP-derived values during EVD drainage states

Variable	Open 1 (O1)	Closed (C)	Open 2 (O2)
ICP-evd	9.09 (3.00)	12.12 (6.58)*	10.00 (3.56)
ICP-p	8.45 (6.52)	9.26 (6.85)*	9.02 (6.80)
AMP-evd	1.11 (1.10)	1.57 (1.36)*	1.14 (1.14)
AMP-p	1.58 (0.98)	1.81 (1.26)	1.76 (1.06)
RAP-evd	0.51 (0.42)	0.54 (0.45)	0.41 (0.49)
RAP-p	0.66 (0.34)	0.60 (0.37)*	0.64 (0.37)

Values gives as mean (SD); *significant difference defined as $p < 0.05$ between both O1 and O2 versus C

Mean ICP amplitude AMP-evd increased by 0.46 (SD = 0.61, $p < 0.001$) and decreased by 0.43 (SD = 0.75, $p < 0.001$) during the transition from O1 to C and C to O2 respectively. AMP-p increased by 0.22 (SD = 0.38, $p < 0.001$) and decreased by 0.05 (SD = 0.43, $p = 0.059$) during closing and opening of the EVD.

Mean RAP-evd increased by 0.03 (SD = 0.46, $p = 0.243$) and decreased by 0.13 (SD = 0.66, $p = 0.001$). RAP-p decreased by 0.06 (SD = 0.26, $p < 0.001$) and increased by 0.04 (SD = 0.25, $p = 0.005$) (Table 1).

Difference in PRx Between Parenchymal and Ventricular Signals

Mean PRx-evd increased by 0.13 from O1 to C and decreased by 0.09 from C to O2, and both changes were significant ($p < 0.005$). Mean PRx-p increased by 0.02 ($p = 0.38$) from O1 to C and decreased by 0.12 from C to O2 ($p < 0.005$) (Table 2). The mean difference between PRx-evd and PRx-p was 0.12 (SD = 0.30) for O1, 0.02 (SD = 0.27) for C and −0.02 (SD = 0.27) for O2 (Table 3). The coefficient of repeatability below which the absolute differences between two measurements would lie with 95% probability was 0.60 for O1, 0.52 for C and 0.53 for O2. The intraclass correlation coefficient for absolute agreement of single measures using a two-way random model was 0.66 (CI 0.54–0.75) for O1, 0.77 (CI 0.72–0.81) for C and 0.69 (CI 0.63–0.75) for O2.

Repeated-measures ANOVA determined that the mean difference in PRx calculation between parenchymal and ventricular signals differed significantly between different EVD drainage states ($F(2614) = 22.15$, $p < 0.0005$). Post hoc tests for mean PRx differences between EVD drainage states using Bonferroni correction demonstrated a significant difference between O1 versus C ($p < 0.0005$) and O1 versus O2 ($p < 0.0005$) but not between C versus O2 ($p = 0.35$).

Table 2 Mean PRx values during EVD drainage states

Variables	Open 1 (O1)	Closed (C)	Open 2 (O2)
PRx-evd	−0.12 (0.34)	0.01 (0.41)*	−0.08 (0.35)*
PRx-p	0.00 (0.44)	0.02 (0.38)	−0.10 (0.35)*

Values gives as mean (SD); *significant difference defined as $p < 0.05$ between current and previous EVD state

Table 3 Differences and agreement between parenchymal and ventricular signal–derived PRx calculations

PRx	Open 1 (O1)	Closed (C)	Open 2 (O2)
Mean difference (SD)	0.12 (0.30)	0.02 (0.27)	−0.02 (0.27)
Coefficient of repeatability (lower–upper limit of agreement)	0.60 (−0.48 to 0.72)	0.52 (−0.51 to 0.54)	0.53 (−0.55 to 0.52)
Intraclass correlation coefficient (two-way random model, absolute agreement)			
Single measures (95% CI)	0.66 (0.54–0.75)	0.77 (0.72–0.81)	0.69 (0.63–0.75)
Average measures (95% CI)	0.80 (0.70–0.86)	0.87 (0.84–0.90)	0.82 (0.77–0.86)

Discussion

This study demonstrates that the calculation of the PRx using an open and closed ventricular drainage system is in moderate to good agreement with parenchymal-derived calculations in a manipulation-free setting.

ICP

The drainage of CSF significantly reduced the magnitude and amplitude of the ICP signal measured through the EVD. However, this effect on ICP was limited in parenchymal measurements. Changes in ICP magnitude and amplitude are in agreement with the results of a recent study in patients with subarachnoid haemorrhage [7].

PRx

Opening of the EVD system did not necessarily increase the difference in PRx between ventricular and parenchymal calculations. Agreement between both PRx calculations was slightly better with a closed EVD system. One patient in this study showed a large mean difference in PRx calculation

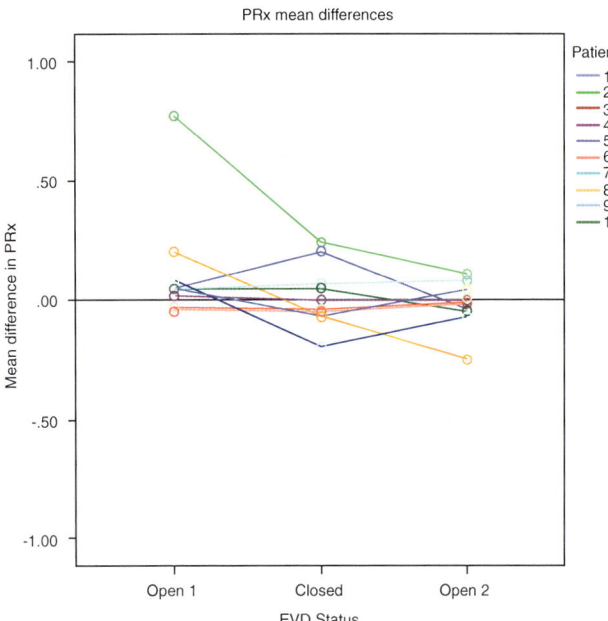

Fig. 1 Mean difference in PRx calculations using parenchymal and ventricular ICP signals

during the first open EVD period, but this difference normalised during the second open EVD period (Fig. 1). Absolute mean differences between both PRx calculation methods were within clinically acceptable limits for most patients. If the results of this current manipulation-free study are confirmed in a regular clinical setting with manipulations, the concept of autoregulation monitoring could potentially be used in all patients requiring an EVD. The fundamental question whether parenchymal and ventricular ICP signals contain the same information regarding the state of autoregulation remains unresolved.

An important limitation of this study is the small group of 10 patients and the lack of manipulations, which could compromise generalisability. These results need to be confirmed in a regular clinical setting which includes patient manipulations to assess for possible confounding effects.

Conclusion

Drainage of CSF reduces both the ICP magnitude and amplitude. This effect is pronounced in measurements through the EVD and marginal in parenchymal ICP measurements. In the manipulation-free circumstances of the present study, agreement of PRx obtained through parenchymal and ventricular measurements was moderate to good depending on the statistical method used, and this was not necessarily influenced by drainage.

Conflicts of interest statement We declare that we have no conflict of interest.

References

1. Stocchetti N, Maas AIR. Traumatic intracranial hypertension. N Engl J Med. 2014;370(22):2121–30. http://www.ncbi.nlm.nih.gov/pubmed/24869722. Accessed 10 Jul 2014
2. Güiza F, Depreitere B, Piper I, Citerio G, Chambers I, Jones P, et al. Visualizing the pressure and time burden of intracranial hypertension in adult and paediatric traumatic brain injury. Intensive Care Med. 2015;41(6):1067–76. http://link.springer.com/10.1007/s00134-015-3806-1
3. Kirkman M, Smith M. Intracranial pressure monitoring, cerebral perfusion pressure estimation, and ICP/CPP-guided therapy: a standard of care or optional extra after brain injury? Br J Anaesth. 2014;112:35–46. http://www.ncbi.nlm.nih.gov/pubmed/24293327. Accessed 7 Dec 2014
4. Czosnyka M, Smielewski P, Kirkpatrick P, Laing RJ, Menon D, Pickard JD. Continuous assessment of the cerebral vasomotor reactivity in head injury. Neurosurgery. 1997;41:11–9. http://www.ncbi.nlm.nih.gov/pubmed/9218290. Accessed 12 Feb 2015
5. Howells T, Elf K, Jones PA, Ronne-Engström E, Piper I, Nilsson P, et al. Pressure reactivity as a guide in the treatment of cerebral perfusion pressure in patients with brain trauma. J Neurosurg. 2005;102:311–7.
6. Steiner L, Czosnyka M, Czosnyka M, Piechnik SK, Piechnik SK, et al. Continuous monitoring of cerebrovascular pressure reactivity allows determination of optimal cerebral perfusion pressure in patients with traumatic brain injury. Crit Care Med. 2002;30:733–8. http://www.ncbi.nlm.nih.gov/pubmed/11940737
7. Aries MJH, de Jong SF, van Dijk JMC, Regtien J, Depreitere B, Czosnyka M, et al. Observation of autoregulation indices during ventricular CSF drainage after aneurysmal subarachnoid hemorrhage: a pilot study. Neurocrit Care. 2015;23(3):347–54. http://link.springer.com/10.1007/s12028-015-0107-z

Visualizing Cerebrovascular Autoregulation Insults and Their Association with Outcome in Adult and Paediatric Traumatic Brain Injury

Marine Flechet, Geert Meyfroidt, Ian Piper, Giuseppe Citerio, Iain Chambers, Patricia A. Jones, Tsz-Yan Milly Lo, Per Enblad, Pelle Nilsson, Bart Feyen, Philippe Jorens, Andrew Maas, Martin U. Schuhmann, Rob Donald, Laura Moss, Greet Van den Berghe, Bart Depreitere, and Fabian Güiza

Abstract *Objective*: The aim of this study is to assess visually the impact of duration and intensity of cerebrovascular autoregulation insults on 6-month neurological outcome in severe traumatic brain injury.

Material and methods: Retrospective analysis of prospectively collected minute-by-minute intracranial pressure (ICP) and mean arterial blood pressure data of 259 adult and 99 paediatric traumatic brain injury (TBI) patients from multiple European centres. The relationship of the 6-month Glasgow Outcome Scale with cerebrovascular autoregulation insults (defined as the low-frequency autoregulation index above a certain threshold during a certain time) was visualized in a colour-coded plot. The analysis was performed separately for autoregulation insults occurring with cerebral perfusion pressure (CPP) below 50 mmHg, with ICP above 25 mmHg and for the subset of adult patients that did not undergo decompressive craniectomy.

Results: The colour-coded plots showed a time-intensity-dependent association with outcome for cerebrovascular autoregulation insults in adult and paediatric TBI patients. Insults with a low-frequency autoregulation index above 0.2 were associated with worse outcomes and below −0.6 with better outcomes, with and approximately exponentially decreasing transition curve between the two intensity thresholds. All insults were associated with worse outcomes when CPP was below 50 mmHg or ICP was above 25 mmHg.

Conclusions: The colour-coded plots indicate that cerebrovascular autoregulation is disturbed in a dynamic manner, such that duration and intensity play a role in the determination of a zone associated with better neurological outcome.

M. Flechet • G. Meyfroidt • G.V. den Berghe • F. Güiza (✉)
Department of Intensive Care Medicine, University Hospitals Leuven, Leuven, Belgium

Klinik für Neurochirurgie, Universitätsklinikum Tübingen, Tübingen, Germany

School of Mathematics and Statistics, University of Glasgow, Glasgow, UK

Department of Clinical Physics and Bioengineering, NHS Greater Glasgow & Clyde, Glasgow, UK

Department of Neurosurgery, University Hospitals Leuven, Leuven, Belgium
e-mail: fabian.guiza@kuleuven.be

I. Piper
Department of Clinical Physics, Southern General Hospital, Glasgow, UK

G. Citerio
San Gerardo Hospital, Monza, Italy

I. Chambers
Medical Physics, James Cook University Hospital, Middlesbroughnza, UK

P.A. Jones
Department of Paediatric Neurology, Royal Hospital for Sick Children, Edinburgh, UK

T.-Y. M. Lo
Department of Paediatric Intensive Care, Royal Hospital for Sick Children, Edinburgh, UK

P. Enblad • P. Nilsson
Neurosurgery, Department of Neuroscience, Uppsala University, Uppsala, Sweden

B. Feyen • A. Maas
Department of Neurosurgery, Antwerp University Hospital, Edegem, Belgium

P. Jorens
Department of Intensive Care Medicine, Antwerp University Hospital, Edegem, Belgium

M.U. Schuhmann
Klinik für Neurochirurgie, Universitätsklinikum Tübingen, Tübingen, Germany

R. Donald
School of Mathematics and Statistics, University of Glasgow, Glasgow, UK

L. Moss
Department of Clinical Physics and Bioengineering, NHS Greater Glasgow & Clyde, Glasgow, UK

B. Depreitere
Department of Neurosurgery, University Hospitals Leuven, Leuven, Belgium

Keywords Traumatic brain injury · Cerebrovascular autoregulation · Autoregulation index · Visualization · Adults · Children

Introduction

Traumatic brain injury (TBI) is one of the most important health care problems worldwide [1, 2]. The management of severe TBI is primarily aimed at avoiding secondary brain damage, which mainly manifests as brain ischemia.

Cerebrovascular pressure autoregulation (CAR) is the capacity of the cerebral vasculature to maintain a constant cerebral blood flow (CBF) through varying cerebral perfusion pressure (CPP). It is well known that autoregulation is often deficient in severe TBI [3], although the degree and range of this dysfunction can vary among patients, and in time within the same patient [4]. Figaji et al. [5] have demonstrated the validity of the autoregulation concept in children with TBI.

Continuous monitoring of cerebrovascular autoregulation through parameters such as the Pressure Reactivity Index (PRx) [6] or Low frequency Autoregulation Index (LAx) [7] has enabled the identification of CPP ranges in which autoregulation is more active. In retrospective analyses, higher percentages of time of actual CPP contained within these ranges were associated with better outcomes [7–9].

PRx and LAx can be used to continuously identify episodes of potentially impaired CAR in TBI patients. A cut-off value for each index differentiates between episodes of active and disturbed autoregulation [10, 11]. However, as was demonstrated for intracranial pressure (ICP) [11], it is unlikely that a static threshold would capture the complexity of the association between autoregulation and outcome.

The aim of the present study is to assess the effect of CAR insults, according to varying definitions of intensity and duration, on functional outcome at 6 months based on prospectively collected data from continuously monitored adult and paediatric patients with severe TBI. In addition, the impact of ICP, CPP and decompressive craniectomy (DC) on the capacity to tolerate CAR insults is investigated.

Materials and Methods

Patients and Data

The adult cohort consisted of 259 patients with severe TBI aged 16 years and older: 164 patients were included from the Brain-IT database [12], which collected data from 22 centres between March 2003 and July 2005. The Multi-Centre Research Ethics Committee for Scotland (MREC/02/0/9) granted the use of these data for scientific purposes on 14 February 2002. The data of the remaining 95 adult patients were collected from four centres: 38 from the San Gerardo Hospital in Monza, Italy, between March 2010 and April 2013; 25 from the University Hospitals Leuven, Belgium, between September 2010 and September 2013; 20 from the University Hospital Antwerp, Belgium, as part of the 'Individualized targeted monitoring in neurocritical care' (NEMO) project [13], between May 2010 and June 2013; and 12 from the University Hospital Tübingen, Germany, between February and December 2009. Local ethics committee approval to use the anonymized data for this analysis was obtained at all centres.

The paediatric cohort consisted of 99 TBI patients, aged between 2 and 16 years: 81 patients were part of a study on TBI in children, recruited during 62 non-consecutive months up to July 2003, from two paediatric centres in Edinburgh and Newcastle, UK [14]. The study had local ethics committee and management approval at both centres, and informed consent was obtained before enrolment. The remaining 18 paediatric patients were part of the Brain-IT database.

Patients were managed according to Brain Trauma Foundation guidelines. Data collection included baseline risk factors (age, gender, admission Glasgow Coma Scale (GCS), admission pupil reactivity), minute-by-minute ICP and mean arterial blood pressure (MAP) monitoring data, and Glasgow Outcome Score (GOS) at 6 months. For the paediatric patients, a modified GOS was used, as described in the original paper [14]. Monitoring data in the NEMO database were recorded and stored every second; the median value of each minute interval was taken to obtain a minute-by-minute value. Signals from all data sets were reviewed independently by two senior clinicians in Leuven (GM, BD), and obvious artefacts at visual inspection were removed. A correction of the CPP values for arterial blood pressure transducer height was made based on the information obtained on the centre-specific protocol. For patients from centres where the transducer was at the atrium level and who were nursed with the head of the bed elevated at 30°, 10 mmHg was subtracted from the registered CPP. This was the case in 101 of 259 (39.0%) of the adult patients. No corrections were made in the paediatric cohort.

Visualization Method

The method for visualizing the univariate association between insult and outcome used to assess the pressure and time burden of intracranial hypertension in Güiza et al. [11] was applied in the current analysis to investigate the relationship between CAR and outcome. A LAx value was calculated every minute during the monitoring period as the moving median of the Pearson correlation coefficients between ICP and MAP for the past time intervals of 3, 5, 10, 20, 30, 60 and 90 min, using minute-by-minute resolution data [7]. CAR insults were defined as a LAx value exceeding a certain intensity for a certain duration of time. Finally, the Pearson correlation coefficient between GOS and the average number of CAR insults (of a certain intensity and duration) was calculated where supported data were available and was expressed by a graded colour code: negative correlations in red and positive correlations in blue. The contour for zero correlation was highlighted in black and defined as the 'transition curve' as in the original study.

The relationship between CAR insults and outcome was visualized separately for insults for which CPP < 50 mmHg, those for which ICP > 25 mmHg and for the subset of adult patients that did not undergo DC ($n = 214$).

All analyses were done in MATLAB 2014b® (The MathWorks, Natick, MA, USA).

Results

Demographic and outcome data of the studied cohorts are presented in Table 1.

The colour-coded plots visualizing the correlations between GOS at 6 months and the average number of different types of CAR insults are shown in Fig. 1a–c. In each plot, two clear overall regions emerge: one with negative correlations (blue), indicating types of CAR insults that occur more frequently in patients with higher GOS, and one with positive correlations (red), indicating types of CAR insults that occur more frequently in patients with lower GOS. The transition curves between the two zones are approximately exponential in all cohorts: for higher insult intensities, the transition occurs at shorter insult durations, and, conversely, for lower insult intensities the transition occurs at longer insult durations. In all cases, regardless of duration, CAR insults of LAx above 0.2 were associated with worse outcomes and below −0.6 with better outcomes. Figure 1d shows the overlaid transition curves for adults, adults without decompressive craniectomy and children; insults of LAx above 0 could be tolerated for 13, 19 and 35 min. The plots for insults where CPP < 50 mmHg or for ICP > 25 mmHg were uniformly associated with worse outcomes (coloured red) for all studied cohorts (data not shown).

Discussion

In this study, the univariate relationship between 6-month neurological outcome and CAR insults is summarized in colour-coded plots. These plots do not represent the cumulative time/pressure dose per patient, but per type of insult, characterized by duration and intensity. The main finding is the emergence of regions of positive and negative association between CAR insults and outcome that were separated by transition curves, which had an exponential course similar to that seen in [11] for ICP. The higher the LAx, the shorter the time this insult type could be tolerated. Although the association appears stronger for the case of adults without decompressive craniectomy, remarkably the transition curves for the three studied cohorts lie very close together, hinting at the universal applicability of the CAR

Table 1 Demographic and outcome data

	Adult cohort	Adult cohort without DC	Paediatric cohort
Number of patients (n)	259	214	99
LOS days, median (IQR)	15 (7–24·25)	14 (7–23)	4 (2–6·75)
Age, median (IQR)	42 (26–58)	42 (26–58)	11·4 (7.9–14.88)
Gender (%male)	79.9	80.4	74.7
Pupil reactivity			
None (%)	12.7	11.2	7.1
One (%)	11.2	11.2	11.1
Two (%)	70.7	71.5	74.7
Unknown, untestable or missing (%)	5.4	6.1	7.1
GCS total, median (IQR)	7 (4–10)	7 (4–10)	7 (5–8)
Unknown, untestable or missing (%)	6 × 6	6 × 1	1 × 0
GCS motor, median (IQR)	4 (1–5)	4 (1 × 5–5)	4 (2–5)
Unknown, untestable or missing (%)	4 × 3	2 × 8	0 × 0
Decompressive craniectomy (%)	17 × 4	0 × 0	Unknown
GOS at 6 months, median (IQR)	4 (3–5)	4 (3–5)	4 (4–5)
GOS 1 = death (n; %)	46; 17 × 8	36; 16 × 8	12; 12 × 1
GOS 2 = vegetative (n; %)	10; 3 × 9	7; 3 × 3	0; 0 × 0
GOS 3 = severe disability (n; %)	70; 27	58; 27 × 1	7; 7 × 1
GOS 4 = moderate disability (n; %)	49; 18 × 9	44; 20 × 6	39; 39 × 4
GOS 5 = low disability (n; %)	84; 32 × 4	69; 32 × 2	41; 41 × 4

IQR = 25–75th percentile

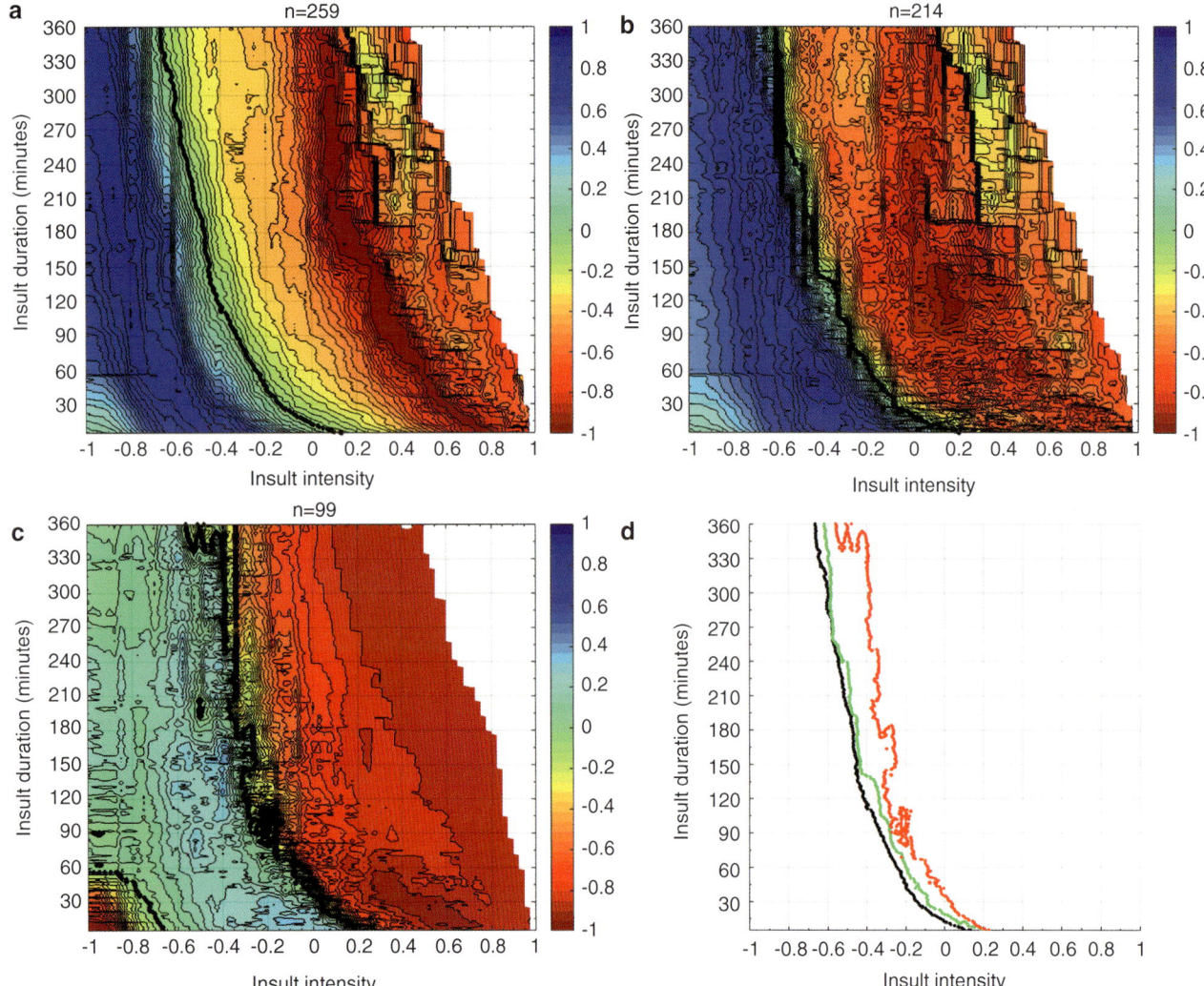

Fig. 1 Visualization of correlation between GOS and average number of CAR insults per GOS category: (**a**) adults ($n = 259$) (**b**) adults without decompressive craniectomy ($n = 214$) (**c**) children ($n = 99$). Each *colour-coded point* in the plot refers to a number of CAR insults, defined by a LAx intensity threshold (*X*-axis) and a duration threshold (*Y*-axis). The univariate correlation of each CAR insult (characterized by LAx intensity and duration thresholds) with outcome is colour-coded according to the scale ranging from −1 to 1. *Negative numbers* indicate CAR insults associated with worse outcomes (lower GOS categories); positive numbers indicate CAR insults associated with better outcomes (higher GOS categories). The contour of zero correlation is highlighted in *black* and is called the transition curve. (**d**) Overlaid transition curves for adults, adults without decompressive craniectomy and children respectively from left to right

insult concept, regardless of age. Insults when CPP <50 or ICP > 25 mmHg were associated with poor outcome regardless of CAR status, which mirrors the findings of Güiza et al. [11].

This study supports previous work reporting on the dynamic aspect of autoregulation impairment in TBI [4, 6]. Furthermore, together with a previous analysis on ICP insults [11], the current study further advocates the need to bring patients to a state of functional autoregulation in adult and paediatric TBI management.

This study has the following limitations. First, the sample size remains relatively small, noticeably so for the paediatric cohort, where the lack of data likely precluded the generation of a smoother transition curve. Second, because the data were available in minute-by-minute resolution, only LAx could be studied to define CAR insults. Third, the data incorporate therapeutic influences, which cannot be removed. Fourth, artefacts in the monitoring data were manually removed by two clinical experts, and we cannot exclude that some artefacts went unnoticed. Lastly, we cannot exclude an influence on results from confounders that were not analysed.

Conclusions

Following TBI, CAR is disturbed in a dynamic manner, such that duration and intensity play a role in the determination of a safe CAR zone. Insults of impaired CAR can only be sustained provided that they are of short duration. Hence, episodes of disturbed CAR should be considered as brain-endangering secondary insults in their own right, regardless of ICP and CPP. The current findings need to be validated with other CAR indexes, and the relative weight of ICP and CAR insults needs to be further explored.

Acknowledgments M.F. receives funding from the Research Foundation Flanders (FWO) as a Ph.D. fellow (11Y1116N). G.M. receives funding from FWO as senior clinical investigator (1846113N). G.V.dB., through the KULeuven, receives long-term research financing via the Flemish government Methusalem programme. Brain-IT was funded by the European Framework Program (FP5-QRLI-2000-00454, QLGT-2002-00160 and FP7-IST-2007-217049). The NEMO project in the University Hospital Antwerp was funded by the Flemish Government Agency for Innovation by Science and Technology (IWT). The authors wish to acknowledge the non-author steering group members of Brain-IT: Barbara Gregson, Tim Howells, Karl Kiening, Arminas Ragauskas, Juan Sahuquillo and Jan Oliver Neumann.

Conflicts of interest statement We declare that we have no conflict of interest.

References

1. Hydera AA, Wunderlich CA, Puvanachandra P, Gururaj G, Kobusingye OC. The impact of traumatic brain injuries: a global perspective. NeuroRehabilitation. 2007;22:341–53.
2. Peeters W, van den Brande R, Polinder S, Brazinova A, Steyerberg EW, Lingsma HF, Maas AI. Epidemiology of traumatic brain injury in Europe. Acta Neurochir. 2015;157:1683–96.
3. Bouma GJ, Muizelaar JP, Bandoh K, Marmarou A. Blood pressure and intracranial pressure-volume dynamics in severe head injury: relationship with cerebral blood flow. J Neurosurg. 1992;77:15–9.
4. Sviri GE, Aaslid R, Douville CM, Moore A, Newell DE. Time course for autoregulation recovery following severe traumatic brain injury. J Neurosurg. 2009;111:695–700.
5. Figaji AA, Zwane E, Fieggen AG, Argent AC, Le Roux PD, Siesjo P, Peter JC. Pressure autoregulation, intracranial pressure, and brain tissue oxygenation in children with severe traumatic brain injury. J Neurosurg Pediatr. 2009;4(5):420–8.
6. Czosnyka M, Smielewski P, Kirkpatrick P, Laing RJ, Menon D, Pickard JD. Continuous assessment of the cerebral vasomotor reactivity in head injury. Neurosurgery. 1997;41:11–7.
7. Depreitere B, Güiza F, Van den Berghe G, Schuhmann MU, Maier G, Piper I, Meyfroidt G. Pressure autoregulation monitoring and cerebral perfusion pressure target recommendation in patients with severe traumatic brain injury based on minute-by-minute monitoring data. J Neurosurg. 2014;120:1451–7.
8. Aries MJ, Czosnyka M, Budohoski KP, Steiner LA, Lavinio A, Kolias AG, Hutchinson PJ, Brady KM, Menon DK, Pickard JD, Smielewski P. Continuous determination of optimal cerebral perfusion pressure in traumatic brain injury. Crit Care Med. 2012;40:2456–63.
9. Güiza F, Meyfroidt G, Lo TY, Jones PA, Van den Berghe G, Depreitere B. Continuous optimal CPP based on minute-by-minute monitoring data: a study of a pediatric population. Acta Neurochir Suppl. 2016;122:187–91.
10. Sorrentino E, Diedler J, Kasprowicz M, Budohoski KP, Haubrich C, Smielewski P, Outtrim JG, Manktelow A, Hutchinson PJ, Pickard JD, Menon DK, Czosnyka M. Critical thresholds for cerebrovascular reactivity after traumatic brain injury. Neurocrit Care. 2012;16(2):258–66.
11. Güiza F, Depreitere B, Piper I, Citerio G, Chambers I, Jones PA, Lo TY, Enblad P, Nillson P, Feyen B, Jorens P, Maas A, Schuhmann MU, Donald R, Moss L, Van den Berghe G, Meyfroidt G. Visualizing the pressure and time burden of intracranial hypertension in adult and paediatric traumatic brain injury. Intensive Care Med. 2015;41:1067–76.
12. Piper I, Citerio G, Chambers I, Contant C, Enblad P, Fiddes H, Howells T, Kiening K, Nilsson P, Yau YH. The Brain-IT group: concept and core dataset definition. Acta Neurochir (Wien). 2003;145:615–28.
13. Feyen BFE, Sener S, Jorens PG, Menovsky T, Maas AI. Neuromonitoring in traumatic brain injury. Minerva Anestesiol. 2012;78:949–58.
14. Chambers IR, Jones PA, Lo TY, Forsyth RJ, Fulton B, Andrews PJ, Mendelow AD, Minns RA. Critical thresholds of intracranial pressure and cerebral perfusion pressure related to age in paediatric head injury. J Neurol Neurosurg Psychiatry. 2006;77(2):234–40.

Assessing Cerebral Hemodynamic Stability After Brain Injury

Bianca Pineda, Colin Kosinski, Nam Kim, Shabbar Danish, and William Craelius

Abstract *Objective*: Following brain injury, unstable cerebral hemodynamics can be characterized by abnormal rises in intracranial pressure (ICP). This behavior has been quantified by the RAP index: the correlation (R) between ICP pulse amplitude (A) and mean (P). While RAP could be a valuable indicator of autoregulatory processes, its prognostic ability is not well established and its validity has been questioned due to potential errors in measurement. Here, we test (1) whether RAP is a consistent measure of intracranial hemodynamics and (2) whether RAP has prognostic value in predicting hemodynamic instability following brain injury.

Materials and Methods: RAP was tested in seven brain injured patients treated in a surgical intensive care unit. A sample of ICP data was randomly chosen and segmented into 1 hour periods. Hours were then categorized as either stable, which contained no sharp rises in ICP, or unstable, which contained ≥ 1 sharp rise—where a sharp rise is defined as ICP exceeding a mean slope of 0.15 mmHg/s. Equal numbers of stable and unstable segments were then selected for each patient. RAP was calculated as the Pearson's correlation coefficient between ICP pulse amplitude (AMP) and mean (mICP), determined in 6 second windows, according to established methods.

Results: Results showed that (1) average AMP and ICP levels were similar between stable and unstable periods and (2) unstable periods were identified by RAP values exceeding 0.6 with an average positive predictive value of 74%.

Conclusions: We conclude that RAP can provide a valid measure of ICP dynamics, is not affected by sensor drift, and can better distinguish periods of instability than ICP or AMP alone.

Keywords Intracranial pressure (ICP) · Compensatory reserve · Pressure-volume relationship · Cerebral hemodynamics · Autoregulation · Brain injury · Pulsatility

Introduction

Ensuring adequate cerebral blood flow following brain injury involves a delicate balance between cerebral perfusion pressure (CPP) and safely low intracranial pressure (ICP) to prevent secondary brain injury. ICP is considered the more critical parameter because its elevation can quickly trigger a cycle of brain swelling, reduced cerebral blood flow, and ischemic tissue damage which can affect outcome after brain injury [1, 2]. Swelling-induced damage may be understood in terms of the Monro-Kellie doctrine [3, 4] which formalizes the concept that cranial volume consists of three compartments—brain tissue (parenchyma), cerebrospinal fluid (CSF), and intracranial blood—where

$$V_{Cranium} = V_{Parenchyma} + V_{CSF} + V_{Blood}.$$

Following brain injury, influxes from CSF or blood volume can sharply increase ICP [5–7]. The relationship between ICP and volume (PV) has been variously modeled as exponential [8, 9], sigmoidal [5, 10, 11], or a combination of linear and exponential [12, 13], where the PV curve is separated into two zones by a breakpoint. While these models differ somewhat dynamically, they all predict the same two interrelated phenomena: (1) PV slope (i.e., intracranial elastance) steepens with increasing volume and (2) ICP pulse amplitude increases with rising mean pressure [5, 14–17]. Therefore, unstable periods are defined here as segments with steep rises in ICP (ICP slope > 0.15 mmHg/s).

The index of compensatory reserve (RAP) was formulated according to PV relationships and is defined as the correlation (R) between ICP pulse amplitude (A) and mean (P) [14]. Observations on patients have indicated that low RAP values are associated with intact compensatory reserve and subcritical ICP while high RAP may be associated with poor patient outcomes [5, 10, 11, 14, 18]. However, the reliability of RAP as a clinical prognosticator has been questioned because its accuracy can be degraded by spurious baseline drifts of ICP [19, 20].

Materials and Methods

Continuous recordings of ICP were collected from patients with primary diagnosis of brain injury admitted to the surgical intensive care unit of Robert Wood Johnson University Hospital. Subjects for this study were retrospectively selected based on the following criteria: age >18 years old, diagnosis of traumatic brain injury (TBI), cerebrovascular accident (CVA), or subarachnoid hemorrhage (SAH), >18 hours of ICP recordings, and outcome to rehab. The study was approved by the Rutgers IRB, and all data were de-identified to eliminate risks of unauthorized disclosure of personal identifiers in accordance with Health Insurance Portability and Accountability Act guidelines. Informed, written consent was obtained from family members to obtain demographic information.

ICP was monitored with intraparenchymal microtransducers (Camino Direct Pressure Monitor-2, Camino Laboratories, San Diego, CA) and sampled at 50 Hz as previously described [21]. Following removal of artifacts, an event finder was used to separate data into two categories of 1 hour periods: stable, which contained no sharp rises in ICP, or unstable, which contained ≥1 such events. The event finder marked times when the slope of the filtered ICP record exceeded a 0.15 mmHg/s threshold. RAP, consisting of the Pearson's correlation coefficient between ICP pulse amplitude (AMP) and mean (mICP), was computed for every 40 values (240 s) of AMP and mICP using a first-in, first-out method.

Cumulative distributions of AMP, mICP, and RAP were used to compare stable and unstable periods for all patients. Additionally, the Mann–Whitney U (a.k.a. Wilcoxon rank sum) and the paired t-test were applied to find differences between stable and unstable RAP data. These tests were repeated on downsampled data to remove bias due to oversampling. Furthermore, the positive and negative predictive values (PPV and NPV), sensitivity, and specificity were calculated for an arbitrary RAP threshold of 0.6.

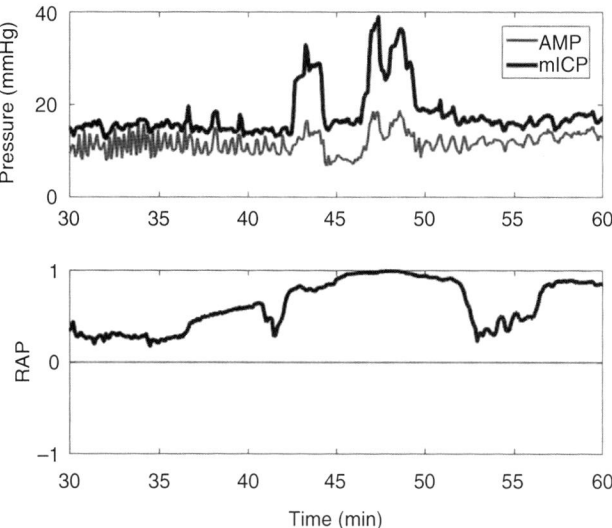

Fig. 1 AMP, mICP, and RAP during a 1 hour timespan. Note the close temporal correspondence between mICP and AMP as well as the rise in RAP coinciding with the sharp rises in ICP

Results

AMP-mICP Correlation

Strong correlations between mICP and AMP were noted during both stable and unstable periods for all patients—with a close temporal correspondence between mICP and AMP (Fig. 1). The average Pearson correlation between AMP and mICP for all seven patients was 0.62, while the average linear slope was 0.13.

Stable vs. Unstable Data Distributions

While distributions of stable vs. unstable AMP and ICP (Fig. 2) are similar, RAP distributions differed substantially between the two periods ($p < 0.001$, t-test, Mann–Whitney U) even though ICP exceeded 20 mmHg in 41.3% and 45.2% of measurements for stable vs. unstable periods respectively. An arbitrary RAP threshold shows that RAP >0.6 identifies unstable periods with an average PPV of 74.0%, NPV of 12.0%, sensitivity of 11.9%, and specificity of 74.1% for all patients. Downsampling the data by a factor of 100 did not substantially diminish the significant difference between stable and unstable RAP periods ($p < 0.001$).

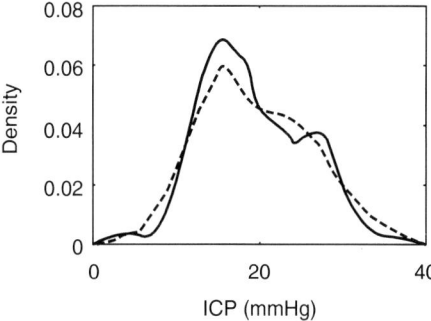 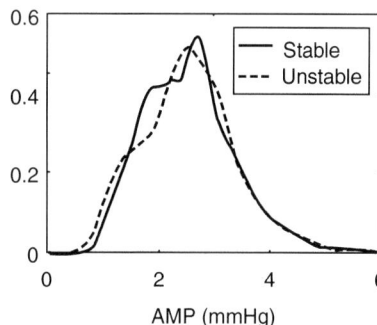 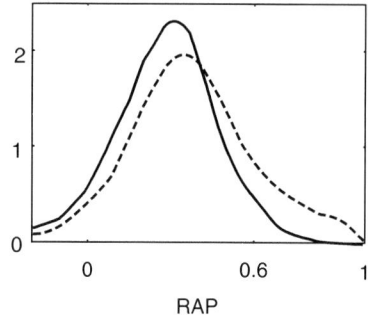

Fig. 2 Distributions of AMP, ICP, and RAP. Nonparametric distribution fits comparing stable vs. unstable periods for AMP, ICP, and RAP distributions (all patients), where RAP $p < 0.001$ (*t*-test, Mann–Whitney *U*)

Longitudinal AMP-mICP

Scatter plots of AMP vs. mICP from an exemplar patient (Fig. 3) show the change in the spread of data over 315 hours of continuous recording. Note that the early hours are characterized by wider scatter compared to later hours and a similar trend was observed in the other six patient data. A longitudinal plot of hour-by-hour mICP-AMP slope for the same patient (Fig. 3) shows that while values were highly variable in the first 200 hours, slope variability lessened over time.

Discussion

Since our study was not designed to characterize a patient group, find differences in patients' clinical status, or assess treatment, we evaluated RAP as a predictor of hemodynamic instability in a small patient sample. In the seven patients studied, our results showed RAP to have a PPV for hemodynamic instability of 74%. Since RAP calculation is highly dependent upon the recording accuracies of both AMP and mICP, it is important to determine the reliability of this prediction. In particular, previous studies found inaccuracies in ICP measurements by sensors similar to the one used herein (Camino) due to drift [19, 20]. However, drift can be ruled out as a source of error in our results since (1) the significant differences in RAP distribution between stable and unstable periods could not have been caused by drift unless it differed systematically between those hours and (2) AMP and mICP corresponded closely temporally (Fig. 1), a phenomenon that cannot be explained by drift [22, 23].

Studies have shown that AMP and mICP become decoupled/uncorrelated during the nonlinear portions of a PV curve (either at safely low or critically high ICP) while showing correlation during linear portions [5]. We observed a similar phenomenon wherein AMP-mICP becomes progressively linear with increasing values of ICP. This supports RAP as a measure of the linearity of AMP vs. mICP (Pearson's correlation coefficient) and indicator of the state of pressure-volume compensation [23, 24].

Our observed mean slope of AMP vs. mICP = 0.13 for all patients is lower than that found in most studies, but it still falls within the range of expected values for patients with good outcome [12, 13, 25, 26]. It is possible that better predictive accuracies could be established by testing a range of thresholds for defining instability and by stratifying unstable periods according to the number and magnitude of pressure rises occurring over the course of an hour.

Conclusions

By providing some predictive value on future behavior of ICP, RAP contains more information than monitoring ICP levels alone. This could be clinically useful because hemodynamic instability and the total duration of ICP elevation during acute treatment are strongly associated with poor outcomes after TBI [27, 28]. Additionally, as more direct monitoring of the Monro-Kellie doctrine becomes possible, RAP could become useful in guiding acute interventions such as a closed-loop ventricular drainage protocol [3].

Acknowledgements We thank Sandia Royal, R.N., Mary Ann Brookes, R.N., and Susette Coyle, R.N., for help with patient selection/records and Martin Barboza for technical help.

Conflicts of interest statement The authors declare that they have no financial or academic conflicts of interest.

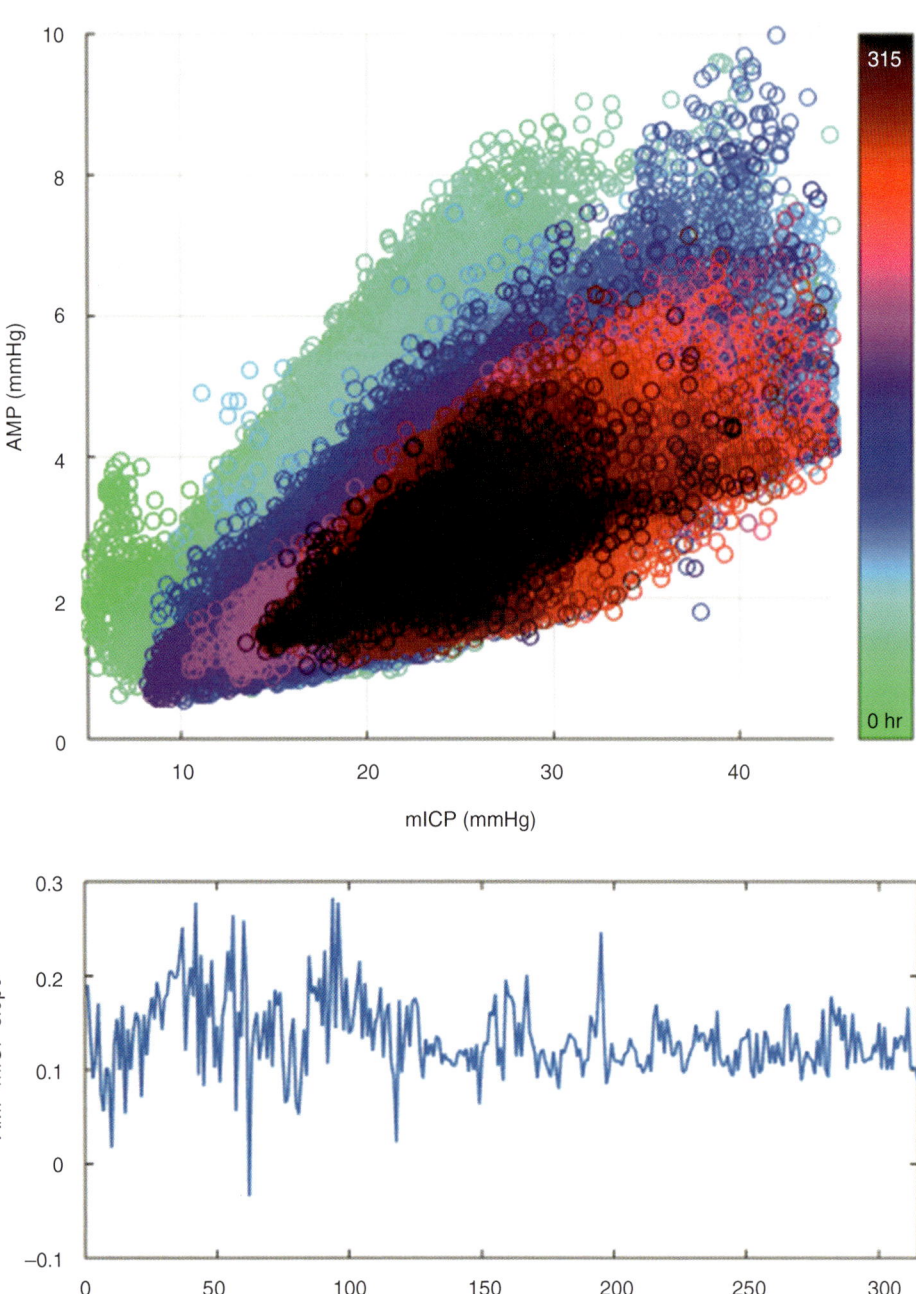

Fig. 3 Longitudinal AMP-mICP. The *top panel* shows a scatter plot of AMP vs. mICP over a time period of 315 hours for an exemplar patient where the *darkest portion* denotes the end of the recording. The *bottom panel* is a plot of the average AMP-mICP slope for every hour. The later time points indicate a narrowing of the ICP range, a decrease in average slope, and possible stabilization

References

1. Kawoos U, McCarron RM, Auker CR, Chavko M. Advances in intracranial pressure monitoring and its significance in managing traumatic brain injury. Int J Mol Sci. 2015;16(12):28979–97. doi:10.3390/ijms161226146
2. Chesnut R, Videtta W, Vespa P, Le Roux P, Int Multidisciplinary C. Intracranial pressure monitoring: fundamental considerations and rationale for monitoring. Neurocrit Care. 2014;21:64–84. doi:10.1007/s12028-014-0048-y
3. Kim D-J, Czosnyka Z, Kasprowicz M, Smieleweski P, Balédent O, Guerguerian A-M, et al. Continuous monitoring of the Monro-Kellie doctrine: is it possible? J Neurotrauma. 2012;29(7):1354–63. doi:10.1089/neu.2011.2018
4. Kim MO, Adji A, O'Rourke MF, Avolio AP, Smielewski P, Pickard JD, et al. Principles of cerebral hemodynamics when intracranial pressure is raised: lessons from the peripheral circulation. J Hypertens. 2015;33(6):1233–41. doi:10.1097/hjh.0000000000000539
5. Balestreri M, Czosnyka M, Steiner LA, Schmidt E, Smielewski P, Matta B, et al. Intracranial hypertension: what additional informa-

tion can be derived from ICP waveform after head injury? Acta Neurochir. 2004;146(2):131–41. doi:10.1007/s00701-003-0187-y
6. Barie PS, Ghajar JBG, Firlik AD, Chang VA, Hariri RJ, Ross SE, et al. Contribution of increased cerebral blood-volume to posttraumatic intracranial hypertension. J Trauma Injury Infect Crit Care. 1993;35(1):88–96. doi:10.1097/00005373-199307000-00015
7. Kim D-J, Kasprowicz M, Carrera E, Castellani G, Zweifel C, Lavinio A, et al. The monitoring of relative changes in compartmental compliances of brain. Physiol Meas. 2009;30(7):647–59. doi: 10.1088/0967-3334/30/7/009
8. Shulman K, Marmarou A. Pressure volume considerations in infantile hydrocephalus. Dev Med Child Neurol. 1971;25:90–5.
9. Shapiro K, Marmarou A, Shulman K. Characterization of clinical CSF dynamics and neural axis compliance using the pressure-volume index: I. The normal pressure-volume index. Ann Neurol. 1980;7(6):508–14.
10. Timofeev I, Czosnyka M, Nortje J, Smielewski P, Kirkpatrick P, Gupta A, et al. Effect of decompressive craniectomy on intracranial pressure and cerebrospinal compensation following traumatic brain injury. J Neurosurg. 2008;108(1):66–73. doi:10.3171/jns/2008/108/01/0066
11. Kim DJ, Czosnyka Z, Keong N, Radolovich DK, Smielewski P, Sutcliffe MP, et al. Index of cerebrospinal compensatory reserve in hydrocephalus. Neurosurgery. 2009;64(3):494–501.
12. Avezaat CJ, van Eijndhoven JH, Wyper DJ. Cerebrospinal fluid pulse pressure and intracranial volume-pressure relationships. J Neurol Neurosurg Psychiatry. 1979;42(8):687–700.
13. Szewczykowski J, Sliwka S, Kunicki A, Dytko P, Korsak-Sliwka J. A fast method of estimating the elastance of the intra cranial system a practical application in neuro surgery. J Neurosurg. 1977;47(1):19–26. doi:10.3171/jns.1977.47.1.0019
14. Czosnyka M, Guazzo E, Whitehouse M, Smielewski P, Czosnyka Z, Kirkpatrick P, et al. Significance of intracranial pressure waveform analysis after head injury. Acta Neurochir. 1996;138(5):531–41. doi:10.1007/bf01411173
15. Czosnyka M, Pickard JD. Monitoring and interpretation of intracranial pressure. Neurosci Neurol. 2006;2006:285–313. doi:10.1142/9781860948961_0011
16. Qvarlander S, Malm J, Eklund A. The pulsatility curve-the relationship between mean intracranial pressure and pulsation amplitude. Physiol Meas. 2010;31(11):1517–28. doi:10.1088/0967-3334/31/11/008
17. Kosteljanetz M. Intracranial pressure: cerebrospinal fluid dynamics and pressure-volume relations. Acta Neurol Scand Suppl. 1987;111:1–23.
18. Petrella G, Czosnyka M, Keong N, Pickard JD, Czosnyka Z. How does CSF dynamics change after shunting? Acta Neurol Scand. 2008;118(3):182–8.
19. Eide PK, Sorteberg A, Meling TR, Sorteberg W. The effect of baseline pressure errors on an intracranial pressure-derived index: results of a prospective observational study. Biomed Eng Online. 2014;13:99. doi:10.1186/1475-925x-13-99
20. Eide PK, Sorteberg W. An intracranial pressure-derived index monitored simultaneously from two separate sensors in patients with cerebral bleeds: comparison of findings. Biomed Eng Online. 2013;12:14. doi:10.1186/1475-925x-12-14
21. Kim N, Krasner A, Kosinski C, Wininger M, Qadri M, Kappus Z, et al. Trending autoregulatory indices during treatment for traumatic brain injury. J Clin Monit Comput. 2015;30:821–31. doi:10.1007/s10877-015-9779-3
22. Eide PK, Holm S, Sorteberg W. Simultaneous monitoring of static and dynamic intracranial pressure parameters from two separate sensors in patients with cerebral bleeds: comparison of findings. Biomed Eng Online. 2012;11:66. doi:10.1186/1475-925x-11-66
23. Eide PK, Rapoport BI, Gormley WB, Madsen JR. A dynamic nonlinear relationship between the static and pulsatile components of intracranial pressure in patients with subarachnoid hemorrhage. J Neurosurg. 2010;112(3):616–25. doi:10.3171/2009.7.jns081593
24. Czosnyka M, Smielewski P, Piechnik S, Schmidt EA, Al-Rawi PG, Kirkpatrick PJ, et al. Hemodynamic characterization of intracranial pressure plateau waves in head-injury patients. J Neurosurg. 1999;91(1):11–9.
25. Czosnyka M, Wollk-Laniewski P, Batorski L, Zaworski W. Analysis of intracranial pressure waveform during infusion test. Acta Neurochir. 1988;93(3–4):140–5.
26. Avezaat CJJ, Vaneijndhoven JHM. The role of the pulsatile pressure variations in intracranial-pressure monitoring. Neurosurg Rev. 1986;9(1–2):113–20. doi:10.1007/bf01743061
27. Majdan M, Mauritz W, Wilbacher I, Brazinova A, Rusnak M, Leitgeb J. Timing and duration of intracranial hypertension versus outcomes after severe traumatic brain injury. Minerva Anestesiol. 2014;80(12):1261–72.
28. Marmarou A, Anderson RL, Ward JD, Choi SC, Young HF, Eisenberg HM, et al. Impact of icp instability and hypotension on outcome in patients with severe head trauma. J Neurosurg. 1991;75:S59–66.

Systolic and Diastolic Regulation of the Cerebral Pressure-Flow Relationship Differentially Affected by Acute Sport-Related Concussion

Alexander D. Wright, Jonathan D. Smirl, Kelsey Bryk, and Paul van Donkelaar

Abstract *Objective*: To determine whether acute sports-related concussion (SRC) exerts differential effects on cerebral autoregulatory properties during systole versus diastole.

Materials and methods: One hundred and thirty-six contact-sport athletes tested preseason; 14 sustained a concussion and completed follow-up testing at 72 hours, 2 weeks, and 1 month post-injury. Five minutes of repetitive squat-stand maneuvers induced blood pressure (BP) oscillations at both 0.05 and 0.10 Hz. Beat-by-beat peak-systolic and end-diastolic BP (sysBP/ diasBP) and middle cerebral artery blood velocity (sysMCAv/diasMCAv) were recorded using finger photoplethysmography and transcranial Doppler ultrasound, respectively. Relationships between sysBP-sysMCAv and diasBP-diasMCAv were quantified using transfer function analysis to estimate *coherence* (correlation), *gain* (response magnitude), and *phase* (response latency).

Results: Significant main effects of the cardiac cycle were observed across all outcome metrics. A significant main effect of SRC was observed for 0.10 Hz phase: systolic and diastolic *phases* were reduced at 72 h (21.8 ± 5.2%) and 2 weeks (22.7 ± 7.1%) compared to preseason but recovered by 1 month. Concussion significantly impaired diastolic, but not systolic, *gain*: 0.10 Hz diastolic *gain* was increased (27.2 ± 7.7%) at 2 weeks, recovering by 1 month.

Conclusions: Impairments in autoregulatory capacity, observed for a transient period following SRC that persist beyond symptom resolution and clinical recovery, appear to be differentially affected across the cardiac cycle. Similar patterns of impairment were observed for systolic and diastolic *phases* (response latency); however, normalized *gain* (response magnitude) impairments were identified only in diastole. These findings may explain the increased cerebral vulnerability as well as exercise-induced symptom exacerbation observed post-SRC.

Keywords Sports-related concussion · Mild TBI · Cerebral blood flow · Cerebral autoregulation · Blood pressure · Autonomic dysfunction · Transfer function analysis

Introduction

Sports-related concussion (SRC)—a mild form of traumatic brain injury (TBI)—is a major public health concern, with recent reports estimating incidences of 1.1–1.9 million injuries each year in US youth alone [1]. Whereas the majority of patients recover clinically within 2 weeks [2], recent data suggest physiological recovery may take longer; for example, recovery of cerebral blood flow (CBF) [3], myelin content [4], and cerebral metabolism [5] may take 1 month or more. Concussed brains are characterized by a temporal window of vulnerability to additional trauma following injury [5]. While it has been suggested that this may result from impairments in cerebral autoregulation (CA) [6], this hypothesis has not been confirmed experimentally.

Myogenic, autonomic, and metabolic mechanisms are known to be involved in CA, which must function to protect the brain from high systolic pressures during surges in blood pressure (BP) and from hypoperfusion during BP reductions [6, 7]. CA function is impaired following moderate and severe TBI [8] and is a significant predictor of poor outcome following severe TBI [9]. The extent to which the dynamic

A.D. Wright (✉)
MD/PhD Program, University of British Columbia,
Vancouver, BC, Canada

Southern Medical Program, Reichwald Health Sciences Centre,
University of British Columbia Okanagan, Kelowna, BC, Canada

Experimental Medicine Program, Faculty of Medicine, University of British Columbia, Vancouver, BC, Canada

School of Health and Exercise Sciences, University of British Columbia Okanagan, Kelowna, BC, Canada
e-mail: adwright@alumni.ubc.ca

J.D. Smirl • K. Bryk • P. van Donkelaar
School of Health and Exercise Sciences, University of British Columbia Okanagan, Kelowna, BC, Canada

BP-CBF relationship is affected by SRC is unknown [6]. Previous reports suggested peak-systolic and end-diastolic components of CBF may contain valuable information on CA function [10].

The aim of this study was to prospectively evaluate whether the acute effects of SRC on indices of dynamic CA differ for systolic and diastolic components of the cardiac cycle.

Materials and Methods

Participants

Preseason testing of 136 male contact-sport athletes was completed; 14 were subsequently diagnosed with a concussion [2] and underwent additional testing at 72 hours, 2 weeks, and 1 month post-injury. All subjects underwent familiarization of testing procedures and abstained from exercise, caffeine, and alcohol for at least 12 hours prior to all testing sessions. Written informed consent, approved by the University of British Columbia Clinical Research Ethics Board, was obtained prior to participation.

Instrumentation and Data Analysis

A three-lead electrocardiogram (ECG) was used to collect R-R intervals. Cerebral blood velocity in the middle cerebral artery (MCAv) was indexed using transcranial Doppler ultrasound (ST3, Spencer Technologies, Seattle, WA, USA). Beat-to-beat BP was recorded using finger photoplethysmography (Finometer PRO, Finapres Medical Systems, Amsterdam, The Netherlands), and partial pressure of expired carbon dioxide ($P_{ET}CO_2$) was monitored using an online gas analyzer (ML206, AD Instruments, Colorado Springs, CO, USA). All data were sampled at 1000 Hz (PowerLab 8/30 ML880, AD Instruments) and stored for offline analysis using commercially available software (LabChart version 7.1, AD Instruments).

Participants completed repetitive squat-stand maneuvers for 5 min at each of two different frequencies (0.05 and 0.10 Hz) [11]. Beat-to-beat values of systolic (sysBP) and diastolic blood pressure (diasBP), systolic (sysMCAv) and diastolic MCAv (diasMCAv), and $P_{ET}CO_2$ were determined from each R-R interval. All data were processed and analyzed with custom-designed software in LabView 14 (National Instruments, Austin, TX, USA), as outlined previously [11]. Data were analyzed in accordance with best practice guidelines for transfer function analysis [12] to determine sysBP-sysMCAv and diasBP-diasMCAv coherence, phase, and normalized gain. Metrics were sampled at the point estimate of the driven frequency (0.05 or 0.10 Hz), selected to fall within the very-low-frequency (0.02–0.07 Hz) and low-frequency (0.07–0.20 Hz) ranges of CA. Phase wraparound was not present for any point estimates.

Statistical Analyses

All statistical analyses were performed using SPSS Statistics for Macintosh (Version 22.0, IBM Corp., Armonk, NY). A 2 (cardiac cycle) by 4 (time) two-way repeated-measures (RM) ANOVA was used to evaluate the effect of acute SRC on each metric at each driven frequency. When omnibus tests indicated significant main effects, preplanned t-tests with Bonferroni correction were used to evaluate specific pairwise contrasts (i.e., each post-injury time point relative to preseason).

Results

Demographic characteristics, time to medical clearance to return to play, and resting physiological data across testing sessions and groups are outlined in Table 1. Representative traces of MAP, MCAv, and $P_{ET}CO_2$ are shown in Fig. 1. Two-way RM-ANOVA indicated significant main effects of cardiac cycle for coherence, phase, and gain (Fig. 2). At both driven frequencies, coherence (0.05 Hz: $F_{1,13} = 42.989$, $p < 0.001$, partial eta^2 = 0.768; 0.10 Hz: $F_{1,13} = 40.052$, $p < 0.001$, partial eta^2 = 0.755) and gain (0.05 Hz: $F_{1,13} = 171.86$, $p < 0.001$, partial eta^2 = 0.93; 0.10 Hz:

Table 1 Demographics, symptom profiles, and resting physiological parameters during each test session for acutely concussed athletes

Metric	Preseason	72 H	2 Week	1 Month
Age (years)	19.0 (1.4)			
BMI (kg/m^2)	24.7 (1.7)			
RTP (days)	median = 14, range 7-35 days			
No. of symptoms	3.7 (5.8)	11 (5.7)	3.5 (3.0)	1.3 (2.3)
Symptom severity	3.5 (3.4)	24.8 (20.3)	4.6 (3.4)	1.5 (2.5)
MAP (mmHg)	95.3 (14.8)	88.2 (19.2)	91.1 (18.1)	91.0 (16.6)
MCAv (cm/s)	53.8 (7.0)	52.3 (8.1)	52.7 (9.0)	53.6 (8.0)
HR (bpm)	79.4 (8.3)	80.2 (13.3)	80.0 (10.7)	79.1 (10.6)
$P_{ET}CO_2$ (mmHg)	37.7 (3.2)	36.8 (4.0)	37.6 (4.4)	37.4 (4.7)

Data are presented as mean (SD) unless otherwise noted. *BMI* body mass index, *RTP* time to medical clearance to return to play, *HR* heart rate, *PETCO2* end-tidal partial pressure of carbon dioxide; note that symptom severity scores are the sum of 22 symptoms that were ranked on a scale of 0–6 (0 = none, 6 = severe)

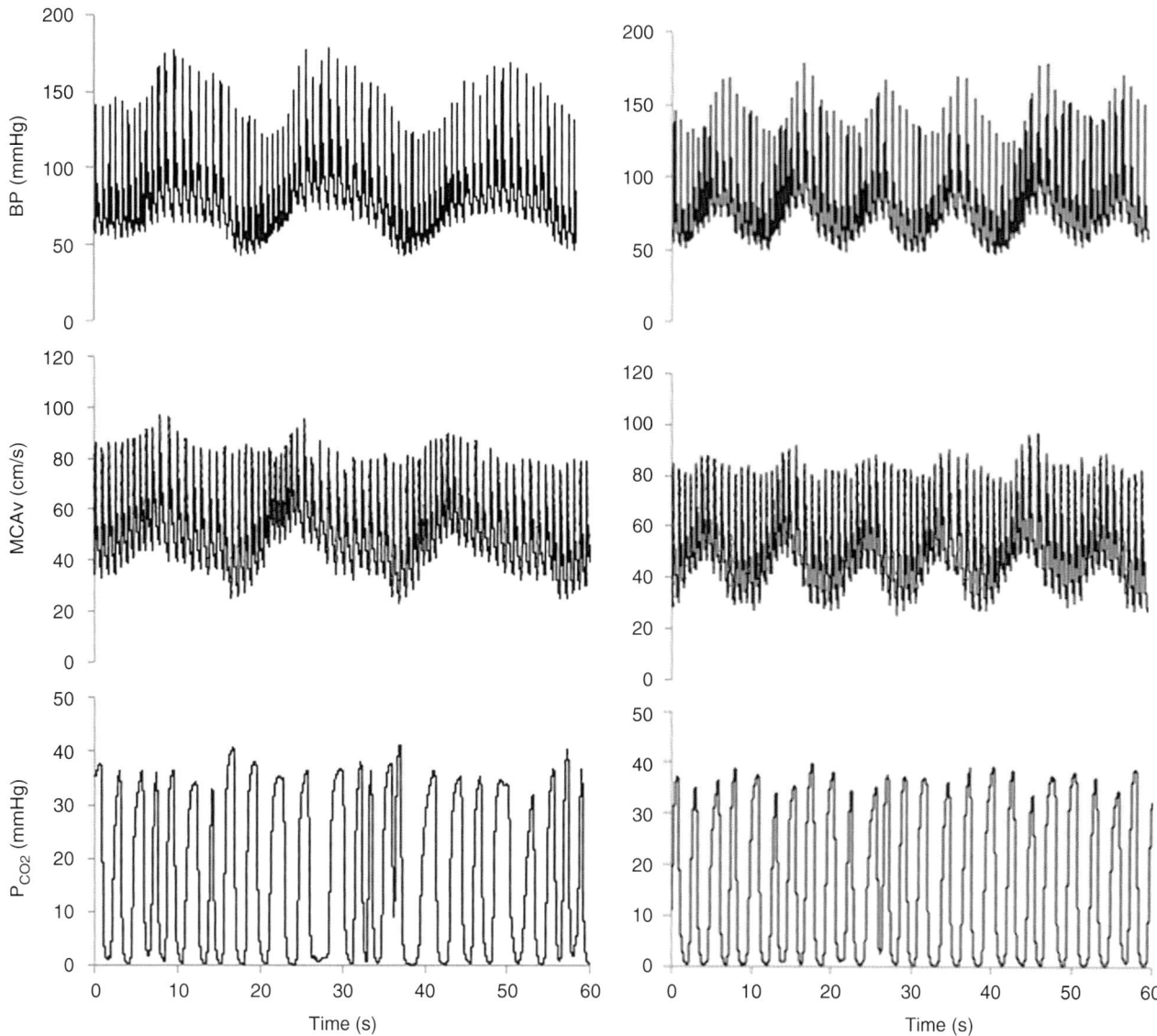

Fig. 1 Representative time series for blood pressure (BP, *top*), middle cerebral artery blood velocity (MCA*v*, *middle*), and expired carbon dioxide (P_{CO2}, *bottom*) during 60 s of squat-stand maneuvers performed at 0.05 Hz (*left*) and 0.10 Hz (*right*)

$F_{1,13} = 126.732$, $p < 0.001$, partial eta$^2 = 0.907$) were significantly higher in diastole than in systole, while phase (0.05 Hz: $F_{1,13} = 46.912$, $p < 0.001$, partial eta$^2 = 0.783$; 0.10 Hz: $F_{1,13} = 12.981$, $p = 0.003$, partial eta$^2 = 0.5$) was lower in diastole, suggesting the high-pass-filter behavior of the cerebrovasculature was preserved following injury. A main effect of time was observed for 0.10 Hz phase ($F_{3,39} = 3.971$, $p = 0.015$, partial eta$^2 = 0.234$). Relative to preseason, preplanned contrasts revealed a 21.8% decrease in 0.10 Hz phase at 72 h post-injury (95% CI: −0.08 to −0.26 rad, $t_{13} = 4.209$, adjusted $p = 0.003$) and 22.7% at 2 weeks (95% CI: −0.06 to −0.30 rad, $t_{13} = 3.186$, adjusted $p = 0.021$). Interaction terms between cardiac cycle and time were significant for gain at 0.10 Hz only ($F_{1.785,23.2} = 3.938$, $p = 0.038$, partial eta$^2 = 0.233$), with subsequent analyses of simple effects revealing a significant effect of time for diastolic gain. Relative to preseason, planned contrasts revealed a 27.2% relative increase in diastolic *gain* at 2 weeks (95% CI: +0.185 to +0.783%/% adjusted $p = 0.012$), suggesting that a greater magnitude of diasBP was passed to the cerebrovasculature following SRC.

Discussion

SRC appears to exert differential effects on systolic versus diastolic regulation of the cerebral pressure-buffering system. Transient impairments in indices of CA were more pronounced in diastole—both the latency and the magnitude of

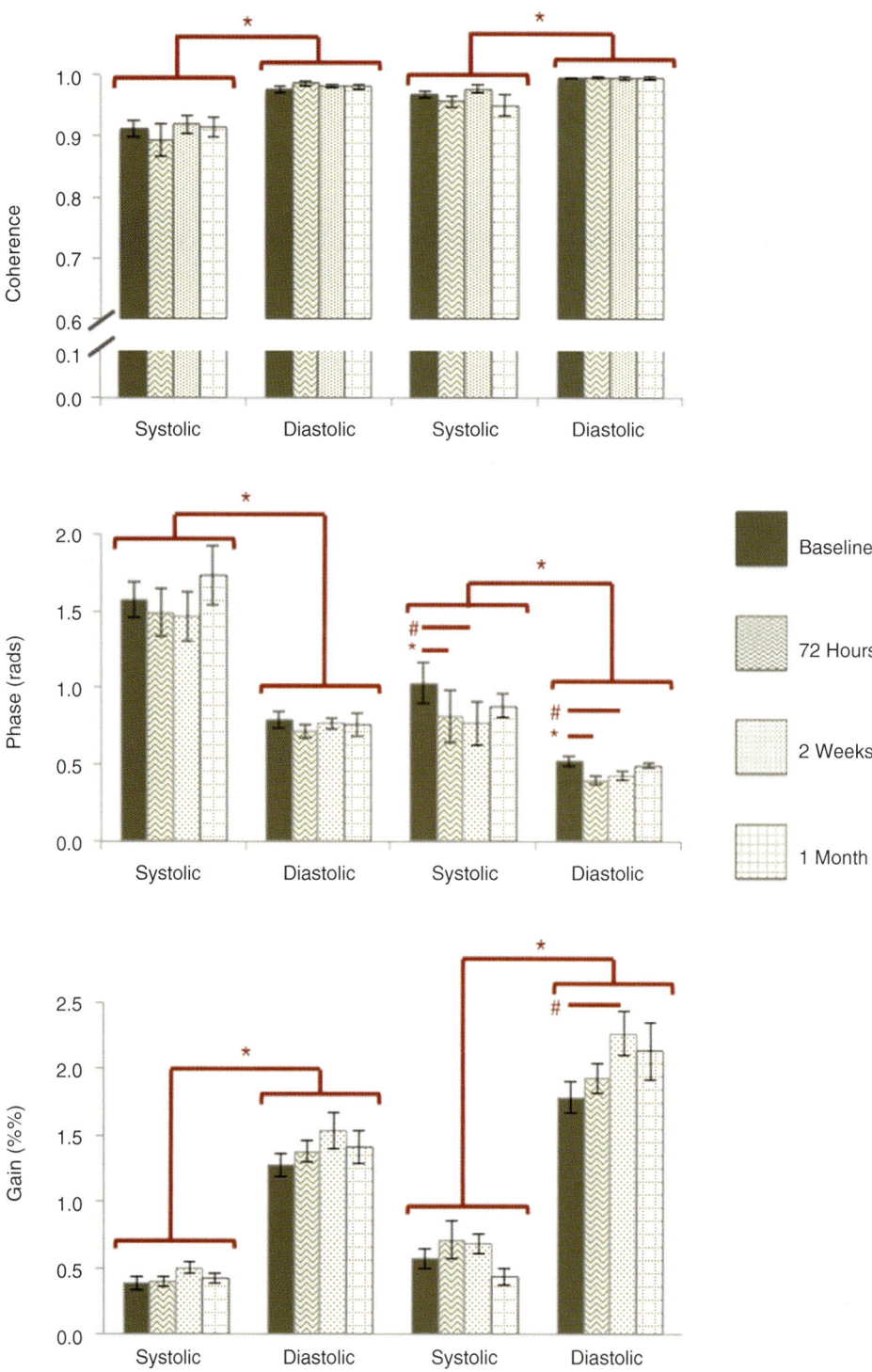

Fig. 2 Transfer function analysis outcome metrics (mean ± SE) in systole and diastole for squat-stand maneuvers performed at 0.05 Hz (*left*) and 0.10 Hz (*right*). *Asterisk* indicates $p \leq 0.003$; *hash* indicates $p \leq 0.025$

the response were impaired, whereas only response latency was impaired during systole—and persisted for at least 2 weeks (Fig. 2). Importantly, in many cases these impairments lasted beyond medical clearance time for return to full participation in contact sports but recovered 1-month post-injury. This highlights an important distinction between clinical and physiological recovery. Although the clinical relevance of this finding cannot be discerned from this data set, it may explain the increased vulnerability of the concussed brain to additional trauma during this period.

Impairments in transfer function analysis metrics at 0.10 Hz only implies an alteration in autonomic regulation of the cerebrovasculature [13], adding to an emerging story within the literature of SRC-induced autonomic dysfunction [14–16]. Increased sympathetic drive has been shown to effect a transient "stiffening" of peripheral vessels following SRC [15], which would alter responsiveness to changes in BP. Pharmacological studies have shown that partial sympathetic blockade dramatically alters the CA phase response at frequencies including 0.10 Hz [13, 17]. Phase impairments present within 3 days, with additional impairment in gain at 2 weeks, are in accordance with the suggestion that impairment of CA likely first affects the latency of the response before affecting the efficiency [18]. These results collectively demonstrate that SRC induces an autonomic dysregulation that affects cerebral hemodynamics for at least 2 weeks post-SRC, with resolution by 1 month (Fig. 2).

Our data suggest that the brain remains relatively more efficient at buffering surges in BP than reductions in BP following SRC. Interestingly, this pattern of impairment has also been observed during exercise in otherwise healthy individuals; with increased exercise intensity, gain of the diastolic CA response gradually increased in the low-frequency range (0.07–0.20 Hz), whereas systolic CA performance remained intact [7]. Furthermore, compromised regulation of diastolic MCAv has been suggested as a precipitating factor in the onset of syncope [19]. Combined with additional SRC-induced CA impairments, this may explain the exercise-induced exacerbation of symptoms—including headache and dizziness—commonly observed following SRC. That such impairments persisted beyond symptom resolution and clinical recovery raises concerns about prematurely returning athletes to competitive contact sports prior to recovery of cerebrovascular function.

To mitigate both the incidence and severity of SRC, a better understanding of the neurobiological underpinnings is needed. Although not yet ready for clinical use, assessments of CA appear to be a promising approach to better understanding the autonomic pathophysiology underlying SRC. Significant impairments were detected in the latency and magnitude of CA responses, more pronounced in diastole than in systole, for at least 2 weeks following injury, which recovered by 1 month. While validation is required in a larger number of subjects, these results imply a transient autonomic disruption following SRC that may outlast symptom resolution and clinical recovery, encouraging the development of further prospective investigations into the effects of SRC on mechanisms controlling CBF. The exploration of the relationships between age, sex, impact biomechanics, and CA function on susceptibility to injury is warranted.

Conflicts of interest statement We declare that we have no conflict of interest.

References

1. Bryan MA, Rowhani-Rahbar A, Comstock RD, Rivara F, Seattle Sports Concussion Research Collaborative. Sports- and recreation-related concussions in US youth. Pediatrics. 2016;138(1):e20154635.
2. McCrory P, Meeuwisse WH, Aubry M, Cantu B, Dvorák J, Echemendia RJ, et al. Consensus statement on concussion in sport: the 4th international conference on concussion in sport held in zurich, november 2012. Br J Sports Med. 2013, Apr;47(5):250–8.
3. Maugans TA, Farley C, Altaye M, Leach J, Cecil KM. Pediatric sports-related concussion produces cerebral blood flow alterations. Pediatrics. 2012, Jan;129(1):28–37.
4. Wright AD, Jarrett M, Vavasour I, Shahinfard E, Kolind S, van Donkelaar P, et al. Myelin water fraction is transiently reduced after a single mild traumatic brain injury – a prospective cohort study in collegiate hockey players. PLoS One. 2016;11(2):e0150215.
5. Vagnozzi R, Signoretti S, Tavazzi B, Floris R, Ludovici A, Marziali S, et al. Temporal window of metabolic brain vulnerability to concussion: a pilot 1 h-magnetic resonance spectroscopic study in concussed athletes—part III. Neurosurgery. 2008;62(6):1286–95. discussion 1295–6
6. Tan CO, Meehan WP, Iverson GL, Taylor JA. Cerebrovascular regulation, exercise, and mild traumatic brain injury. Neurology. 2014;83(18):1665–72.
7. Ogoh S, Fadel PJ, Zhang R, Selmer C, Jans Ø, Secher NH, Raven PB. Middle cerebral artery flow velocity and pulse pressure during dynamic exercise in humans. Am J Physiol Heart Circ Physiol. 2005, Apr;288(4):H1526–31.
8. DeWitt DS, Prough DS. Traumatic cerebral vascular injury: the effects of concussive brain injury on the cerebral vasculature. J Neurotrauma. 2003, Sep;20(9):795–825.
9. Kirkness CJ, Mitchell PH, Burr RL, Newell DW. Cerebral autoregulation and outcome in acute brain injury. Biol Res Nurs. 2001, Jan;2(3):175–85.
10. Budohoski KP, Reinhard M, Aries MJ, Czosnyka Z, Smielewski P, Pickard JD, et al. Monitoring cerebral autoregulation after head injury. Which component of transcranial doppler flow velocity is optimal? Neurocrit Care. 2012, Oct;17(2):211–8.
11. Smirl JD, Hoffman K, Tzeng YC, Hansen A, Ainslie PN. Methodological comparison of active and passive driven oscillations in blood pressure; implications for the assessment of cerebral-pressure flow relationships. J Appl Physiol (1985). 2015;119:487.
12. Claassen JA, Meel-van den Abeelen AS, Simpson DM, Panerai RB, International Cerebral Autoregulation Research Network (CARNet). Transfer function analysis of dynamic cerebral autoregulation: a white paper from the international cerebral autoregulation research network. J Cereb Blood Flow Metab. 2016, Apr;36(4):665–80.
13. Hamner JW, Tan CO, Lee K, Cohen MA, Taylor JA. Sympathetic control of the cerebral vasculature in humans. Stroke. 2010, Jan;41(1):102–9.
14. Blake TA, McKay CD, Meeuwisse WH, Emery CA. The impact of concussion on cardiac autonomic function: a systematic review. Brain Inj. 2016;30(2):132–45.
15. La Fountaine MF, Toda M, Testa AJ, Hill-Lombardi V. Autonomic nervous system responses to concussion: Arterial pulse contour analysis. Front Neurol. 2016;7:13.
16. Abaji JP, Curnier D, Moore RD, Ellemberg D. Persisting effects of concussion on heart rate variability during physical exertion. J Neurotrauma. 2016;33(9):811–7.

17. Hilz MJ, Wang R, Marthol H, Liu M, Tillmann A, Riss S, et al. Partial pharmacologic blockade shows sympathetic connection between blood pressure and cerebral blood flow velocity fluctuations. J Neurol Sci. 2016;365:181–7.
18. Tiecks FP, Lam AM, Aaslid R, Newell DW. Comparison of static and dynamic cerebral autoregulation measurements. Stroke. 1995, Jun;26(6):1014–9.
19. Ogoh S, Fisher JP, Purkayastha S, Dawson EA, Fadel PJ, White MJ, et al. Regulation of middle cerebral artery blood velocity during recovery from dynamic exercise in humans. J Appl Physiol (1985). 2007, Feb;102(2):713–21.

Induced Dynamic Intracranial Pressure and Cerebrovascular Reactivity Assessment of Cerebrovascular Autoregulation After Traumatic Brain Injury with High Intracranial Pressure in Rats

Denis E. Bragin, Gloria L. Statom, and Edwin M. Nemoto

Abstract *Objective*: In previous work we showed that high intracranial pressure (ICP) in the rat brain induces a transition from capillary (CAP) to pathological microvascular shunt (MVS) flow, resulting in brain hypoxia, edema, and blood-brain barrier (BBB) damage. This transition was correlated with a loss of cerebral blood flow (CBF) autoregulation undetected by static autoregulatory curves but identified by *induced* dynamic ICP (iPRx) and cerebrovascular (iCVRx) reactivity. We hypothesized that loss of CBF autoregulation as correlated with MVS flow would be identified by iPRx and iCVRx in traumatic brain injury (TBI) with elevated ICP.

Methods: TBI was induced by lateral fluid percussion (LFP) using a gas-driven device in rats. Using *in vivo* two-photon laser scanning microscopy, cortical microcirculation, tissue oxygenation (NADH autofluoresence), and BBB permeability (fluorescein dye extravasation) were measured before and for 4 h after TBI. Laser Doppler cortical flux, rectal and brain temperature, ICP and mean arterial pressure (MAP), blood gases, and electrolytes were monitored. Every 30 min, a transient 10 mmHg rise in MAP was induced by i.v. bolus of dopamine. iPRx = ΔICP/ΔMAP and iCVRx = ΔCBF/ΔMAP.

Results: We demonstrated that iPRx and iCVRx correctly identified more severe loss of CBF autoregulation correlated with a transition of blood flow to MVS after TBI with high ICP compared to TBI without an increase in ICP.

Conclusions: In TBI with high ICP, high-velocity MVS flow is responsible for the loss of CBF autoregulation identified by iPRx and iCVRx.

Keywords Traumatic brain injury · Cerebral blood flow autoregulation · Microvascular shunts · Intracranial pressure · Induced cerebrovascular reactivity · Induced intracranial pressure reactivity · Rats

Introduction

Cerebrovascular autoregulation is the ability of the brain to maintain cerebral blood flow (CBF) despite changes in cerebral perfusion pressure (CPP), a difference between mean arterial pressure (MAP) and intracranial pressure (ICP). The critical CPP is the pressure at which CBF begins to fall after maximum cerebrovascular dilation has occurred and historically has been determined at ~50 mmHg by decreasing arterial pressure to lower CPP while tracking changes in CBF [1]. However, clinically CPP often decreases owing to an increase in ICP as in traumatic brain injury (TBI).

To test that, several animal studies used increased ICP to decrease CPP instead of decreasing arterial pressure and reported a loss of autoregulation at ~30 mmHg [2–5]. The reason for an "apparently" better preserved autoregulation at a lower CPP was unclear, until we showed that in a normal rat brain, that high ICP induced a transition of capillary blood flow to high-velocity, nonnutritive microvascular shunt (MVS) flow that was associated with brain hypoxia, edema, and blood-brain barrier (BBB) damage [6, 7]. This transition was correlated with a loss of CBF autoregulation undetected by static autoregulatory curves but identified by *induced* dynamic ICP (iPRx) and cerebrovascular (iCVRx) reactivity [8]. More recently, we proved the existence of MVS flow in cerebral microcirculation following TBI with high ICP [9].

In this study we determined whether iPRx and iCVRx accuratelys identifys a loss of CBF autoregulation correlated with the transition of blood flow to MVS after TBI with high ICP.

D.E. Bragin (✉) · G.L. Statom · E.M. Nemoto
Department of Neurosurgery, University of New Mexico School of Medicine, University of New Mexico, Albuquerque, NM, USA
e-mail: dbragin@salud.unm.edu

Materials and Methods

The animal protocol was approved by the Institutional Animal Care and Use Committee of the University of New Mexico Health Sciences Center and carried out in accordance with the National Institutes of Health Guide for the Care and Use of Laboratory Animals. The procedures used in this study are described in our earlier publications [6–9].

Experimental Paradigm

Two groups of ten rats each were used in this study:

1. TBI resulting in a permanent increase in ICP of 30 mmHg.
2. TBI without an ICP increase (ICP = 10 mmHg).

We used *in vivo* two-photon laser scanning microscopy (2PLSM) through a cranial window over the pericontusion area of the parietal cortex to measure microvascular red blood cell flow velocity, visualized by serum labeled with tetramethylrhodamine dextran (TMR), and tissue oxygenation, reflected by nicotinamide adenine dinucleotide (NADH) autofluorescence, for 4 h after TBI. BBB permeability was measured by TMR extravasation. Doppler cortical flux, MAP, ICP, blood gases, electrolytes, hematocrit, pH, and rectal and cranial temperatures were monitored throughout the study. Every 30 min, a transient 10 mmHg rise in MAP was induced by an i.v. bolus of dopamine:

$$iPRx = \Delta ICP / \Delta MAP \text{ and } iCVRx = \Delta CBF / \Delta MAP.$$

Surgery

Acclimated Sprague–Dawley male rats (Harlan Laboratories, Indianapolis, IN, USA), weighing between 300 and 350 g, were intubated and mechanically ventilated on 2% isoflurane/30% oxygen/70% nitrous oxide. Rectal and temporal muscle temperature probes were inserted. Femoral venous and arterial catheters were inserted for intravenous injections, arterial pressure monitoring, and blood sampling. A catheter was inserted into the cisterna magna for ICP monitoring and manipulation. For imaging and TBI, a craniotomy 5 mm in diameter was made over the left parietal cortex, filled with 2% agarose/saline, and sealed with a cover glass.

TBI was induced by fluid percussion injury (FPI) using a gas-driven device in rats resulting in (1) no ICP increase (1.5 atmosphere of air pressure absolute (ATA), 50 ms pulse duration) and (2) persistent ICP increase for up to 6 h (1.5 ATA, 150 ms pulse duration).

Microscopy

An Olympus BX51WI upright microscope (Olympus, Tokyo, Japan) and a water-immersion LUMPlan FL/IR 20×/0.50 W objective were used. Excitation (740 nm) was provided by a Prairie View Ultima multiphoton laser scan unit (Prairie Technologies, Inc., Middleton, WI, USA) powered by a Millennia Prime 10 W diode laser source pumping a Tsunami Ti: sapphire laser (Spectra-Physics, Mountain View, CA, USA). Blood plasma was labeled by i.v. tetramethylrhodamine isothiocyanate dextran (155 kDa) in physiological saline (5% wt/vol). All microvessels in an imaging volume (500 × 500 × 300 μm) were scanned at each study point, measuring the diameter and blood flow velocity in each vessel (3–20 μm Ø). Tetramethylrhodamine fluorescence was band-pass-filtered at 560–600 nm and NADH autofluorescence at 425–475 nm. Imaging data processing and analysis were carried out using the NIH ImageJ.

Statistical Analyses

Statistical analyses were carried out using Student's *t*-test or the Kolmogorov–Smirnov test where appropriate. Differences between groups were determined using two-way analysis of variance (ANOVA) for multiple comparisons and post hoc testing using the Mann–Whitney *U* test. The statistical significance level was set at $P < 0.05$. Data are presented as mean ± standard error of the mean (SEM).

Results

As in our previous report, FPI in group I resulted in a sustained increase in ICP to 30.9 ± 4.4 mmHg from the pre-injury level of 10.1 ± 2.7 mmHg ($P < 0.01$); in group II, ICP was not changed (10.8 ± 3.6 mmHg). Arterial pressure in both groups was unaltered.

Table 1 Monitored cerebral variables (mean ± SEM)

Groups	mCBF, mm/s	MVS/CAP ratio	Perfused capillaries, %	NADH, %	BBB, ΔF/Fo	iCVRx	iPRx
Baseline	0.74 ± 0.09	0.41 ± 0.07	100	100	0	−0.02 ± 0.05	−0.02 ± 0.07
TBI—I	0.53 ± 0.94**	1.41 ± 0.32**	46.9 ± 16.5***	172.8 ± 9.6**	12.43 ± 1.02**	0.61 ± 0.03**	0.35 ± 0.02*
TBI—II	0.48 ± 0.08**	0.25 ± 0.02	72.3 ± 14.6*	154.5 ± 8.3*	9.15 ± 0.98*	0.37 ± 0.02*	0.26 ± 0.02

*$P < 0.05$; **$P < 0.01$; ***$P < 0.001$

In group I, the rise in ICP was associated with an increase in the MVS/CAP ratio from 0.41 ± 0.07 at baseline to 1.41 ± 0.32 at 4 h after TBI (Table 1, $P < 0.01$). The percentage of perfused capillaries decreased to 46.9 ± 16.5% compared to baseline ($P < 0.001$), and microvascular CBF (mCBF) fell from 0.74 ± 0.09 at baseline to 0.53 ± 0.94 (Table 1, $P < 0.05$ from baseline). Impairment of microcirculation in group I led to tissue hypoxia, reflected by NADH accumulation (172.8 ± 9.6%, $P < 0.01$), and increased BBB permeability, reflected by an increase in perivascular tissue fluorescence ($\Delta F/F_{0[\text{pre-injury}]} = 12.43 \pm 1.02$, Table 1, $P < 0.01$), both compared to a baseline.

In group II, *without* an ICP increase, microvascular CBF fell to 0.48 ± 0.08 mm/s (Table 1, $P < 0.05$), and the percentage of perfused capillaries decreased to 72.3 ± 14.6% ($P < 0.05$) compared to baseline. Tissue hypoxia and BBB damage were less prominent than in group I with high ICP (Table 1, $P < 0.05$ for both) with (NADH = 154.5 ± 8.3%, $P < 0.05$) and increased tissue fluorescence ($\Delta F/F_{0[\text{pre-injury}]} = 9.15 \pm 0.98$, np < 0.05) from baseline.

An evaluation of dynamic cerebrovascular reactivity in TBI group I with high ICP showed impaired CBF autoregulation as iCVRx increased to 0.61 ± 0.03 from −0.02 ± 0.05, respectively ($P < 0.01$ from baseline); in group II, iCVRx increased only to 0.37 ± 0.02 (Table 1, $P < 0.05$ from baseline and group I).

Dynamic ICP reactivity also revealed higher impairment in group I with high ICP than in group II without ICP increase: iPRx values were 0.35 ± 0.02 vs. 0.26 ± 0.02, $P < 0.02$, compared to −0.02 ± 0.07 at baseline, respectively (Table 1, $P < 0.05$ for both).

Discussion

Our results show that despite apparently similar CBF reductions as measured by Doppler, CBF autoregulation was more impaired in the TBI group with increased ICP, suggesting that high ICP induced a transition from capillary to MVS flow involved in the loss of CBF autoregulation in the injured brain. In fact, 2PLSM showed that capillary flow in TBI with high ICP was more damaged than in TBI without an ICP rise, and the apparently preserved CBF in group I was due to high-velocity nonnutritive MVS flow. Passive CBF autoregulation curves fail to identify the correct critical CPP threshold because they passively decrease CPP and measure the decrease in CBF based upon the overall average flow rate through the microvasculature flow compartments. In the induced dynamic method, an arterial transient into the cerebral microvasculature differentially impacts capillaries and MVS, and the response in ICP and CBF depends upon the degree of MVS or the MVS/CAP ratio, which we suggest correlates with the degree of loss of autoregulation as a fraction of capillary flow. As the MVS/CAP ratio increases, so does the proportion of tissue with loss of autoregulation, as reflected by the increase in iPRx and iCVRx (Fig. 1).

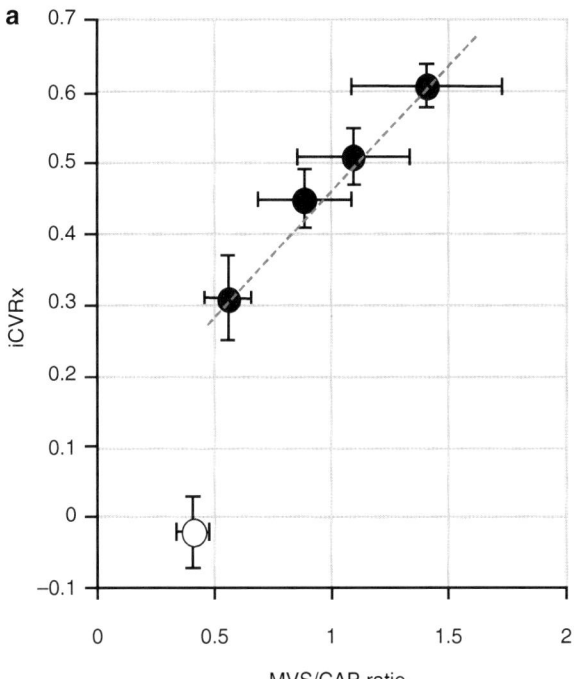 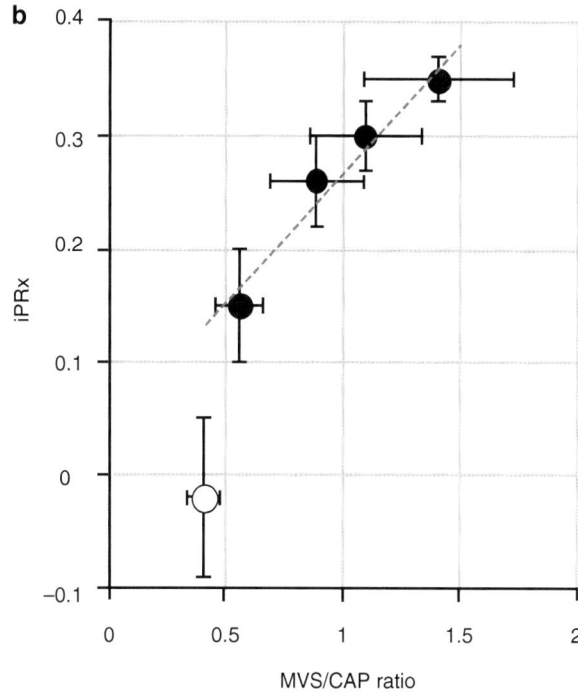

Fig. 1 Correlation between MVS/CAP flow ratio and iCVRx (**a**) and iPRx (**b**) plotted for every hour after TBI with high ICP. *Open circles*—baseline; *red dotted line*—linear fit

Conclusion

Dynamic iPRx and iCVRx accurately identified impaired CBF autoregulation following TBI with and without an increase in ICP.

Acknowledgments This work was supported by American Heart Association 14GRNT20380496, National Institutes for Health P20GM109089 and RSF #17-75-20069. The pneumatic percussion device was custom made at UNM Physics and Astronomy Department Machine Shop by John DeMoss, Anthony Gravagne, and John Behrendt.

Conflicts of interest statement We declare that we have no conflict of interest.

References

1. Rapela CE, Green HD. Autoregulation of canine cerebral blood flow. Circ Res. 1964;15(Suppl):205–12.
2. Miller JD, Stanek A, Langfitt TW. Concepts of cerebral perfusion pressure and vascular compression during intracranial hypertension. Prog Brain Res. 1972;35:411–32.
3. Grubb RL Jr, Raichle ME, Phelps ME, Ratcheson RA. Effects of increased intracranial pressure on cerebral blood volume, blood flow, and oxygen utilization in monkeys. J Neurosurg. 1975;43:385–98.
4. Johnston IH, Rowan JO, Harper AM, Jennett WB. Raised intracranial pressure and cerebral blood flow. I. Cisterna magna infusion in primates. J Neurol Neurosurg Psychiatry. 1972;35:285–96.
5. Hauerberg J, Juhler M. Cerebral blood flow autoregulation in acute intracranial hypertension. J Cereb Blood Flow Metab. 1994;14:519–25.
6. Bragin DE, Bush RC, Müller WS, Nemoto EM. High intracranial pressure effects on cerebral cortical microvascular flow in rats. J Neurotrauma. 2011 May;28(5):775–85.
7. Dai X, Bragina O, Zhang T, Yang Y, Rao GR, Bragin DE, Statom G, Nemoto EM. High intracranial pressure induced injury in the healthy rat brain. Crit Care Med. 2016;44(8):e633–8.
8. Bragin DE, Statom GL, Yonas H, Dai X, Nemoto EM. Critical cerebral perfusion pressure at high intracranial pressure measured by induced cerebrovascular and intracranial pressure reactivity. Crit Care Med. 2014;42(12):2582–90.
9. Bragin DE, Thomson S, Bragina O, Statom G, Kameneva MV, Nemoto EM. Drag-reducing polymer enhances microvascular perfusion in the traumatized brain with intracranial hypertension. Acta Neurochir Suppl. 2016;122:25–9.

Prediction of the Time to Syncope Occurrence in Patients Diagnosed with Vasovagal Syncope

Kyriaki Kostoglou, Ronald Schondorf, Julie Benoit, Saharnaz Balegh, and Georgios D. Mitsis

Abstract *Objective*: In this study we aimed to predict the time to syncope occurrence (TSO) in patients with vasovagal syncope (VVS), solely based on measurements recorded during the supine position of the head-up tilt (HUT) testing protocol.

Methods: We extracted various time and frequency domain features related to morphological aspects of arterial blood pressure (ABP) and the electrocardiogram (ECG) raw signals as well as to dynamic interactions between beat-to-beat ABP, heart rate, and cerebral blood flow velocity. From these we identified the most predictive features related to TSO.

Results: Specifically, when no orthostatic stress is involved, TSO in VVS patients can be predicted with high accuracy from a set of only five ECG features.

Keywords Vasovagal syncope · Head-up tilt · Random forest · Feature selection

Introduction

Head-up tilt (HUT) testing [1] is a common diagnostic tool in the workup of vasovagal syncope (VVS). The procedure initially involves the patient lying supine on a tilt table and then being gradually tilted to an angle between 60° and 80°. Physiological signals like arterial blood pressure (ABP), electrocardiogram (ECG), and cerebral blood flow velocity (CBFV) are monitored throughout the protocol. At some point during HUT, VVS may be induced if the patient is susceptible at that time. On other occasions VVS patients may not faint during HUT. The VVS response is poorly understood, in particular those processes that convert a seemingly normal response to orthostatic stress [2] to one where ABP and heart rate (HR) decline abruptly, reducing cerebral perfusion and causing transient loss of consciousness. This study represents a first attempt to identify markers of VVS that predict the "state" of the patient many minutes before the actual VVS occurrence.

Recordings acquired during HUT are at present the main source of information in terms of understanding the mechanisms underlying VVS. In the majority of VVS studies, the obtained signals are usually preprocessed in order to reflect mean hemodynamic changes that occur beat-to-beat (i.e., HR, R-R intervals) [3–6], omitting, however, the importance of the morphology of raw waveforms. For example, it has been shown that ABP waveforms exhibit prominent features that can provide crucial information about the cardiovascular status of a patient [7]. In [8], the authors identified a significant difference in the aortic pressure waveform between VVS patients and healthy controls, whereas in [9] the authors were able to discriminate VVS from healthy middle-aged subjects using features derived from finger arterial pressure waves. Transthoracic impedance waveforms, which allow the computation of ventricular ejection variation and ECG features, have also been deemed predictive of positive HUT tests [10–12]. Physiological changes that eventually lead to syncope may be reflected on the dynamic interactions of a variety of physiological signals, suggesting that univariate and multivariate system identification techniques could also elucidate the mechanisms underlying VVS.

Based on the foregoing discussion, we analyzed recordings obtained from 71 VVS patients undergoing HUT and extracted various time and frequency domain features, as well as features that are related to dynamic interactions. With the help of machine learning techniques, we aimed to identify the most informative features and predict the time to syncope occurrence (TSO). We focused only on supine position measurements with the hope of extracting robust baseline

K. Kostoglou
Department of Electrical and Computer Engineering, McGill University, Montreal, QC, Canada

R. Schondorf • J. Benoit • S. Balegh
Department of Neurology, McGill University, Montreal, QC, Canada

G.D. Mitsis (✉)
Department of Bioengineering, McGill University, Montreal, QC, Canada
e-mail: georgios.mitsis@mcgill.ca

VVS markers that would indicate the likelihood of syncope at a time when physiologic processes appear to be indistinguishable from normal.

Methods

Seventy-one subjects undergoing HUT (10 min resting period in the supine position and a maximum of 40 min of 80° tilt) in the Jewish General Hospital, Autonomic Reflex Laboratory, Montreal, Canada, were diagnosed as VVS patients. The HUT test protocols were approved by the hospital internal review board, and informed consent was obtained from all subjects. We analyzed recordings acquired solely during baseline (the initial 10 min in supine position). Beat-to-beat HR, systolic, diastolic, and mean ABP and CBFV were derived off-line. Initially we focused only on the ABP and ECG time series. We divided the recordings into smaller windows and extracted various time and frequency domain indices that were previously used in the literature (e.g., mean and standard deviation of R-R intervals, root mean square of successive differences, power and coefficient of variation in different frequency bands, geometrical indices). We also computed morphological characteristics of the raw waveforms (e.g., area under curve, pulse root mean square error, full width at half maximum, wavelet coefficients, energy and entropy). TSO was defined as the absolute difference between the time point where subjects were stabilized in the HUT position and the time point just before BP started dropping abruptly.

Dynamic interactions between ABP and HR variability (HRV) (reflecting autonomic nervous activity [AA] and baroreflex function [BF]) or ABP and CBFV (reflecting cerebral autoregulation [CA] and cerebrovascular resistance [CVR]) were modeled using both transfer function analysis (TFA) [13–15] and multivariate autoregressive (MVAR) models [16, 17] (eMVAR and eGC MATLAB toolbox [17]). TFA provides a simple representation of a linear time-invariant filter in the frequency domain. The characteristics of this filter can be described by its gain and phase lag in different frequency bands. In our case, we focused on the very low (VLF: 0.005–0.04 Hz), low (LF: 0.04–0.15 Hz), and high (HF: 0.15–0.4 Hz) frequency bands [18]. Clinicians usually apply TFA thanks to its ease of use; however, this method assumes that the system under consideration is single input–single output (omitting the contributions of other inputs). MVAR models, on the other hand, are usually used to capture linear interdependencies and couplings among multiple time series and to identify causality in the time and frequency domains. The most popular measures extracted by MVAR models are the coherence (Coh) (describing coupling in the frequency domain), partial coherence (PCoh) (describing direct coupling), directed coherence (DC) (describing causality), partial directed coherence (PDC) (describing direct causality), and other related measures such as the directed transfer function (DTF), generalized PDC, and granger causality (GC). We retained features from both TFA and MVAR methods.

To predict TSO, we used random forests (RFs) [19, 20] in a regression context. RFs are an ensemble of decision trees that can handle highly nonlinear interactions, and they can cope with a small number of observations and a large number of features. However, their most important characteristic is that they can assess feature importance. RF trees are trained by selecting random observations from an initial data set and taking into account a specific set of random features. All the remaining observations are used as a validation set, known also as an out of bag (OOB) set. As the forest building progresses, it generates an internal unbiased estimate of the generalization error (OOB error), which is then used to extract the most important features. The prediction of a target value is given either by averaging over all trees in regression or by majority voting in classification, making the ensemble less sensitive to noise. RF feature importance (FI) is defined as the increase in the predicted OOB error if the values of that feature are permuted across the OOB observations. This measure is computed for every tree, subsequently averaged, and divided by the standard deviation over the entire forest. The idea behind this procedure is that if a feature is important, rearranging its values will have a negative impact on the prediction accuracy. Conversely, if a feature is noninformative, the predictive performance of the model will not be altered. To acquire the optimal set of features for our problem, we applied a backward selection scheme [21], where in each iteration of the algorithm we discarded the least important RF features until we reached a minimum normalized mean square error (NMSE) and maximum Pearson's Correlation Coefficient (ρ) between actual and predicted TSO.

Results

The highest predictive performance (ρ: 0.952) (Table 1) was acquired using baseline ECG time series divided into 30 s windows. Five features were found to be important: the entropy of the coefficients extracted by applying wavelet decomposition (Daubechies, second order) on the ECG waveforms, the mean difference between the timing of the P and Q peaks and the P and R peaks, the coefficient of variation of the skewness of the T waves, and, lastly, the power band ratio of the HRV signal in the range 0.2–0.3 Hz (pr0.2_0.3) (activity in this range is usually related to respiratory sinus arrhythmia). All features, except pr0.2_0.3, were positively correlated with TSO. Based on the baseline ABP time series, the achieved prediction (ρ: 0.882) was inferior to that obtained from the ECG signal. As previously, five features were found to be important: full width at half maximum, the log energy of the initial and normalized (between 0 and 1) BP waveforms, the number of pairs of adjacent R-R intervals (R in this case is the systolic ABP), where the first R-R interval exceeds the second R-R interval by more than 20 ms, and the area under the curve of the normalized (between 0 and 1) BP waveforms. All aforementioned features exhibited a positive correlation with TSO. Mean ECG and ABP waveforms from all subjects for different TSO values can be found in Fig. 1. Features related with interactions between ABP and HRV had a low predictive performance (ρ: 0.352). On the other hand, features expressing the relationship between ABP and CBFV exhibited better performance (ρ: 0.771). Five features were found to be informative: DC and PDC from CBFV to mean ABP in the LF range (negative correlation with TSO), the mean CVR, defined as MABP divided by CBFV (positive correlation with TSO), and the TFA gain and phase in the LF range (negative correlation with TSO). These results indicate possible differences in CA and CVR in VVS patients, which ultimate lead to different TSO values.

Table 1 Pearson's correlation coefficient between actual and predicted TSO using different types of features

Feature used for prediction	Pearson's Correlation Coefficient (ρ) between actual and predicted TSO
ECG features	0.957
ABP features	0.882
Features related to interactions between ABP and HRV (reflecting AA or BF)	0.313
Features related to interactions between ABP and CBFV (reflecting CA or CVR)	0.771

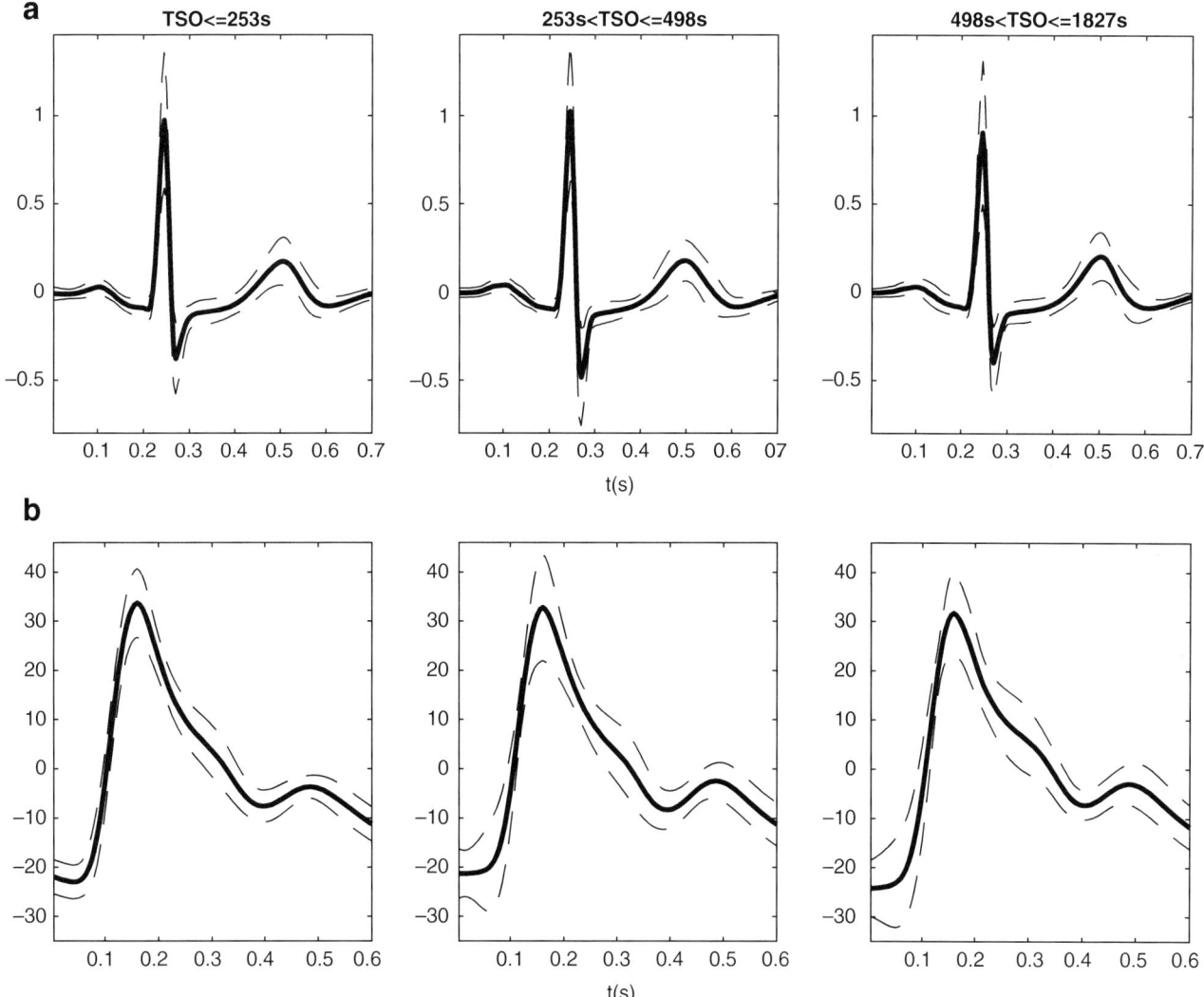

Fig. 1 Mean ± standard deviation of the demeaned (**a**) ECG and (**b**) ABP waveforms for patients with TSO less than or equal to 253 s (*left panel*), between 253 and 498 s (*middle panel*), and between 498 and 1827 s (*right panel*)

Conclusions

We have found that TSO in VVS patients can be predicted with high accuracy from a set of five ECG features, even when no orthostatic stress is involved. This is a first step toward using a feature detection approach for the diagnosis and warning of impending syncopal events. Extracted features related to the interactions between various recorded signals may help in shedding additional light on the underlying mechanisms of VVS.

Conflicts of interest statement We declare that we have no conflict of interest.

References

1. Kenny RA, Bayliss J, Ingram A, Sutton R. Head-up tilt: a useful test for investigating unexplained syncope. Lancet. 1986;327(8494):1352–5.
2. van Lieshout JJ, Wieling W, Karemaker JM, Eckberg DL. The vasovagal response. Clin Sci (London 1979). 1991;81(5):575–86.
3. Mallat Z, Vicaut E, Sangaré A, Verschueren J, Fontaine G, Frank R. Prediction of head-up tilt test result by analysis of early heart rate variations. Circulation. 1997;96(2):581–4.
4. Virag N, Sutton R, Vetter R, Markowitz T, Erickson M. Prediction of vasovagal syncope from heart rate and blood pressure trend and variability: experience in 1,155 patients. Hear Rhythm. 2007;4(11):1375–82.
5. Pruvot E, Vesin JM, Schlaepfer J, Eromer M, Kappenberger L. Autonomic imbalance assessed by heart rate variability analysis in vasovagal syncope. Pacing Clin Electrophysiol. 1994;17(11):2201–6.
6. Bellard E, Fortrat J-O, Vielle B, Dupuis J-M, Victor J, Lefthériotis G. Early predictive indexes of head-up tilt table testing outcomes utilizing heart rate and arterial pressure changes. Am J Cardiol. 2001;88(8):903–6.
7. Avolio AP, Butlin M, Walsh A. Arterial blood pressure measurement and pulse wave analysis—their role in enhancing cardiovascular assessment. Physiol Meas. 2009;31(1):R1.
8. Simek J, Wichterle D, Melenovsky V, Malik J, Svobodova J, Svacina S. Pulse wave analysis during supine rest may identify subjects with recurrent vasovagal syncope. Clin Sci. 2005;109(2):165–70.
9. Pecha S, Hakmi S, Wilke I, Yildirim Y, Hoffmann B, Reichenspurner H, Willems S, von Kodolitsch Y, Aydin A. Pulse wave analysis of the aortic pressure waveform in patients with vasovagal syncope. Heart Vessel. 2016;31(1):74–9.
10. Bellard E, Fortrat J-O, Schang D, Dupuis J-M, Victor J, Lefthériotis G. Changes in the transthoracic impedance signal predict the outcome of a 70 head-up tilt test. Clin Sci. 2003;104(2):119–26.
11. Schang D, Feuilloy M, Plantier G, Fortrat J-O, Nicolas P. Early prediction of unexplained syncope by support vector machines. Physiol Meas. 2006;28(2):185.
12. Schang D, Bellard E, Plantier G, Dupuis JM, Victor J, Leftheriotis G. Comparison of computational algorithms applied on transthoracic impedance waveforms to predict head-up tilt table testing outcome. Comput Biol Med. 2006;36:225–40.
13. Hamilton JD. Time series analysis, vol. 2. Princeton, NJ: Princeton University Press; 1994.
14. Zhang R, Zuckerman JH, Giller CA, Levine BD. Transfer function analysis of dynamic cerebral autoregulation in humans. Am J Physiol Circ Physiol. 1998;274(1):H233–41.
15. Schondorf R, Stein R, Roberts R, Benoit J, Cupples W. Dynamic cerebral autoregulation is preserved in neurally mediated syncope. J Appl Physiol. 2001;91(6):2493–502.
16. Lütkepohl H. New introduction to multiple time series analysis. New York, NY: Springer Science & Business Media; 2005.
17. Faes L, Porta A, Nollo G. Testing frequency-domain causality in multivariate time series. IEEE Trans Biomed Eng. 2010;57(8):1897–906.
18. Mitsis GD, Zhang R, Levine BD, Marmarelis VZ. Cerebral hemodynamics during orthostatic stress assessed by nonlinear modeling. J Appl Physiol. 2006;101:354–66.
19. Breiman L. Random forests. Mach Learn. 2001;45(1):5–32.
20. Kostoglou K, Michmizos KP, Stathis P, Sakas D, Nikita KS, Mitsis GD. Prediction of the Unified Parkinson's disease rating scale improvement in deep brain stimulation. IEEE Trans Biomed Engin. 2017;64(5):1123–30.
21. Guyon I, Elisseeff A. An introduction to variable and feature selection. J Mach Learn Res. 2003;3:1157–82.

Statistical Signal Properties of the Pressure-Reactivity Index (PRx)

Sophie Kelly, Steven M. Bishop, and Ari Ercole

Abstract *Objectives*: The pressure-reactivity index (PRx) is defined in terms of the moving correlation coefficient between intracranial pressure (ICP) and mean arterial pressure (MAP) and is a measure of cerebral autoregulation ability. Plots of PRx against cerebral perfusion pressure (CPP) show a U-shaped behaviour: the minimum reflecting optimal cerebral autoregulation (CPPopt). However U-shaped behaviour may also occur by chance. To date there has been no evaluation of the statistical properties of these signals.

Materials and Methods: We simulated PRx/CPP distributions using synthetic ICP and MAP signals from Gaussian noise with known cross-correlation and calculated the statistical distribution of extrema in the PRx/CPP relationship.

Results: The calculation of PRx on random data is statistically biased to show a U-shaped behaviour when the signals are positively cross-correlated (equivalent to PRx > 0). For PRx < 0, the bias is towards an inverse U-shaped behaviour. We demonstrate that this bias is eliminated by Fisher transforming the PRx data before CPPopt analysis.

Conclusions: Cross-correlated signals are biased to show a U-shaped distribution. A CPPopt-like behaviour will be observed more often than not even from random ICP and MAP signals that do not exhibit autoregulation, unless PRx is Fisher transformed. Care must be taken in interpreting CPPopt in terms of physiology calculated from untransformed data.

Keywords Cerebral autoregulation · Traumatic brain injury · PRx · Statistical properties · Bias · Fisher transform.

S. Kelly
Clinical School, Addenbrooke's Hospital,
University of Cambridge, Cambridge, UK

S.M. Bishop • A. Ercole (✉)
Division of Anaesthesia, University of Cambridge,
Cambridge, UK
e-mail: ae105@cam.ac.uk

Introduction

Traumatic brain injury (TBI) is a leading cause of death and disability [1]. Intracranial pressure (ICP) and cerebral perfusion pressure (CPP) monitoring is fundamental to the intensive care of patients with TBI in order to prevent secondary brain injury. Current guidelines for the management of severe TBI recommend maintaining ICP below 22 mmHg and CPP between 60 and 70 mmHg [2]. However, TBI is highly heterogeneous, and fixed thresholds do not account for this. Therapies to sustain cerebral perfusion can also be associated with harm. In particular, excessive CPP may exceed autoregulatory capacity, increasing intracranial blood and oedema volumes.

Management of patients based on the state of their cerebral autoregulation has been suggested. Cerebral autoregulation may remain intact over a narrowed range of CPP or be abolished after TBI [3, 4]. It has been suggested that such individualised CPP therapy is more appropriate [3, 5].

One attractive method for quasi-continuous autoregulation assessment is the cerebrovascular pressure reactivity (PRx). PRx is defined as the moving Pearson correlation coefficient between 30 consecutive 10 s averaged values (=5 min window) of mean arterial pressure (MAP) and ICP. Averaging suppresses pulse and respiratory transients [5]. PRx can provide a useful approximation of the state of autoregulation validated against both TCD and PET studies [6, 7]. Software is available for the continuous determination of PRx at the bedside [4].

Disturbed pressure reactivity leads to a more positive PRx and is of interest. PRx has been shown to be a more reliable predictor of mortality than ICP thresholds [6, 8]. Plotting mean PRx over a moving 4 h window against 5 mmHg bins of CPP reveals a U-shaped relationship [4]. The point at which PRx is the lowest is determined by curve fitting. This point defines the optimal CPP (CPPopt), representing the CPP for which autoregulation is best preserved.

CPPopt appears to be clinically significant. Retrospective observational studies have demonstrated patients managed away from CPPopt were associated with worse clinical outcome [3]. Recent data suggested excess mortality for patients managed below CPPopt and excess severe disability for those managed above it [4]. True causality is not yet established; nevertheless, the concept of autoregulation-personalised treatment is attractive. The technique is technically feasible. Whilst CPPopt can be identified approximately 70% of the time [4], improved curve fitting heuristics and novel visualisation techniques can aid appreciation of trends and overcome gaps in the data [9].

PRx is a derived parameter obtained from relatively complex calculations. The statistical properties of PRx measurements are not immediately obvious, but it is important to be sure that there are no biases that might affect subsequent analyses. Successive PRx/CPP measurements form a distribution. However, if MAP and ICP are correlated/anti-correlated, this distribution moves because mean PRx increases/decreases. Because PRx is limited to values between −1 and +1, the distribution becomes asymmetrical because of a ceiling effect, and this may introduce spurious apparent U-shaped relationships between PRx and CPP.

Furthermore, the distribution of PRx with CPP depends on the statistical signal properties of the MAP/ICP waveforms. Statistical fluctuations in these signals can have a complex long-range autocorrelation, and it is known that the spectral properties (or, equivalently, degree of self-similarity/signal complexity) of physiological recordings reflect the underlying homeostatic burden/reserve. This can vary with physiological stress or manipulation [10] and so may vary with time and can be highly prognostic [11]. This signal autocorrelation further distorts the distribution of PRx/CPP measurements and could be another source of bias.

A common (but not universal) heuristic is to first Fisher transform PRx to "normalise" its distribution before assessing for a CPPopt minimum. However, the use of the Fisher transformation to remove the ceiling effect of correlated data has not been investigated. This simulation investigates whether the Fisher transformation is necessary to remove the distribution bias of data and to produce a curve from which a meaningful CPPopt can be calculated.

In this study, we present Monte Carlo simulations characterising the statistical properties of PRx as a function of CPP looking for potential sources of U-shaped bias that may confound/distort any true underlying autoregulation behaviour. In particular, we examine the effect of different levels of correlation between MAP and ICP. Furthermore, we examine the influence of autocorrelation on bias. Finally, we study the effect of Fisher transformation on any such bias.

Materials and Methods

MAP and ICP signals were synthesised from white noise. A degree of first-order lagged autocorrelation was then introduced into both the MAP and ICP signals according to Eq. 1:

$$y(t) \mapsto (1-\phi) \times y(t) + \phi \times y(t-1). \qquad (1)$$

The parameter ϕ was tuneable, simulating different degrees of memory in the signal varying between −1 (anti-persistent) and +1 (persistent).

Correlation was subsequently added to ICP according to Eq. 2:

$$\text{ICP} \mapsto \rho \times \text{MAP} + \sqrt{1-\rho^2} \times \text{ICP}. \qquad (2)$$

Thus ρ represents an underlying correlation between the two signals. Crucially, this correlation does not imply any autoregulation; ρ is not a function of CPP. Thus, whilst we expect PRx to be non-zero for non-zero ρ, there should be no U-shaped behaviour in the PRx/CPP relationship if the CPPopt calculation is unbiased.

To test this null hypothesis, we calculated PRx as the moving window Pearson correlation coefficient from our synthetic signals analogously with clinical practice. PRx values so obtained were evenly binned against the mean CPP for the window period and a quadratic fit performed to this mean PRx/CPP data (Eq. 3, where U, V and W are fitted parameters):

$$\text{PRx} = U \times \text{CPP}^2 + V \times \text{CPP} + W. \qquad (3)$$

We extracted the quadratic parameter, U, from the fit as a measure of the curvature of the PRx/CPP relationship with 1000-fold repetition to obtain a mean/standard deviation. This was repeated for different values of $\rho \in [-1,+1]$ and $\phi \in [-1,+1]$.

To examine the effect of the Fisher transformation on the statistical properties of PRx, we additionally transformed the calculated PRx values before our quadratic fit using Eq. 4:

$$\text{PRx} \mapsto \frac{1}{2} \ln\left(\frac{1+\text{PRx}}{1-\text{PRx}}\right). \qquad (4)$$

Calculations were carried out using MATLAB Release 2015b (The MathWorks Inc., Natick, MA, USA) on Linux. Code was optimised to run in parallel on 16 × 3.3 GHz Intel Xeon cores with a total of 32 GB RAM (typical runtime ~23 h).

Results

Figure 1 shows how the quadratic parameter, U, varies with the correlation parameter ρ for white noise ICP/MAP ($\phi = 0$). For $\rho = 0$, U is close to zero. For increasing positive ρ (ICP

Statistical Signal Properties of the Pressure-Reactivity Index (PRx)

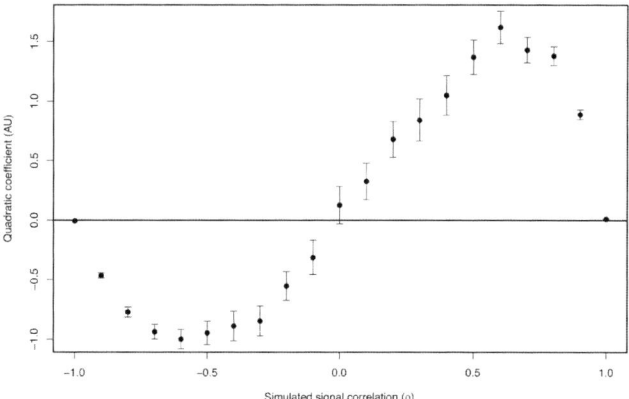

Fig. 1 Plot of fitted quadratic parameter U (arbitrary units × 10^{-5}) against ICP/MAP correlation strength ρ. Positive values of U suggest a U-shaped tendency between ICP and CPP; negative values represent an inverted U-shape

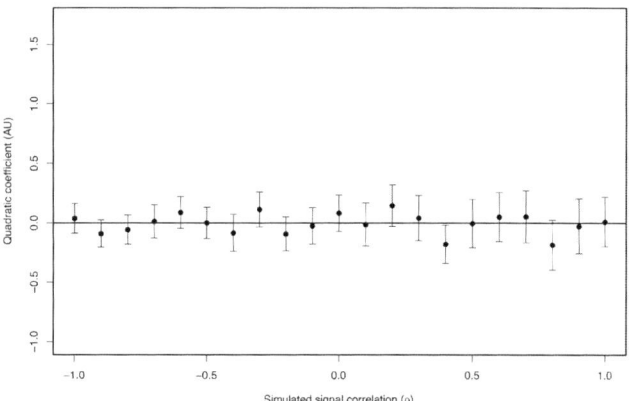

Fig. 2 Equivalent plot to Fig. 1 for Fisher-transformed PRx. Unlike the untransformed case, there is no longer a demonstrable U-shape bias for any value of ρ

and MAP are correlated) U becomes positive and non-zero, demonstrating a U-shaped tendency to the PRx/CPP relationship. Since the ICP and MAP signals are simulated from correlated noise only, without any autoregulation behaviour, this represents a U-shaped bias.

For ρ below zero, U is negative/non-zero, meaning that there is, on average, an inverted U-shaped bias for situations where PRx is negative. For $\rho = \pm 1$ U becomes zero since PRx is exactly ± 1 for all CPP.

Figure 2 shows analogous data to Fig. 1, but in this case, the simulated PRx values were first Fisher transformed before the fitting of a quadratic curve against CPP. Within errors, the relationship of U against ρ is seen to be abolished.

Figure 3 shows the effect of changing the degree of autocorrelation ϕ for a fixed $\rho = 0.6$ (chosen so that U is approximately maximal in Fig. 1). The U-shaped bias is seen to reduce slightly with increasing positive autocorrelation. For negative autocorrelation, U is found to increase dramatically.

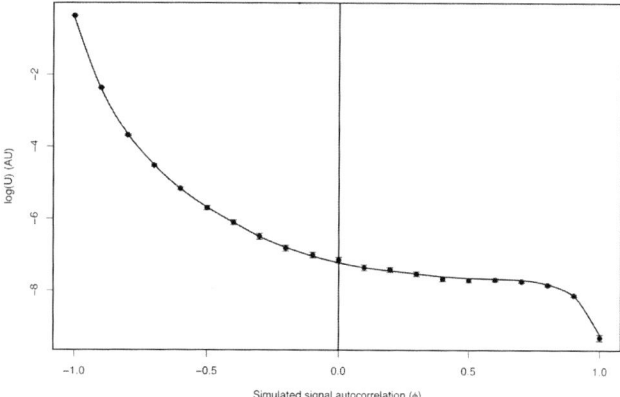

Fig. 3 Parameter U (logarithmic scale) as a function of autocorrelation ϕ for simulated ICP/MAP data with fixed $\rho = 0.6$. For zero autocorrelation, this corresponds to a value of U near the maximum seen in Fig. 1. The bias is reduced slightly for increasing positive autocorrelation (persistence). However, with negative autocorrelation (anti-persistent data), the U-shaped bias increases dramatically

Discussion

Our simulations demonstrate that PRx is statistically biased to display U-shaped behaviour, centred on the mean value of CPP, in the absence of autoregulation. The direction and magnitude of this U-shape depends on the degree and sign of the cross-correlation between MAP and ICP. This consideration is important: For positively correlated signals (such as occurs with a generally pressure-passive ICP/MAP relationship), this could distort the true autoregulatory minimum or even introduce a spurious CPPopt. For negatively correlated ICP/MAP (as might be expected on average for an autoregulating system), the U-shaped bias is inverted, which may serve to distort or abolish the true autoregulatory minimum.

In Fig. 1, it is noteworthy that the relationship is not symmetrical, $\rho = \pm 1$, the maximum U being greater than the minimum. This results from an inherent correlation between ICP and CPP since CPP = MAP-ICP. Repeating the simulations for the ICP/MAP relationship (as opposed to the clinically important case of ICP/CPP) removes the asymmetry.

Conclusions

We show that PRx/CPP is statistically biased, and this applies to any similar parameter from two correlated time series. Furthermore, this bias is exacerbated if the signals are autocorrelated with anti-persistence. Since changes in autocorrelation and signal complexity are known to occur in the face of physiological perturbation, the U-shaped bias is therefore expected to be dependent on physiological stress. We recommend that the Fisher transformation always be used before analysing such data. This rescales the Pearson correlation coefficient in such a way as to normalise its distribution.

Acknowledgements The authors would like to acknowledge M. Czosnyka and P. Smielewski for support and useful discussions.

Conflicts of interest statement We declare that we have no conflict of interest.

References

1. Maas AI, Menon DK, Steyerberg EW, Citerio G, Lecky F, Manley GT, Hill S, Legrand V, Sorgner A, CENTER-TBI Participants and Investigators. Collaborative European NeuroTrauma Effectiveness Research in Traumatic Brain Injury (CENTER-TBI): a prospective longitudinal observational study. Neurosurgery. 2015;76(1):67–80.
2. Brain Trauma Foundation. Brain Trauma Foundation guidelines. 4th ed. Campbell, CA: Brain Trauma Foundation; 2016. https://braintrauma.org/uploads/03/12/Guidelines_for_Management_of_Severe_TBI_4th_Edition.pdf. Accessed 31 Oct 2016
3. Steiner LA, Czosnyka M, Piechnik SK, Smielewski P, Chatfield D, Menon DK, Pickard JD. Continuous monitoring of cerebrovascular pressure reactivity allows determination of optimal cerebral perfusion pressure in patients with traumatic brain injury. Crit Care Med. 2002;30:733–8.
4. Aries MJH, Czosnyka M, Budohoski KP, Steiner LA, Lavinio A, Kolias AG, Hutchinson PJ, Brady KM, Menon DK, Pickard JD, Smielewski P. Continuous determination of optimal cerebral perfusion pressure in traumatic brain injury. Crit Care Med. 2012;40:2456–63.
5. Czosnyka M, Brady K, Reinhard M, Smielewski P, Steiner LA. Monitoring of cerebrovascular autoregulation: facts, myths, and missing links. Neurocrit Care. 2009;10:373–86.
6. Czosnyka M, Smielewski P, Kirkpatrick P, Laing RJ, Menon D, Pickard JD. Continuous assessment of the cerebral vasomotor reactivity in head injury. Neurosurgery. 1997;41:11–9.
7. Steiner LA, Coles JP, Johnston AJ, Chatfield DA, Smielewski P, Fryer TD, Aigbirhio FI, Clark JC, Pickard JD, Menon DK, Czosnyka M. Assessment of cerebrovascular autoregulation in head-injured patients: a validation study. Stroke. 2003;34:2404–9.
8. Lazaridis C, DeSantis SM, Smielewski P, Menon DK, Hutchinson P, Pickard JD, Czosnyka M. Patient-specific thresholds of intracranial pressure in severe traumatic brain injury. J Neurosurg. 2014;120:893–900.
9. Aries MJ, Wesselink R, Elting JW, Donnelly J, Czosnyka M, Ercole A, Maurits NM, Smielewski P. Enhanced visualization of optimal cerebral perfusion pressure over time to support clinical decision making. Crit Care Med. 2016;44(10):e996–9.
10. Bishop SM, Yarham SI, Navapurkar VU, Menon DK, Ercole A. Multifractal analysis of hemodynamic behavior: intraoperative instability and its pharmacological manipulation. Anesthesiology. 2012;117(4):810–21.
11. Gao L, Smielewski P, Czosnyka M, Ercole A. Cerebrovascular signal complexity six hours after intensive care unit admission correlates with outcome after severe traumatic brain injury. J Neurotrauma. 2016. https://doi.org/10.1089/neu.2015.4228.

Author Index

A
Adams, H., 209
Agarkova, D., 25
Agarwal, S., 179
Agbeko, R., 39
Agrawal, S., 7, 29, 147
Ainslie, P.N., 47, 263
Alperin, N., 215
Andrade, R.A.P., 75, 107
Aries, M.J.H., 55, 209

B
Bagci, A.M., 215
Balardy, L., 163, 247
Balédent, O., 221, 233, 237, 247, 255
Balegh, S., 313
Baroncini, M., 221, 237
Benoit, J., 313
Bertuccio, A., 69
Bertuetti, R., 69
Birch, A.A., 103
Bishop, S.M., 189, 317
Boehme, A.K., 179
Bouzerar, R., 237
Bragin, D.E., 21, 93, 309
Bragina, O.A., 93
Brunelli, R., 75, 107
Bruyninckx, D., 287
Bryk, K., 303
Budohoski, K., 139
Bulman, M., 69
Bulters, D.O., 103

C
Cabeleira, M., 7, 29, 69, 121, 143, 147
Cabella, B., 209
Callebaut, I., 287
Calviello, L., 17
Campbell-Bell, C.M., 103
Capel, C., 237
Cardim, D., 7, 29, 47, 69, 79, 209
Cardim, D.A., 75, 107
Carew, M., 7, 29
Chacón, M., 159
Chambers, I., 3, 291
Citerio, G., 3, 291
Claassen, J., 179
Craelius, W., 297

Czosnyka, M., 7, 17, 29, 47, 55, 69, 79, 129, 133, 139, 143, 209, 229, 233, 237, 247
Czosnyka, Z., 69, 133, 163, 229, 233, 237

D
Danish, S., 297
Davis, P., 39
de Korte, C., 115
Deken Delannoy, V., 221
den Berghe, G.V., 291
Dentinger, A., 97
Depreitere, B., 3, 39, 51, 201, 287, 291
Despres, J., 167
Dias, C., 59, 107
Dimitri, G.M., 147
Dobrzeniecki, M., 21
Donald, R., 3, 291
Donnelly, J., 7, 17, 29, 47, 55, 69, 129, 143, 147, 209
Duhamel, A., 221
Durduran, T., 39

E
Ebert, D., 97
Ebrahimi Ardi, C., 221
Elting, J.W.J., 55
Enblad, P., 3, 39, 291
Engel, D.C., 197
Ercole, A., 55, 121, 189, 209, 317
Eyding, J., 115

F
Fanelli, A., 85, 173
Fernandes, D., 59
Fernandes, H.M., 7, 29
Feyen, B., 3, 291
Filippidis, A., 173
Flechet, M., 291
Frigieri, G., 75, 107

G
Garcia, K., 97
Garnett, M., 129, 229
Garnett, M.R., 7, 29
Garnotel, S., 247, 255
Gondry-Jouet, C., 237
Grigoryeva, V., 25

Grzanka, A., 133
Guilfoyle, M.R., 7, 29
Güiza, F., 3, 201, 291

H
Hagberg, S., 93
Hamilton, R.B., 269
Harland, S., 47
Haubrich, C., 7, 29, 147
Hawthorne, C., 89, 183, 205
Heldt, T., 85, 173
Hockel, K., 281
Hodel, J., 221
Hoedemaekers, C.W.E., 115
Holsapple, J., 173
Hutchinson, P.J., 7, 29, 147, 209

J
Jaishankar, R., 173
Jara, J.L., 153, 159
Jones, P.A., 3, 291
Jorens, P., 3, 291

K
Kaczmarska, K., 133
Kalentyev, G., 25
Karaseva, O.V., 11
Kasprowicz, M., 133
Kelly, S., 317
Kennedy McConnell, F.A., 275
Keong, N.C., 229
Kiening, K., 39
Kim, D.-J., 233
Kim, N., 297
Kinsella, J., 89, 183, 205
Klein, S.P., 51, 287
Klingelhöfer, J., 79
Kosinski, C., 297
Kostoglou, K., 313
Krakauskaite, S., 269
Krause, M., 243
Kuchcinski, G., 221
Kurtcuoglu, V., 243

L
Lafitte, P., 163
Lalou, D.A., 129, 133, 229
Landerretche, J., 159
LaVangie, J., 269
Lavinio, A., 129
Lee, H.-S., 111
Lejeune, J.-P., 221
Levin, R., 39
Lio, P., 147
Liu, X., 7, 29, 47, 143, 147, 209
Lo, T., 39
Lo, T.-Y.M., 3, 291
Lokossou, A., 247
Lopes, L., 75
Lukianov, V.I., 11, 35

M
Maarek, O., 167
Maas, A., 3, 291
MacDonald, M., 97
Marchbanks, R.J., 103
Martin, A., 179
Martinez, L., 269
Mascarenhas, S., 75, 107
Matta, B., 69
Matthews, J.M., 85
Maurits, N.M., 55
McLeod, D.D., 79
Megjhani, M., 179
Meixensberger, J., 243
Menon, D.K., 17, 209
Meshcheryakov, S.V., 11, 35
Meyfroidt, G., 3, 39, 201, 291
Mitsis, G.D., 313
Monteiro, E., 59
Moreira, M., 59
Morris, K., 39
Moss, L., 3, 89, 183, 205, 291

N
Nabbanja, E., 229
Nemoto, E.M., 93, 309
Ngai, K., 63
Nilsson, P., 3, 39, 291
Noh, S.-H., 159

O
O'Brien, M., 269

P
Page, G., 247
Panerai, R.B., 153
Park, C., 39
Park, S., 179
Pascoa, R., 59
Payne, S.J., 275
Payoux, P., 247
Pereira, E., 59
Pickard, J.D., 17, 129, 229
Pietersen, J., 69
Pietrangelo, S.J., 111
Pineda, B., 297
Piper, I., 3, 39, 89, 183, 205, 291
Poca, M., 39
Poon, W.S., 63
Puppo, C., 139

R
Ragauskas, A., 39
Rasulo, F., 69
Risser, L., 167
Robba, C., 47, 69, 209
Robinson, T.G., 153
Roh, D., 179
Roshal, L.M., 35
Rouzaud-Laborde, C., 163

Author Index

S
Saeed, N.P., 153
Sahuquillo, J., 39
Salmon, S., 255
Sargsyan, A., 97
Scalzo, F., 269
Scheidt, M., 269
Schmidt, B., 79
Schmidt, E., 247
Schmidt, E.A., 163, 167, 233
Schmidt, J.M., 179
Schondorf, R., 313
Schuhmann, M.U., 3, 281, 291
Schürer, L., 197
Seifert, B., 243
Semenova, Z.B., 11, 35
Seth-Hunter, D., 269
Sharif, S.J., 103
Shaw, M., 89, 183, 205
Slump, C.H., 115
Smielewski, P., 7, 17, 29, 47, 55, 69, 121, 133, 139, 143, 147, 179, 209, 233
Smirl, J.D., 263, 303
Sodini, C.G., 111
Sorokina, E.G., 11
Soto Ares, G., 221
Spavieri, D.L. Jr., 75, 107
Spiegelberg, A., 243
Statom, G.L., 309
Steiner, L., 139
Steiner, L.A., 209
Streif, S., 79

T
Tajsic, T., 69
Terilli, K., 179
Thibeault, C., 269
Trofimov, A.O., 21, 25
Trofimova, S., 25
Tzeng, Y.-C., 263

V
Van den Berghe, G., 3
van der Hoeven, J.G., 115
van Donkelaar, P., 263, 303
Varsos, G.V., 47, 133, 139
Velazquez, A., 179
Verdier, M., 167
Verzola, R.M.M., 75, 107
Vinke, E.J., 115
Voennov, O., 25

W
Wang, C.C., 75, 107
Weinhold, M., 79
Weitz, J., 39
Wesselink, R., 55
Wilk, S.J., 269
Wolf, S., 197
Wong, G.K.C., 63
Wright, A.D., 263, 303
Wu, A., 269

X
Xiuyun, L., 69

Y
Young, A., 147
Young, A.M.H., 7, 29
Yu, C., 63
Yuriev, M., 25

Z
Zabołotny, W., 133
Zheng, V.Z.Y., 63

Subject Index

A

ABP, *see* Arterial blood pressure
Acute brain injury, 115
Acute respiratory distress syndrome (ARDS), 5
Adjusted linear modelling approach, 91
Air-pouch-based parenchymal ICP monitor, 285
Akaike information criteria (AIC), 91, 207
Algorithm's false-positive yield rate, 146
Alzheimer's disease, 221
Amplitude of arterial blood pressure (ABPamp), 22
Analysis of variance (ANOVA), 13
    cerebral pressure-flow dynamics, 264–265
    dCA, 160–161
    ICP, 289
Anatomical Therapeutic Chemical (ATC) system, 163
Anonymisation process, 42, 43
Antihypertensive drugs, 163–165
ARI, *see* Autoregulation index
Arterial blood pressure (ABP), 8, 56, 139, 163, 210
Arterial circulation, 240
Arterial network model, 276
Arterial occlusion, 275
Arterial pressure pulsatility, 236
AR threshold (ART) testing, 104
Artifact filters, 180
Autonomic dysfunction, 307
Autoregulation, 210
Autoregulation index (ARI), 159, 161

B

Bedmaster, 179–180
Big-data, 40
Bioelectrical impedance analysis (BIA), 89
Bioelectrical spectroscopy, 90
Blood-oxygen-level-dependent (BOLD), 153
BMEYE Nexfin device, 174, 175
BMx, 179–182
Brain edema therapy, 23
Brain injury, 297
    acute
        ischemia, 115
        management, 181
        PRx reflects illness severity, 179
    cerebral hemodynamic stability after, 297–300
Brain-IT database, 4
Brain microcirculation, 21
Brain tissue hypoxia, 90
Brain Trauma Foundation (BTF) guidelines, 3, 201–203
B-waves
    computerized methods, 243
    ICP, 243
    See also Slow waves

C

Callosal angle, 225, 227
Cardiac cycle (CC), 248, 249, 257, 264
Causation, 167
CCH, *see* Chronic communicating hydrocephalus
Cephalad vascular fluid shift, 215
Cerebral arterial compliance (cAC), 21–23
Cerebral autoregulation (CA), 263, 275, 303, 317
    arterial network model, 276
    and collateral flow, 276
    collateral flow routes, 278
    CPPopt, 57
    extraventricular drainage ICP monitoring and assessment, 282–283
    LICA occlusion, 277
    negative feedback, 276
    network model, 277
    neuromonitoring parameters and, 283–284
    passive cerebral vascular territories, 276
    simulations, 277
Cerebral blood flow (CBF), 303
    autoregulation, 25, 141
    TFA, 263
Cerebral blood flow velocity (CBFV), 111, 159
Cerebral hemodynamics, 25, 50, 234
Cerebral hemodynamic stability after, brain injury, 297–300
Cerebral macro-and microcirculation, UPI, 115–120
Cerebral microcirculatory bed, 25
Cerebral perfusion pressure (CPP), 8, 25, 179, 201, 292, 317
    acute respiratory distress syndrome, 3
    autoregulation, 210
    beneficial/nonbeneficial effects, 202
    Brain-IT database, 4
    in BTF guidelines, 3
    CPPopt, 210–212
    data acquisition and analyses, 210
    gravity, 203
    hydrostatic pressure gradient, 202
    Local Ethics Committee approval, 4
    management, 59
    measurement method, 201
    methods, 202
    non-beneficial effect, 3

Cerebral perfusion pressure (cont.)
  patients, 210
  per-centre CPP, 4
  per-patient CPPs, 4, 5
  physiological markers, 210
  post hoc analysis, 3
  PRx, 210–212, 317–320
  publications, 202
  retrospective studies, 211
  spin-off, 5
  statistical analysis, 211
  variability, 4, 5
Cerebral pressure-buffering system, 306
Cerebral pressure-flow dynamics, 263–268
Cerebrospinal compensatory reserve index, 18
Cerebrospinal fluid (CSF)
  CCH, 221–222
  drainage, 287
  space, 216
  stroke volume, 222
Cerebrospinal system modeling, 255–259
Cerebrovascular autoregulation, 43, 44, 309–312
Cerebrovascular impedance model, 133
Cerebrovascular pressure autoregulation (CAR), 292–295
Cerebrovascular (iCVRx) reactivity, 309–312
Cerebrovascular resistance (CVR), 314, 315
  in CTBI, 25–27
Channel, MFER waveform, 185
CHART-ADAPT project, 183–184, 187
Chi-squared deviance test, 207
Chronic communicating hydrocephalus (CCH), 221–227
Circle of Willis, 275–278
Classification matrix, 12
Cluster analysis, 13
Coefficient of variation (CoV), 160
Cognitive domain deficit, 64
Cognitive neuroimaging studies, 153
Color Trails Test (CTT), 64
Combined traumatic brain injury (CTBI), 25–27
Computed tomography (CT), 29–33
Computerised infusion test, 229
Continuous wavelet transform (CWT), 148
Contrast-to-noise ratio (CNR), 154
Correlation, 167
CPP, see Cerebral perfusion pressure
CPPopt, see Optimal cerebral perfusion pressure
CrCP, see Critical closing pressure
Critical closing pressure (CrCP), 48
  Aaslid's equation, 135
  cerebral blood flow autoregulation, 141
  intracranial pressure, 133–136
  mild hypocapnia, effect, 139–142
  vascular wall tension (WT), 133
Cross-correlation function, 148
CSF, see Cerebrospinal fluid
Custom-designed LabView interface, 174, 175
CVR, see Cerebrovascular resistance

D
Data-acquisition system, 173–176
  collecting and archiving waveform data, 174, 175
  GE Solar 8000i, 173–174
  time-stamping, 173
  waveform signals, 174–176
Data block, 185
dCA, see Dynamic cerebral autoregulation

Decompressive craniectomy, 36
Denoising method, 154
Diastolic closing margin (DCM), 141
Digital Imaging and Communications in Medicine (DICOM) standard, 187
Dimensionality reduction, 108, 109
Dirac Impulse Response (DIR), 80
Discrete prototype electronic system, 112
Discriminant function analysis, 12, 13
Dislocation syndrome, 35
Doppler mapping procedure, 113
Drugs, 163–164
Dural venous stenosis, 237
DWL Doppler-BoxX, 174, 175
Dynamic adaptive target of active cerebral autoregulation (DATACAR), 43
Dynamic cerebral autoregulation (dCA), 159–162
  ANOVA, 160–161
  CBFV, 159
  linear and nonlinear models, 160
Dynamic helical computed tomography angiography (DHCTA), 22

E
Edge artefact, 192
Elastance, 164
Electric circuit analog model, 85
Electrocardiography (ECG)-gated duration of the diastole (T_{dia}), 22
Electrocardiography (ECG)-gated duration of the systole (T_{sys}), 22
Electronic medical record systems, 121
European Data Format (EDF), 187
Evans' index, 222–224, 226, 227
EVD, see Extraventricular drainage
Excel software, 250
Extraventricular drainage (EVD), 281–287
  cerebral autoregulation, 282–283, 286
  CSF drainage and intermittent closure, 283

F
Filtering method, 154
Finger photoplethysmography, 264
Finite-element-method, 256
Finometer MIDI Finapres, 160
Fisher's exact test, 222–223
Fisher transformation, 318
Fluid-coupled ICP monitoring, 285
Fluid percussion injury (FPI), 310
Fluid-structure interaction, 255–259
  ICP, spatial distribution, 258–259
  linear elasticity, 258
Frame information, 184–185
Friedman test, 116
Frontal lobe syndrome, 40

G
Gamma Index, 13
GE Solar 8000i, 173–174
GE Tram Rac 4A unit, 174–176
Glasgow Coma Scale (GCS), 12–16, 18
Glasgow Outcome Scale (GOS), 12, 13, 18, 52
Globe flattening (GF), 216–218
Gradient-echo EPI sequences, 154
Gunshot wounds, 13

H

Haemodynamic parameters, 141
HDF5, 121–125
Head-up tilt (HUT) testing, 313
Health screen questionnaire, 104
Heuristic algorithm, 180
High-energy trauma, 12
High-frequency pulsed electromagnetic field (PEMF), 93–95
HL7, 186–187
Hong Kong List Learning Test (HKLLT), 64
Hydrocephalus, 229–231, 247
Hypertension, 163–165
Hypoperfusion episodes, 23
Hypotension, 14, 15
Hypoxia, 14, 15

I

ICP, see Intracranial pressure
ICP-derived infusion test, 229–231
ICU, see Intensive care unit
Idiopathic intracranial hypertension (IIH), 216, 237–241
Idiopathic normal pressure hydrocephalus (INPH) guidelines, 243
IIH, see Idiopathic intracranial hypertension
Impaired autoregulation, 276
Impedimed SFB7 Bio-impedance Spectroscopy Unit, 90
Index Table, 122, 125
Induced dynamic ICP (iPRx), 309–312
Informatics approach, 43
Infusion test, 248
Injury Severity Score (ISS), 11, 15
Intensive care unit (ICU)
    AIC, 207
    factors, 205
    LOS, 205
    modelling variable estimates and corresponding standard errors, 207
    multi-factorial model, 207
    pilot study, 206
    poisson regression, 206
    Poisson regression modelling strategy, 207
    PTI, 206
    threshold value, 207
International Space Station (ISS), 97
Intracranial arterial pressure, 4, 5
Intracranial compliance, ICP monitoring and PCMRI, 247–252
Intracranial pressure (ICP), 163, 297, 317
    animals and ethics, 48
    B-wave, 243
    causation, 167
    cerebral autoregulation, 47
    cerebral hemodynamic stability after brain injury, 297–300
    clinical factors, 8, 9
    clinical features, 7–8
    complex data analysis, 168
    correlation, 167
    cross-correlation values, 244
    Cushing vasopressor response, 49
    data acquisition and analysis, 8, 48
    haemodynamic consequences, 48, 49
    and heart rate, 147–151
    histograms, 168
    ICU, 205–207
    implications, 9
    infusion studies, 164
    limitations, 9, 50
    linear relations, 168
    Mann–Whitney test, 244
    MAP and, 201
    mean values, SD and p-values, 245
    monitoring, 7
    parameters, 164
    partial correlations, 168–170
    patients, 8
    peak detection, 189
    Pearson-based correlations, 168, 169
    vs. pre-hospital hypotension, 8, 9
    prognostic value, TBI, 35–37
    protocol, 48
    PRx and, 287–290
    PSS, 164
    pulsatile cerebrospinal fluid flow, 234
    recordings, 298
    slow waves, 129–132
    statistical analysis, 8, 48, 164
    study population, 164
    subpopulation characteristics, 164
    SVWs, 243–246
    vascular wall tension, 49
    wavelet analysis, 148
Intracranial pressure (ICP) monitoring, 247, 281
    air-pouch-based technique, 285–286
    assessment and display, 282
    EVD, 281–286
    intracranial compliance, 247–252
Ischemia, 115, 275, 276
IxTrend Netserver system, 185
iXtrends software, 90

K

KidsBrainIT, 39–45
    anonymisation process, 42, 43
    big-data, 40, 43
    cerebrovascular autoregulation, 43, 44
    frontal lobe syndrome, 40
    ICP visualisation plot analyses, 43–45
    low-frequency autoregulation index, 40
    multi-national paediatric brain monitoring, 41
    network and non-network monitors, 42
    pressure reactivity index method, 43
Kiefer score, 244
Kolmogorov–Smirnov test, 94

L

LabView-based graphical user interface, 174, 175
Lamé's coefficients, 256
Left internal carotid artery (LICA) occlusion, 276, 277
Length of stay (LOS), 205–207
Licox® probes, 198
Linear correlation coefficient, 76
Linear regression, 117
Local maxima scalogram (LMS), 190–192
Log-regression analysis, 13
Low-frequency autoregulation index (LAx), 40, 43, 292
Lumbar infusion, 230
Lumped-parameter physiological model, 85

M

Magnetic resonance imaging (MRI), 153–156
Manipulation-free period (MFP), 288
Mann–Whitney test, 94, 222, 244, 271
Marchbanks Measurement Systems-14 Cerebral and Cochlear Fluid Pressure (CCFP) Analyser, 104
Marshall CT scale, 12
Mathematical model approach, 12, 13
MATLAB, 180, 217
MATLAB Release 2015b, 190–191, 318
Mean arterial blood pressure (MAP), 4, 5, 8, 9, 201–203, 317
Mean cerebral blood flow velocity (mCBFV), 269–272
Mean index (Mx), 141
Mechanical extensometers, 107
Medical Information Bus (MIB), 186–187
Medical Waveform Format Encoding Rules (MFER), 184–186
MFER, *see* Medical Waveform Format Encoding Rules
Microvascular shunt (MVS), 309–311
Microvascular vasospasm, 27
Minimally invasive ICP method (ICPMI), 75–77
Mini-Mental State Examination (MMSE), 64
Modified Boston Naming Test (mBNT), 64
Modified Scholkmann algorithm, 190–194
Monitoring brain tissue oxygenation (pbtO2), 197–199
Montreal cognitive assessment (MoCA), 64
MRICP method, 216
Multifactor prognosis models, 11, 12
Multi-modality monitoring, 173
Multi-planar reconstructions (MPRs), 98
MX800 monitor, 185

N

Navier-Stokes equations, 256
Neonatal piglet model, 90
Neurointensive care units, 183–188
Neuron specific enolase (NSE) levels, 12, 15
NHS network, 184
Nicotinamide adenine dinucleotide (NADH) autofluorescence, 310
NI DAQ 6218, 175
Non-invasive intracranial pressure (nICP)
    assessment model, 69–72, 79–82
    monitoring methods, 107–110
Non-normal pressure hydrocephalus (NNPH), 244–245
Non-parametric analysis, 14
Nonparametric comparison tests, 17
Non-parametric Kruskal–Wallis test, 60
Non-parametric statistic methods—Spearman's Rank Correlation Index, 13
Non-parametric Wilcoxon test, 31, 135
Normal pressure hydrocephalus (NPH), 229, 243–244

O

Olympus BX51WI upright microscope, 94
Optic nerve protrusion, 215
Optic nerve sheath (ONS), 71
Optimal cerebral perfusion pressure (CPPopt), 179
    algorithm, 144
    arterial blood pressure, 56
    artifact filters and lower frequency sampling, 180
    autoregulation-guided CPP therapy, 56
    calculation, 144–145, 180, 181
    cerebral autoregulation, 57, 58
    CPP, 210–212
    definition, 55
    future evaluation and implementation, 57
    heuristic algorithm, 180
    0.2-Hz (5 s) data, 180
    intraparenchymal probe, 56
    landscape, 56, 57
    methodology, 56
    and PaO_2/FiO_2, 59–61
    patient management, 143
    Pearson's R correlation, 181, 182
    pressure reactivity index, 143
    protocol, 144
    recording, 56, 57
    sensitivity analysis, 146
    statistical analysis, 180
    study population and data collection, 180
    subarachnoid hemorrhage, 180
    time (horizontal) axis, 56
    U-shaped curves, 144–146
    visualisation method, 56
Optimum cerebral perfusion, 25
Oscillatory process, 36
Osirix Lite software, 222
Otoscopy, 104
Out of bag (OOB), 314

P

Paediatric intensive care unit (PICU), 40
Paired *t* test, 140
Papilledema, 237
Partial correlations, 168–170
Partial least squares discriminant analyses (PLS-DA), 60, 61
Patient data module (PDM), 174
Peak detection, 189–194
Peak intensity (PI), 116
Pearson's correlation coefficient, 135, 168, 169, 292–293
    CPPopt, 181, 182
    ICP monitoring, 251
    PRx, 181, 182
    TSO, 315
PFart, 239
PFvein, 239
Phase-contrast magnetic resonance imaging (PCMRI), 221–222
    ICP monitoring, 248–252
    IIH, 238
    intracranial compliance, 248–252
Philips Medical ICCA bedside e-Record system, 186, 187
Poisson regression modelling strategy, 206, 207
Post hoc analysis, 3
Post-processing vascular subtraction technique, 105
Power spectrum densities (PSDs), 108, 109, 267
Pressure in the sagittal sinus (PSS), 164
Pressure reactivity index (PRx), 8, 18, 30, 31, 43, 59, 141, 143, 179, 287, 317
    artifact filters and lower frequency sampling, 180
    calculation, 180, 181
    correlation, 318
    CPPopt and, 318
    distribution, 318
    Fisher transformation, 318–320
    heuristic algorithm, 180
    0.2-Hz (5 s) data, 180
    and ICP, 287–290
    MATLAB Release 2015b, 318
    Monte Carlo simulations, 318
    parameter, 318–319
    Pearson's R correlation, 181, 182, 317
    statistical analysis, 180

statistical properties, 318
study population and data collection, 180
subarachnoid hemorrhage, 180
U-shaped bias, 319–320
Pressure time index (PTI), 206
Pressure times time dose, 37
Pressure volume index (PVI), 164
Program Statistica 7.0, 22
PRx, see Pressure reactivity index
Pulsatile cerebrospinal fluid flow, 233–236
Pulsatile flow, 236
Pulsatility index (PI), 70, 80, 240, 269–272

Q
Quality Table, 122, 125

R
RAP index, 297–299
Real-time nICP estimation, 85–88
Receiver operating characteristics (ROC) curve, 223
Regions of interest (ROIs), 116
Resistive resistance, 90
The Rey Osterrieth Complex Figure Test, 64
Rheoencephalography (REG), 90
Room air readings, 198–199
Root mean square (RMS), 244
Rout, 229–231
200-run Monte Carlo simulation, 190–191

S
Sampling information, 184–185
S-100β protein level, 12, 15
Scheffe test, 36, 37
Scholkmann algorithm, 189–190
Sequence, MFER waveform, 185
Shapiro–Wilk test, 60, 135, 160
Sheep model, 90
Sit-to-stand maneuver, 160
Sliding window approach, 148
Slow vasogenic waves (SVWs), 243, 244
Slow waves, 129–132
Smart Neuro ICU, 188
SmartPLS 3 software, 52
Spearman's correlation coefficients (SCCs), 53, 60, 130, 217
Spencer ST³ transcranial Doppler (TCD) ultrasound system, 87
Spontaneous variations, 161
Sports-related concussion (SRC), 303–307
SPSS 20, 52
Squat-stand manoeuvres, 264
SRC, see Sports-related concussion
Standard intraparenchymal microtransducer, 108
Stimulus offset, 104
Stroke volume, 227
Student's t test, 48, 94, 222
Subarachnoid hemorrhage (SAH), 180, 269
Support vector regression (SVR), 160
SVWs, see Slow vasogenic waves
Symbol-Digit Modalities Test, 64

T
TBI, see Traumatic brain injury
Thigh cuff maneuvers, 160
3-D acquisition hardware, 98

Three-dimensional ophthalmic ultrasound imaging, 97–101
Time to peak (TTP), 116
Time to peak intensity (T_{PI}), 116
Time to syncope occurrence (TSO), 313–316
Total cerebral blood flow (tCBF), 249, 250
Transcranial bioimpedance (TCB) measurement, 89–92
Transcranial Doppler (TCD) ultrasound, 269
   algorithmic vessel location, 111
   beamforming, 112
   CBFV, 111
   comprehensive study, 271
   cross-sectional study, 271
   discrete prototype electronic system, 112
   Doppler mapping procedure, 113
   flow phantom experiments, 114
   human subject test data, 113
   limitations, 111, 113
   Mann–Whitney test, 271
   mCBFV, 269–272
   middle cerebral artery, 112
   monitoring process, 272
   vs. MRI, CT and PET, 269
   multiethnic populations, studies in, 273
   PI, 269–272
   prerequisite, 272
   side-to-side differences, lack of, 272
   SRC, 304
   technical difficulties, 272
   two traditional TCD metrics, 269
   vessel search and identification, 114
   vessel tracking, 111, 112
   wearable prototype form factor, 111
Transfer function analysis (TFA), 263, 265–267, 306–307
Transtemporal acoustic window (TAW), 112
Transverse sinus, 237–238
Traumatic bifrontal contusions, 63–65
Traumatic brain injury (TBI), 201, 203, 206, 292, 317
   ABP, 17, 19
   adult cohort, 292
   baseline neurological status, 18
   blood pressure transducer, 18
   CAR and, 292–295
   cerebral arterial compliance, 21–23
   cerebrospinal compensatory reserve index, 18
   clinical outcome, 18
   computed tomography, 29–33
   CPP, 3–6, 209–212
   CPP/ICP-oriented protocol, 18
   CPPopt, 55–58
   with high intracranial pressure, 309–312
   intracranial pressure, 7–9, 47–50
   KidsBrainIT, 39–45
   lower and upper threshold of CPP, 17
   MAP monitoring, 18
   mortality rate, 11
   NCCU management protocol, 18
   nonparametric comparison tests, 17
   optimal cerebral perfusion pressure and PaO_2/FiO_2, 59–61
   outcomes, 51–53
   paediatric cohort, 292
   pressure reactivity index, 18, 19
   prognosis, 11–16
   slow vasogenic ICP waves, 18, 20
   TCD, 269, 271
   with traumatic bifrontal contusions, 63–65
   vegetative state (VS), 17–18

Traumatic Coma Data Bank, 30
TSO, *see* Time to syncope occurrence
t-test, 22, 304
Tukey's method, 160
Two-photon laser scanning microscopy (2PLSM), 94, 310
Two-tailed Mann-Whitney U test, 52
Tympanic membrane displacement (TMD), 103–106
Tympanometry, 104
Type II diffuse brain injury, 14

U
Ultrasound contrast agents (UCAs), 115
Ultrasound perfusion imaging (UPI), 115–120
Univariate tests, 140

V
Vascular disturbances, 25
Vascular pulse, 104
Vascular wall tension (WT), 133
Vasovagal syncope (VVS), 313, 315–316
Ventricular area, 222
Ventriculomegaly, 221, 227
Ventriculo-peritoneal shunt, 222
Visual impairment/intracranial pressure (VIIP) syndrome, 215–219

W
Wavelet analysis, 148
Wavelet coherence method, 148
Wilcoxon signed rank sum test, 116–117
Windkessel model, 140
Withdrawal criteria, 36

Printed by Printforce, the Netherlands